LASERS
and Energy Devices in Aesthetic Dermatology Practice

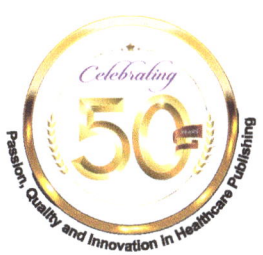

LASERS
and Energy Devices in Aesthetic Dermatology Practice

Editor
Kabir Sardana
MD DNB MNAMS
Professor
Dr Ram Manohar Lohia Hospital
and
Postgraduate Institute of Medical Education and Research
New Delhi, India

Forewords
Ganesh S Pai
Anil Ganjoo
Apratim Goel

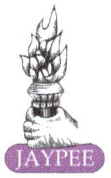

JAYPEE BROTHERS MEDICAL PUBLISHERS
The Health Sciences Publisher
New Delhi | London | Panama

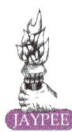 **Jaypee Brothers Medical Publishers (P) Ltd.**

Headquarters
Jaypee Brothers Medical Publishers (P) Ltd.
4838/24, Ansari Road, Daryaganj
New Delhi 110 002, India
Phone: +91-11-43574357
Fax: +91-11-43574314
Email: jaypee@jaypeebrothers.com

Overseas Offices
J.P. Medical Ltd.
83 Victoria Street, London
SW1H 0HW (UK)
Phone: +44 20 3170 8910
Fax: +44 (0)20 3008 6180
Email: info@jpmedpub.com

Jaypee-Highlights Medical Publishers Inc.
City of Knowledge, Bld. 235, 2nd Floor, Clayton
Panama City, Panama
Phone: +1 507-301-0496
Fax: +1 507-301-0499
Email: cservice@jphmedical.com

Jaypee Brothers Medical Publishers (P) Ltd.
Bhotahity, Kathmandu, Nepal
Phone: +977-9741283608
Email: kathmandu@jaypeebrothers.com

Website: www.jaypeebrothers.com
Website: www.jaypeedigital.com

© 2019, Kabir Sardana

The views and opinions expressed in this book are solely those of the original contributor(s)/author(s) and do not necessarily represent those of editor(s) of the book.

All rights reserved. No part of this publication may be reproduced, stored or transmitted in any form or by any means, electronic, mechanical, photocopying, recording or otherwise, without the prior permission in writing of the publishers.

All brand names and product names used in this book are trade names, service marks, trademarks or registered trademarks of their respective owners. The publisher is not associated with any product or vendor mentioned in this book.

Medical knowledge and practice change constantly. This book is designed to provide accurate, authoritative information about the subject matter in question. However, readers are advised to check the most current information available on procedures included and check information from the manufacturer of each product to be administered, to verify the recommended dose, formula, method and duration of administration, adverse effects and contraindications. It is the responsibility of the practitioner to take all appropriate safety precautions. Neither the publisher nor the author(s)/editor(s) assume any liability for any injury and/or damage to persons or property arising from or related to use of material in this book.

This book is sold on the understanding that the publisher is not engaged in providing professional medical services. If such advice or services are required, the services of a competent medical professional should be sought.

Every effort has been made where necessary to contact holders of copyright to obtain permission to reproduce copyright material. If any have been inadvertently overlooked, the publisher will be pleased to make the necessary arrangements at the first opportunity. The **CD/DVD-ROM** (if any) provided in the sealed envelope with this book is complimentary and free of cost. **Not meant for sale.**

Inquiries for bulk sales may be solicited at: jaypee@jaypeebrothers.com

Lasers and Energy Devices in Aesthetic Dermatology Practice

First Edition: **2019**

ISBN: 978-93-5270-530-6

THE SECRET OF JOY

The *Isha Upanishad*, in its first verse, takes us at once to the secret of this Truth:

ईशावास्यमिदं सर्वं यत्किञ्च जगत्यां जगत् ।
तेन त्यक्तेन भुञ्जीथा मा गृधः कस्यस्विद्धनम् ॥

īśāvāsyamidaṃ sarvaṃ yatkiñca jagatyāṃ jagat |
tena tyaktena bhuñjīthā mā gṛdhaḥ kasyasviddhanam ||

'Whatever there is in this ephemeral world, all is enveloped by the Lord. The renunciation, of the world is the key to happiness. Do not covet the wealth of anyone.'

It is said that when a Western journalist asked Mahatama Gandhi the key to happiness in three words, he said, "Renunciation is Joy", which is derived from the *Isha Upanishad* (तेन त्यक्तेन). Thus, it is important to know that there is little-lasting joy in the exterior aspects of the world as they are transient and unecessary attachment always ends in grief as these embodiments are always lost. Longer the attachment more the sorrow. Thus those who renunciate the attachment to the exterior aspects attain bliss. But most are already caught up in the "rat race" of life, wherein the evergreen truth as espoused by Sri Raman Maharishi stands in good stead, "Destiny cannot be changed." Thus work, without attachment to the results of your action, which paraphrases the essence of the *Bhagwad Gita* teachings

The last aspect of the verse मा गृधः कस्यस्विद्धनम् means whatever you have gained by your honest labor, say all moral and spiritual teachers, that alone belongs to you; enjoy life with that, and do not covet what belongs to others. As a corollary try not to harm others as, I assure you, it comes back with interest—sooner or later!

Contributors

Aastha Gupta MD
Senior Resident
Postgraduate Institute of Medical
Education and Research and
Dr Ram Manohar Lohia Hospital
New Delhi, India

Ajay Deshpande MBBS DVD DNB
Consultant Dermatologist
Maharashtra Medical Foundation
Joshi Hospital
Pune, Maharashtra, India

Ananta Khurana MD DNB MNAMS
Associate Professor
Postgraduate Institute of Medical
Education and Research and
Dr Ram Manohar Lohia Hospital
New Delhi, India

Anil Aggrawal MD Forensic Medicine (AIIMS)
Director–Professor (Forensic Medicine)
Maulana Azad Medical College
New Delhi, India

Anil Ganjoo MD DVD FAAD
Director
Skinnovation Clinics, New Delhi, India
President, South Asian Association for
Regional Cooperation–Association of
Aesthetic Dermatology (SAARC–AAD)
Vice President, Indian Association of
Dermatologists, Venerologists and
Leprologists (IADVL)—National (2016)
Scientific Chair, Aesthetics
Past President, IADVL, New Delhi, India

Apratim Goel MD (Skin) DNB (Skin) FAGE
Consultant Dermatologist and CEO
Cutis Skin Solution
Mumbai, Maharashtra, India

Ashraf Badawi MD
Assistant Professor of Dermatology
Laser Institute, Cairo University, Egypt
Visiting Professor of Dermatology and
Laser Applications
Szeged University, Hungary
Vice President
The European Society for Lasers and
Energy-based Devices (ESLD)

Avitus John Raakesh Prasad MD
Managing Director
SP Derma Center
Madurai, Tamil Nadu India

Ganesh S Pai MD DVD FAAD
Medical Director
DERMA-CARE
Skin and Cosmetology Centre
The Trade Centre
Mangaluru, Karnataka, India

Kabir Sardana MD DNB
Professor
Dr Ram Manohar Lohia Hospital and
Postgraduate Institute of Medical
Education and Research
New Delhi, India

Khushbu Goel MD
Consultant Dermatologist
Kubba Skin Clinic and Max Hospital
New Delhi, India

Masuma Molvi MD
Dermatologist
Minal Medical Centre
Dubai, UAE

Niteen V Dhepe MD FAAD Fellow ASDS ASLMS EADV ISHRS IADVL ACSI
Medical Director
Skin City
The Postgraduate Institute of Dermatology
Pune, Maharashtra, India

Pooja Arora Mrig MD DNB MNAMS
Associate Professor
Postgraduate Institute of Medical Education and Research and
Dr Ram Manohar Lohia Hospital
New Delhi, India

Preeti Kothari MD
Dermatologist
Radiant Aesthetics
Mumbai, Maharshtra, India

Red Alinsod MD
Gynecologist
South Coast Urogynecology
Alinsod Institute for Aesthetic Vulvovaginal Surgery (AIAVS)
Laguna Beach, California

Seema Rani MD DNB
Associate Professor
Postgraduate Institute of Medical Education and Research and
Dr Ram Manohar Lohia Hospital
New Delhi, India

Shikha Bansal MBBS MD MNAMS
Associate Professor
Department of Dermatology
Vardhman Mahavir Medical College and Safdarjung Hospital
New Delhi, India

Shilpa Garg DNB Dermatology Venereology & Leprosy
Consultant
Department of Dermatology
Sir Ganga Ram Hospital
New Delhi, India

Shivani Bansal MD DNB
Consultant Dermatologist
Kaya Skin Clinic, New Delhi, India
Associate Consultant
Max Hospital Panchsheel
New Delhi, India

Shruti Dewan MBBS DDVL MD (AM)
Dermatologist
New Delhi and NCR

Sidharth Tandon MD
Assistant Professor (Dermatology)
Santosh Medical College
Ghaziabad, Uttar Pradesh, India

Soni Nanda MD DNB
Consultant Dermatologist
Shine n Smile Skin Clinic
New Delhi, India

Sujay Khandpur MD DNB MNAMS
Professor
Department of Dermatology and Venereology
All India Institute of Medical Sciences
New Delhi, India

Sumit Gupta MD
Consultant Dermatologist
Skinnovation Clinics
New Delhi, India

Surabhi Sinha MD DNB
Specialist
Dr Ram Manohar Lohia Hospital
New Delhi, India

Tanvi Pal MD (Dermatology)
Consultant Dermatologist
Kubba Skin Clinic and
BLK Superspecialty Hospital
New Delhi, India

Tarang Goyal MD
Professor and Head
Department of Dermatology, Venerology
and Leprosy
Muzaffarnagar Medical College
Meerut, Uttar Pradesh, India

Vallari Gatne MD
Dermatologist
Skin City
Pune, Maharashtra, India

V Dhir DVD
Consultant Dermatologist
Dr Ram Manohar Lohia Hospital
New Delhi, India

Vivek Mehta MD
Consultant Dermatologist and
Medical Director
Pulastya Cadle
New Delhi, India

Vivek Nair MD FAAD (USA) FISD (USA)
Consultant Dermatologist and
Hair Transplant Surgeon
Gurugram, Haryana, India
www.drnairsskinclinic.com

Foreword

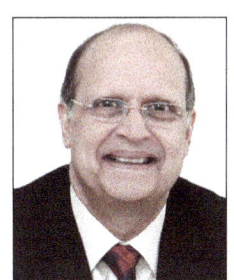

Work gives meaning and purpose to our profession; sustained work with a relentlessly focused mind, attending to the smallest detail creates something exceptional, in this case, a book edited by Professor Kabir Sardana. Since we are what we repeatedly do, excellence is not an isolated act but a sustained habit, a quality possessed by the author.

From his previous book to this, there are greater details, clinical and technological updates. Joe Girard had said that "the elevator to success is out of order. You have to use the stairs one by one". Between the two books, it is been a long climb.

"We know what we are, but know not what we may be" said William Shakespeare. We know now that Dr Kabir Sardana has become an accomplished author and the reader has much to gain by possessing the book.

Ganesh S Pai MD DVD FAAD
Medical Director,
DERMA-CARE
Skin and Cosmetology Centre
The Trade Centre
Mangaluru, Karnataka, India

Foreword

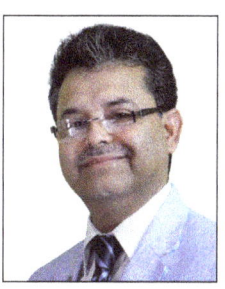

The advent of lasers has come as a welcome boon to numerous patients suffering from various laser amenable conditions. Since the concept of lasers was introduced in the late 1950s, the lasers have come a long way. From the initial days of Ruby laser being used for all kinds of lesion to the present day of multiple wavelengths being used for every single condition, the world of lasers has seen a sea change in the last few decades. Also the tremendous advances in the understanding of the laser physics over the recent past has improved our knowledge of laser-tissue interactions, and has helped us to improve outcomes in various laser amenable conditions.

Most of the literatures available on lasers have been from the west and is based on their use on the Caucasian skins. There has always been a need to publish data from our part of the world with experiences of uses of lasers on our kind of skins of color.

This publication will go a long way in plugging the gap in our knowledge about uses of lasers in dark skins.

The book is a wonderful compilation of chapters from the pioneers in the world of lasers and is a must read for all those who aspire to be successful laser surgeons, and also for the seniors as a very useful reference guide.

I congratulate Dr Kabir Sardana and his team of editors for this stupendous effort and wish this book a grand success.

Anil Ganjoo MD DVD FAAD
Director
Skinnovation Clinics, New Delhi
President
South Asian Association for Regional Cooperation–
Association of Aesthetic Dermatology (SAARC–AAD)
Vice President
Indian Association of Dermatologists,
Venerologists and Leprologists (IADVL)—National (2016)
Scientific Chair
Aesthetics
Past President
IADVL, New Delhi, India

Foreword

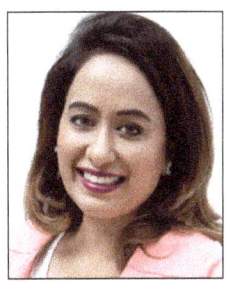

It is an honor and pleasure to write this foreword for this unique textbook on lasers by Dr Kabir Sardana. I am sure that contents will fill few lacunae in the cosmetic practice. Since most of the information about lasers and aesthetic procedures is evolving constantly, it is important to amalgamate this information with already existing knowledge and that is the main aim of this textbook. The topics chosen are all those that apply to the current times and trends.

I am very pleased to be able to contribute also as an author for a few chapters in this textbook. My dear friend and colleague, Dr Kabir has picked up so many stars from the galaxy by choosing the best experienced doctors as authors from the industry. All the authors are aesthetic practitioners themselves, and hence the book gives many practical points that will help those who wish to enhance their practice. This book is compact, easy-to-carry and comfortable-to-use. This book will fill the gap provided by the operating information on devices provided by laser manufacturers and other available information.

However, books are not a replacement for practical experience and training with hands on experience on the technology. So please use this as a guide and source of updated information. I would be happy to know what you feel about the book and my chapters in particular.

Enjoy reading.

Apratim Goel MD (Skin) DNB (Skin) FAGE
Consultant Dermatologist and CEO
Cutis Skin Solution
Mumbai, Maharashtra, India

Preface

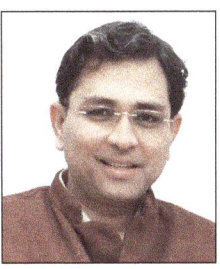

I have always been amazed at the confidence shown by speakers at conferences when they show results with lasers in conditions that rarely respond completely and within three months of the machine being bought! Acne scars, for example, nevus of ota and a lot more. Equally audacious is the confidence by which the laser companies sell their wares, when they themselves have little knowledge of what they sell. Herein lies the genesis of this book, which aims at rising above the mechanistic approach where we learn which buttons to push, in courses provided by the more reputable device manufacturers just after a laser is purchased. This approach is foolish beyond words, and can harm patients, and worse create medicolegal hazards. My aim was to make the practicing dermatologist, make a reliably educated guess, without influences!

The book answers the three basic questions, what to do, why to do it and how to do it? But our basic target is the dermatologists who need a step-by-step approach to the technology commonly used and not the laser that a speaker in most conferences uses, which as a thumb rule is expensive, the reason why the company sponsors the talk in the first place! Though the Food and Drug Administration (FDA) gives clearance of a device for a particular labeled indication, this cannot be taken as any assurance that it will work safely and effectively enough to satisfy the patients. Tragically, it may not be an understatement that a majority of lasers bought in this country are not US-FDA approved in the first place!

The book also gives a frank assessment of technology and does not gloss over their results. In fact we have covered many other aspects in the treatment of common disorders so that the clinician has a rounded view of therapy beyond lasers. We have experts in the field of interest so that "many wise minds" come together for this book.

We have also covered other energy devices beyond lasers and brought them all together in this book. A dedicated **Index of Therapeutic Indications** is provided for the busy practitioner.

But this is not a "Cook Book" and only a guide on the best approach is provided. Individual laser parameters can vary, thus there is no substitute for hands-on training, which cannot be obtained in this book or sitting in a lecture hall more so when there are hundreds sitting in it!

Hope you like the effort. More will follow soon…

But remember the famous adage

"Lasers are not Erasers" thus do not expect or promise the sky.

Kabir Sardana

Acknowledgments

I would like to thank my wife and practicing dermatologist, Dr Supriya Mahajan for standing by me and tolerating my tapping on my "TVS Gold Bharat" keyboard late into the night. Those who know about it will know the staccato, it can make!

I would like to thank my colleagues residents in my former institution Maulana Azad Medical College (MAMC) and present workplace Dr Ram Manohar Lohia Hospital, New Delhi, India, for their role in my interest in Lasers

A special thanks to the team at M/s Jaypee Brothers Medical Publishers (P) Ltd, New Delhi, India, especially Shri Jitendar P Vij (Group Chairman) and Mr Ankit Vij (Managing Director), for latching on to the project, the ever persistent Ms Chetna Malhotra Vohra (Associate Director–Content Strategy), who kept persisting on to the project despite delayed deadlines, mails and copyright tweaks, Ms Madhuri Aggarwal (Development Editor) who has been silently tolerating my busy schedules, Mr Ankush Sharma (Artist) and Mr Manver Singh (Typesetter).

The book went through numerous schedules, and luckily it was delayed as since May 2018 when it was supposed to be launched lots new has happened in this field.

And lastly, our tributes to the countless patients who have taught us dermatology and helped us to learn and relearn lasers!

Contents

SECTION 1: Laser and Energy-based Technologies

Chapter 1. Laser–tissue Interactions and its Clinical Correlates 3
Kabir Sardana, Sidharth Tandon

Chapter 2. Ablative Lasers 50
Kabir Sardana

Chapter 3. Pigmented Lesions and Tattoos 132
Kabir Sardana, Seema Rani, Pooja Arora Mrig

Chapter 4. Fractional Photothermolysis 241
Kabir Sardana, Sumit Gupta

Chapter 5. Vascular Lasers 320
Tanvi Pal, Sujay Khandpur, Kabir Sardana

Chapter 6. Lasers for Hair Removal 353
Shivani Bansal, Soni Nanda, Kabir Sardana,
Shikha Bansal, Tarang Goyal

Chapter 7. Cosmetic Use of Radiofrequency in Dermatology 387
Vivek Nair, Kabir Sardana, Apratim Goel

Chapter 8. High Intensity and/or Microfocused
Ultrasound with/without Visualization 434
Apratim Goel, Vallari Gatne, Preeti Kothari

Chapter 9. Noninvasive Body Contouring and Lipolysis 447
Shruti Dewan, Vivek Nair, Kabir Sardana

Chapter 10. Combination Laser Therapy:
Rationale and Indications 482
Kabir Sardana

Chapter 11. Laser Toning in Dermatology 500
Vivek Mehta, Kabir Sardana

SECTION 2: Therapeutic Indications

Chapter 12. Clinical Indications 515
Shilpa Garg, Kabir Sardana, Niteen V Dhepe, Ashraf Badawi,
Aastha Gupta, Ananta Khurana, Sidharth Tandon, Khushbu Goel,
Red Alinsod, Avitus John Raakesh Prasad, Ajay Deshpande,
Surabhi Sinha

- 12A. Acne Scars 516
  Shilpa Garg, Kabir Sardana, Niteen V Dhepe

- 12B. Lasers for Scars, Keloids, and Stretch Marks 532
  Kabir Sardana, Niteen V Dhepe

- 12C. Striae Distensae 550
  Kabir Sardana

- 12D. Cellulite, Fat Reduction, Laxity, and Body Contouring 557
  Kabir Sardana, Niteen V Dhepe

- 12E. Miscellaneous Laser Responsive Disorders 572
  Kabir Sardana, Ashraf Badawi, Aastha Gupta, Ananta Khurana,
  Sidharth Tandon, Khushbu Goel, Red Alinsod, Niteen V Dhepe,
  Avitus John Raakesh Prasad, Ajay Deshpande, Surabhi Sinha

SECTION 3: Practical Aspects and Complications

Chapter 13. How to Setup a Laser Center in a Private Setup? 699
Apratim Goel, Masuma Molvi

Chapter 14. How to Setup a Laser Clinic in a Public Funded Institution 712
V Dhir, Kabir Sardana, Ananta Khurana

Chapter 15. Why, When, and How to Buy a Laser? 728
Anil Ganjoo, Kabir Sardana

Chapter 16. Medicolegal Aspects of Lasers in Dermatological Practice 741
Anil Aggrawal, Kabir Sardana

Chapter 17. Complications and their Management 769
Kabir Sardana, Ganesh S Pai

Index *791*

Index of Therapeutic Indications

Acne Keloidalis Nuchae 91
Acne Scars 87, 281, 419
Acne Vulgaris 572
Actinic Cheilitis 91
Adenoma Sebaceum 104
Aging, Skin 483
Alopecia 625
Amyloidosis 196, 603
Angiokeratomas 647
Angiolymphoid Hyperplasia with Eosinophilia 598
Basal Cell Carcinoma/Squamous Cell Carcinom 663
Becker's Nevus 159
Benign Tumors 104
Café-au-lait Macules 155
Cellulite 450, 557
Cherry Angioma 644
Darier's Disease 114, 598
Eczema 599
Elastosis Perforans Serpiginosa 599
Epidermal Nevi/Nevus Comedonicus 95
Erythroplasia of Queyrat 664
Fat 450, 557
Fibrous Papule 578
Freckles 158
Glomus Tumor 650
Granuloma Faciale 600
Granuloma Annulare 600
Hailey-Hailey 114
Hair Gray 379
Hair Removal 353
Hair Transplant 120
Hemangiomas 340
Hirsutism 356
Hori's Macules 188

Hyperhidrosis 667
Hypertrichosis 357
Infraorbital Hyperpigmentation 191
Keloids 120, 532
Keratosis Pilaris 594
Koenen Tumors 578
Labial Melanotic Macules 153
Leg Veins 346
Lentigines 150
Lichen Planus Pigmentosus 194
Lichen Sclerosus 601
Lupus Erythematosus 602
Lymphangioma Circumscriptum 121
Melanocytic Nevi, Congenital 168
Melanocytic Nevi 100, 163
Melasma 171, 306, 504, 607
Minocycline Pigmentation 193
Molluscum Contagiosum 595
Mongolian Spots 190
Nail Disorders 634
Nail Matrixectomy 118
Neurofibromas 105, 579
Nevi (Epidermal and Dermal) 94, 590
Nevus Lipomatosus Superficialis 591
Nevus of Ota/Ito 183
Nevus Sebaceous 100
Nevus Spilus 153
Paget's Disease 664
Parapsoriasis/Mycosis Fungoides 665
Pearly Penile Papules 106
Photodamage Skin 297
Poikiloderma of Civatte 344, 617
Pores 679
Port-wine Stains 330
Postinflammatory Hyperpigmentation 182, 615

Pseudofolliculitis 379, 631
Psoriasis 604
Pyogenic Granuloma 345, 657
Redness, Facial 343
Rejuvenation 419, 503, 684
Rhinophyma 92
Rosacea 344
Sarcoidosis 603
Scars, Atrophic 540
Scars, Chickenpox 88
Scars, Post-traumatic 89, 301, 544
Scars, Surgical 544
Sebaceous Hyperplasia 108, 582
Seborrheic Keratoses 107, 159, 579
Skin Tightening 313
Steatocystomas 109
Striae 305, 419, 550
Syringoma 106
Tattoo removal 123, 201
Telangiectasia, Facial 343
Telangiectasia 651
Trichoepitheliomas 109, 578
Venous Lake 345, 655
Vitiligo Surgery 122, 310, 619
Vulval, Rejuvenation 686
Vulval, Tightening 420
Warts 115, 595
Wound Healing 660
Xanthelasma 109, 584
Xanthoma Disseminatum 114
Zoon's Balanitis 662

Section 1
Laser and Energy-based Technologies

CHAPTER 1

Laser–Tissue Interactions and its Clinical Correlates

Kabir Sardana, Sidharth Tandon

BASICS OF LASER–TISSUE INTERACTIONS

Light can be divided into the ultraviolet (UV) (200–400 nm), visual (VIS; 400–760 nm), near infrared (NIR; 760–1,400 nm), mid-infrared (MIR; 1.4–3 µm), and far infrared (FIR; 3 µm and beyond) and these also constitute the important wavelength ranges in laser dermatology (Grossweiner L et al.).

Light behavior conforms to some basic elements, which are modified while traversing the skin (Grossweiner L et al.). Normally, the percentage of incident light reflected from the skin surface is determined by the index of refraction mismatch between the skin surface (stratum corneum, n = 1.55) and air (n = 1) (Hillenkamp FR et al. and Neimz M et al.). The *Fresnel equation* can be used to describe how much light will be reflected from the skin. Depending upon the angle between the light beam and the skin surface, this value varies considerably. More light is reflected at "grazing" angles of incidence (Fig. 1.1) (Hillenkamp FR et al. and Neimz M et al.).

Clinical Applications

- While performing laser surgery, it is necessary to deliver light approximately perpendicular to the skin to minimize reflective losses. This regular reflectance is about 4–7% for light incident at right angles to the skin (Fig. 1.1). One can reduce interface losses by applying an alcohol solution (n = 1.4) or even water (n = 1.33). This allows for optical coupling. The light that is not reflected at the skin surface penetrates into the epidermis (Welch AJ et al.).

  At this point, further light propagation in the skin is determined by wavelength-dependent localized absorption and scattering (Figs. 1.1 and 1.2A). Overall, because of the scattering, much of the incident light is remitted (remittance refers to the total light returned to the environment due to multiple scattering in the epidermis and dermis, as well as the regular reflection from the surface) (Figs. 1.1 and 1.2).

4 SECTION 1: Laser and Energy-based Technologies

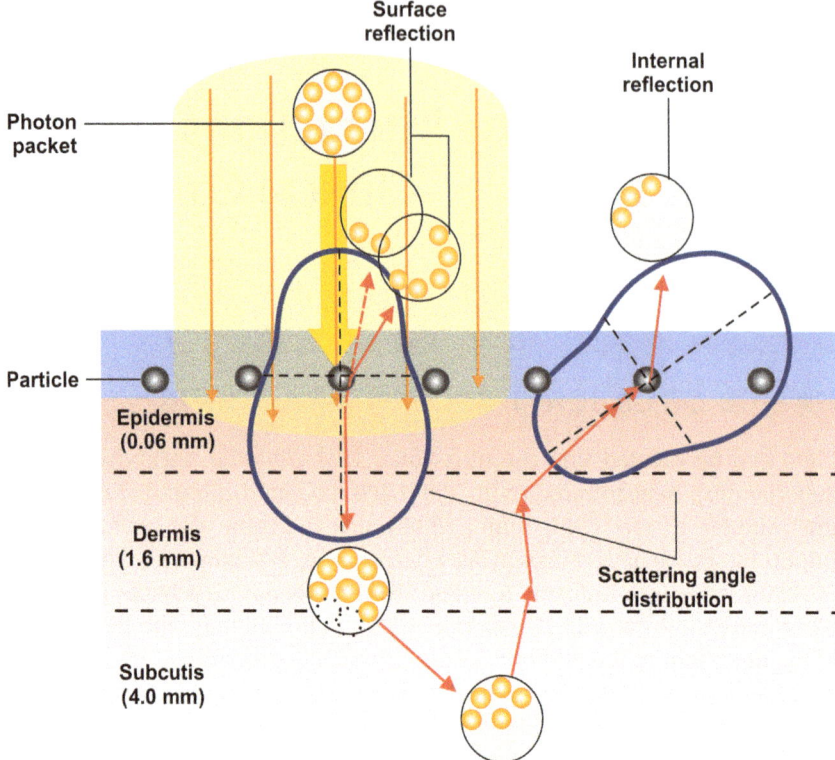

Fig. 1.1: Schematic diagram of the skin showing the simulation of laser beam interaction.

- From a therapeutic point of view, light reflected from the surface is "wasted" energy. The amount of light wasted because of *remittance* varies from 15% to as much as 70%, depending upon the wavelength and skin type (Neimz M et al., Welch AJ et al., and Anderson RR et al.).

    For example, with the 1,064 nm, 60% of an incident laser beam may be remitted. One can easily verify this by holding a finger just adjacent to the beam near the skin surface. Considerable warmth will be felt with higher fluences, all of which is due to a remitted portion of the beam (Welch AJ et al.).

TYPES OF LIGHT DEVICES

Lasers contain four main components: (1) the lasing medium, (2) the excitation source, (3) feedback apparatus, and (4) an output coupler. The amplifier of a laser is the laser material that can be a solid, a gas, or a liquid. The feedback mechanism is produced by the resonator, where the light is reflected by two mirrors so that the photons pass several times through the laser material. The number of photons within the resonator increases exponentially due to the stimulated emission (Fig. 1.2B).

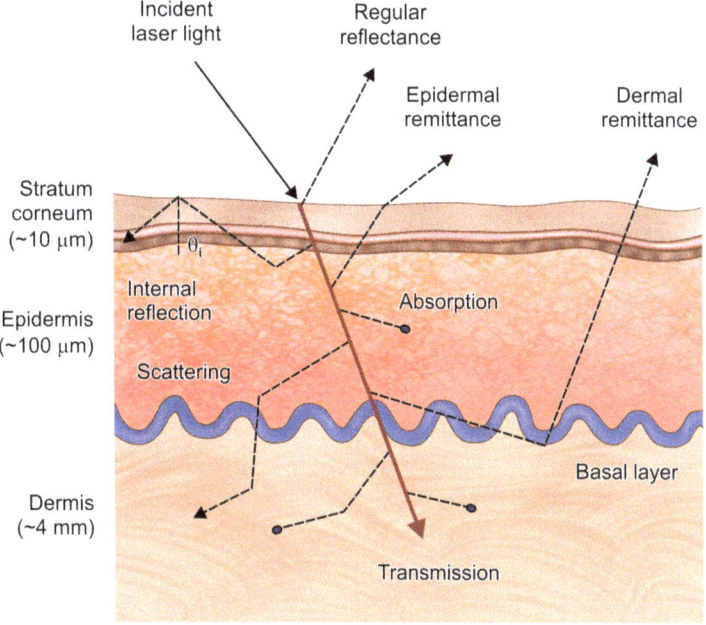

Fig. 1.2A: A diagram showing the fate of an incident light beam. The ideal straight uninterrupted beam is never achieved in vivo

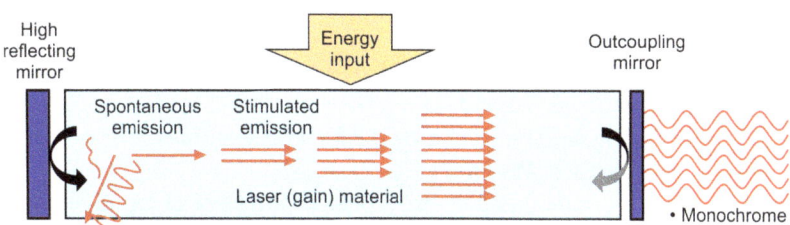

Fig. 1.2B: A diagram depicting the components of a conventional laser.

With respect to lasing media, there are diode lasers, solid-state lasers, dye, and gas lasers.

Solid-state lasers include the neodymium-doped yttrium aluminum garnet (Nd:YAG) laser, erbium-doped yttrium aluminum garnet (Er:YAG) laser, alexandrite laser, and the ruby laser. The *gas lasers* include the carbon dioxide (CO_2) laser, argon ion laser, and the excimer lasers, while the *diode* and *dye lasers* are singular in their respective classes.

LASER PARAMETERS AND THEIR IMPORTANCE

Basic *parameters* for any laser depend on the type of lasers. For continuous wave (CW) lasers, power, time, and spot size are important while for pulsed lasers the energy per pulse, pulse duration (PD), spot size, fluence, repetition rate, and the total number of pulses are the important factors (Sardana K et al., Boulnois JL et al., and Welch AJ et al.).

- **Energy** is measured in joules (J).

$$Energy\ (J) = Power\ (W) \times Time\ (s)$$

Energy is the ability to do work and is equal to force times the distance over which the force is exerted. Newton's second law states that force is equal to mass times acceleration. Energy can also be defined as a product of power × time. This is relevant to laser surgery in that the power of the laser beam multiplied by the pulse duration determines the total energy delivered to the target area.

- **Fluence:** The amount of energy delivered per unit area is the fluence, sometimes called the dose or radiant exposure, given usually in J/cm^2.

$$Fluency\ (J/cm^2) = Energy\ (J)/Area\ (cm^2)$$

Fluence is best described as the energy density. It is equal to the energy in joules divided by the surface area of the beam (cm^2). This expresses the dose of energy delivered to the site of laser impact and incorporates the concepts of irradiance and time *(fluence = irradiance × pulse width)*.

It has been estimated that when irradiance is greater than 100 W/cm^2, the degree of tissue damage depends directly on *time* of application *(pulse width)* and not on irradiance. It is important to remember that irradiance determines rate of tissue vaporization but that fluence determines the amount of energy deposited and thus the amount of vaporization. The *minimum fluence* needed to affect pure vaporization of tissue with a CO_2 laser is 5 J/cm^2.

The rate of energy delivery is called *power*, measured in watts (W). One watt is one joule per second *(W = J/s)*.

- The power delivered per unit area is called the **irradiance or power density**, usually given in W/cm^2.

Irradiance is calculated as the power of the laser beam divided by its surface (cross-sectional) area.

Thus, for a circular beam of spot size (diameter) d, with power P, the irradiance is equal to $P/\pi (d/2)^2$, or $4P/\pi d^2$.

It is obvious from this equation that a twofold change in d produces a fourfold change in irradiance, while changes in P result in a corresponding linear change in irradiance. In practical terms, irradiance is the *single most important* determinant of the rate of vaporization or ablation of tissue.

Power density determines the action mechanism in cutaneous applications (Fig. 1.2C) (Sardana K et al. and Boulnois JL et al.). For example, a very low irradiance (typical range of 2–10 mW/cm^2) does not markedly increase tissue temperature and is associated with diagnostic applications, photochemical processes, and biostimulation. On the other extreme, a very short nanosecond (ns) pulse can generate high peak power densities which are associated with photomechanical effects and even plasma formation. Plasma is a "spark" due to ionization of matter.

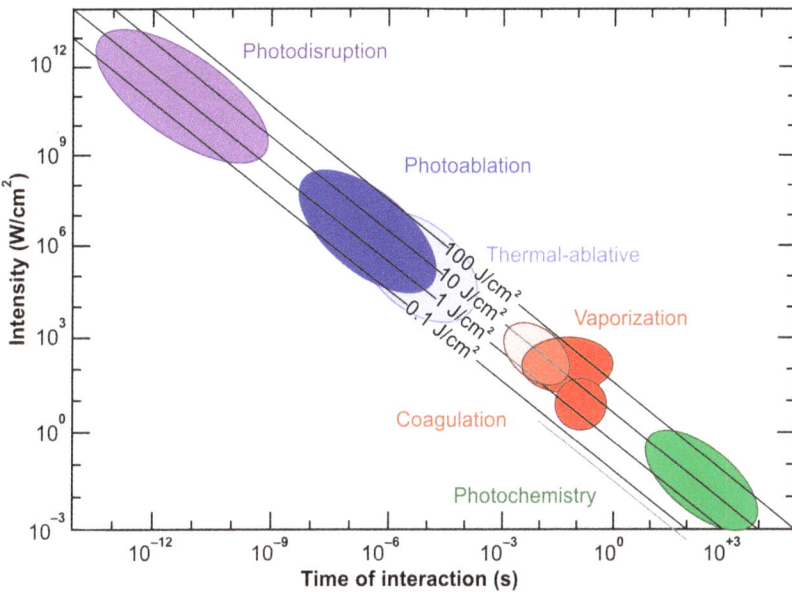

Fig. 1.2C: The tissue effects of laser as a function of power density ranges.
Source: Adapted from Sardana K, Garg VK. Lasers in Dermatological Practice. New Delhi: Jaypee Brothers Medical Publishers (P) Ltd; 2016.

- **Laser exposure duration** (called pulse width for pulsed lasers) is the time over which energy is delivered. Dermatology uses electronic medical record (EMR) exposures ranging from many seconds to nanoseconds. This is a very crucial parameter and is useful in pulsed lasers.

  Shorter the PD less is the wastage of energy and if it is less than the thermal relaxation time (TRT) of the target organelles less is the thermal damage. Thus, an ultrapulse laser is better than a CW laser, in terms of thermal damage (Sardana K et al.).

  For a given pulse energy, a shorter pulse delivers more of its total energy above the threshold power needed to perform material removal and/or transformation (Fig. 1.3). In contrast, most of the energy of a longer pulse simply goes into heating the material.

Clinical implications (Sardana K et al.): Based on pulse width lasers may be continuous, pulsed, quasi-continuous, and Q-switched (Fig. 1.4, Table 1.1).

The older lasers had pulse durations that varied from seconds to milliseconds (0.01 s/10^{-3} s). Millisecond CO_2 lasers are gated lasers but largely CW in nature. The CO_2 laser is a classic example of a continuous mode laser.

Here it must be understood that based on the principles of TRT, if the epidermis is the target, the laser should have a PD less than 1 ms, which is the TRT of skin (1,000 µs = 1 ms). Thus, to ensure minimum thermal damage the laser should have a PD less than 1 ms. Microsecond lasers

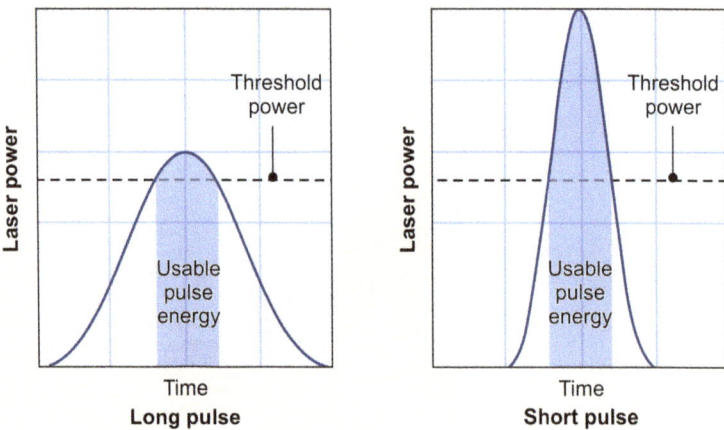

Fig. 1.3: The effect of pulse duration on effective energy used. With longer pulses, much of the usable pulse energy is delivered below the threshold and contributes only to unwanted peripheral thermal effects. With shorter pulses, a higher proportion of the pulse energy is delivered above the threshold power level, maximizing the threshold energy while minimizing peripheral heating.

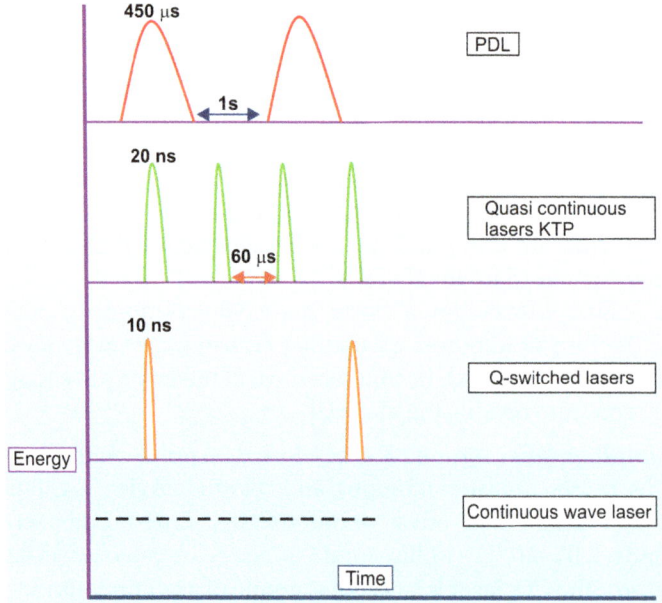

Fig. 1.4: A figurative depiction of the energy pulse duration and pulse width of lasers. (PDL: pulsed dye laser)
Source: Adapted from Sardana K, Garg VK. Lasers in Dermatological Practice. New Delhi: Jaypee Brothers Medical Publishers (P) Ltd; 2016.

Table 1.1: Clinical applications with regard to the pulse-width of lasers.

Long pulses	0.001 s, millisecond (ms), 10^{-3} s	Hair removal, varicose veins
Quasi-CW	0.000001 s, microsecond (µs), 10^{-6} s	Skin rejuvenation
Q-switched	0.000000001 s, nanosecond (ns), 10^{-9} s	Pigmented lesions, tattoo
Mode-locked	0.000000000001 s, picosecond (ps), 10^{-12} s	Pigmented lesions, tattoo
Femto	0.000000000000001 s, femtosecond (fs), 10^{-15} s	Refractive surgery in ophthalmology

(0.000001 s/10^{-6} s) are the ideal lasers (ultrapulse mode) and have a setting of 90–900 µs. Most Er:YAG lasers are also microsecond lasers. Thus, if the aim is to minimize thermal damage the PD should be less than 1 ms.

In the pulsed dye laser (PDL), a single or a train of pulses is emitted. Pseudocontinuous lasers (KTP) have very short pulses of light repeated at very high repetition rates. Extremely short pulses are achieved by Q-switching. These nanosecond lasers (0.000000001 s/10^{-9} s) are used in pigmented lesions (Q-switched lasers). Recently picosecond lasers (0.000000000001 s/10^{-12} s) have been used in tattoos and are discussed in **Chapter 3: Pigmented Lesions and Tattoos**.

Operational modes *(Sardana K et al.):* The operational modes of lasers are CW, pulsed as interrupted radiation (in ms), pulsed free running (in hundreds of ms), Q-switched (in ns), or mode-locked (in fs).

Continuous wave laser may be differentiated from a pulsed laser, which provides bursts of energy. In the CW mode, the laser delivers a continuous beam of light with little or no variation in power output over time (Fig. 1.5A). In CW operation, the physician controls laser output, typically by maneuvering it with a foot pedal.

Interrupted radiation of a CW laser is done by mechanical or electronic switching with modification of the pulse length. The pulse frequency is low to moderate, up to 100 Hz. Flash lamp pumped solid-state lasers in the free-running mode have pulse lengths of 50 ms up to several 100 ms. Pulses of medical dye laser systems can vary from microseconds to 50 ms.

Please note that some of the rudimentary (Chinese/Korean) lasers touted as pulsed laser essentially have gated pulses and are not pulsed.

Superpulse: The next generation of CO_2 lasers used were the so-called "superpulsed (SP) technology". The pulses were of the order of 50–200 mJ and were delivered with varying repetition rates (50–500 Hz). Sometimes they were delivered as couplets spaced very close together temporally. Unlike gated or mechanically shuttered pulses, however, these laser emissions were truly pulsed, that is, they were generated at the electrical source as pulsed exposures. These lasers delivered average powers similar to CW lasers, but the lasers were not "on" all of the time (Fig. 1.5A).

The different modes in the SP laser that we use are (Fig. 1.5B):
- *Mode A:* 1,000 ms pulse width
- *Mode B:* 1,200 ms pulse width
- *Mode C:* 1,400 ms pulse width
- *Mode D:* 1,600 ms pulse width
- *Mode E:* 1,800 ms pulse width
- *Mode F:* 2,000 ms pulse width
- *Mode G:* 2,200 ms pulse width
- *Mode F:* 2,400 ms pulse width.

These settings are studied in sustainable and replicable in vitro, in vivo, and ex vivo studies and the take home message is that a pulse width *less than* **2.5 ms** is good enough for the ideal balance between ablation and coagulation with minimal thermal damage.

These three modes (except pico/ultrashort mode) are included in the CO_2 laser and their different tissue effects are depicted in Figure 1.5C. With CW sources, the user must know the spot size, exposure time, and power density to determine the fluence. In many CW applications (i.e. wart treatment with a CO_2 laser), the fluence is *not* too helpful in characterizing the overall tissue effect. One normally observes tissue vaporization and coagulation in real time and suspends the procedure when an appropriate endpoint is reached. For CW mode, CO_2 lasers are typically used with a focusing (collimated)

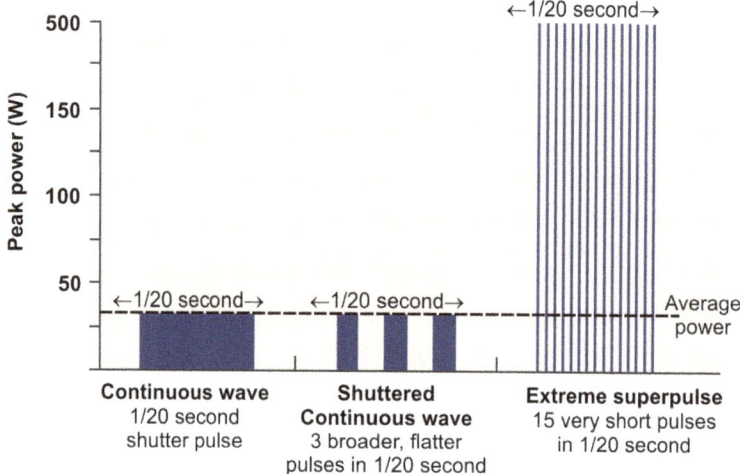

Fig. 1.5A: A display of the various modes of a conventional CO_2 laser, without ultrapulse mode. Note that the average power of a superpulse laser is high, but each pulse is more than the TRT of the skin (1 ms). But in routine surgeries this is a very useful setting. (CO_2: carbon dioxide; TRT: thermal relaxation time)

CHAPTER 1: Laser–Tissue Interactions and its Clinical Correlates   11

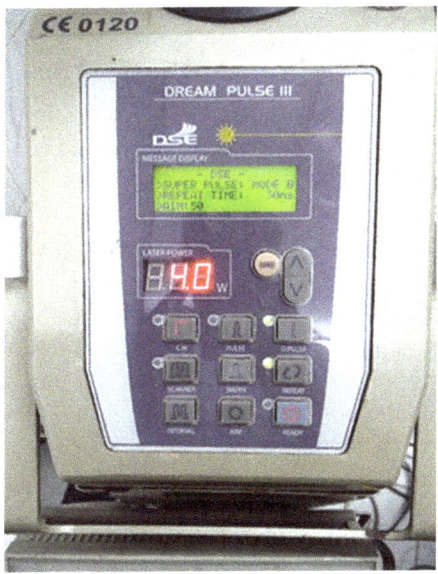

Fig. 1.5B: The superpulse mode, an ideal mode for most benign tumors and nevi, note the three variables, the *dose*, the *mode* which predicts the pulse width, and the *repeat time*. If the repeat time is increased one can achieve higher thermal damage. If it is lowered higher penetration thus, enabling flexibility in ablation.

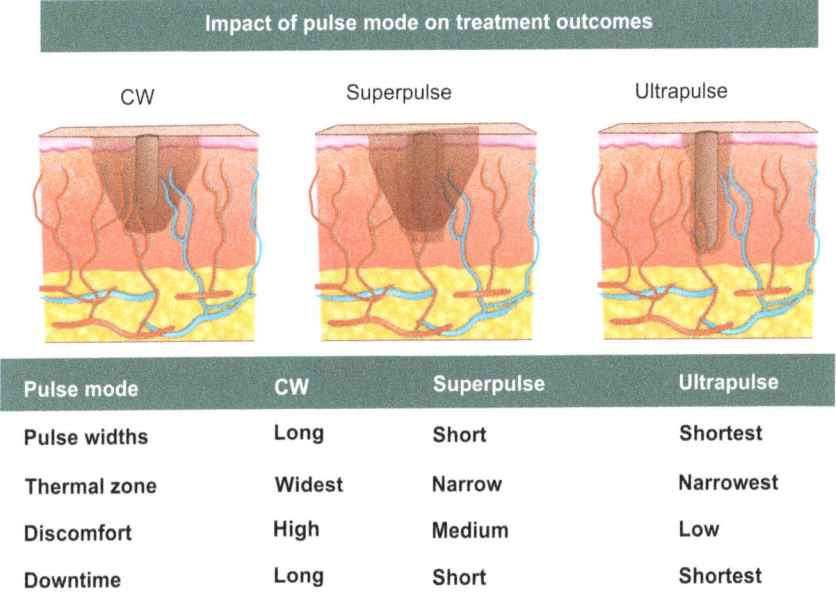

Pulse mode	CW	Superpulse	Ultrapulse
Pulse widths	Long	Short	Shortest
Thermal zone	Widest	Narrow	Narrowest
Discomfort	High	Medium	Low
Downtime	Long	Short	Shortest

Fig. 1.5C: Tissue effects of the three common modes of CO_2 laser. (CO_2: carbon dioxide; CW: continuous wave)

handpiece. This allows the operator to control spot size and tissue effects simply by moving the handpiece tip toward or away from the skin (Fig. 1.6).

Q-switching: Shorter pulses with very high intensities in the nanosecond range are produced by Q-switching of the laser. The single, intense pulse with duration on the order of nanoseconds is produced. It is generally used in crystal lasers such as ruby, alexandrite, and Nd:YAG, described here.

With Q-switching (the Q-factor stands for *quality factor*, used in electronics theory terminology), a fast electromagnetic switch (Pockels cell) in the laser cavity causes excitation of the active medium to buildup far in excess of the level of the medium when the shutter is open. In operation, the flash lamp is turned on and the population inversion gradually grows. Lasing is prevented by the shutter. When the population inversion is at a maximum, the shutter is opened so that lasing occurs and a large burst of energy is emitted as the cavity rapidly depletes the population inversion. The net result is an extremely high peak power (greater than 10^6 W) nanosecond duration pulse or series of pulses.

The Q-switch can be *passive*, when using a crystal called "saturable absorber" that produces rapid pulses, or *active*, when using an electronic modulator crystal called "Pockels cell". The former are the cheaper machines, which can handle power outputs and hence spot size is limited to a few

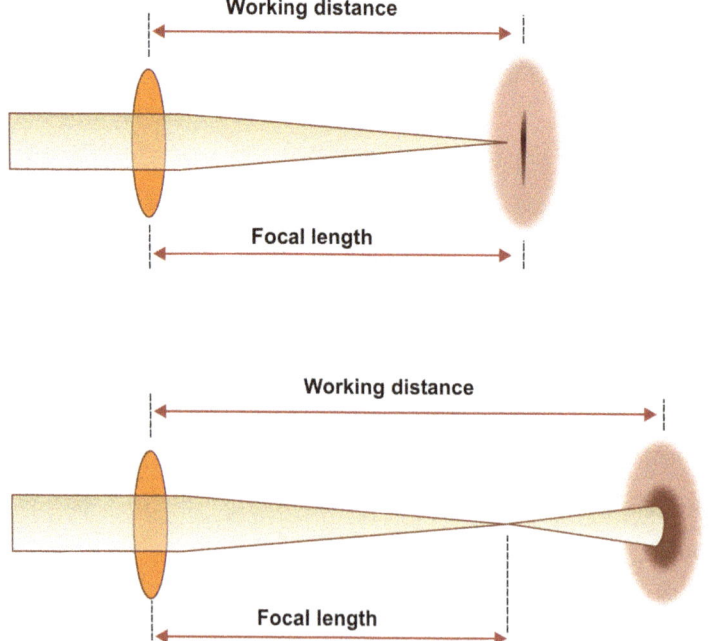

Fig. 1.6: The manual adjustment of the working distance of a carbon dioxide (CO_2) laser and the consequent tissue effect.

millimeters (1-3 mm). They also fail to achieve high repetition rates of pulses (high frequencies), working in a maximum of 2-3 Hz. The active Q-switch uses a Pockels cell which is a crystal subjected to a high electric frequency and is electronically controlled to produce a very fast and stable light switching effect. The result is faster pulses with very high peak powers that are not possible with passive systems. Thus, they can handle high energy, larger spot sizes (10 mm), and faster repetition frequencies of 2-20 Hz. Equipment with active Q-switch allow the device to be turned off, and thus the laser can also work in the quasi-CW mode, with micropulse, giving greater flexibility to the system.

Ultrashort/picosecond laser pulses are generated by mode coupling **(Chapter 3: Pigmented Lesions and Tattoos)** due to the coherent properties of the laser. Compared to Q-switching, where the shortest PDs are in the range of the resonator period, mode coupling can generate even shorter laser pulses.

The picosecond lasers for dermatology provide pulses ranging from 375 ps to 760 ps. The inherent advantages lie in the fact that as the peak power is inversely proportional to PD a shorter PD would generate higher powers for the same energy.

A picosecond laser generates a very high peak power, making the photomechanical fragmentation of the target tissue and consequently the treatment is more efficient. The machine requires lower high-energy levels and thus the treatments are milder with and faster recovery time. For example, in tattoo removal, a picosecond laser needs fewer sessions than a nanosecond system, and applications can be performed every 15 days, while in nanosecond systems, sessions are 45-60 days apart. The faster the system is the milder and more effective is the treatment. But there are other practical issues and not all consider it to be a superior technology (*see* **Chapter 3: Pigmented Lesions and Tattoos**).

Other important factors are the *laser spot size* (which greatly affects intensity inside the skin), whether the incident light is convergent, divergent, or diffuse, and the uniformity of irradiance over the exposure area (spatial beam profile).

Spot size: The spot size in *ablative* lasers is dependent on the distance that the handpiece is held away from the skin surface (Fig. 1.6). There is a Gaussian distribution of irradiance across the beam, with peak intensity in the center and minimal intensity at the beam edges. Therefore, the smaller the beam, the less even is the vaporization due to a very sharp drop in irradiance from center to edge. A larger spot size allows for a more gradual drop in irradiance from center to edge, and thus for more even vaporization (Fig. 1.7).

In general, the spot size should be 3-4 X more than d (penetration depth), as larger spots make it more likely that photons will be scattered back into the incident collimated beam (Anderson R et al. and Ross EV et al.). Photons that are scattered out of the beam are essentially wasted. Traveling "alone", they

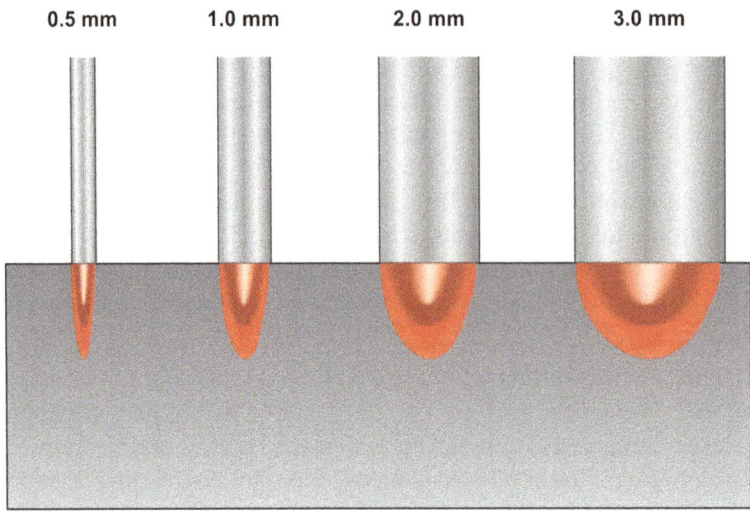

Fig. 1.7: A depiction of the tissue effect of a carbon dioxide (CO_2) laser in relation to the spot size. Note that a larger area is impacted on increasing the spot size. A proportionate increase in the fluence is needed.

carry insufficient energy to cause macroscopic thermal responses in tissue. The consequences of spot size are explained as follows. Basically, for small beams (narrow) scattered photons are carried out of the beam path after only a few scattering events. A good analogy is a highway with exits. With a narrow highway, any movement obliges the car to "take" the exit, and the car does not return to the road. On the other hand, on a superhighway with many lanes, cars can move about and stay within the original boundary of the thoroughfare. Only cars on the extreme left and right are likely to "get" off the road.

By using the aforementioned spot size arguments, one can exploit the properties of small spots to change the way particular wavelengths behave in the skin. For example, one can tailor a 1,064 nm laser to heat progressively larger depths of skin by increasing the spot size (Figs. 1.8A to C).

For shallow penetrating lasers such as CO_2 and erbium where the d << spot size, the diameter of the beam does *not* intrinsically affect the depth of tissue response. Hence, the value of the pulse diameter is not always important in the ablative lasers as far as the depth of penetration is concerned.

Clinical applications:
- As spot size increases, the volume of tissue heated increases and thus the energy required to heat that volume also increases. Therefore, higher power lasers must be used to achieve the minimum fluence (5 J/cm^2) needed for vaporization with larger spot sizes. If one *increases* spot size without a concomitant increase in power, then *slow* heating of tissue occurs with less vaporization and greater thermal injury leading to scarring.

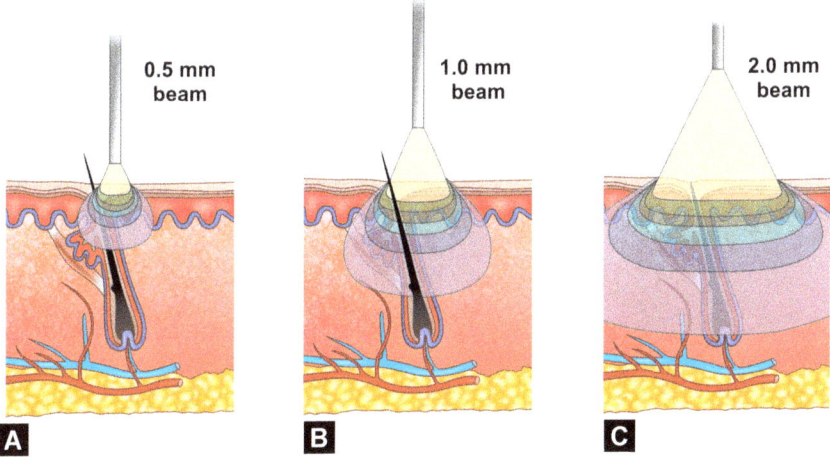

Figs. 1.8A to C: Note how spot size changes impact depth of penetration. Shown are the fluence patterns for 1,064 nm light with beams (A) 0.5 mm; (B) 1.0 mm; and (C) 2.0 mm in diameter on the skin surface.

Large spots increase the dermal/epidermal damage ratio as well as the relative *penetration depth*. However, absolute epidermal damage will be greater with the larger spot with the same fluence. It follows that it is prudent to *reduce* the fluence by 20%, for example, if one *increases* the spot size between treatment sessions in care of a port-wine stain (PWS). Also, one should note that for any turbid medium, even if the spot is "top hat", there will be an accumulation of photons near the center of the beam such that a greater clinical effect will often be noted at the center of the spot.

- The **pulse profile**, that is, the character of the pulse shape in time (instantaneous power versus time) is another feature that can impact the tissue response.
- **Beam profile:** Top hat versus Gaussian (Welch AJ et al., Anderson RR et al., and Welch AJ et al.).

Laser beam profiles can be of various shapes: the Gaussian profile is common. This has the shape of a bell curve and is the fundamental mode of most lasers (Figs. 1.9A and B). One often sees this shape when the beam has been delivered through an articulated arm (with mirrors at the knuckles). For some wavelengths, this is still the most effective way to deliver energy (CO_2 and erbium).

Clinical application: The Gaussian profile is often disparaged as an inferior profile for lasers. In many applications, the criticism is well founded. For example, in treating a lentigo with a typical Q-switched ruby laser, one will often observe complete ablation of the epidermis at the center of the "spot" but only whitening at the periphery. On the other hand, sometimes a bell-shaped profile is desirable, for example, when applying a small spot of FIR

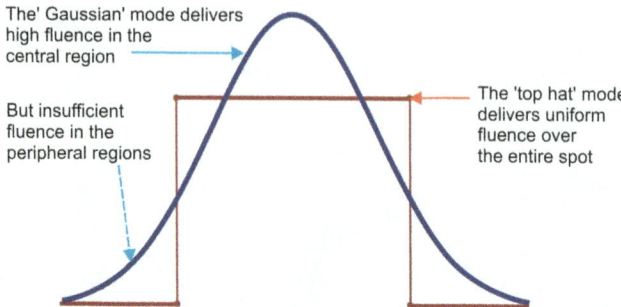

Fig. 1.9A: Gaussian versus top hat: beam shape influences treatment uniformity and efficacy.

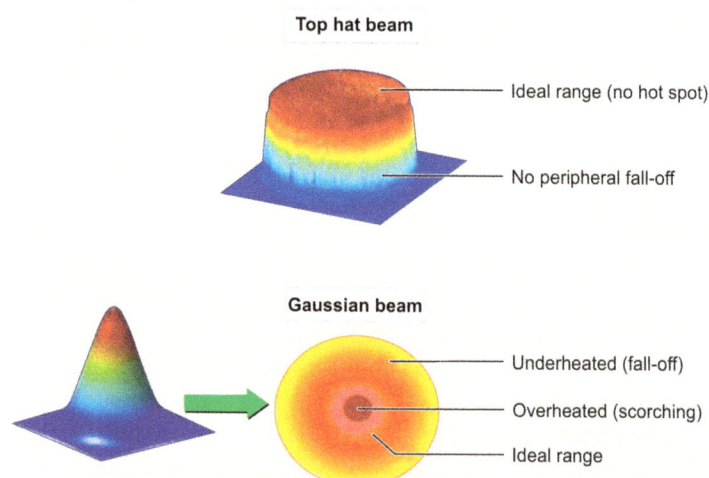

Fig. 1.9B: Comparison of the beam types of lasers. In most indications, the top hat profile is preferred. The lower half of the figure demonstrates the conversion of a Gaussian beam into a top hat beam, which can be achieved in certain laser.

beam with a scanner. In this scenario, the wings of the beam allows for some overlap without delivering "too much" energy at points of overlap.

In most applications, top hat profile is desirable, and with many fiber delivery systems this is the case, as the beam is mixed by the multiple internal reflections within the fiber.

- **Thermal damage time:** In some applications, the immediate chromophore and the final target are not collocated (i.e. hair shaft and hair bulb/bulge). In this case, thermal damage time is defined as the time required for irreversible target damage with sparing of the surrounding tissue. For a nonuniformly absorbing of target structure, the thermal damage time is the time when the outermost part of the target reaches the target damage

temperature through heat diffusion from the heater. In this case, the eventual target and the heater (for example, hair shaft) are different and at a considerable distance from each other. Using this model, the thermal damage time can be many times longer than the TRT.
- **Thermal kinetic selectivity:** Along the same lines is the concept of thermal kinetic selectivity (TKS). In this model, one selects larger or smaller targets based on PD (Fig. 1.10). For example, if one wants to heat larger targets while sparing relatively smaller ones, the pulse duration is extended beyond the TRT of the smaller target. This principle can be theoretically be used while treating PWSs in pigmented skin. In this manner, for example, a melanosome will be heated to a lower temperature than the subjacent vessel.

Extrapolating Parameters to Machines

One of the challenges is understanding all these terms within the context of a specific device and specific clinical situation. When a novice confronts a laser instrument panel, there is often a fear of using lasers with multiple features (Figs. 1.11A to C). Many physicians would prefer to have fewer options and a simpler display, especially early on in their use of a particular laser. Here comes the dependence on the laser manufactures. But knowledge of various parameters can enable a very effective use of lasers and as you pay a tidy sum, it is a shame that we do not ask more.

But there is no harm in understanding the various options so that a wide array of procedures can be attempted. Before initiating a good option is to test the various settings on a wooden tongue depressor to gauge the tissue effects. At the end of the day one can use a particular setting for each indication using the endpoints as a guide.

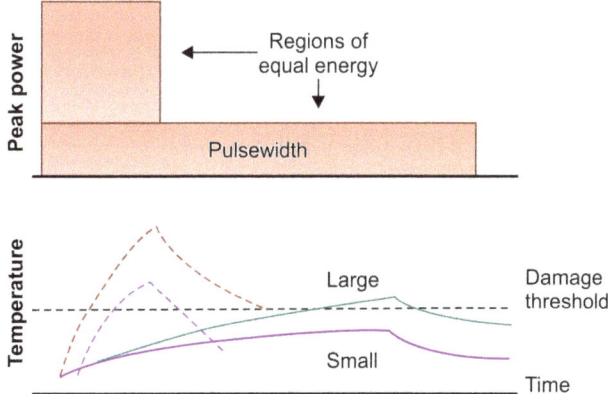

Fig. 1.10: Relationship between size of target and pulse duration to peak temperature. The longer pulse favors heating of the larger target (blood vessel) versus the smaller melanosome.

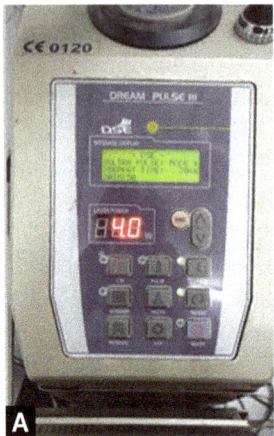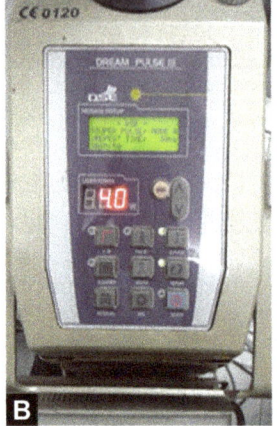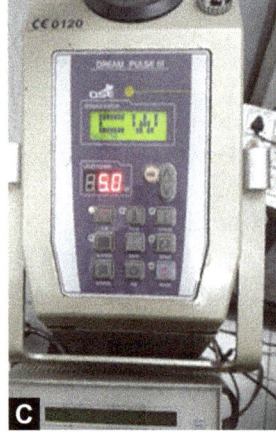

Figs. 1.11A to C: Depicts the three modes of CO_2 laser namely: (1) Ultrapulse; (2) Superpulse; and (3) Continuous wave. The laser also has a scanner mode that can be used for larger areas with rapid ablation in pulsed mode. The number of pulses impacted depends on the repeat mode and the interval can be varied to increase the depth. This is the ideal panel that can help the clinician to vary the ablation. There are fixed modes as well which can be good for starters. The last mode has no lit up parameters on the panel as it is the CW-CO_2 mode. (CO_2: carbon dioxide; CW: continuous wave)

ABSORPTION SPECTRUM AND PRINCIPLE OF SELECTIVE PHOTOTHERMOLYSIS

What makes a light source a good choice for a given application is the ability of its emitted light to interact with the tissue so as to achieve the desired effect. This is known as selective photothermolysis (SPT) (Ross EV et al. and Anderson RR et al.). Although Dr Leon Goldman argued for color as a means to selectively damage dermal targets as early as 1963, SPT offered an elegant and mathematically rigorous rationale for developing different tissue selective lasers. As described by Dr Anderson, extreme localized heating achieved with SPT relies on:

- A *wavelength* that reaches and is preferentially absorbed by the desired target structures.
- An exposure *duration* less than or equal to the time necessary for cooling of the target structures, and
- Sufficient *energy* to damage the target.

The heterogeneity of the skin allows for very selective injury in thousands of microscopic targets.

Selectivity is accomplished by matching a specific wavelength of light to a chromophore—that is, the light absorbent part of a molecule—in the tissue. The energy directed into the target area produces sufficient heat to damage or alters the target while allowing the surrounding area to remain relatively untouched.

Thus to reiterate, the crucial parameters for achieving ideal SPT are: *wavelength, PD,* and *energy level* (Hillenkamp FR et al., Neimz M et al., Anderson RR et al., and Sardana K et al.).

Absorption Spectrum

(Neimz M et al., Anderson RR et al., Sardana K et al., Boulnois JL et al., Welch AJ et al., and Anderson R et al.)

The absorption spectra of major skin chromophores dominate laser tissue interactions in dermatology. The *absorption coefficient* is the probability per unit path length that a photon at a particular wavelength will be absorbed (Neimz M et al. and Anderson RR et al.). It is, therefore, measured in units of 1/distance and is typically designated as μ_a, given as cm^{-1}.

The absorption coefficient depends on the concentration of chromophores present. Skin contains pigments and distinct microscopic structures that have different absorption spectra. Common tissue chromophores targeted in dermatology applications are water (which makes up 70% of tissue), hemoglobin (blood), melanin (in the epidermis, pigmented lesions, and hair), lipids (subcutaneous fat and sebaceous glands), and protein (specifically, collagen) (Neimz M et al. and Anderson RR et al.). Each of these has a specific absorption spectra that corresponds to a semiconductor laser material able to produce the matching wavelength (Fig. 1.12A). Because penetration depth depends highly on the wavelength of light, it must be considered when determining the energy needed for a particular application (Fig. 1.12B).

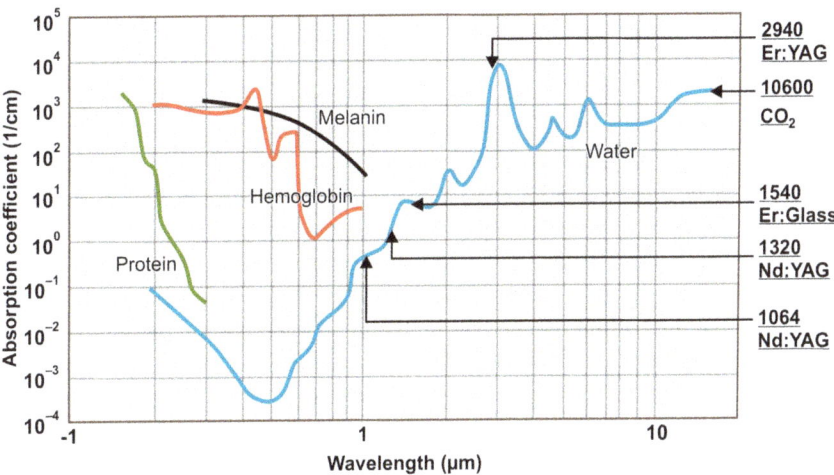

Fig. 1.12A: Each of the major biological chromophores has an absorption spectra. The wavelength of light needed to activate each of these correlates with a semiconductor laser material. Above are shown typical solid-state lasers used for these wavelengths. Penetration depth of light is strongly dependent on wavelength, and must be considered when determining the energy for a particular application.

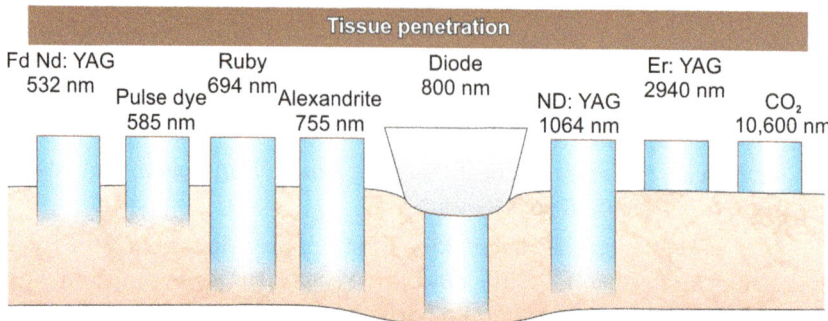

Fig. 1.12B: Tissue penetration. (CO_2: carbon dioxide; Er:YAG: erbium-doped yttrium aluminum garnet; Nd:YAG: neodymium-doped yttrium aluminum garnet)

If tissues were clear, then only absorption would be required to characterize light propagation in skin (Neimz M et al., Anderson RR et al., and Sardana K et al.). However, the dermis is white because of light scatter. Scattering is responsible for much of the light's behavior in the skin (beam dispersion, spot size effects, etc.). The main scattering wavelengths are between 400 nm and 1,200 nm, where the average distance a photon travels between two scattering events is between 0.05 mm and 0.2 mm.

- *Hemoglobin:* There is a large oxyhemoglobin (HbO_2) peak at 415 nm, followed by smaller peaks at 540 nm and 577 nm. An even smaller peak is found at 940 nm. For deoxyhemoglobin (deoxyHb), the peaks are at 430 nm and 555 nm. Because of the discrete peaks of hemoglobin absorption, the laser physician can optimize heating of the vessel with excellent protection of the surrounding structures (Neimz M et al., Welch AJ et al., Anderson RR et al., and Sardana K et al.).
- *Melanin:* Most pigmented lesions result from "too" much melanin in the epidermis. By choosing almost any wavelength (<800 nm), one can preferentially heat epidermal melanin (Fig. 1.12A). Shorter wavelengths will tend to create very high superficial epidermal temperatures, whereas longer wavelengths tend to bypass epidermal melanin (i.e. 1,064 nm).

The melanin present in the top layers of the skin acts as a window curtain. Energy absorption by this **melanin "curtain"** will increase with darker skin patients or with patients at the higher positions of the skin types on the Fitzpatrick scale. The absorbed energy will generate local heat, which when excessive can generate unpleasant adverse effects such as burns, hypochromic spots, or stimulate melanocytes producing hyperchromic spots.

This is why for deeper pigmented disorders 1,064 nm is used like in nevus of Ota, but in Indian skin the poor response is as the epidermis is not an optical window and scattering of light occurs. Also, there are variations in color of the nevus of Ota and thus possibly multiple laser wavelengths may be needed to help in an adequate result (Sardana K et al.).

- *Water:* Water makes up about 65% of the dermis and lower epidermis. There is some water absorption in the UV. Between 400 nm and 800 nm, water absorption is quite small (which is consistent with our real-world experience that light propagates quite readily through a glass of water). Beyond 800 nm, there is a small peak at 980 nm, followed by larger peaks at 1,480 nm and 1,060 nm. The water maximum is 2,940 nm (Er:YAG). Thus, the Er:YAG is ideally suited for ablation but as it has lesser coagulation than CO_2 laser it is not preferred for deeper ablation (Fig. 1.12A).
- *Carbon:* Carbon is not per se a chromophore but rather a product of prolonged skin heating. Once carbon is formed at the skin surface, the skin become "opaque" to most laser wavelengths (that is, most energy will be absorbed very superficially). It follows that the dynamics of surface heating changes immediately once carbon is formed. This can be used creatively as an advantage. For example, one could use a layer of carbon paper to convert a deeply penetrating laser to one that would only affect the surface.
- *Collagen:* Dry collagen shows absorption peaks near 6 µm and 7 µm. With a free electron laser, these peaks can be exploited for selective molecular targeting. In this manner, collagen is directly heated rather than relying on heat conduction due to its close bonds to tissue water (where Er:YAG and CO_2 lasers work). Ellis et al. found that this approach provided more efficient resurfacing and might allow for less tissue irradiation and less thermal damage than CO_2 lasers (Ellis DL et al.).

  The *clinical applications* of these are multiple:
- Firstly the practice of combining different lasers, say for treating melasma or nevus of Ota, makes little sense as the lasers have different absorption spectrum. The practice of treating pigmented lesions with synergistic lasers is a classic example of lack of science as, if a ablative laser even in a fractional mode is used followed by a pigment-specific laser, the former will create a tissue reaction that may obviate the effects of the pigment-specific laser as the chromophores involved may have a change in their absorption spectrum, their size, and depth. If combinations are to be done it is better to do a sequential combination with a gap of a few days to weeks. The one exception may be nevus of Ota, where three or more lasers may be used, as nevus of Ota has variations in color. But this is after test spots are done to decide the appropriate wavelength.
- In Indian skin, specially for pigmented lesions, the implications are obvious a longer wavelength is better as it minimizes damage to the epidermis and there is less scatter, hence, the popularity of the 1,064 nm Nd:YAG for pigmented skin.

Thermal Relaxation Time

For effective treatment and to prevent interaction with the surrounding area, the pulse width should be sufficiently shorter than the TRT of the targeted chromophore (Neimz M et al., Welch AJ et al., Anderson RR et al., Sardana K et al., and Anderson RR et al.).

For most tissue targets, a simple rule of thumb can be used.

"The TRT in seconds is about equal to the square of the target dimension in millimeters".

For a flat object, such as lentigines, the TRT can be estimated by the ratio:
$$TRT = d^2/4a$$
where "d" is the thickness of the material and "a" is the thermal conductivity of the material.

For a cylindrical object, such as hair or vein:
$$TRT = d^2/16a$$

Thus, a 0.5 mm **melanosome** (5×10^{-4} mm) should cool in about 25×10^{-8} s, or **250 ns**, whereas an 0.1 mm **PWS vessel** should cool in about 10^{-2} s, or **10 ms**. While there is no substitute for testing and experimentation, Figure 1.13, which provides guidance for determining approximate pulse width, can serve as a starting point.

Clinical applications:

- The popularity of the 1,540 nm laser, in rejuvenation is based on the fact that entire epidermis and large portions of the dermis are heated, and TRT is on the order of seconds, because d is several 100 mm.
- For calculating the TRT of the epidermis with the melanosome as the immediate chromophore, one can consider either the entire *epidermis* as the target (thickness of 80–100 μm), or the *dermal–epidermal junction* (10 μm), or finally, the *melanosome* itself (1 μm diameter) when using melanin as chromophore. Each skin "unit" will have its own respective TRT.

Thermal relaxation time of some potential targets

Target	Thermal relaxation time
Erythrocyte	2 μm hair follicle
200 μm hair follicle	40 ms
0.5 μm melanosome	0.25 μs
10 μm nevus cell	0.1 ms
0.1 mm diameter vessel	10 ms
0.4 mm diameter vessel	80 ms
0.8 mm diameter vessel	300 ms

Fig. 1.13: For effective treatment, the pulse duration should be sufficiently **shorter** than the thermal relaxation time (TRT) of the targeted chromophore to allow selectivity from surrounding tissue. Typical optical fluence needed for effective treatment targeting is between 1 J/cm² and 100 J/cm²; the corresponding spot size ranges from 0.1 cm² to 10 cm². Typical durations for common treatments include 0.001 ms for a melanosome (the organelle responsible for melanin in animal cells) to 1 minute for 5 mm of subcutaneous fat.

A Q-switched laser pulse will confine high temperatures to the melanosome. The upper epidermis is heated only after postpulse heat conduction away from the dermis–epidermis (DE) junction. On the other hand, in treating with a 10 ms 532 nm pulse, heat will diffuse freely from the melanosome during the pulse, resulting in more uniform epidermal heating. This diffuse and gentle epidermal heating may be desirable or undesirable depending on the specific clinical indication. Most importantly, the physician can titrate the degree of epidermal heating by manipulation of the PD.

The TRT explains the *futility* of using lasers in *melasma* where there are three variables: (1) size of the target is variable as the melanosome, melanocytes, clumps of melanocytes, and that too at, (2) variable levels, and then we have (3) pigmented skin wherein the epidermis is not an optical window. So, what is needed is a laser that has *variable* PD, variable depths, and also minimum thermal damage, a combination that is impossible to achieve by any single laser. Hence, it is obvious that as a monotherapy lasers are of little use in melasma even in the so-called laser toning mode (Sardana K et al.).

- The wide variability of results in conditions like hyperhidrosis and lipolysis is because there is very little corroborative data on these indications. Though we have detailed these in chapters in this book lets examine the clinical applicability of lasers for lipolysis.

Goldman had proposed that two properties must be considered to determine the effectiveness of laser lipolysis: (1) wavelength, and (2) the energy employed. According to the theory of SPT, these chromophores (fat, collagen, and blood vessels) preferentially absorb the laser energy based on the specific absorption coefficient, according to the wavelength. Many wavelengths, including 924 nm, 968 nm, 980 nm, 1,064 nm, 1,319 nm, 1,320 nm, 1,344 nm, and 1,440 nm, have been evaluated by their interaction with these chromophores. Many authors suggest that certain wavelengths are more effective for lipolysis (DiBernardo BE et al.).

Parlette and Kaminer have documented that the 924 nm wavelength has a higher selectivity to absorb *fat,* but it is *not effective* to induce cutaneous retraction, thus it is not useful for improving *laxity*. They showed that 1,064 nm wavelength has a good penetration in the tissue but *low absorption* by fat. However, its distribution of heating is superior with good cutaneous retraction effect. Finally, the 1,320 nm wavelength has demonstrated great absorption by *fat,* but with low penetration in the tissue, so it is safe for treating more fragile skins, such as in the neck and arm areas (Parlette EC et al.).

So, here is a classical example where different wavelengths have been used as the target is not just the fat, but one of the aims is heat generation also. What are we achieving by lasers here, selective damage or heat generation?

The same is true for lasers for hyperhidrosis, hence, the use of "target blind" energy devices, like radiofrequency (RF) **(For such indications *see* Chapter 12D: Laser Responsive Disorders)**.

HEAT GENERATION AND COOLING

All laser–tissue interactions are guided by the same energy balance rules that guide all of physics. Heat generation can occur in one of two ways. Firstly, it can occur at the site of the chromophore (Anderson R et al.). In this case, there is very precise localized heating consistent with the theory of SPT (Anderson R et al.). These hotspots under the skin allow a specific damage to the target chromophore while the normal skin is spared, so long as the ratio of absorption coefficients (i.e. blood vs. bloodless dermis) is high enough (optimally > 10).

When treating by heating tissue water, the injury is typically from "top to bottom", the exception being deeper penetrating NIR and MIR wavelengths coupled with surface cooling. In this scenario, one can coordinate heating and cooling to damage specific slices of subsurface skin. Spatially selective temperature elevation is possible when: (1) the absorption coefficient of the target exceeds that of collateral tissue (SPT), or (2) when the "innocent bystander" tissues are cooled so their peak temperatures do not exceed some damage threshold.

Visible light technologies [especially green-yellow light sources such as intense pulsed light (IPL), KTP laser, and PDL] are popular in cutaneous laser surgery especially in vascular disorders. They are also the wavelength ranges where epidermal damage is most likely. The epidermis is an innocent bystander in cutaneous laser applications where the intended targets, such as hair follicles or blood vessels, are located in the dermis. Specifically, absorption of light by epidermal melanin causes epidermal heating. Melanin is distributed throughout the epidermis but is especially concentrated in the basal cell layer. Melanin absorption of visible light causes heating of melanosomes and through thermal diffusion, subsequent damage to the entire epidermis. This is especially true for green-yellow light, but the risk of selective DE junction-derived epidermal injury extends to wavelengths as long as 1,064 nm. This also a reason why the results of PDL in Indian skin are so poor as the abundant melanin competes with the laser wavelength.

Beyond visible light (green, yellow, and red) sources, surface cooling also has been employed in *NIR and MIR* lasers. With NIR lasers, surface cooling is important, but not only because of DE junction-derived epidermal heating. In addition, deep beam penetration may cause catastrophic bulk heating. With MIR lasers (1.32 mm, 1.45 mm, and 1.54 mm), the chromophore is water. It follows that with even very low fluences, surface cooling is imperative. Without cooling, the ubiquitous nature of water in the skin causes laser-induced top to bottom injury. There is no discrete heating. All of the techniques are susceptible to operator error and device failure. It follows that as physicians rely more heavily on cooling devices, any lack of their proper deployment unveils the dark side of cooling.

Before the availability of surface cooling, fluence thresholds for efficacy and epidermal damage were often close. The *timing* of the cooling relative to the laser pulse is important. Cooling can be pre, during the pulse (parallel), or after the pulse (post) (Aguilar G et al.). All three cooling periods are important. For example, postcooling may prevent retrograde heating (i.e. from the vessel back to the epidermis) from damaging the skin surface.

Clinical Applications

- The first goal of surface cooling is preservation of the epidermis. Unintentional heating of the basal cell layer can lead to vesiculation, crusting, and at times, scarring.
- The second and related goal of surface cooling is to allow for delivery of higher fluences to the intended target (i.e. the hair bulb and/or bulge or a subsurface blood vessel). Often, the highest fluence that can be used in targeting hair and/or subsurface vessels is limited by heating of the epidermis (Paithankar D et al.). By cooling the epidermis, higher fluences and, therefore, higher temperature elevations are possible in the targeted structures in the dermis.
- Another benefit of surface cooling is analgesia, as almost all cooling strategies will provide some pain relief (Hohenleutner U et al., Greve B et al., Chan HH et al., and Raulin C et al.).
- Besides protection of the DE junction from pigment "unfriendly" wavelengths, bulk cooling is sometimes required because the volume heated is large and there is a risk for large volume overheating and catastrophic scarring (i.e. with 1,064 nm).

    Overall, shorter wavelengths pose a greater risk to the skin surface, because the ratio of epidermal to dermal heating is higher. This ratio derives from: (1) a higher absorption of melanin by shorter wavelengths, and (2) a tendency for photon scatter to limit penetration of shorter wavelengths. This leads to an accumulation of energy near the DE junction (Aguilar G et al., Choi B et al., and Zenzie HH et al.).
- There are some scenarios where cooling is *unlikely* to prove beneficial: (1) when the absorption of the wavelength is very strong by water (i.e. Er:YAG and CO_2), here the cooling and heating zone are overlapping so that preservation of epidermal viability is unfeasible (also because there is no concomitant cooling with ablative lasers), also (2) when using Q-switched lasers in the range from 532 nm to 1,064 nm, cooling achieves pain reduction but will only modestly reduce the high peak temperatures generated by these ultrashort pulses in melanin and exogenous inks (tattoos).

LASER SKIN OPTICS RELEVANT TO DERMATOLOGIST

The optical properties of human skin determine the penetration, absorption, and internal dosimetry of laser light in skin. The cosmetic surgeon can divide the skin into two main components: (1) the epidermis (primarily an absorber of visible light due to melanin), and (2) the dermis.

One of the most important preconditions to using lasers is to **memorize** the **absorption** spectra of the main chromophores in planning the procedure but it is also crucial to remember that the optical properties of the skin are not static.

Light–tissue interactions can be broken down into:
- The *transport* of light in tissue
- *Absorption* of light and heat generation in tissue
- Localized *temperature elevation* in the target tissue (and denaturation of proteins), and
- *Heat diffusion* away from the target (Neimz M et al., Welch AJ et al., Sardana K et al., and Anderson R et al.).

In any light–tissue interaction, the thermal or photochemical effects depend on the local energy density at the target. Surface fluence represents the energy per unit area incident on the skin. Once the light penetrates the surface, it undergoes a complex series of *absorbing* and *scattering* events (Figs. 1.1, 1.2 and 1.14). Characterization of the light pathways is best understood by thinking of the incident beam in terms of its constituent photons, where the photons statistically are either scattered or absorbed in a wavelength-dependent fashion (Jacques SL et al.). The probabilities of absorption or scattering (designated μ_a and μ_s, respectively) are determined by experiment.

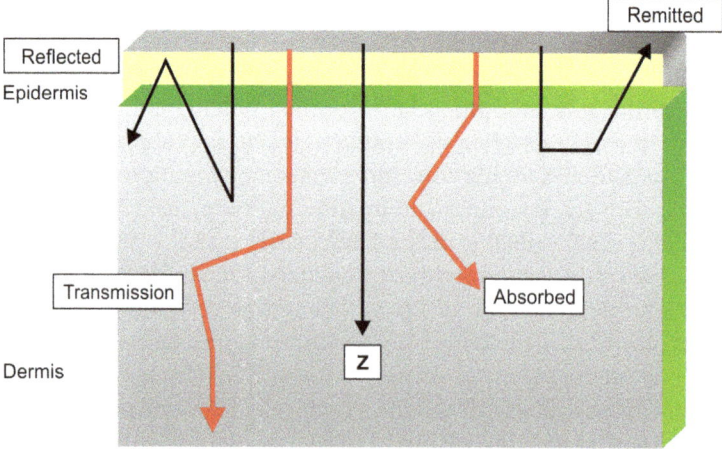

Fig. 1.14: Laser–tissue interaction. Ideal laser penetration is a straight line (z) which is not normally seen as the skin is not an optical window.

For most visible light, there are typically 100 scattering events before a photon is absorbed. As it turns out, the photon scatters roughly 10 times before it loses its orientation with respect to the initial direction as it migrates in a random walk. With scattering, there is **backscattered light** that augments the delivered irradiance to yield a higher fluence beneath the tissue than at the tissue surface (Fig. 1.15) (Jacques SL et al.).

While the absorption spectrum is detailed earlier we will also dwell on the scattering in this section. The scattering behavior of biological tissue is important because it determines the volume distribution of light intensity in the tissue. This is the primary step for tissue interaction, which is followed by absorption and heat generation. Scattering of a photon is accompanied by a change in the propagation direction without loss of energy. Scattering leads to an increase in the light intensity directly below the tissue surface being enhanced by a factor of 2-4 as compared with the intensity of the incident beam. The increased fluence rate is caused by scattered photons overlapping with the incident photons.

Clinical Implications
(Sardana K et al.)

- It has been shown that the light intensity directly below the tissue surface is enhanced by a factor of 2-4 as compared with the intensity of the

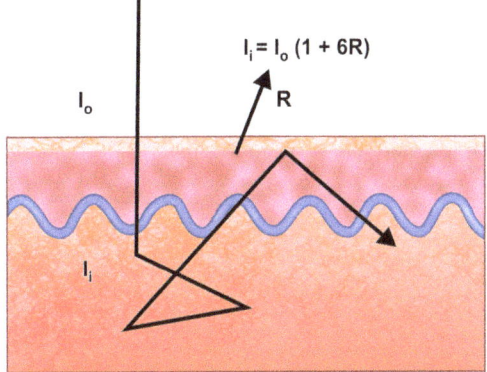

λ (nm)	R	I_i/I_o
585	0.3	2.8
694	0.6	4.6
1064	0.7	5.2

Fig. 1.15: If I_o is the surface fluence and I_i is the fluence in the dermis and the R is the reflected energy, the ratio determines the effective fluence. Longer the wavelength more the effective fluence. This explains the disastrous PIH due to the *so-called* low fluence Nd:YAG for melasma in Indian skin. (Nd:YAG: neodymium-doped yttrium aluminum garnet; PIH: postinflammatory hyperpigmentation)

incident beam, as explained earlier. Because of the scattering effect, the penetration depth depends on the irradiated area. Thus, the penetration depth will double if for the same irradiance, the beam diameter increases from 1 mm to 5 mm. Thus, for treating PWSs or for hair removal, 10–15 mm spot diameters of the laser are recommended as it increases the depth of the laser beam. In tattoos and nevus of Ota in case there is inadequate response, it is wise to increase the diameter of the probe to increase the depth.

- An often-used term is "penetration depth" (d), which describes the path length that causes light to be reduced to 37% of its surface irradiance. For a clear solution, d accurately conveys the depth-dependent fluence attenuation. However, for turbid tissue like the dermis, where backscattering can be considerable, the "real" penetration depth can be more than d. This value may be 2–3 X d for example, with 1,064 nm (Zenzie HH et al. and Jacques SL et al.).
- Jacques notes that a typical bloodless tissue value for μ_a in the visible range is 1 cm^{-1}. But in real life scenario, the scattering leads to an augmented energy and depth.

One should consider the choice of laser within the context of the application and the respective absorption and scattering coefficients. If the absorption coefficient is μ_a more than 200 cm^{-1}, one typically is looking at a "what you see is what you get" laser (examples are Er:YAG and CO_2). Between 1 cm^{-1} and 200 cm^{-1}, are the green-yellow lasers (i.e. PDL, KTP, and alexandrite). Finally, when one considers μ_a less than 1 cm^{-1}, we are typically dealing with deeply penetrating light sources where you can injure the skin without obvious surface changes, a "what you do not see can hurt you" laser (an example is Nd:YAG).

Beyond 600 nm, the increase in penetration and a brisk cutoff in hemoglobin (Hgb) absorption makes for a therapeutic window between 600 nm and 1,200 nm. In this range, radiation penetrates biological tissues at a lower loss thus enabling treatment of deeper tissue structures.

RELEVANT WAVELENGTH RANGES AND CLINICAL APPLICATION

An overview of the absorption spectrum and depth of various lasers is depicted here (Fig. 1.16 and Table 1.2). Based on this, we will dwell on the clinical utility of various lasers used in clinical practice (Sardana K et al.).

Green Yellow

These wavelengths are highly absorbed by Hgb and melanin and are especially useful in treating epidermal pigmented lesions and superficial vessels (Angermeier MC et al., West TB et al., Chan H et al., Kauvar AN et al., and Lee MW et al.).

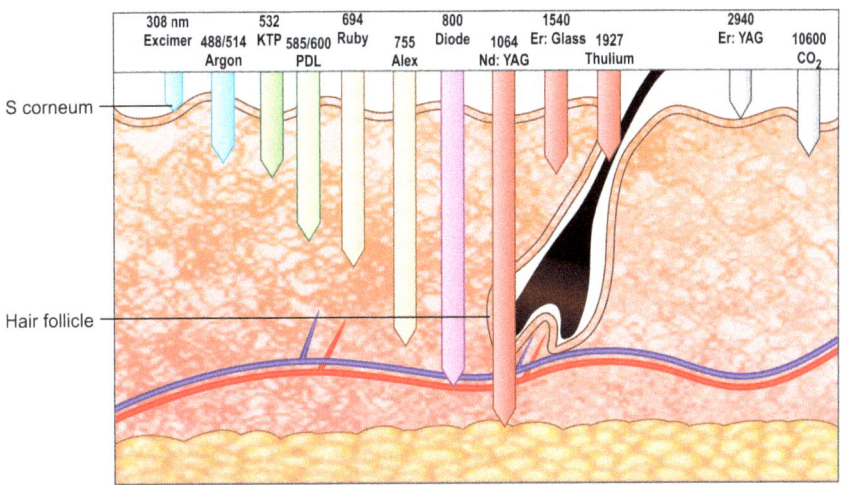

Fig. 1.16: Optical penetration depth of common lasers used in dermatology. (CO_2: carbon dioxide; Er:YAG: erbium-doped yttrium aluminum garnet; Nd:YAG: neodymium-doped yttrium aluminum garnet; PDL: pulsed dye laser)

Table 1.2: Depth of light penetration into tissue depends on wavelength and is limited by scattering and absorption.

Wavelength (nm)	410	532	595	694	755	810	940	1064
OxyHb (40% Hct)	1990	187	35	1.2	2.3	3.6	5.2	2.2
DeoxyHb	1296	138	96	6.6	5.2	2.7	3.0	0.6
Melanin*	140	56	38	23	17	13	7	5.7
Water	6.7×10^{-5}	0.00044	0.0017	0.005	0.03	0.02	0.27	0.15
Bloodless dermis	10	3	2	1.2	0.8	0.6	0.5	0.4
OPD in skin (μm)	100	350	550	750	100	1200	1500	1700

*Moderately pigmented adult: 10% melanin volume fraction in epidermis (DeoxyHb: deoxyhemoglobin; Hct: hematocrit; OPD: optical penetration depth; OxyHb: oxyhemoglobin)

There are two issues concerning these lasers, one is their *poor penetration* in skin (and the even poorer penetration in blood) which makes them poor choices for treatment of deeper pigmented lesions or deeper larger vessels. Similarly, they are not useful for permanent hair reduction [with the possible exception of very large spots (i.e. IPL)] that enhances light depth. The effective portions of many IPL spectra include the green yellow (GY) range. By the proper manipulation of a laser delivery device, one can optimize parameters for selective heating of pigmented versus vascular lesions as given here (Sardana K et al.). Applying a compression handpiece without cooling with 595 nm, blood is depleted (due to blanching) as a target and pigment is preferentially heated.

If the pulse duration is reduced to the nanosecond range, melanosomes are preferentially heated over vessels. For example, extremely short Q-switched 532 nm pulses will cause fine vessels to rupture, but inadequate heat diffusion to the vessel wall precludes long-term vessel destruction. On the other hand, melanosomes are sufficiently heated for single-session lentigo destruction. By choosing specific wavelengths with respect to Hgb and melanin, one can achieve some degree of selective melanin or Hgb heating.

Red and Near Infrared (I) (630 nm, 694 nm, 755 nm, and 810 nm)

(Neimz M et al., Welch AJ et al., Anderson RR et al., and Sardana K et al.)

Deeply penetrating red light (630 nm) CW devices are efficient activators of protoporphyrin after topical application of aminolevulinic acid (ALA). The 694 nm (ruby) laser is optimized for pigment reduction and hair reduction in lighter skin types. The 810 nm diode and 755 nm alexandrite laser, depending on spot size, cooling, pulse duration, and fluence can be configured to optimize outcomes for hair reduction, lentigines, or blood vessels. They are positioned in the absorption spectrum for blood and melanin between the GY wavelengths and 1,064 nm (Fig. 1.16 and Table 1.2). They will penetrate deeply enough in blood to coagulate vessels up to 2 mm; also, they are reasonably tolerant of epidermal pigment in hair reduction (with surface cooling) as long as very dark skin is not treated. By decreasing the pulse width into the nanosecond range, the alexandrite laser is a first-line treatment for many tattoo colors.

Near Infrared (II) 940 nm and Neodymium-doped Yttrium Aluminum Garnet (1,064 nm)

These two wavelengths have been used for a broad range of vessel sizes on the leg and face (Passeron T et al., Kaudewitz P et al., and Major A et al.). They occupy a unique place in the absorption spectrum of the "3" chromophores, that is blood, melanin, and water. Because of the depth of penetration (on the order of mm), they are especially useful for hair reduction and coagulation of deeper blood vessels. By varying fluence and spot size, reticular ectatic veins, as well as those associated with nodular PWSs or hemangiomas, can be safely targeted. On the other hand, they are not well-suited for epidermal pigmented lesions.

Mid-infrared Lasers and Deeply Penetrating Halogen Lamps

These lasers and lamps heat tissue water. The absorption coefficients for the 1,320 nm, 1,450 nm, and 1,540 nm systems are 3 cm^{-1}, 20 cm^{-1}, and 8 cm^{-1}, respectively and the corresponding penetration depths are 1,500 µm, 300 µm, and 700 µm (Trelles MA et al. and Paithankar DY et al.). It follows that for equal surface cooling and equal fluences, the most superficial heating will occur with the 1,450 nm laser, followed by the 1,540 nm and 1,320 nm lasers.

The MIR spectral subset have become the mainstay for fractional nonablative technologies.

Far Infrared Systems

The major lasers are the CO_2 and Er:YAG lasers. Using models, as well as experiments, one can determine relative rates of ablation and heating. Overall, the ratio of ablation to heating is much higher with the Er:YAG laser. However, one can extend the thermal field of the Er:YAG laser by extending the pulse or increasing the repetition rate, and likewise one can decrease the thermal field of CO_2 laser by decreasing pulse width or decreasing fluence (Smith KJ et al. and Majaron B et al.).

It follows that for applications where precision is required in ablation, Er:YAG is preferred. On the other hand, depending on settings, the CO_2 laser combines an enviable blend of ablation and heating. The depth of residual thermal damage (RTD) is typically more uniform with CO_2 than the depth of ablation with Er:YAG, such that the CO_2 laser is more useful for global skin improvement (fine or moderate wrinkle without severe contour defects) on the face. The thresholds for ablation for CO_2 and erbium lasers vary inversely with their optical penetration depths in tissue (20 µm and 1 µm, respectively). This assumes thermal confinement (this presumes that there is no dissipation of energy). It follows that less surface fluence is required for ablation with the erbium laser. With the CO_2 laser, we are operating at ablation threshold in typical resurfacing applications, so a large fraction of energy is invested in tissue heating. This results in low ablation efficiency, and only a small mass of dermal tissue is ablated. In contrast, the erbium laser operates well above threshold (approximately 8–10 X for a fluence of 5 J/cm^2), resulting in greater ablation and less thermal denaturation. The CO_2 laser at typical operating parameters performs self-limited controlled heating of the skin, whereas the erbium laser operates in an almost purely ablative regime.

Comparison of Two Common Ablative Technologies (Carbon Dioxide vs. Erbium-doped Yttrium Aluminum Garnet)

The key to successful applications of soft tissue lasers and their advantages over other surgical tools is their ability to accurately cut and efficiently coagulate the soft tissue at the same time. However, not all lasers are efficient at both cutting and coagulating. Some laser wavelengths (such as those of erbium lasers) are great at cutting but are not as efficient at coagulating, as explained earlier.

Photothermal ablation and laser pulsing: The most efficient soft tissue laser ablation (and incision and excision) is a process of vaporization of intra and extracellular water heated by the laser light within the irradiated soft tissue. Water vapors, rapidly steaming out of the intensely laser-heated soft tissue, carry with them cellular ashes and other byproducts of this fast boiling and vaporization process. Because of very strong absorption by the soft tissue, mid-infrared erbium (circa 3,000 nm) and infrared CO_2 laser (circa 10,000 nm) wavelengths are highly efficient and spatially accurate laser ablation tools.

The rate of how fast the irradiated tissue diffuses the heat away is defined by TRT, which equals approximately 1.5 ms for 75% water rich soft tissue irradiated by 10,600 nm CO_2 laser.

Practical implications of the TRT concept are simple and yet very powerful for appropriate application of laser energy. The most efficient *heating* of the irradiated tissue takes place when laser pulse energy is high and its duration is much *shorter* than TRT. The most efficient *cooling* of the tissue adjacent to the ablated zone takes place if time duration between laser pulses is much *greater* than TRT. Such laser pulsing is referred to as *superpulse* and is a must have feature of any state-of-the-art soft tissue surgical CO_2 laser that minimizes the depth of coagulation. It is a very useful tool for most dermatological ablative tools (Fig. 1.17).

Photothermal coagulation: Coagulation occurs as a denaturation of soft tissue proteins that occurs in 60–100°C temperature range leading to a significant reduction in bleeding (and oozing of lymphatic liquids) on the margins of

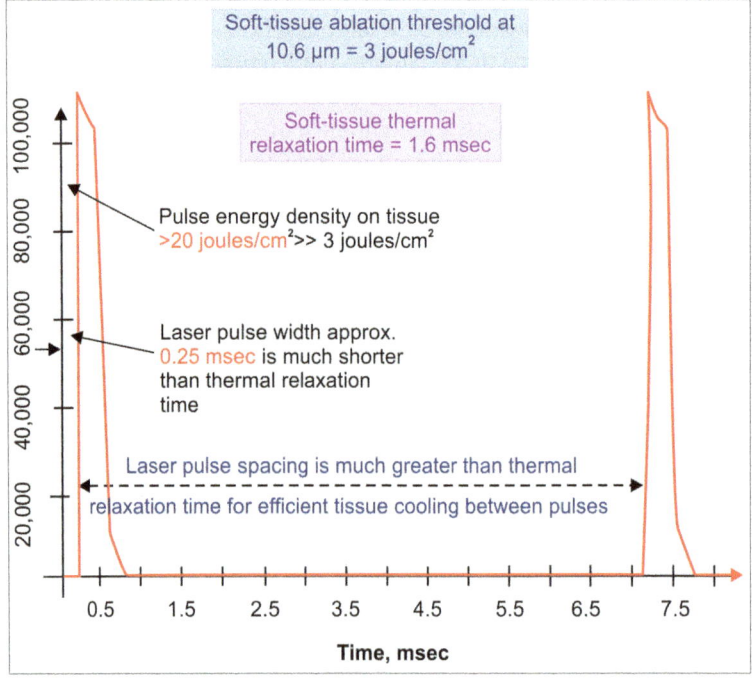

Fig. 1.17: A depiction of tissue fluence and pulse duration settings for efficient soft tissue ablation (superpulse: high-power short pulse).

ablated tissue during laser ablation (and excision/incision) procedures. This can be of use in case dermal depth is needed.

Since blood is contained within and transported through the blood vessels, the diameter of blood vessels B (estimated to range from 21 µm to 40 µm) is a highly important spatial parameter that influences the efficiency of photocoagulation process. Photothermal coagulation is also accompanied by hemostasis due to shrinkage of the walls of blood vessels (and lymphatic vessels) due to collagen shrinkage at increased temperatures. The coagulation depth H (for 60-100°C temperature range inside the ablation margins) is proportional to the absorption depth A (an inverse of absorption coefficient) (Fig. 1.18).

- The coagulation depth H relative to the blood vessel diameter B is an important measure of coagulation and hemostasis efficiency. For $H>>B$ (diode laser wavelengths), optical absorption (near IR attenuation) and coagulation depths are significantly greater than blood vessel diameters; coagulation takes place over extended volumes.
- For H more than or equal to B (CO_2 laser wavelengths in Figure 1.18), coagulation extends just deep enough into a severed blood vessel to stop the bleeding. In another words, the CO_2 laser's excellent coagulation efficiency is due to the close match between the photothermal coagulation depth of approximately 50 µm, and soft tissue blood capillary diameters of approximately 20-40 µm. The key to the success of the soft tissue CO_2 laser is its ability to cut and coagulate the soft tissue simultaneously.

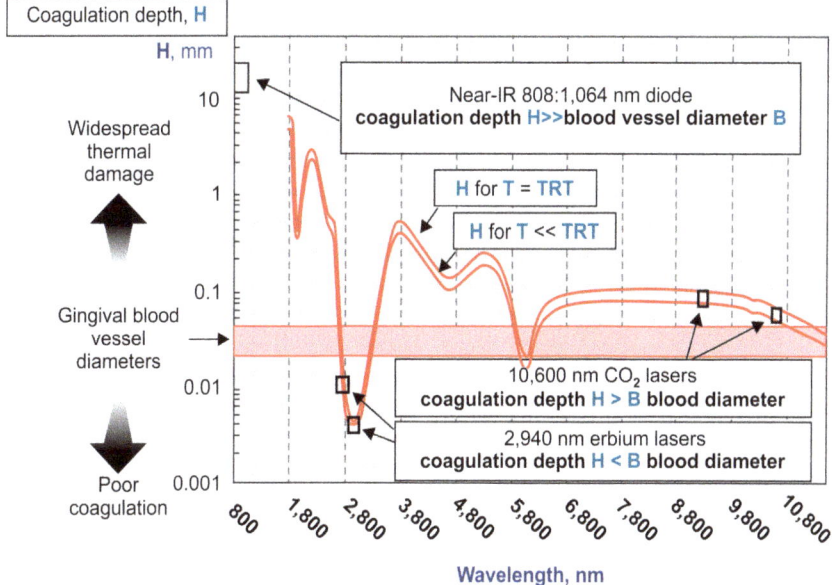

Fig. 1.18: Coagulation depth spectrum for pulsed laser ablation; TRT is thermal relaxation time. Logarithmic scale is in use.

- For $H<<B$ (see erbium laser wavelengths in Figure 1.18), optical absorption and coagulation depths are significantly smaller than blood vessel diameters; coagulation takes place on relatively small spatial scale and cannot prevent bleeding from the blood vessels severed during tissue ablation.
- *Implications:* In the cutting and coagulation mode, unlike the resurfacing mode, the pulsed CO_2 is better, but in fine surgeries where coagulation is not required the Er:YAG is a superior mode.

Fractional Technology (Sardana K et al.): Pixilated Injury (Aka Fractional Photothermolysis)

One can create a "pixilated" injury with water as a chromophore in what is called fractional photothermolysis. Thus, the MIR and FIR lasers are commonly used in this technology.

Roughly 100 µm spots have been used with 250–500 µm spacing. The tissue can recover from this fractional injury without the widespread epidermal loss observed after traditional resurfacing applications (Fig. 1.19A). Depending on the technology used two forms are described and though initial enthusiasm was favored toward the ablative fractional lasers, this has been replaced with the fractional radiofrequency (FRF). But it must be remembered that even with these technologies the deeper ice pick scars do not completely respond.

Ablative and Nonablative Lasers

By definition, an ablative laser is one that removes the skin surface and produces controlled coagulation of the tissue underneath. Nonablative systems produce only tissue coagulation, keeping the skin surface intact. At the NIR range, the absorption of melanin reduces drastically. Moreover, the absorption of water increases exponentially. Thus, through appropriate selection of

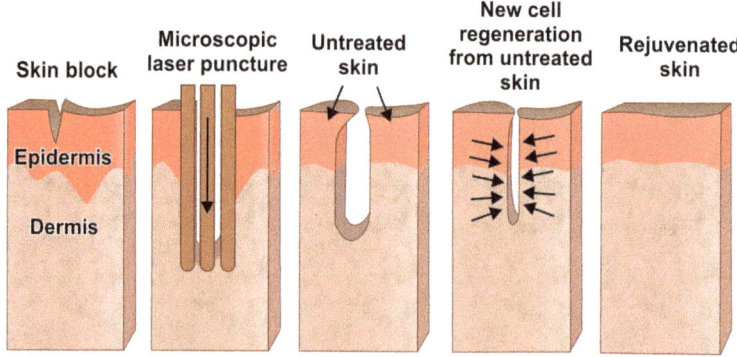

Fig. 1.19A: Diagram illustrating the process of rapid skin regeneration produced by carbon dioxide (CO_2) fractional laser.

wavelength and pulse duration, it is possible to vary the intensity of the heat generated in the skin changing from nonablative to an ablative interaction.

Therefore, the difference from a nonablative to an ablative laser is simply its wavelength and consequent intensity of interaction with the water in the chromophore. The graph (Fig. 1.19B) shows the curve of absorption of the water in the chromophore for two lasers used in skin rejuvenation: (1) Er:Glass (1,540 nm), and (2) CO_2 (10,600 nm).

As the absorption coefficient of Er:Glass is lesser than CO_2 it will heat less and also as water is the main chromophore in the skin, will get less absorbed and penetrate deeper. Hence, it will be a gentler on the skin with dermal remodeling and less downtime. The CO_2 will achieve high thermal effects and will penetrate less as it is more absorbed by water. The Er:YAG with a higher absorption coefficient will have even a lesser absorption as most of the skin is water and would be gentler than the CO_2 laser.

A summary of the various technologies is given here in the Table 1.3.

Radiofrequency Technology

Radiofrequency skin interactions are fundamentally different than optical ones. Rather than "optical" fluence and absorption coefficients, local heat generation depends on the local resistance and the local current density. With most RF systems, there is a rapidly alternating current that, given the impedance of the skin, generates heat. The distribution of the current density is determined by the configuration of the electrodes relative to the skin anatomy (Fig. 1.20A). Depending on the type of surface cooling, one can create various zones of heating under the skin. There are two types of

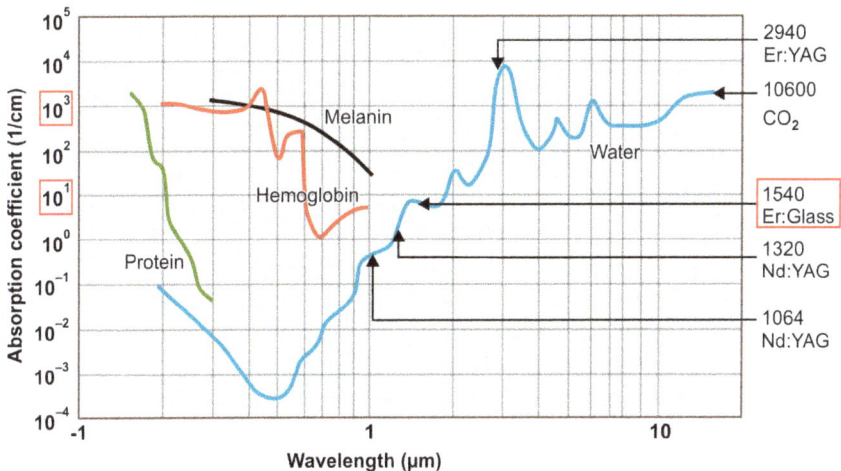

Fig. 1.19B: A comparison of various technologies for rejuvenation. (CO_2: carbon dioxide; Er:YAG: erbium-doped yttrium aluminum garnet; Nd:YAG: neodymium-doped yttrium aluminum garnet)

Table 1.3: Summary of the various ablative and nonablative lasers.

CO_2 (10,600 nm)	Balanced mixture of ablation and coagulation of the tissue leading to a complete rejuvenation result that is still the gold standard of the market but may cause PIH in Indian skin
Er:YAG (2,940 nm)	It has a high water absorption, causes less ablation, safer than CO_2, but achieves less depth, with less collagen remodeling in the dermis
Nd:YAG (1,064 nm and 1,320 nm)	It has nonablative effect only in the coagulation of the dermis
Tm:YAG	Very superficial laser
Diode	A compact system with wavelength of 1,450 nm; nonablative effect
Er:Fiber or Er:Glass	It has the wavelength of 1,550 nm or 1,540 nm. Both are nonablative

(CO_2: carbon dioxide; Er:YAG: erbium-doped yttrium aluminum garnet; Nd:YAG: neodymium-doped yttrium aluminum garnet)

electrode deployment with variations therein (Koch RJ et al. and Sadick NS et al.):

1. In one scenario, *bipolar electrodes* are combined with either a diode laser or IPL device. In this configuration, there is so-called synergy between the two applications. With the bipolar electrode configuration, electrical field density is intrinsically confined fairly superficially (the field intensity reaches about as deep as one-half the distance between the electrodes) (Fig. 1.20A).

   If both positive and negative electrodes are placed in the contact tip (bipolar electrode), current density tends to flow superficially (path of least resistance from electrode to electrode, and therefore, temperature elevation is confined to superficial skin). By placing the electrodes further apart, the current density depth will increase. The control of the tissue heating is determined by variations in electrode type, power, and cooling times.

2. In *monopolar configurations*, the dispersive electrode is located at a distant point on the body. Monopolar skin rejuvenation systems tend to create large volumes of heating. They disperse the electrical energy over the breadth of the electrode through a concept known as capacitive coupling. This type of coupling helps to prevent the natural accumulation of electrical energy at the electrode edge (Fig. 1.20C).

3. *Fractional treatment:* In contrast to lasers where the thermal effect is limited to the periphery of the ablation crater, RF energy flows through the whole dermis, adding volumetric heating to fractional treatment. This volumetric heating adds a skin tightening effect. RF fractional technologies can be administered from the surface, using a grid of electrodes, or intradermally, using a grid of microneedles which deliver the

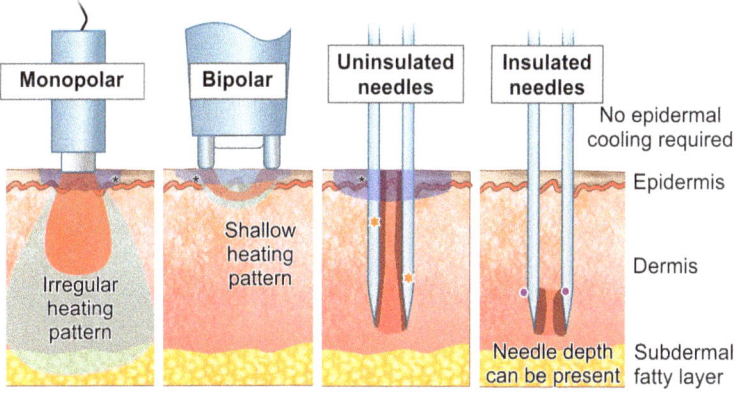

Fig. 1.20A: An overview of the varied radiofrequency (RF) technologies in use in dermatology.

RF energy within the dermis (Lapidoth M et al.). The surface electrodes provide a more superficial effect improving texture and fine lines (Man J et al.) while longer needles penetrate deeper, providing deeper dermal remodeling (Mulholland RS et al.).

The adjustable microneedles allow the depth of delivery of the RF energy to be set depending on the desired result, which allows for the energy to be targeted directly at the tissue being treated with minimal impact on the surrounding tissue and skin. The varying depth of delivery allows the procedure to be precisely customized to address specific problem areas with minimal downtime. The treatment depth can also be varied to allow for resurfacing of the skin, leading to improvement in fine lines, wrinkles, and acne scars (Fig. 1.20B).

Microneedle RF treats the skin in a minimally invasive manner. Dielectric coated needles have become popular in delivering aggressive heating to the reticular dermis without thermal damage to the skin's surface (Willey A et al.). By heating deep dermal collagen at a higher temperature than could be safely used at the epidermal level, a much stronger collagen contraction effect can be achieved in order to improve deep wrinkles and enhance skin tightening. The combination of deep dermal treatment with superficial fractional treatment has a high potential for complete skin improvement while avoiding skin excision.

By introducing larger needle electrodes into the deep dermis, for example in RF-assisted liposuction, RF can be used to address tightening of the fibroseptal network of the adipose layer with subsequent accommodation of the overlying skin during local fat removal. When energy is applied under the skin, the dermis and epidermis are relatively protected. More aggressive heating up to 60–70°C can be applied during treatment, creating immediate

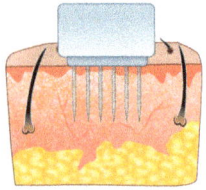
1. Drive a needle into a target area

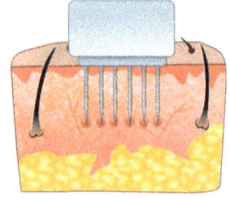
2. Apply RF energy from a lower end of the needle

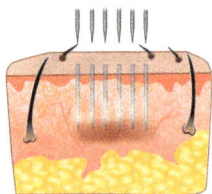
3. Remove the needle if application of RF energy is completed

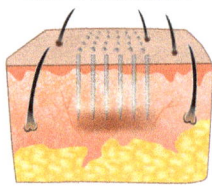
4. Collagen, elastic tissue rejuvenation and healing

Fig. 1.20B: A diagrammatic depiction of the microneedle RF.

and more pronounced collagen contraction. In some clinical studies (Paul M et al. and Duncan D et al.) up to 42% area skin contraction was achieved after RF-assisted lipolysis.

It is often said that FRF is safe for all skin types because of its "color blind" characteristic. However, it should be noted that, while the RF interaction with skin does not depend on the presence of melanin or any other chromophore, darker skin types and tanned skin are still susceptible to postinflammatory hyperpigmentation (PIH). The FRF will heat and induce a wound healing process response in the skin; therefore, it is wise to treat these high-risk skin types with greater caution.

PRACTICAL APPLICATIONS OF LTI (LASER-TISSUE INTERACTIONS)

Though there are various applications of LTI, a few examples relevant to common situations are mentioned here. I would like to emphasize that the use of two or more lasers in the *same* sittings may not have a proportionate additive effect as the LTI of a single laser can be reliably predicted, but the tissue changes that ensue can change the tissue dynamics of the second laser. Thus, concomitant "cocktail" lasers have little scientific basis, even though may be practiced by clinicians. The exceptions include skin conditions which have multiple elements to treat. A classic example is photoaging, though Asian skin, does not age like Caucasian skin. But an aging skin has lentigines, freckles, seborrheic keratosis (SK), laxity of skin, and melanocytic nevi. Here the first measure should be to treat the pigmented lesions by a Q-switched laser, then the nevi by a Er:YAG/CO_2 and then the laxity by a fractional/

microinvasive RF. But combining in the same sessions is not only illogical can be a painful experience for the patient.

Pulse Duration of Lasers
(Sardana K et al. and Anderson R et al.)

With very short pulse widths (pw), lasers vaporize targets but can side effects that may not be desirable. For example, in treating blood vessels, rapid heating results in acute vessel wall damage and petechial hemorrhage (with Q-switched 532 nm). With intermediate length pulses (0.1–1.5 ms), one can gently heat targets without immediate rupture of the vessels. But intravascular thrombosis can create purpura and delayed hemorrhage. With longer pulses (6–100 ms), the ratio of contraction to thrombosis increases and side effects are less likely.

Too long pulses with very small targets can create two problems. With highly absorbing targets (i.e. tattoo inks), the heat generation is so great and long-lived that significant diffusion occurs to the surrounding dermis. On the other hand, using a long pulse YAG for a nevus of Ota results in an insufficient temperature rise as the pigmented nevus cells cool off too fast during the delivery of the pulses (also melanin absorption is much weaker than black ink).

With ablative lasers, the ideal numbers are a fluence of about 4–5 J/cm^2 applied in less than or equal to 1 ms, the TRT of human skin. When the pulse width exceeds the TRT of skin, the surrounding tissue undergoes prolonged, less efficient heating that may result in unexpected and undesired effects including superheating of tissue and char formation. For the CO_2 laser the ideal pulse duration to achieve ablation without superheating the surrounding tissue is approximately 0.7 ms.

In order for any ablative device to reach a given depth, the length of exposure is increased in the CW laser, or the number of pulses is increased in the pulsed laser. When the pulse duration is increased beyond the TRT of skin and the thermal effect of the laser–tissue interaction outpaces the velocity of ablation, the result is wider zones of thermal injury. This unseen effect of prolonged pulse width alters treatment density and can lead to complications (Fig. 1.20C).

Selective Photothermolysis of Tattoos
(Hillenkamp FR et al., Neimz M et al., Sardana K et al., and Anderson R et al.)

Amorphous carbon, graphite, India ink, and organometallic dyes, typically found in dark blue-black amateur and professional tattoos, have a broad absorption in the visible and NIR portions of the spectrum. At visible wavelengths longer than 600 nm, hemoglobin and melanin light absorption is minimized and tattoo dyes can be targeted selectively.

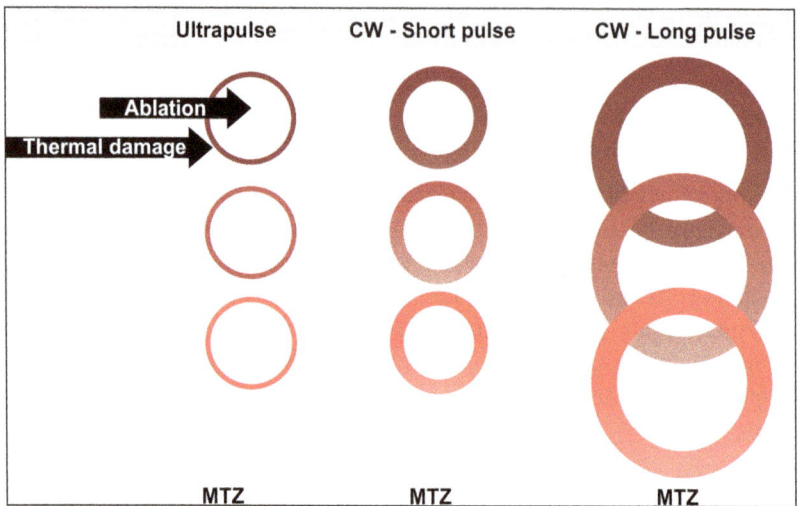

Fig. 1.20C: The effect of pulse duration on treatment density in fractional carbon dioxide (CO_2) laser resurfacing. Each circle represents a microthermal wound created by the fractional laser beam. The pulse duration is shortest with the ultrapulse and longest with the long-pulse continuous wave (CW) laser. The circumferential lines represent the areas of thermal damage (i.e. thick lines denote greater thermal damage than thin lines). As the pulse duration increases, the circumferential lines become thicker, the areas of thermal damage increase, and the treatment density increases. At the long pulses the wound areas begin to overlap, resulting in further increases in thermal damage. At this stage the treatment has become fully ablative (i.e. 100% density). This effect is believed to account for the unexpected adverse effects at long pulse durations of fractional resurfacing procedures.
Source: Duplechain JK. Neck rejuvenation; surgical and non-surgical. Facial Plast Surg Clin of North Am. 2014;22(2):2003-16.

The pigment granules characteristically found in tattoos have diameters of 0.5–100 mm, which correspond to TRT of 20 ns to 3 ms. With the development of the Q-switched ruby (694 nm), alexandrite (755 nm), and Nd:YAG (1.06 mm) lasers, tattoo removal without scarring can be achieved. The frequency-doubled, Q-switched Nd:YAG laser (KTP laser) emits at a wavelength of 532 nm, which provides improved removal of red dye. Recently picosecond lasers have been used for tattoos.

But there is an issue of competing pigment in the Indian skin and also the problem of slow results, as the ultimate results are based on the capacity of the macrophages to digest the tattoo pigment. Hence, modified methods have been used to remove the surface epidermis with faster results that can be applied to difficult tattoos (Sardana K et al. and Sardana K et al.).

Selective Photothermolysis of Pigmented Lesions
(Sardana K et al. and Anderson R et al.)

Pigmented lesions can be divided into epidermal and dermal. Although highest in the UV portion of the spectrum, melanin absorption is also significant in the visible and NIR wavelengths. The diameters of individual melanosomes (0.5–1.0 µm) and melanocytes (7 µm) correspond to TRT of 20–1,000 ns.

Static epidermal pigmented lesions such as lentigos tend to be straightforward to treat. Q-switched green, red, and NIR wavelengths have been utilized for this indication. Though Q-switched lasers are used most commonly the gentle heating by the millisecond laser can also treat epidermal disorders. With longer pulses (ms), the dermal melanocyte does not become hot enough to achieve pigment reduction, thus ensuring selective epidermal damage.

The geometry (and therefore the microscopic characteristics) of pigmented lesions is important. In the treatment for a nevus versus a lentigo, it must be noted that the nevus is composed of melanocytes in aggregates as (collectively of a size of 100 µm in diameter) whereas the lentigo is a mere sheet of melanocytes some 10 µm thick. So, the TRT of the nevus cell is about 10 ms while that of the lentigo is about 0.1 ms. Thus, in treating nevus with a long-pulsed alexandrite laser with a high fluence, the TRT will approach a second. More importantly, the thick slab of melanocytes will take long to cool, such that there will be considerable heat diffusion away from the target. On the other hand, the lentigo represents a slab only tens of microns thick; there will be heat diffusion during the long pulse and rapid cooling after the pulse.

Thus, with microsecond-domain fluences, the nevus might result in scarring and a lighter lentigo might not become hot enough for clearance. If one applies nanosecond pulses to the two lesion types, the lentigo shows a good response with possibly complete clearing, whereas the nevus will require multiple sessions, as each laser application will result in heat confined to the most superficial part of the lesion. Conversely a microsecond laser might work for nevi.

Thus, the known laser principles of pigment specific lasers do *not apply* to all pigmented lesions especially melanocytic nevi, where ablative lasers are more effective (Sardana K et al).

"Dermal" static pigmented lesions such as nevus of Ota respond best to Q-switched lasers. With longer pulses (ms domain), the dermal melanocytes, which are of relatively low concentration (compared to melanocytic nests in compound nevi or highly pigmented basal cell layers in lentigos), simply do not become hot enough to achieve pigment reduction (Anderson R et al.).

Selective Photothermolysis and Laser-assisted Hair Removal
(Ross EV et al.)

The human hair follicle is a complex structure derived from both epidermal and dermal components. The target chromophores, primarily melanin-rich hair shafts, are located deep in human skin (bulge around 1.5 mm and bulb at 2–7 mm). At this depth, only red and NIR wavelengths are useful (690–900 nm). The follicular structure responsible for regeneration has not been conclusively identified and, therefore, current systems target the entire follicle. As a result, long pulse widths on the order of milliseconds and high fluences capable of heating large volumes of tissue are required.

Millisecond-domain ruby, alexandrite, diode, and Nd:YAG lasers using high light doses can produce selective injury to human hair follicles resulting in prolonged growth delay and in some cases, permanent hair loss after a single treatment.

Selective Photothermolysis of Cutaneous Blood Vessels

The pulsed dye lasers at 577–595 nm wavelengths well absorbed by the targeted hemoglobin molecule relative to other optically absorbing structures, cause selective thermal damage to dermal blood vessels while minimizing epidermal melanin absorption. Furthermore, because the TRT for cutaneous blood vessels varies between 10 ms and 300 ms, a variable pulse duration is required for optimal results.

By varying the pulse duration, treatments can be performed purpurically (with bruising) by rupturing the blood vessel, or subpurpurically by slowly heating the vessel causing coagulation of the blood vessel. The V beam PDL lasers have 0.45 ms, 1.5 ms, 3 ms, 6 ms, 10 ms, 20 ms, 30 ms, and 40 ms pulsed durations. The shorter the pulse duration, the more destructive the energy becomes, while with the longer pulse durations, the energy is more gentle thus causing coagulation of the target without harming structures around the treated area (Fig. 1.20D).

For coagulation and treatments without purpura, the laser pulse duration should be shorter than the TRT of the target absorbing the laser radiation in order to confine the thermal damage and spare surrounding tissue. The relaxation time of a target is determined by the target's size (milliseconds or greater for vascular lesions).

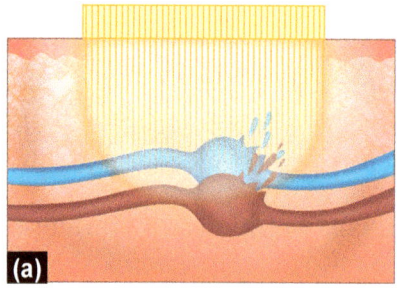 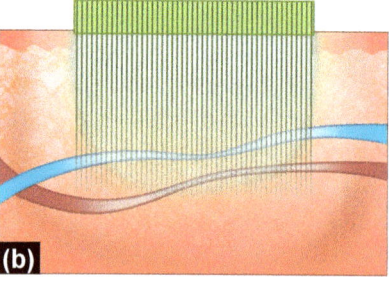

Fig. 1.20D: Longer wavelengths allow treatment of vascular lesions without purpura, as seen with traditional pulsed dye lasers. (a) Short-pulsed, yellow-light treatment of vascular lesion with vessel rupture versus; (b) Longer-pulsed, green-light treatment with vessel shrinkage and avoidance of purpura.

But there are numerous variations in pulse duration and absorption of various chromophores (bloodless dermis, HbO_2, and deoxyHb) that can complicate this simplistic interpretation. Moreover, remember that shorter wavelength are absorbed in the epidermis and the epidermal pigment in Indian skin can complicate the laser physics and thus, in Indian skin the results are far from satisfactory.

Fractional Lasers and Penetration Depth—Site Variations

Most data is extrapolated from abdominoplasty specimens. But the depth achieved in the abdomen is not same as in the face. This is important for clinicians who extrapolate data from pilot ex vivo studies. Also while performing fractional lasers clinicians often give multiple passes on a single site. These can have clinical implications:

Site Variation

The depth achieved on the facial skin is about 28% less than on the abdominal skin (Fig. 1.21A). The 28% correction factor formula, when applied to abdominal MTZ depths, corrects for the differences between abdominal and facial skin and allows greater accuracy in simulating/predicting facial skin laser column depths (Bailey SH et al.).

Abdominal MTZ (μm) - (28% × Abdominal MTZ) = Face MTZ

This is primarily as the histology of the face is different from the abdominal skin (Fig. 1.21B). Thus, on the face the thermal energy from the laser beam is dissipated along the blood vessels, and thus the energy required is higher than what is predicted on the abdominal skin. The markedly higher density

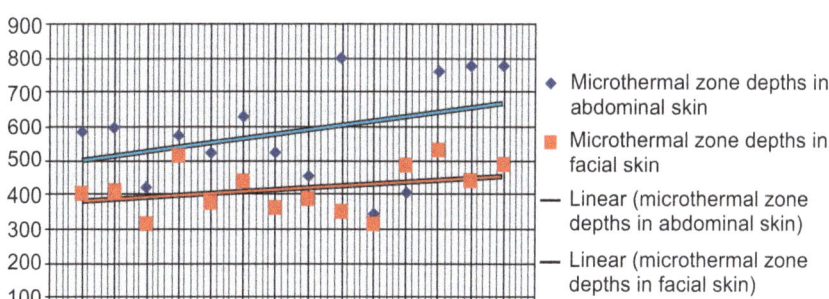

Fig. 1.21A: Graph representing the depths of microthermal zone (MTZ) in the facial and abdominal tissue. Note the difference between the depths of the MTZ between abdominal and facial tissue. Calculated mean difference = 28%.

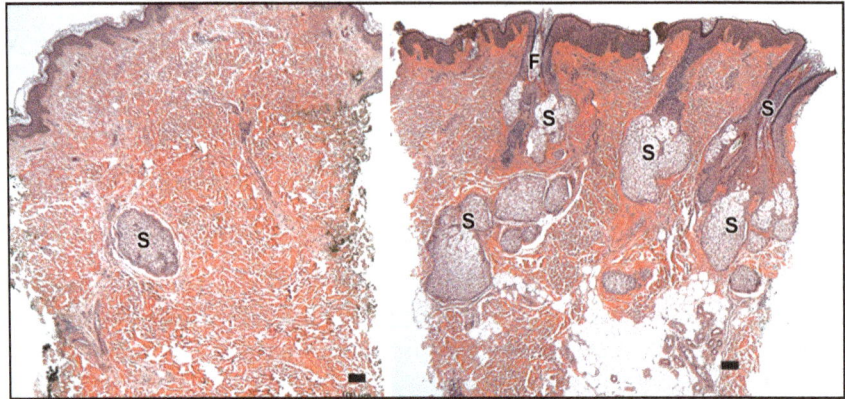

Fig. 1.21B: A comparison of the histology of the facial and abdominal skin. (S: sebaceous glands, F: hair follicle)

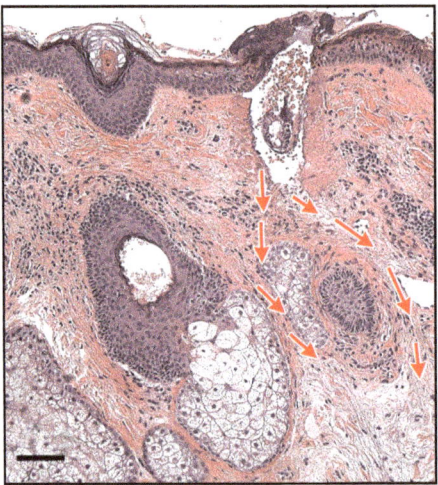

Fig. 1.21C: The abundant pilosebaceous units cause divergence of the laser energy.

of pilosebaceous units found in the face creates variation in the distribution of energy in the dermis. Therefore, instead of dispersing energy in a straight line from the epidermis to the dermis, the laser energy may travel around the blood vessels, diverge around sebaceous glands, or possibly travel down a hair shaft without damaging the surrounding skin (Fig. 1.21C).

Pulsing

Double pulsing is defined as two discrete pulses of laser energy to be delivered to the same treatment area within quick succession, at less than 1 ms between the pulses. Using the theory of SPT the thermal heat has not had sufficient time to dissipate following the first pulse before the second has

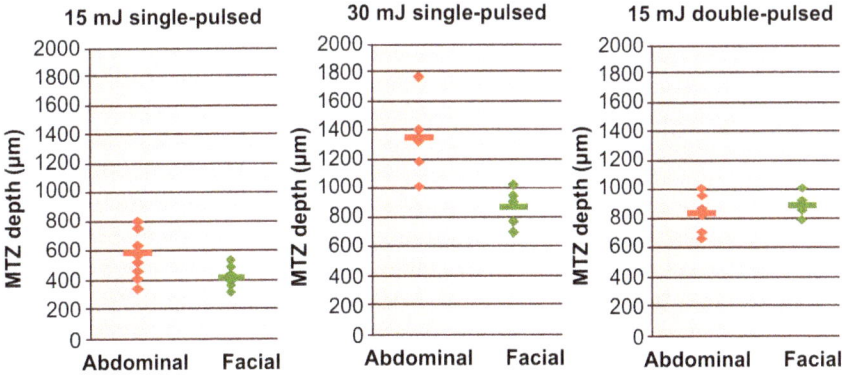

Fig. 1.21D: Comparison of the MTZ depths at each laser setting by treatment site (abdominal vs. facial).

been delivered. The net effect, therefore, is greater coagulation of the tissue (Fig. 1.21D).

With a single pulse at *15 mJ, depths* of injury of facial and abdominal skin (415 µm and 582 µm, respectively) were similar. With *double pulsing at 15 mJ*, injury to abdominal skin (822 µm) was more superficial than with a single pulse at 30 mJ (1,345 µm). The difference in depths was 523 µm.

A similar comparison for facial skin shows a much smaller difference (881 µm – 854 µm = 27 µm), suggesting that laser injury patterns in facial and abdominal skin are not the same.

The *widths* of laser-induced injury in the face and abdomen were also measured. The data showed that for facial skin, the widths of injuries induced by double and single pulses (493 µm and 312 µm, respectively) at 15 mJ differed by 181 µm, much larger than the 27 µm observed for facial injury depths. When facial injuries induced by single pulses at 30 mJ and 15 mJ were compared, the difference in widths was even larger (534 µm –312 µm = 222 µm).

Thus, though it was expected that double pulse treatments at energy of 15 mJ would deliver exactly twice the energy as a single pulse 15 mJ treatment and the same energy as a single pulsed 30 mJ treatment this was not seen on histopathology. Thus, double pulsing is of little use as the thermal effects were actual more attenuated then expected with double pulsing. Essentially, it is better to increase the pulse energy than give multiple pulses (Oni G et al.).

Fundamental Principles of Laser Tissue Interactions

The vast amount of data is of little meaning if not used correctly. Thus, in practice, *four principles* have to be remembered on which most laser applications are based:
1. **Absorption spectra of various chromophores:** It is important to understand the wavelength that is absorbed by the target chromophore.

This is especially relevant in tattoos, thus accounting for the use of 532 nm (*green*) for a *red* tattoo and 1,064 nm (*blue*) for a *black* pigment. This also accounts for the use of Er:YAG as an ablative tool for dermal tumors where the target chromophore is water.
2. **Pulse duration of the lasers:** This is directly dependent on the size of the target. This explains, why a Q-switched laser is used for a nanosized tattoo and this also explains the logic of using a microsecond laser (Er:YAG) is for epidermal ablation (TRT 10 ms). The use of picosecond lasers for tattoos is claimed to be a cutting edge discovery, but this was discovered many years back. Even for tattoos, it is not vastly superior to Q-switched lasers as, laser tattoo interaction is a small part of the story, more important is host response that removes the pigment.
3. **Penetration depth of laser:** The optical penetration depth is an important consideration especially in pigmented skin. As melanin has a wide range of absorption spectrum, most lasers can be used for pigment disorders. The reason most of us use the Q-switched Nd:YAG 1,064 nm is as it penetrates deeper and thus would not interact with the competing epidermal pigment, which is a competing factor in pigmented skin (Issa MC et al.).
4. **Modulation of lasers in pigmented skin:** A *fourth* aspect is the *PIH* that Indian skin is prone for and thus high impact lasers with increases thermal damage should be avoided as they may cause more harm than good. The use of lasers for melasma is an example where the patient has a worsening of the disorder, specially in pigmented skin. In fact the nonjudicious use of lasers, like Nd:YAG has led to disastrous results.

CONCLUSION

The concepts discussed may seem extensive and tedious, but they have two important clinical implications. *Firstly* the concept of simultaneous combination or sequential use of lasers for a single pathology defy lasers physics as most of the concepts laid earlier are based on a single laser. Hence, the combination of various lasers achieves little, except to add a sense of novelty in conferences discourses. The *second* problem that has been borne out by numerous practitioners is that excessive and inordinate laser use without understanding the skin type can lead to PIH that tends to spoil results. This is especially true in melasma and cases of PIH treated by lasers in pigmented skin. *Third* and most important is that clinicians should ask for in vitro or ex vivo dose parameter studies published in indexed journals. That way one can use conservative doses. As a thumb rule use a dose or density lesser than what is recommended for Caucasian skin. But do not tweak the pulse duration.

It is also useful if laser users also publicize what can go wrong with lasers especially in Indian skin without bandying the results in fairer skin types, where the laser optics can be predicted as the epidermis is largely an optical window. A chapter on laser complications mirrors these sentiments (Chapter 17).

Do not learn lasers from company sales people as they have little knowledge of laser physics. I am surprised by some who learn laser physics from company representatives who know very little beyond marketing.

I conclude by the famous adage that, that it is sensible to be *"wiser by learning from others mistakes, than be foolish by learning by one's own mistakes".* A working knowledge of LTI would be the first step in following this principle and the detailed applications follow in the forthcoming chapters.

BIBLIOGRAPHY

1. Aguilar G, Majaron B, Karapetian E, et al. Experimental study of cryogen spray properties for application in dermatologic laser surgery. IEEE Trans Biomed Eng. 2003;50:863-9.
2. Anderson R, Ross E. Laser–tissue interactions. In: Fitzpatrick R, Goldman M (Eds). Cosmetic Laser Surgery. St Louis: Mosby; 2000. pp. 1-30.
3. Anderson RR, Parrish JA. Selective photothermolysis: precise microsurgery by selective absorption of pulsed radiation. Science. 1983;220:524-7.
4. Anderson RR, Parrish JA. The optics of human skin. J Invest Dermatol. 1981;77:13-9.
5. Angermeier MC. Treatment of facial vascular lesions with intense pulsed light. J Cut Laser Ther. 1999;1:95-100.
6. Bailey SH, Brown SA, Kim Y, et al. An intra-individual quantitative assessment of acute laser injury patterns in facial versus abdominal skin. Lasers Surg Med. 2011;43:99-107.
7. Boulnois JL. Photophysical processes in recent medical developments: a review. Lasers Med Sci. 1986;1:47-66.
8. Chan H. The use of lasers and intense pulsed light sources for the treatment of acquired pigmentary lesions in Asians. J Cosmet Laser Ther. 2003;5:198-200.
9. Chan HH, Lam LK, Wong DS, et al. Role of skin cooling in improving patient tolerability of Q-switched alexandrite (QS Alex) laser in nevus of Ota treatment. Lasers Surg Med. 2003;32:148-51.
10. Choi B, Pearce JA, Welch AJ. Modeling infrared temperature measurements: implications for laser irradiation and cryogen cooling studies. Phys Med Biol. 2000;45:541-57.
11. DiBernardo BE, Reyes J. Evaluation of skin tightening after laser-assisted liposuction. Aesthet Surg J. 2009;29:400-7.
12. Duncan D. Improving outcomes in upper arm liposuction: adding radio-frequency-assisted liposuction to induce skin contraction. Aesthet Surg J. 2012;32:84-95.
13. Ellis DL, Weisberg NK, Chen JS, et al. Free electron laser infrared wavelength specificity for cutaneous contraction. Lasers Surg Med. 1999;25:1-7.
14. Greve B, Hammes S, Raulin C. The effect of cold air cooling on 585 nm pulsed dye laser treatment of port-wine stains. Dermatol Surg. 2001;27:633-6.
15. Grossweiner L. The Science of Phototherapy. Boca Raton: CRC Press; 1994. p. 217.

16. Hillenkamp FR. Interaction between laser radiation and biological systems. In: Hillenkamp FR, Sacchi C (Eds). Lasers in Medicine and Biology. New York: Plenum; 1980. pp. 37-68.
17. Hohenleutner U, Walther T, Wenig M, et al. Leg telangiectasia treatment with a 1.5 ms pulsed dye laser, ice cube cooling of the skin and 595 vs 600 nm: preliminary results. Lasers Surg Med. 1998;23:72-8.
18. Issa MC, Tamura B. Lasers, lights and other technologies. In: Issa MC, Tamura B (Eds). Clinical Approaches and Procedures in Cosmetic Dermatology. New York: Springer; 2018.
19. Jacques SL. Laser–tissue interactions. Photochemical, photothermal, and photomechanical. Surg Clin North Am. 1992;72:531-58.
20. Jacques SL. Simple optical theory for light dosimetry during PDT. In: Tuchin V (Ed). Selected Papers on Tissue Optics. Bellingham: International Society for Optical Engineering (SPIE); 1992. p. 655.
21. Kaudewitz P, Klovekorn W, Rother W. Effective treatment of leg vein telangiectasia with a new 940 nm diode laser. Dermatol Surg. 2001;27:101-6.
22. Kauvar AN, Frew KE, Friedman PM, et al. Cooling gel improves pulsed KTP laser treatment of facial telangiectasia. Lasers Surg Med. 2002;30:149-53.
23. Koch RJ. Radiofrequency nonablative tissue tightening. Facial Plast Surg Clin North Am. 2004;12:339-46.
24. Lapidoth M, Halachmi S. Radiofrequency in cosmetic dermatology. Aesthet Dermatol. 2015;2:1-22.
25. Lee MW. Combination 532-nm and 1064-nm lasers for noninvasive skin rejuvenation and toning. Arch Dermatol. 2003;139:1265-76.
26. Majaron B, Verkruysse W, Kelly KM, et al. Er:YAG laser skin resurfacing using repetitive long-pulse exposure and cryogen spray cooling: II. Theoretical analysis. Lasers Surg Med. 2001;28:131-38.
27. Major A, Brazzini B, Campolmi P, et al. Nd:YAG 1064 nm laser in the treatment of facial and leg telangiectasias. J Eur Acad Dermatol Venereol. 2001;15:559-65.
28. Man J, Goldberg DJ. Safety and efficacy of fractional bipolar radiofrequency treatment in Fitzpatrick skin types V-VI. J Cosmet Laser Ther. 2012;14:179-83.
29. Mulholland RS, Ahn DH, Kreindel M, et al. Fractional ablative radiofrequency resurfacing in Asian and Caucasian skin: a novel method for deep radiofrequency fractional skin rejuvenation. J Cosmet Dermatol Sci Appl. 2012;2:144-50.
30. Neimz M. Laser–tissue Interactions, 2nd edition. Berlin: Springer; 2002. p. 303.
31. Oni G, Robbins D, Bailey S, et al. An in vivo histopathological comparison of single and double pulsed modes of a fractionated CO(2) laser. Lasers Surg Med. 2012;44:4-10.
32. Paithankar D, Ross E. Comparison of cryogen spray and surface contact cooling through heat transfer modeling. Laser Exp. 2000;1:1-14.
33. Paithankar DY, Clifford JM, Saleh BA, et al. Subsurface skin renewal by treatment with a 1450-nm laser in combination with dynamic cooling. J Biomed Optics. 2003;8:545-51.
34. Parlette EC, Kaminer ME. Laser-assisted liposuction: here's the skinny. Semin Cutan Med Surg. 2008;27:259-63.
35. Passeron T, Olivier V, Duteil L, et al. The new 940-nanometer diode laser: an effective treatment for leg venulectasia. J Am Acad Dermatol. 2003;48:768-74.
36. Paul M, Blugerman G, Kreindel M, et al. Three-dimensional radiofrequency tissue tightening: a proposed mechanism and applications for body contouring. Aesthet Plast Surg. 2011;35:87-95.

37. Raulin C, Greve B, Hammes S. Cold air in laser therapy: first experiences with a new cooling system. Lasers Surg Med. 2000;27:404-10.
38. Ross EV, Grossman MC, Duke D, et al. Long-term results after CO_2 laser skin resurfacing: a comparison of scanned and pulsed systems. J Am Acad Dermatol. 1997;37:709-18.
39. Ross EV, Ladin Z, Kreindel M, et al. Theoretical considerations in laser hair removal. Dermatol Clin. 1999;17:333-55.
40. Sadick NS, Makino Y. Selective electrothermolysis in aesthetic medicine: a review. Lasers Surg Med. 2004;34:91-7.
41. Sardana K, Chakravarty P, Goel K. Optimal management of common acquired melanocytic nevi (moles): current perspectives. Clin Cosmet Investig Dermatol. 2014;7:89-103.
42. Sardana K, Chugh S, Garg VK, et al. Laser tissue interactions. In: Sardana K, Garg VK (Eds). Lasers in Dermatological Practice, 1st edition. New Delhi: Jaypee Brothers Medical Publishers (P) Ltd; 2014.
43. Sardana K, Chugh S, Garg VK. Are Q-switched lasers for nevus of Ota really effective in pigmented skin? Indian J Dermatol Venereol Leprol. 2012;78:187-9.
44. Sardana K, Garg VK, Arora P, et al. Histological validity and clinical evidence for use of fractional lasers for acne scars. J Cutan Aesthet Surg. 2012;5:75-90.
45. Sardana K, Garg VK, Bansal S, et al. A promising split-lesion technique for rapid tattoo removal using a novel sequential approach of a single sitting of pulsed CO(2) followed by Q-switched Nd:YAG laser (1064 nm). J Cosmet Dermatol. 2013;12:296-305.
46. Sardana K, Garg VK. Lasers are not effective for melasma in darkly pigmented skin. J Cutan Aesthet Surg. 2014;7:57-60.
47. Sardana K, Ranjan R, Kochhar AM, et al. A rapid tattoo removal technique using a combination of pulsed Er:YAG and Q-switched Nd:YAG in a split lesion protocol. J Cosmet Laser Ther. 2015;17:177-83.
48. Sardana K. The science, reality, and ethics of treating common acquired melanocytic nevi (moles) with lasers. J Cutan Aesthet Surg. 2013;6:27-9.
49. Smith KJ, Skelton HG, Graham JS, et al. Depth of morphologic skin damage and viability after one, two, and three passes of a high-energy, short-pulse CO_2 laser (Tru-Pulse) in pig skin. J Am Acad Dermatol. 1997;37:204-10.
50. Trelles MA, Allones I, Levy JL, et al. Combined nonablative skin rejuvenation with the 595 and 1450-nm lasers. Dermatol Surg. 2004;30:1292-8.
51. Welch AJ, van Gemert MJ, Starr JC, et al. Definitions and overview of tissue optics. In: Welch AJ, van Gemert MJ (Eds). Optical-thermal Response of Laser-irradiated Tissue. New York: Plenum; 1995. pp. 15-46.
52. Welch AJ, van Gemert MJ. Overview of optical and thermal interaction and nomenclature. In: Welch AJ, van Gemert MJ (Eds). Optical-thermal Response of Laser-irradiated Tissue. New York: Plenum; 1995. pp. 1-14.
53. West TB, Alster TS. Comparison of the long-pulse dye (590-595 nm) and KTP (532 nm) lasers in the treatment of facial and leg telangiectasias. Dermatol Surg. 1998;24:221-6.
54. Willey A, Kilmer S, Newman J, et al. Elastometry and clinical results after bipolar radiofrequency treatment of skin. Dermatol Surg. 2010;36:877-84.
55. Zenzie HH, Altshuler GB, Smirnov MZ, et al. Evaluation of cooling methods for laser dermatology. Lasers Surg Med. 2000;26:130-44.

CHAPTER 2

Ablative Lasers

Kabir Sardana

INTRODUCTION

The advent of ablative lasers was heralded by the use in 1964 of the carbon dioxide (CO_2) laser with a wavelength of 10,600 nm in the far-infrared region, which was used for surgical applications in 1967. The high absorption of the 10,600 nm wavelength by intracellular water (Fig. 2.1) led to the development of a number of applications, including the use of the CO_2 laser as a scalpel for excisional surgery, as a destructive instrument for cutaneous malignancies (similar to electrodesiccation and curettage), in cutaneous laser resurfacing,

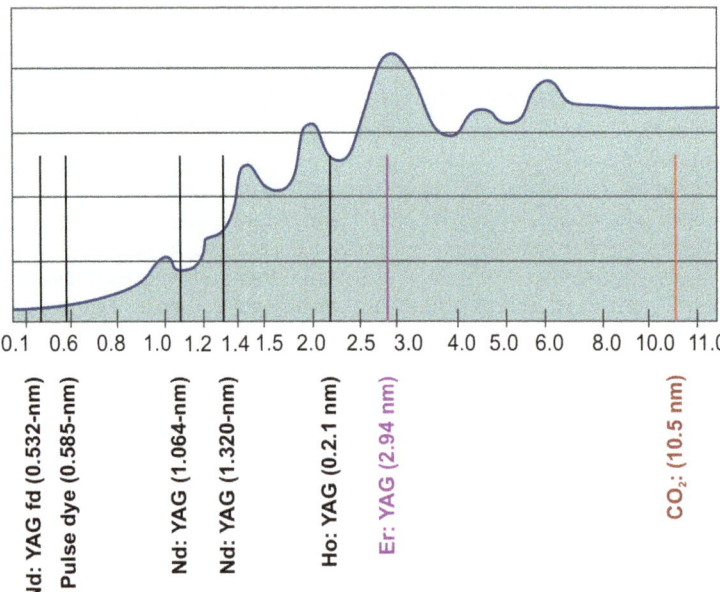

Fig. 2.1: Absorption spectrum of the commonly used lasers highlighting the two commonly used wavelenghths CO_2 and Er:YAG.

and in the ablation of various dermal and epidermal lesions. For many years the continuous wave CO_2 laser became more convenient than a cold steel scalpel in certain instances where there was a greater need for *hemostasis*, since the laser instantly coagulates blood vessels up to 0.5 mm in diameter. A very small spot size (0.1–0.2 mm) is needed to use the laser in this manner. In addition to the coagulation and sealing of small vessels, small cutaneous nerve endings and lymphatics are also sealed, offering a distinct advantage with less postoperative pain and edema.

Though in India most practitioners use the CO_2 lasers in its various forms another precise and superlative tool is the erbium (Er):YAG laser. This is especially true for epidermal and superficial dermal indications. In my own experience with the Dermablate, the erbium:YAG laser was successful in treating innumerable conditions and can be combined by CO_2 to enable hemostasis. The unique tissue dynamics of the erbium:YAG laser, is such with its wavelength of 2,940 nm, it is absorbed by water 10 times more readily than the carbon dioxide laser (wavelength, 10,600) (Fig. 2.1). Consequently, it is absorbed more superficially within the skin, leading to extremely precise ablation of the epidermis and dermis. The threshold of fluence required for clean ablation is 1.5 J/cm^2, compared with 4-5 J/cm^2 for the carbon dioxide laser. The thermal relaxation time is 50 μsec for the erbium:YAG laser; the carbon dioxide laser's time is 1 msec. The thermal injury is 5–10 μm for the erbium:YAG and 20–60 μm for the CO_2 laser. Thus, this makes it a safer ablative tool.

At present, three lasers are used for ablative indications and in all chromophore in water, the difference lies in their relative affinity for water. As shown in the Figure 2.1, the Er:YAG has a higher affinity than CO_2 thus it is absorbed more and as the skin is made up largely of water, it has the least thermal damage.

CARBON DIOXIDE LASERS

The continuous-wave carbon dioxide laser, producing infrared light with a wavelength of 10,600 nm, was the first to be used for resurfacing procedures. Its wavelength is strongly absorbed by water, which is the most abundant chromophore in the skin and comprises approximately 70% of its total volume. This seemed to make it an ideal tool for generalized superficial ablation. But its tissue-dwell time could not be precisely controlled and far exceeded the 1 ms thermal relaxation time of the 20–30 μm of cutaneous tissue that absorbs CO_2 light. Excessive thermal diffusion and concomitant unintended tissue damage were the common results.

However, in the early 1990s, new pulsed and scanning CO_2 lasers were developed that could deliver very high peak fluences of at least 5 J/cm^2 high enough to vaporize cutaneous tissue in less than 1–2 milliseconds (Fig. 2.2). For the thickness of the tissue **(20–60 μm)**, the TRT is about **800 μs**. This is

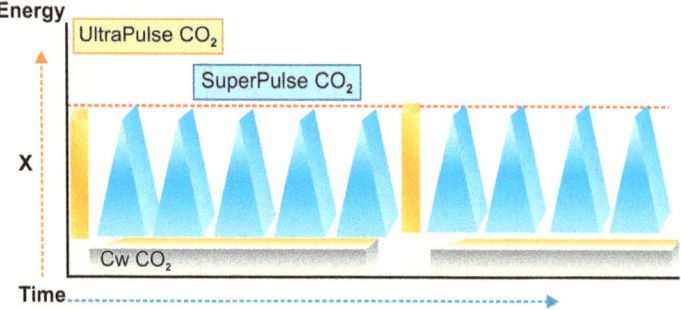

Fig. 2.2: A comparison of the waveform of various modes of CO_2 laser. Note that for the same energy (X) generated by an ultraPulse (<1 ms) waveform, 5 SuperPulse waves are generated. A continuous wave is seven times longer than the UltraPulse for the same energy.

achieved by the *ultrapulse lasers* where a 250-mJ pulse using a 2.5-mm probe size achieves much higher fluencies in a shorter time as compared to the continuous wave (Cw) CO_2. The *superpulse laser* is a mechanically shuttered laser whose peak power is higher than Cw lasers but the average power over time is the same.

Histology shows that with one pass, the CO_2 laser vaporizes 20–30 µm of tissue and creates a zone of thermal damage measuring 40–120 µm. With continuous heating, the target water is removed, tissue desiccation occurs, and heat accumulates creating a widespread zone of nonselective thermal necrosis. Thermal necrosis more than 100 µm thick interferes with wound healing and carries a significant risk of scarring.

Thus, the newer pulsed systems can precisely and safely remove thin layers of skin, between 20 µm and 30 µm with each pass, while leaving an acceptably narrow zone of residual thermal damage (RTD): 25 µm to 70 µm, in contrast to the 200–600 µm zone produced by the continuous-wave CO_2 laser.

The main difference between the conventional Cw CO_2 and pulsed lasers lies in the depth of ablation and the consequent thermal damage. As can be seen in Figure 2.3, with pulsed lasers the coagulation is minimal and most of the depth is due to the ablation while in case of Cw CO_2, the coagulation is more accounting for more side effects.

Principles of Carbon Dioxide Lasers

R Rox Anderson and Parrish coined the term "selective photothermolysis" in 1983 to describe the process by which a chromophore is heated by laser light absorption in a time period shorter than its thermal relaxation time. The latter is the amount of time required for a material to lose 50% of its heat by conduction to its surroundings. Thus, when a chromophore is heated by selective photothermolysis, only the intended target is damaged and there

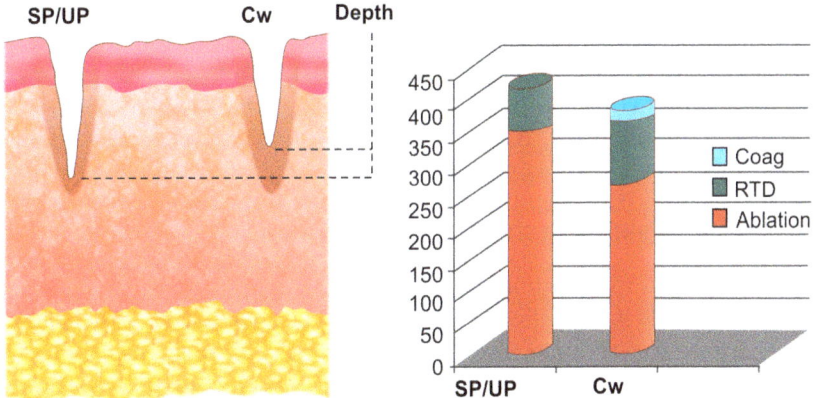

Fig. 2.3: A comparison of the tissue effects of pulsed and Cw CO_2 laser. There is a marked difference in the coagulation profile of Cw and pulsed CO_2 lasers.

is minimal diffusion of heat and no consequent injury to the surrounding structures. The mechanism of injury involves both thermal coagulation and/or photoacoustic injury in the form of supersonic high pressure shock waves.

For both the CO_2 and Er:YAG lasers, the predominant mechanism is photothermal. The pulse fluence necessary to achieve vaporization and thus ablation of skin tissue with the CO_2 laser is **5 J/cm²** with a calculated TRT of **800 μs**. The unique aspect of CO_2 laser is that for each 20 μm that is ablated, 3-4 times this amount is damaged. It is this latter effect that allows for the purported collagen remodeling and wound healing. This zone of coagulation is modest compared to 1,000 μm layer of damage that results from Cw CO_2 lasers. The flip side is that this damage can also cause side effects.

Types of CO_2 Lasers (Table 2.1)

Most clinicians use the ***superpulsed CO_2*** lasers, which deliver pulse energies in the 10-50 mJ range. The peak power per pulse is 2-10 times higher than Cw CO_2 lasers, but the average power over time is similar (*see* Fig. 2.2).

The UltraPulse laser introduced by Coherent (now Lumenis) solved the problem of having to create second (duty cycles pulses of pulses) with the superpulsed lasers. This was the first laser capable of delivering very high fluence pulses (~200-500 mJ) with large spot sizes capable of tissue vaporization with a single pulse. The depth of vaporization with an UltraPulse laser was studied in pig skin using pulses of 250-450 mJ. In human skin, the depth of thermal damage using the UltraPulse laser was 20 μm after one pass, 40 μm after two passes, and 70 μm after three passes.

Various modifications have been used with the CO_2 laser. The *Nova-Pulse* can generate 7 J/cm² of fluence by rapidly moving a small spot size through a computer pattern generator. The *TruPulse* (Tissue Technologies) laser can produce peak powers up to 10,000 watts at very short pulse durations

(65-125 μs). Another laser system that can achieve results similar to those of the UltraPulse is the *Sharplan SilkLaser*. This device offers two modes: the FeatherTouch and SilkTouch. This scanned laser uses a *continuous wave CO_2 laser beam* that is scanned over a defined pattern so rapidly that the tissue dwell time in any given spot is less than 1 ms. Thus, the effect is essentially the same as that of a high-energy pulsed system.

How do the Different CO_2 Lasers Compare?

Alster et al. compared four resurfacing lasers and found that they were similar in histologic and clinical outcomes. Kauvar et al. studied the histology of superpulsed, SilkTouch, and UltraPulse lasers in human skin and found that after three passes, the SP and SilkTouch RTDs (residual thermal damage) were both 150 μm, the UltraPulse RTD was 70 μm, and the Cw laser RTD (10 W and 0.2 s exposure) was 400 μm. Many investigators have compared the various levels of RTD after three passes in LSR: a summary of which is provided in Table 2.1. The important aspect to note is the variation in the thermal coagulation as shown in Table 2.2.

Table 2.1: Comparison of available CO_2 lasers.

Lasers	Typical "settings"	Typical safe fluence (J/cm²)	Typical RTD after two to three passes (μm)
UltraPulse	Density 6, 300 mJ	7.5	90–110
NovaPulse	Computer scanner E16, 7 W	6–7	60–80
Silk Laser	18 W/36 W (with 200 mm handpiece)	15/8	110/70
TruPulse	500 mJ	5	50
UniPulse	16–18 W/20% overlap	14	70

Table 2.2: Comparison of UltraPulse and Cw CO_2.

Lasers	UltraPulse	SilkTouch*	FeatherTouch**
1st pass	Epidermal vaporization +20 μm of dermal necrosis	Epidermal vaporization +70 μm of dermal necrosis	Epidermal vaporization +10 μm of dermal necrosis
2nd pass	Epidermal vaporization +40 μm of dermal necrosis	Epidermal vaporization +100 μm of dermal necrosis	Epidermal vaporization +30 μm of dermal necrosis
3rd pass	Epidermal vaporization +60 μm of dermal necrosis		Epidermal vaporization +50 μm of dermal necrosis

300 mJ, 2.25 mm spot, 100 W, density 6
*28 J/cm², **10 J/cm²

VARIATIONS IN LASER SETTINGS AND TISSUE EFFECT

As CO_2 is still the workhorse of most laser practitioners in India we will dwell on it. It should be appreciated that the conventional pulsed CO_2 lasers can be tweaked to give optimal coagulation and residual thermal damage, which can enable the surgeon to use the laser for varying indications with minimal damage.

Most CO_2 lasers have **three** options Cw (continuous wave), R mode (repeat mode) and S mode (single mode). It should be remembered that all three are *essentially Cw modes.* Plus there is a superpulsed mode where a train of pulses are used which approximate the effect of the UltraPulse laser. Possibly the most important aspect to differentiate them is the pulse duration of the laser, which conventionally has a setting that is in seconds. Thus, they start from *0.01 second to 0.99 seconds.* This means that the minimum is 10 milliseconds, thus most lasers used in clinical practice are *not* UltraPulse lasers. An ideal $SpCO_2$ laser should have a pulse duration of 1-10 ms but this aspect is covered after this section.

A basic principle of minimizing thermal damage is to use *pulses over a range of 0.25-10 ms (0.01 sec), with a maximum dose of 10 J/cm². * The various modes are depicted in Figure 2.4 and are detailed further.

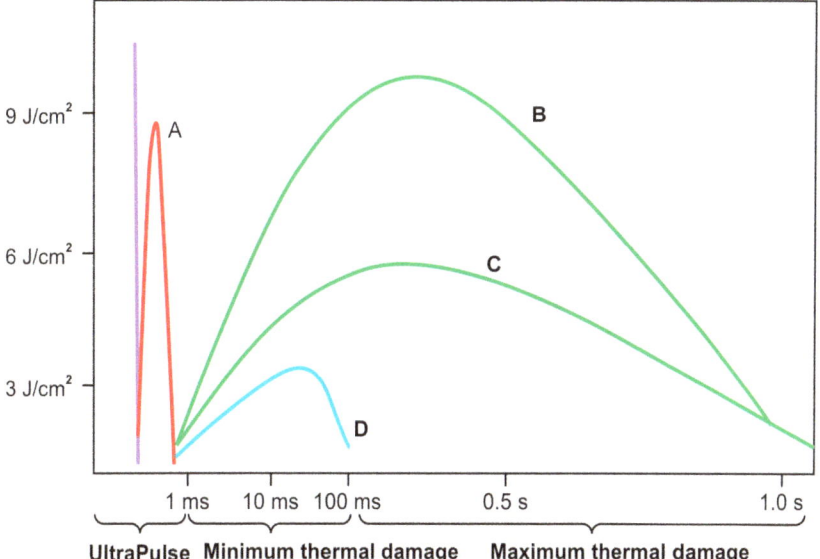

Fig. 2.4: A comparison of the various modes of CO_2 lasers with their tissue effect. (A) Ultrapulse mode; (B) Cw repeat/vaporization mode; (C) Cw repeat mode (more thermal damage); (D) Minimum thermal damage (low fluence, low pulse duration).

High Power Density (PD)/Short Exposure Time (Resurfacing Mode)

Ideal: UltraPulse mode (Fig. 2.5A)

Principle: The aim of the therapy is to reduce the zone of thermal damage, which is the result of both: (1) Subablative localized energy densities (at the base of the wound, as the beam is rapidly attenuated) and (2) Heat conduction during and after the pulse. This is usually done best by ultraPulse lasers where the pulse duration is less than 1 ms.

First pass: The entire epidermis is ablated with a fluence of 5–8 J/cm^2 with a 1 ms (0.001 s) domain laser, the depth of ablation is 10–40 mm.

At this point, the epidermis is normally wiped away with wet gauze, and the papillary dermis is exposed. However, there is a case to be made for not wiping. If one knows the extent of the injury after one pass and is confident that this level of injury will successfully reverse the skin pathology, wiping only serves to increase patient discomfort and prolong healing. More importantly, there appears to be a level of dermal thermal injury beyond which long-term hypopigmentation is almost inevitable in selected patients, especially appearing along the lateral cheeks and extending to the jawline. Thus, one can titrate the injury according to the level of desired injury with one pass if one reliably knows the laser end points.

Second pass: With the CO_2 laser, once the denatured friable epidermis is wiped off, it takes many pulses to ablate the residual acellular dermis. With the typical Gaussian beam of the CO_2 laser, there will be some ablation at

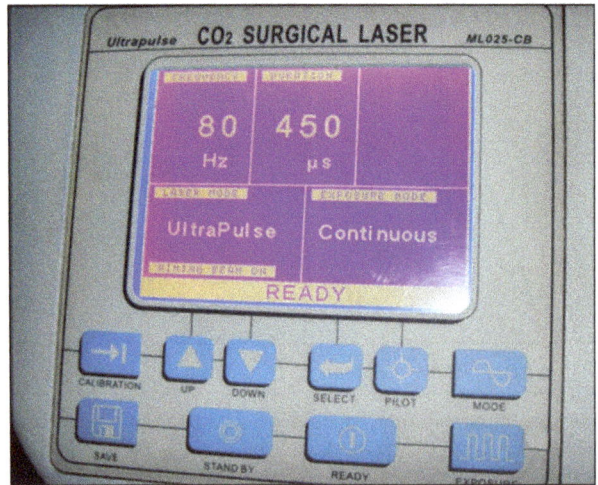

Fig. 2.5A: High power/short exposure (450 μs) UltraPulse mode. Indication: All epidermal and most dermal disorders. Note the pulse duration <1 ms

7 J/cm² average fluence at the center of the spot, but very little at the perimeter. Overall, using this average fluence, the ablation is about 10-15 μm per pass. As the average fluences reach 10 J/cm², 15 J/cm², and 20 J/cm², the relative ratio of ablation to tissue heating will increase. That is, roughly the same RTD will result, but the amount of ablation per pass will increase.

What to Look for?

Depending on the patient's pathology and age, one sees different surface characteristics after wiping the denatured epidermis.

Younger patient: For younger patients with modest photodamage, normally a pink to red dermis is exposed.

Older patient: For an older patient with severe solar elastosis, one sees yellowing immediately.

Low–Medium Pulse Duration (PD)/Long Exposures in Cw (Defocused Mode)

Ideal settings: 5-10 J/cm², 50 ms (0.10 sec-1 sec) (Fig. 2.5B)
Cw (repeat mode)

Principle: This is the so-called **vaporization mode**, which is actually a combination of simultaneous heating and vaporization. Most conventional CO_2 lasers can be used in this mode. As normally the lasers are kept at a distance that is beyond the focus length, thus it is called as **defocused** mode.

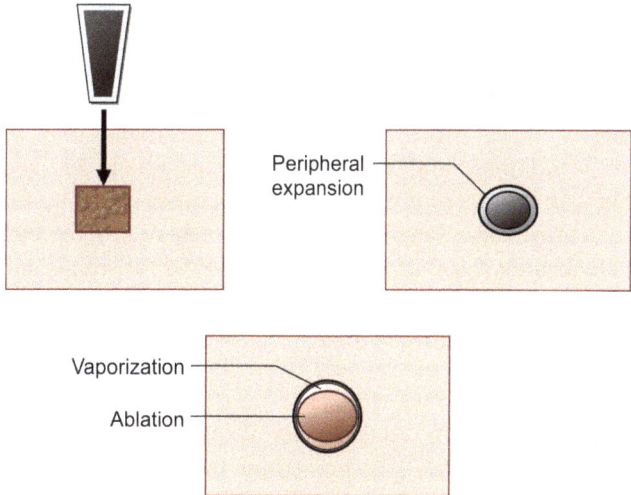

Fig. 2.5B: Sequence of tissue change due to Cw CO_2 set in a defocused vaporization mode (8 J/cm²; 0.5–1 sec).

Use: This is used for treating *warts* and *other exophytic lesions* where some tissue heating at the base of the wound is tolerated. Usually, one will encounter vaporization at the center of the spot and charring at the periphery.

Method: To decrease char, one must move in a "pirouetting" motion so that the char is not continuously heated. When the CO_2 laser burns a hole in the skin, the mechanism for ablation is the rapid conversion of water to steam. In the epidermis, the fragility of this layer provides for easy ablation, as the water vapor easily escapes the intracellular space, typically carrying with it a solid residue of exploded cells. This debris will continue to be heated as it is carried off, thus one sees "burning" or combustion. The sequence as proposed by Verdaasdonk et al. is shown in Figure 2.5B, which explains the tissue effect of CO_2 lasers (as below).

1. Initially, there is slight tissue discoloration. Coincident with a "pop", the surface lifts suggesting boiling bubbles underneath. The sound is due to the rapid ejection of air through the ablation front (nozzle effect), like bursting a balloon.
2. This is followed by a small black spot in center of the beam, due to the carbonization of the dehydrated tissue. Within a few tenths of a second, this charred zone expanded and a ring was formed.
3. Next, the char combusts, unveiling a new hydrated surface.
4. Then there are cyclical rings of carbonization and vaporization, following each other in rapid succession as a progressively deeper crater was formed.

Important Caveats

Though this is the mode *most often used* (5 J/cm^2, 0.5-1 seconds (Fig. 2.5C) it must be emphasized that this setting has issues with the residual thermal damage (RTD). If the "char" is never "blown off" (either by vaporization of water below the char or by combustion), and there is deep heating beneath the skin surface, which is the case as temperatures higher than 1000°C this may lead to heat damage and consequent scar formation. This is seen in the treatment of warts where prolonged application times of greater than 0.5-1 s can result in a brownish color and finally deep blackening of the surface. With increased blackening, the char acts as a nearly perfect absorber, and the char becomes hotter and hotter.

Thus, remember using lower PDs for prolonged periods is usually not advisable, as it simply results in very deep "invisible" tissue heating. It is advisable in these cases to wipe the char, thus exposing hydrated tissue, so that additional vaporization can take place. If charring does take place and is not removed by wiping, *STOP* the procedure. In all likelihood, the char will fall off and remove the lesion in about 7 days time.

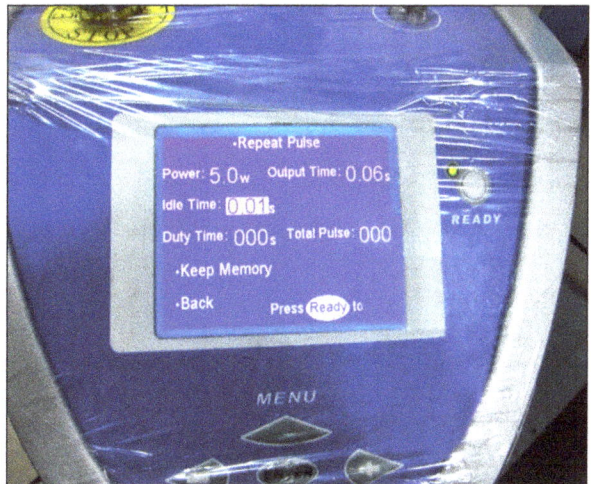

Fig. 2.5C: Low power (<6 J/cm^2; high exposure >0.10 s) leads to more coagulation. Use: Lymphatic and vascular tumors.

Very Low Pulse Durations and Short Exposures

Cw (single pulse, super pulse mode) (Fig. 2.5D)

Principle: Although the thermal gradient is not steep, that is, the temperature decay as a function of depth is small, there is so little total heat that this is safe as long as one pass is made, and this application will typically restrict residual thermal damage (RTD) to the epidermis and superficial papillary dermis. The goal is to use short bursts of subablative PDs to heat a specific thickness

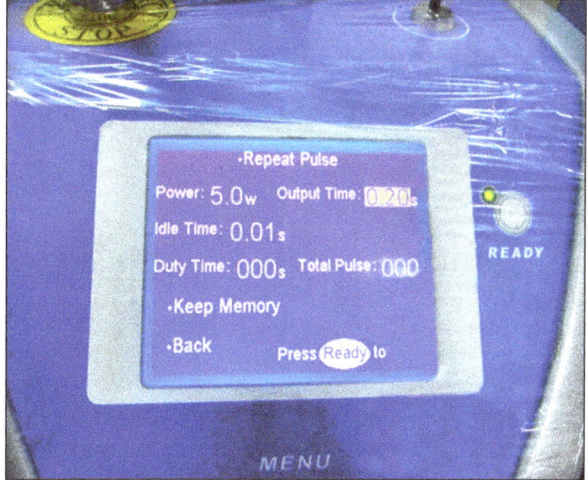

Fig. 2.5D: Low power (<6 J/cm^2; low exposure <0.10 s). Less thermal damage, fine ablation.

of tissue. In the case of dermatosis papulosa nigra (DPN), for example, one can heat the tissue just to a level similar to that of the hyfrecator. The end point is slight whitening of the tissue. This technique is best reserved for those who do not have access to a pulsed CO_2 laser.

Use: It is useful in lentigines and DPN.

Settings: With this technique (also known as ***thermabrasion***), the laser is used in low power mode at 1-5 W with a defocused beam with very short bursts of Cw radiation.

An overview of the principles described above are depicted in vivo in Figure 2.5E in a case of epidermal nevi.

High Pulse Durations with Small Spots (0.1–0.3 mm)

Cutting mode: Used in incisions. Most skin surgeons do not use the CO_2 laser in cutting mode, with the exception of eyelid surgery.

Use

The indications for using CO_2 for cutting regardless of the mode include:
- Bleeding disorders
- Where epinephrine is not indicated
- Vascular lesions (hemangiomas and scalp tumors)
- Infected surgical sites
- In patients with pacemakers or implanted defibrillators.

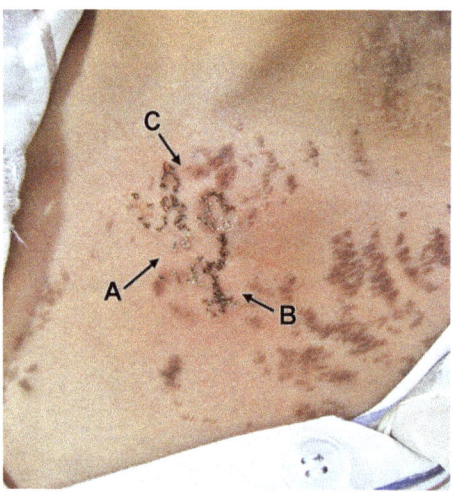

Fig. 2.5E: A depiction of various tissue effects based on the pulse duration and dose (A) 3 J/cm^2; 0.01 sec (whitening effect); (B) 3 J/cm^2; 0.40 sec (coagulation); (C) 9 J/cm^2; 0.50 sec (carbonization).

Clinical Aspects of CO_2 Lasers

Disadvantages

In addition to the cumbersomeness of using the laser as a cutting tool including the need to work around the articulated arm, the need for a smoke evacuator, and the constant vigilance that is required not to inadvertently strike an innocent bystander target, the laser cannot be endorsed as a first choice for incisions because healing is delayed compared with scalpel incisions. It is therefore not recommended for most routine skin surgeries.

Advantages

The advantages, on the other hand, are ease of excision and a relatively bloodless field. The lack of perfect hemostasis is partly explained by the paucity of residual thermal damage (RTD) in a standard excision with CO_2 laser. Because the small spot sizes of 0.1–0.3 mm allow for high PDs, thermal damage is minimal. Microscopically, one finds 90 µm of basophilic change and 100-500 µm of lateral glassy hypereosinophilic change on routine staining. It follows that the high-flow vessels larger than 500 µm are likely to bleed after CO_2 transection. In contrast, without blood flow, vessels up to 2 µm have been coagulated. One should note that minimizing RTD and achieving hemostasis are antagonistic. Ideally, one should choose the laser parameters with the least RTD that still achieves adequate control of bleeding. The amount of bleeding versus other modalities such as diathermy and scalpel has been compared, and it appears that the CO_2 laser performs as well as a cutting electrosurgical current. Another purported advantage of the CO_2 laser is that it seals nerve endings, which presumably results in less postoperative pain than scalpel excision.

Cw Vaporization

In review of the Cw applications described earlier, it becomes clear that most CO_2 laser surgeons somewhat arbitrarily choose the power and pulse duration. Typically, the surgeon repeats the cycle of irradiation and inspection, continuing until almost or no lesional tissue remains. Fleming and Brody proposed a more logical approach to the treatment of lesions with the Cw CO_2 laser. They cited several limitations in the empirical techniques commonly employed:

- In many cases, the surgeon's dependence on visual differentiation of normal from lesional tissue leads to possible overtreatment and scar, or undertreatment and rapid recurrence.
- This technique is slow, because the cycle is repeated for each lesion.

In Fleming and Brody's study, they used a constant power in plotting the depth of the resulting crater as a guide in planning treatments. They noted that crater depth depended on fluence for the powers used (5–18 W and 1 mm spot). They found that the *application time determined the crater depth for constant power and spot size*. For example, a *10-W pulse delivered with a 1-mm spot and application time of 1 s can achieve a depth of 2,500 μm.*

Cw Cutting Mode

The reader should note that 15–25 W will give a cutting depth of 3–5 mm with a hand movement rate of 1.5 mm/s with a 0.3-mm spot. Also, wet gauze should always be used as a backstop so that the beam does not injure unintended targets.

BIBLIOGRAPHY

1. Fleming MG, Brody N. A new technique for laser treatment of cutaneous tumors. J Dermatol Surg Oncol. 1986;12(11):1170-5.
2. Verdaasdonk RM, Borst C, van Gemert MJ. Explosive onset of continuous wave laser tissue ablation. Phys Med Biol. 1990;35(8):1129-44.

Can a Nonpulsed CO_2 Laser be used like an UltraPulse Laser?

As most laser practitioners rarely acquire a true UltraPulse laser, this is a relevant practical point. It must be understood that the Silk laser and UniPulse (*see* Table 2.1) are essentially Cw lasers but achieve comparable RTD as the UltraPulse. But the importance of setting cannot be overemphasized. This is as a high dose or a high pulse duration can change the profile of the laser completely. Putting simply a higher pulse duration can cause coagulation up to 1,000 μm making it akin to a radiofrequency (RF) device. A comparison is given in Table 2.2 between the UltraPulse and Cw CO_2. This shows that if the optimal settings are used a Cw CO_2 can behave like an UltraPulse CO_2 with little clinical difference.

A simple ***thumb rule*** is that energy levels from 7 J/cm² to 9 J/cm² with a pulse duration of 0.3 ms (0.03 s) can safely replicate the results of most UltraPulse CO_2 lasers. And most importantly, with most CO_2 lasers, there is no advantage of exceeding *three passes*.

As in India a large number of CO_2 lasers have a super-pulsed mode we will dwell on this so that this can be used in clinical practice. The "trick" is to achieve *ablation without carbonization*.
- The correct pulse duration, thus a pulse duration of less than **1 ms** is ideal for an UltraPulse mode most super-pulse lasers have a pulse duration more than 1 ms. Note that the laser panels have a display in seconds! (Thus 1 ms = 0.001 seconds, thus if a laser displays the minimum laser pulse of say 0.01 seconds it is way beyond the requirement.)
- A histological or clinical study of the machine that assesses the clinical effects of carbonization.

The machine that we use is a CO_2 laser with 10.6 μm in different modes of applications (ultra and dream pulse surgical CO_2 laser system, DS-40U, DAESHIN ENTERPRISE Co., Ltd., Korea). The dream pulse is the super-pulse mode. This has an adjustable pulse duration (1-1.7 ms). An in vivo study demonstrates the tissue effects (Figs. 2.6A and B)

The ***principle*** enshrined here, which can be used by anyone with a good super pulse laser, is that "The depth of the incisions *increases* with increasing *fluences*, and *decreases* with increasing the *pulse interval*, while the tissue *carbonization* degree increases with decreasing the *pulse interval*. At pulse interval 50 ms, incisions produced no visible signs of carbonization. The *crucial aspect* is the **pulse interval and duration** and *not* the dose or fluence.

Thus, most good super-pulsed lasers can be used with great cosmesis if the pulse duration of (1-1.7 ms) is used with a 50-ms pulse interval.

What is the Comparison of UltraPulse CO_2 with Conventional Cosmetic Procedures?

A comparison between the ultrapulsed CO_2 laser with various pulse energies and numbers of pass and TCA peeling, dermabrasion, and Baker's phenol peel on a porcine model showed that at typical pulse energies, one to three passes produced a wound depth intermediate between a 35% TCA peel

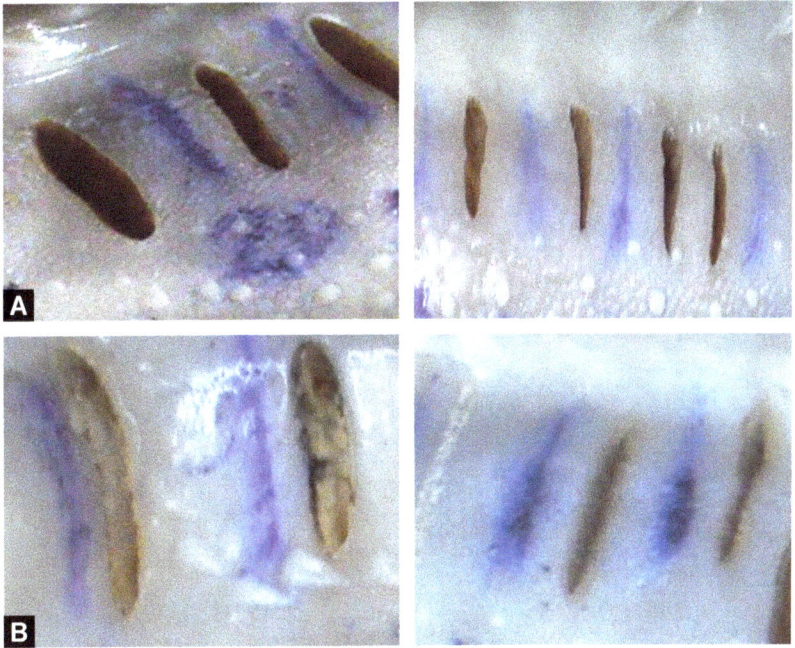

Figs. 2.6A and B: (A) Shows the incisions by the Cw CO_2, note the black residue also known as "carbonization" which is not desirable in fine laser surgeries; (B) Shows the effects with super pulse CO_2 note the "near" clean base.

and dermabrasion, but more superficial than a phenol peel (Fig. 2.7). Thus by varying the dose, epidermal or dermal depth can be achieved to target the condition to be treated. This also highlights the fact that the CO_2 laser, in optimal settings, can match most conventional tools with better precision.

A point that is to be emphasized that the pulse duration of electrocautery and RF is in *seconds* while the most rudimentary CO_2 lasers have a maximum of 0.9 seconds. Thus, the thermal damage and consequent cosmesis of the CO_2 is *superior* to any RF machine or electrocautery device.

Technique Tips

As most of the laser surgeons employ CO_2 to treat dermal tumors, we will focus on this, though a similar principle can be applied to other indications. For individual lesions, the growth is vaporized by using relatively low power settings in the 3 W to 5 W range with a spot size that matches the size of the lesion. The pulse duration should be less than 2 ms (as discussed above). Again *there is no fixed dose as that depends on the machine and the end points.*

1. For individual lesions, the growth is vaporized by using relatively low-power settings in the 3- to 5-W range with a spot size that matches the size of the lesion.

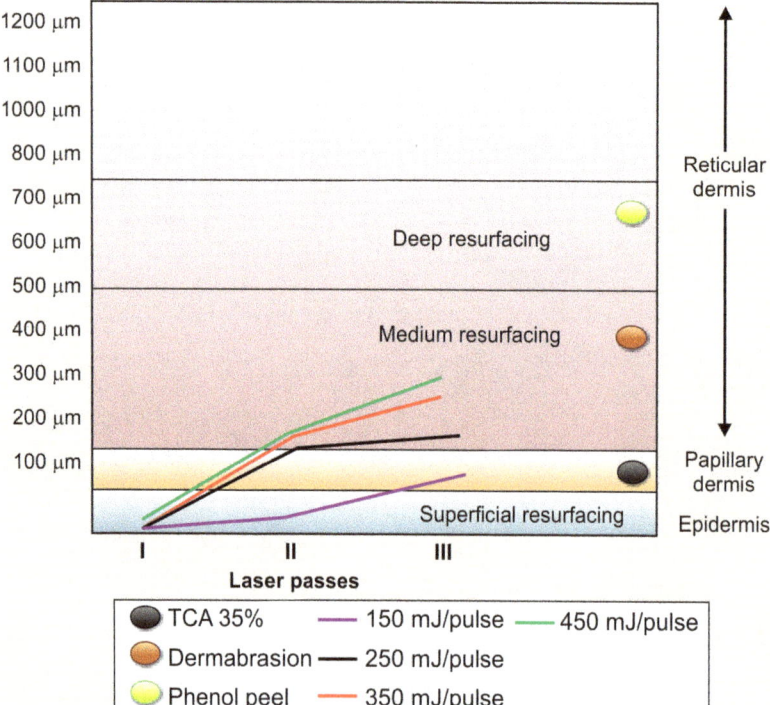

Fig. 2.7: A comparison of the dose depth analysis of UltraPulse CO_2 laser with conventional modalities.

2. Depending upon the depth of the lesion being treated, the entire lesion may not be destroyed. This is especially true for conditions like xanthelasma palpebrarum.
3. Ablation should be carried out to the level of the dermis, but since residual thermal damage will extend 0.5–1 mm beyond the level of ablation, one should not try to remove the entire lesion if there is deep extension.
4. A useful end point is a smooth cutaneous contour.

Patients should be cautioned that some lesions may recur with time and new lesions may develop in the treated areas. Reepithelialization is complete in approximately 2 weeks.

End Points

At the end of the day most surgeons do not use fixed settings but look for end points to reliably ascertain when to stop the ablation procedure. Published reports have correlated clinical signs with anatomic depths of ablation. A *pink* color was found to correlate with superficial papillary dermis, a "*chamois-cloth*" appearance with papillary dermis and "*waterlogged*" *cotton-thread* appearance for reticular dermis. This is true only for deep ablation such as with treatment of plantar warts. When thinner layers of ablation are used, as in resurfacing, these subtle clinical signs are *not seen*. Also it must be understood that this also depends on the laser being used. If an UltraPulse laser is used little residual thermal necrosis (less than 30 µm) exists, thus the thermal reaction will not be sufficient to coagulate fine papillary vessels, and the tissue will be pink because of the visible capillary blood flow. This is typical of the appearance of the tissue after a single laser pass removing the epidermis. After a second or third laser pass, the laser reacting with the dermis leaves almost 70–100 µm of thermal necrosis thus leading to hemostasis, thus giving a whitish appearance. If further passes are given a yellowish brown look will actually indicate thermal injury! Thus, it is advisable as far as CO_2 lasers are concerned, that such signs should be abandoned and the laser surgeon should aim at primarily ablating the dermatological indication, restricting the dose and settings to a maximum of *3–4 passes*.

A few *simple rules* to follow are:
1. Use a pulsed laser or ultrapulse laser at the lowest fluence and pulse duration.
2. Aim for ablation of the tumor first or level it down to the surrounding skin before achieving depth destruction with a CO_2 laser.
3. A low energy and pulse duration will reveal the faint erythema of the papillary dermis, which is a reliable end point.
4. Do not aim for a yellowish discoloration, as that sign in most nonpulsed lasers is a reliable indicator of thermal necrosis!

ERBIUM:YAG LASER

INTRODUCTION

The short pulsed Er:YAG laser is a flashlamp-pumped yttrium-aluminum-garnet (YAG) crystal laser system doped with atoms of the element erbium. Laser energy is generated within a cavity containing the flashlamp-excited YAG crystal rod, mirrors at each end, and a cooling system. On exiting the cavity, the laser light is focused into a beam delivery system that typically incorporates an articulated arm, which allows the use of handpieces capable of producing highly collimated beams.

Erbium:YAG lasers used in cutaneous resurfacing typically have a bell-shaped Gaussian laser beam profile. The erbium:yttrium-aluminum-garnet (Er:YAG) laser produces light in the near-infrared (IR) portion of the electromagnetic spectrum at 2.94 μm. This wavelength was discovered by Soviet researchers in 1975 and its clinical use developed in Europe. The Erbium:YAG laser, with its wavelength of 2940 nm, is absorbed by water 10 times more readily than the carbon dioxide laser (wavelength, 10,600 nm). Consequently, it is absorbed more superficially within the skin, leading to extremely precise ablation of the epidermis and dermis (Fig. 2.8).

The threshold fluence required for clean ablation is 1.5 J/cm, compared with 4-5 J/cm² for the carbon dioxide laser. The thermal relaxation time is

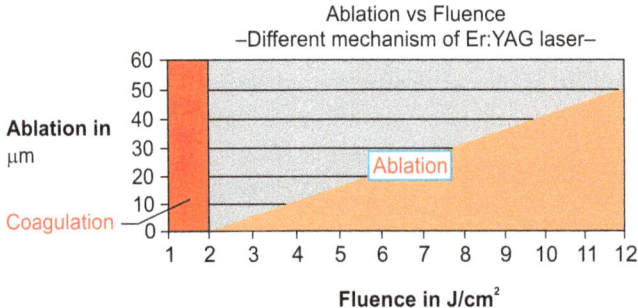

Linear correlation
Constant ablation depth of 5 μm per 1/J/cm² (above ablation treshhold)

Thermal mode
Specs: 1 J/cm², 20 Hz, N = 5...∞
coagulation zone up to 400 μm depth
(with single impulse up to 40 μm)

Recommended parameters
5–6 J/cm² conservative
7–8 J/cm² normal
9–10 J/cm² aggressive treatment

Fig. 2.8: Er:YAG ablation occurs after the threshold dose of about 1.8 J/cm². The dose and settings indicate both linear depth and coagulative effect of modified Er:YAG system.

50 μsec for the Erbium:YAG laser; the carbon dioxide TRT is 1 millisecond. The thermal injury is markedly less for the erbium:YAG lasers. The predictive depth (5 μm/J), the less thermal damage, the progressive depth achieved and faster healing it is preferred, especially for most dermatological indications.

Unlike the CO_2 laser, Er:YAG does not have the typical plateau response with ablation after three passes. Although vaporization does diminish as tissue becomes desiccated, the absorption at 2,940 nm by desiccated tissue is still significant and estimated to be ~2/3 that of hydrated tissue (i.e. 2–2.5 $μm^{-1}$ J/cm^2 of fluence compared to 2–4 $μm^{-1}$/J/cm^2 for hydrated tissue).

Newer modified Er:YAG have been invented to bridge the gap between the tissue effects with added coagulation (Table 2.3) which is consequent to the variable pulse duration. The principle employed is that if the pulse duration is less there is less coagulation while if the pulse duration is increased the coagulation increases. This can lead to various diverse settings (Fig. 2.9) and can closely approximate the CO_2 laser.

Laser-Tissue Interaction

The energy delivered by the Er:YAG laser with a pulse duration of *250–350 μs* is far *below* the 1 millisecond thermal relaxation time calculated for that layer of human skin heated by the pulsed CO_2 laser. However, because of the "short penetration depth" the laser heated tissue is only 1 μm thick and this has a TRT of 1 μm. Thus to minimize thermal damage, the Er:YAG laser emits approximately 20 μs micropulses in a macropulse burst of approximately 200 μs.

Table 2.3: An overview of modulated Er:YAG lasers.

Conventional Er:YAG	*Short-pulsed* (250–350 μs)	1. Derma 20 (ESC Medical Systems Haifa, Israel) 2. Continuum (Continuum Biomedical Dublin, Calif) 3. Dermablate (Asclepion-Meditec Inc, Jena, Germany)
Modulated Er:YAG	*Variable pulse* (500 μs–10 ms)	Contour Sciton Laser Corp
	Combined CO_2 and Er:YAG (50 ms/350 μs)	Derma K ESC/Sharplan
	*Dual Mode** (350 μs/ Thermal mode)	Dermablate MCL 30 (Asclepion-Meditec Inc, Jena, Germany) (1 μs 20 Hz)
	Variable pulse (100–1,000 μs)	Dermablate MCL 31

*In the thermal mode, the frequency is firmly set to 20 Hz, which leads to rapid heating of tissue by subablative pulses 2 (1 J/cm).

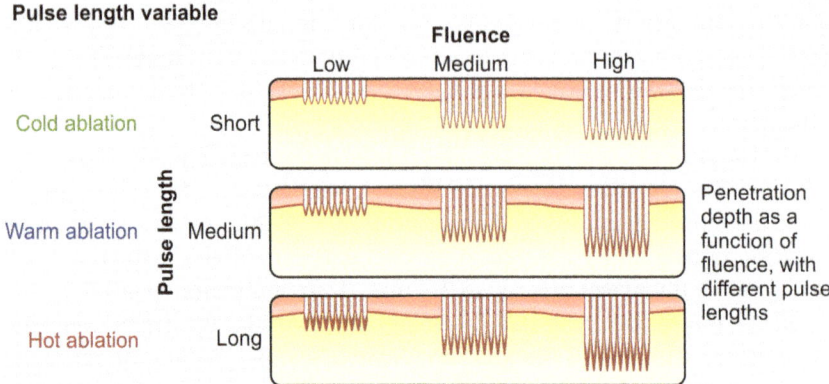

Fig. 2.9: Variable pulse duration and the consequent tissue effect using various modes (Er:YAG Dermablate 31).

In contrast to the CO_2 laser, the Er:YAG laser has 16 times greater affinity for water and a significantly lower tissue ablation threshold (1.6 J/cm^2) which allows the Er:YAG to be operated at 8–10 times above its ablation threshold in most resurfacing applications. Therefore, most of the energy delivered with the Er:YAG laser is used to ablate and the residual thermal damage (RTD) is narrow.

The Er:YAG laser causes vasodilation of dermal blood vessel and causes transudation of fluid that maintains enough water to ensure efficient ablation. The absence of coagulation results in bleeding as the vessels of the superficial dermal plexus are severed.

The unique *advantage* of the laser is minimum thermal damage but the *disadvantage* is minimum coagulation. Though modulated Er:YAG lasers with increasing pulse duration are useful, another option is to give subablative pulses (*see* Fig. 2.8) which will achieve coagulation, but no ablation. Most Er:YAG lasers have an ablation threshold 2 J/cm^2. At this fluence ablation starts. Below 2 J/cm^2 there is no ablation of tissue as the energy is not sufficient to remove tissue, and it remains in the tissue and causes heat generation. In thermal mode, a low energy of 1 J/cm^2 and a pulse repetition rate of 20 Hz is used (*see* Fig. 2.8). Thus, these multiple subablative pulses summate to cause coagulation. These modifications can help close the gap between the Er:YAG and CO_2 lasers.

Technique Tips

The depth of ablation is a function of the pulse energy and spot size or fluence. The *singular advantage* of Er:YAG is that depending on the pathology of the lesion to be removed, the dose can be set, as about **2–5 μm of tissue per J/cm^2** is ablated per pass with currently available Er:YAG laser systems. Thus, say if a syringoma with a depth of 300 µm has to be targeted, a dose of 10 J/cm^2 can be used which can ablate the lesion in about 4 passes (10 J × 4 µm = 40 µm × 5 passes = 200 µm). As there is a concomitant thermal damage of about 15-50 µm/pass, this dose can effectively remove the lesion. Other machines may have a different depth of ablation and a generic depiction is shown in Figure 2.10.

End Point

The removal of the epidermis can be ascertained by the immediate erythema of the papillary dermis. As there is little coagulation, this is the simplest end point to be ascertained. If it is an epidermal or dermal tumor ablation can be achieved but with some concomitant papillary bleeding. But in case of a scar or with dermal irregularities a "tissue-sculpting" mode is needed. This is easily accomplished with a focused handpiece having a focal spot size of 1-2 mm. The ablation is done by holding the handpiece at an *acute* angle to the tissue in a manner such that tissue elevations above the desired plane are preferentially irradiated, thereby decreasing the risk of cutting holes or troughs in the tissue. In case more passes are needed, brisk bleeding occurs which is a reliable indicator of entering the lower dermis. A thermal mode or varying the pulse duration effectively seals the vessels.

But the reliability of depth/energy means that the laser surgeon can predict the depth in most cases by multiplying the energy in J/cm^2 with a

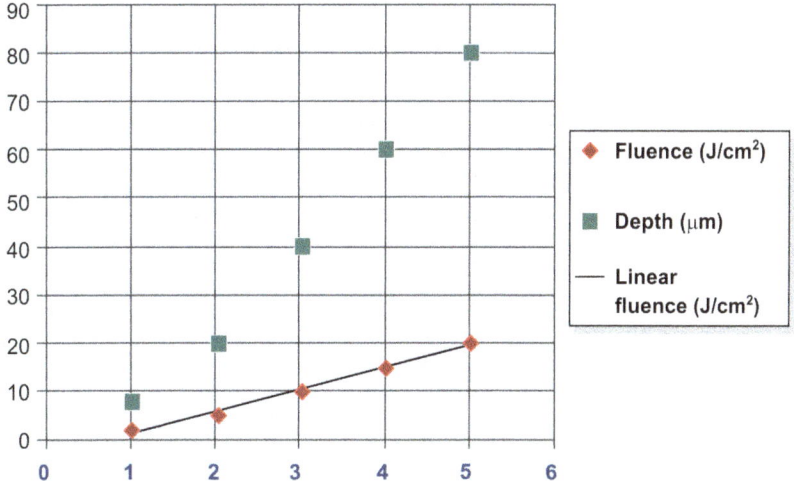

Fig. 2.10: A depiction of the predictable depth and dose equation of Er:YAG after the ablation threshold of about 0.4–1.5 J/cm^2. X-axis fluence in J/cm^2, Y-axis depth in µm.
Source: Sardana K, Ghunawat S. Lasers for lentigines, from Q-switched to erbium-doped yttrium aluminum garnet micropeel, is there a need to reinvent the wheel? J Cutan Aesthet Surg. 2015;8:233-5.

factor of 5, with predictable depth ablation. The end points of the Er:YAG Laser are depicted in Figure 2.11.

COMPARISON OF THE MAJOR ABLATIVE LASERS (CO_2 VERSUS ER:YAG)

According to the theory of selective photothermolysis, *three* criteria must be fulfilled to confine thermal damage to a selected target. *First,* the target tissue must absorb a given wavelength more avidly than the surrounding tissue. *Second,* the time the laser is in contact with the tissue (or pulse duration) must be less than the thermal relaxation time, which is defined as the time needed for a tissue to lose 50% of its heat. The pulse duration must be shorter than the thermal relaxation time (approximately 200–600 µs for skin) to minimize nonspecific lateral thermal damage, which can lead to scarring and pigmentary change. *Third,* sufficiently high levels of energy must be delivered to the target tissue to cause ablation.

The most crucial aspect is the thermal injury below the ablation zone, which is a double-edged sword as, though it induces collagen remodeling through heat-mediated contraction, but can cause damage if not controlled properly. As seen in the Figure 2.12 and Table 2.4, the CO_2 laser tends to reach the dermis with the first pass as compared to the Er:YAG. Also beyond three passes there is little added benefit as the coagulation and concomitant carbonization acts as a heat sink causing more heat damage.

The erbium:yttrium-aluminum-garnet (Er:YAG) laser is characterized by a *thinner* zone of ablation and thermal damage resulting in shorter healing time and a lower rate of post procedure side effects compared with $SPCO_2$ resurfacing lasers. The Er:YAG laser produces a different tissue reaction as compared with the CO_2 laser because of the greater absorption by the target chromophore, water. Because the wavelength of the laser closely approximates the absorption peak of water (3,000 nm), nearly all of the energy is absorbed in the epidermis and papillary dermis, yielding superficial ablation and less

Epidermis	• Yellow-brown, keratinized surface
Epidermal-dermal junction	• Pink upper papillary dermis • Follicle opening small and regular
Papillary dermis (lower)	• Pinpoint bleeding, transudate • Follicle opening wider, "stand out"
Reticular dermis	• Splotchy bleeding, profuse transudate
	• Wide follicle opening: coarse, haphazard collagen bundles
*End points may take seconds to minutes to develop	

Fig. 2.11: End points for Erbium: YAG resurfacing (with magnification).
Source: From Weinstein C. Erbium laser resurfacing: Current concepts. Plast Reconstr Surg. 1999;103(2):602-16.

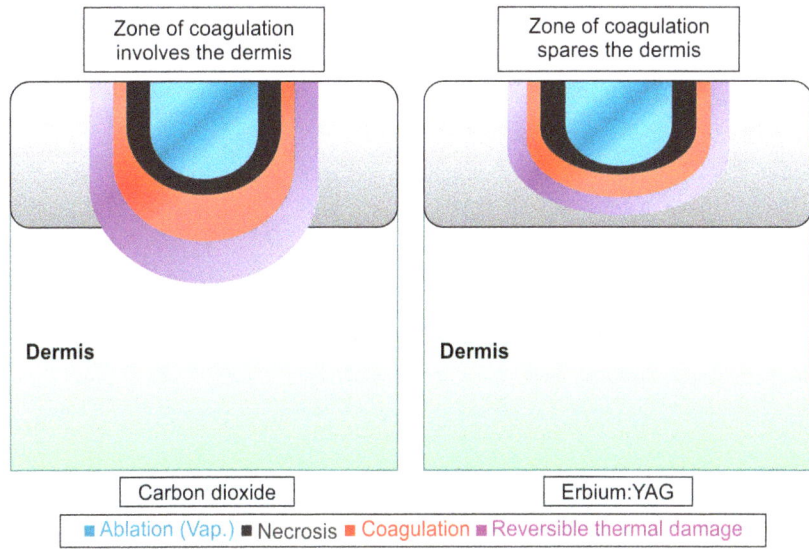

Fig. 2.12: A comparison of the tissue effects of pulsed CO_2 and Er:YAG lasers (ablation, necrosis, coagulation, reversible thermal damage).

underlying thermal damage compared with the CO_2 laser. Vaporization of water by the Er:YAG laser in the ablated epidermis and superficial dermis allows cooling of the tissue as the heat escapes as steam and decreases the heat transferred to the surrounding tissues. This allows the Er:YAG laser to be used for several passes over the ablated area without greatly increasing the zone of thermal damage (Fig. 2.12).

Each pass with the SP Er:YAG laser (250-350 microseconds) ablates approximately 20-25 μm (at 5 J/cm). Depth of thermal damage has been shown to be 30-50 μm at fluencies of 5-8 J/cm^2 compared with 50-200 μm with the CO_2 laser at fluencies of 3.5-6.5 J/cm. In addition, it appears that even with the multiple passes of the Er:YAG laser, the depth of underlying thermal damage is limited to 50 μm. With multiple passes at 5 J/cm^2, it may approach that seen with the pulsed CO_2 laser. No visible contraction of dermal collagen fibers is observed with subepidermal passes of the *SuperPulse* Er:YAG during resurfacing, however, collagen contraction occurs at 55°C to 60°C and relies upon heating of the dermal tissue. Longer-pulse (10 milliseconds) Er:YAG lasers have been shown to increase the zone of underlying thermal damage to approximately 60 μm, which may result in greater skin tightening and wrinkle reduction but increased risk of secondary side effects such as erythema and hyper- and hypopigmentation.

The flip side is a lack of coagulation. This can be adjusted by increasing the pulse duration, which helps achieve coagulation (Fig. 2.13). The advantage though is a clear char free ablation, which in most epidermal and dermal disorders makes an accurate end point of ablation possible.

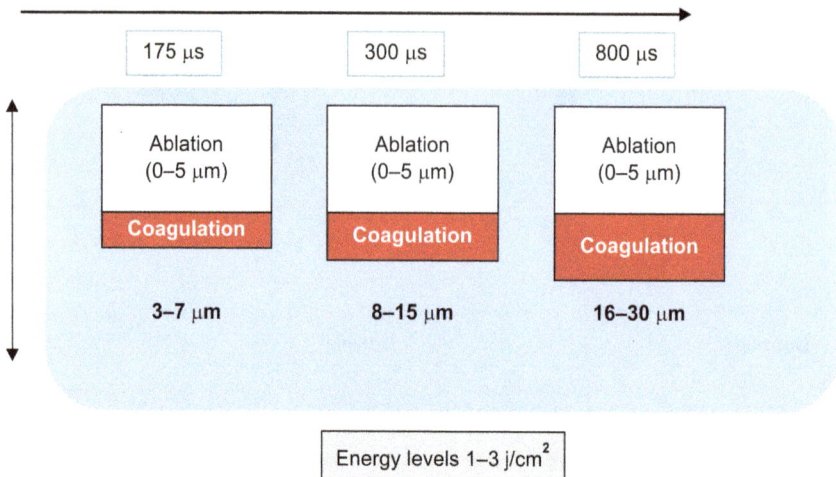

Fig. 2.13: A depiction of the effect of pulse duration on the ablation and thermal effect of Er:YAG laser in the so-called "Er:YAG peel setting". Note that for the same fluence, an increase in the pulse duration leads to more thermal effect.

A comparison of the effects of the two lasers systems is given in Table 2.4. Due to the superior tissue dynamics and side effect profile the variable pulsed Er:YAG is a superior laser system than CO_2 lasers for most dermatological indications *except* vascular and lymphatic tumors.

A comparison of the various technologies is depicted in Figures 2.14A and B.

Combination of ER:YAG/CO_2

For moderate to severe rhytides, a combination of CO_2 and Er:YAG lasers is often used to obtain better clinical results, while minimizing postlaser side effects and complications. The procedure is initiated with flattening of the rhytides or acne scar shoulders first, followed by a single pass over the rest of the cosmetic unit with the Er:YAG laser. The CO_2 laser is then used over the entire treatment area to induce collagen tightening. Often a single pass with the CO_2 is adequate, but on occasion, a second pass is needed.

After the CO_2 laser, the Er:YAG laser is repeated in order to remove some of the thermal damage produced by the CO_2 laser. This sequence minimizes the zone of thermal necrosis, and therefore shortens healing time and decreases posttreatment erythema, while still inducing tissue contraction. Many laser surgeons recommend performing two passes with the CO_2 laser first followed by several passes with the Er:YAG laser. However, by using the Er:YAG laser at the beginning, the epidermis may be ablated with minimal residual thermal necrosis. This serves to eliminate one of the passes performed with the CO_2 laser, which will also decrease the zone of thermal necrosis. Results attained

Table 2.4: A comparison of salient aspects of CO_2 (pulsed) and Er:YAG lasers.

Parameters	CO_2	Er:YAG
OD (Optical penetration)	20 μm	1 μm
Ablation threshold TRT	5 J/cm² 800 μs	0.5–1.5 J/cm² 1 μs/pulse duration 250 μs
Ablation Depth/Pulse	20–60 μm* Plateau at 4th pass	5–50 μm No plateau
Range of thermal injury/pass	75–150 μm**	15–50 μm
Tissue effects	Photothermal	Photomechanical
Tissue levels	Epidermis = an opalescent aspect is obtained Papillary dermis = Pink color Deep papillary dermis = Chamois leather appearance Reticular dermis = Cotton thread appearance due to collagen	Epidermis = Whitening Papillary dermis = Pinpoint bleeding Reticular dermis = Uneven surface (sebaceous glands) brisk bleeding
Histological effect	Coagulation-crater around the ablated area (necrosis, deep thermal effect)	Precise and safe ablation (limited thermal effect)
Safety of treatment	Necrosis makes control of ablation depth difficult	High visibility of treatment range, ablation depth can easily be controlled
Depth of treatment	Treatment is not restricted to the epidermis because of thermal effect. Thus good for dermal disorders	Superficial ablation of epidermal lesions
Thermal effects	Collagen shrinkage because of thermal effect	Less thermal damage
Wound healing	Prolonged wound healing due to necrosis areas	Shorter healing time
Side effects	More	Less

*In human skin the depth of ablation peaks at 225–250 μm after 4 passes using 1–3 pulses, dose of 250–500 mJ (UltraPulse)
**The coagulation varies from 20 μm (1 pass) to 70 μm at 3–4 pass, maximum 100 μm

using this combined method approaches those attained with the CO_2 laser alone, and have a significantly reduced healing time and a lower incidence of complications.

An alternative to switching between two different lasers is to use an Er:YAG laser with a variable pulse width (Contour from Sciton and CO_3 from Cynosure). When used with a longer pulse duration, "CO_2-like" effects may be achieved. The increased pulse duration extends the zone of thermal

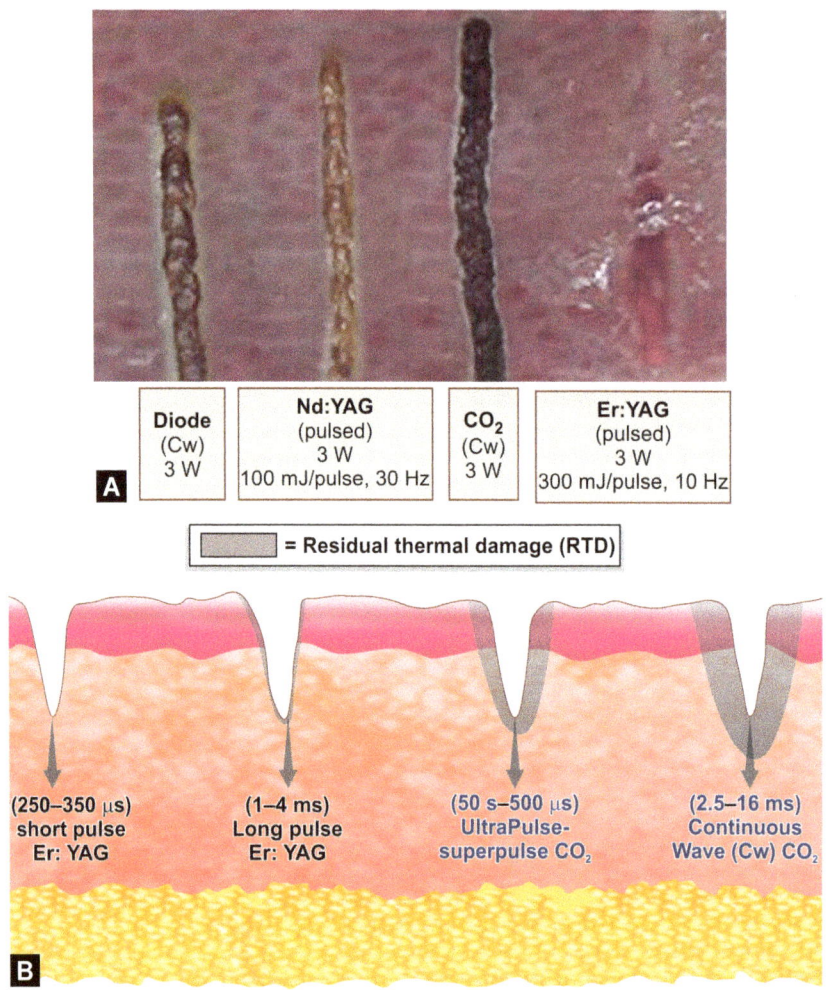

Figs. 2.14A and B: (A) A comparison of the tissue incisions of the major lasers, on soft tissue. Following photothermal ablation caused by lasers, various degrees of thermal denaturation were observed on the irradiated site (chicken liver). The pulsed erbium-doped yttrium-aluminum-garnet (Er:YAG) laser effectively ablates soft tissue, with minimal coagulation and no carbonization. The continuous wave (Cw) carbon dioxide (CO_2) laser also easily ablated soft tissue but carbonization was evident with relatively thin coagulation. The pulsed neodymium-doped yttrium-aluminum-garnet (Nd:YAG) laser produced relatively thick coagulation with moderate carbonization. The Cw diode laser produced the greatest coagulation as well as moderate carbonization. (B) A comparison of thermal damage of the major ablative lasers, note the minimal thermal damage of the Er:YAG laser.

damage, induces collagen contraction, and coagulates small dermal blood vessels. Shortening the pulse duration gives typical "Er:YAG-like" effects with minimal thermal injury and superficial ablation. Therefore, the short pulse mode can be used to initially smooth rhytides and scars, then the long pulse mode can tighten tissue, and finally the short pulse mode used again to remove the layer of necrotic tissue in order to hasten healing. Thus, one can achieve results with one dual mode Er:YAG laser approaching those only previously seen with the use of the CO_2 laser. In addition, due to the wavelength selectivity of the Er:YAG, the longer pulse delivers the "CO_2-like" benefit of thermal damage and subsequent collagen contraction, whereas decreasing risk of deleterious effects seen with the CO_2 laser including hypopigmentation.

BIBLIOGRAPHY

1. Aoki A, Mizutani K, Schwarz F, et al. Periodontal and peri-implant wound healing following laser therapy. Periodontol 2000. 2015;68(1):217-69.

ERBIUM:YSGG LASER RESURFACING

The Er:YSGG laser was approved by the United States FDA in 2008. It generates a wavelength of 2,790 nm and has a water absorption coefficient that lies between that of the Er:YAG (2,940 nm) and CO_2 (10,600 nm) lasers (*see* Fig. 2.1). It was developed in an attempt to provide deeper dermal heating than the traditional Er:YAG laser while still minimizing healing time. Like the Er:YAG laser, the Er:YSGG laser removes a portion of the epidermis with a controlled thermal effect. What makes it unique is that there is only minimal epidermal tissue removal, thus creating a natural protective dressing that diminishes the extent of the recovery process, similar to plasma skin regeneration technology. It is primarily used for pigment, rhytides, and skin tone (Ross EV). A recent study has used it for acne scars (Kim S), though it is the author's opinion that it may not replace the current fractional lasers for this indication.

PLASMA SKIN REGENERATION

Plasma skin regeneration technology uses pulses of ionized nitrogen gas to deliver heat energy directly to the skin. Like other ablative resurfacing lasers, its development came from the desire to approach the results of traditional CO_2 resurfacing without the lengthy recovery time. Unlike lasers, there is no dependence on a specific target such as water, hemoglobin, or melanin.

The system uses energy from an ultrahigh-frequency radiofrequency generator to convert nitrogen gas into plasma within the handpiece. The plasma emerges from a nozzle on the handpiece directly onto the skin's surface, thus transferring energy in a process that is not chromophore-dependent.

At high-energy settings, thermal injury reaches the papillary dermis and extends up to 11.8 μm in depth below the dermal-epidermal junction. In late 2008, the company that produced the only plasma device on the market stopped its production. At the time of writing this chapter, the handpiece nozzles necessary for the plasma treatments were unavailable.

TREATMENT

Preoperative

Patient Selection

- Patient *expectations* are of paramount importance in patient selection and satisfaction. "Before and after" photographs of other patients may be helpful in educating individuals about the degree of improvement one can expect. It must be emphasized that not all lesions will be eliminated and that one must balance the degree of improvement desired with the effects of the postoperative recovery period.
- Traditionally, the major decision as to which laser to use was based on the severity of the lesions to be treated. The traditional **Er:YAG** lasers allow for a much faster recovery time with less posttreatment erythema. However, this occurs at the expense of less clinical improvement. Although the traditional single-mode low-powered Er:YAG laser required several passes to ablate the epidermis and had limited capacity to vaporize beyond papillary dermis due to lack of hemostasis, the introduction of the dual-mode Er:YAG lasers has led to depths of ablation and coagulation comparable to traditional CO_2 lasers.
- *Oral retinoid therapy*: Patients who are taking oral retinoids (e.g. isotretinoin) may have delayed healing and atypical scarring if resurfacing is performed while they are taking the drug. Although the safe time period for performing resurfacing after cessation of oral retinoids is not known, most experts would wait at least 6 months.
- *Lack of skin appendages*: Because the skin reepithelializes by means of the appendages after laser resurfacing, extensive destruction to appendages (e.g. electrolysis, burns, etc.) may cause delayed healing and scarring.
- *Viral diseases*: Erbium:YAG resurfacing produces significant plume. Live viruses may be a hazard to operating room personnel and other patients. It may be hazardous to treat patients with Hepatitis-B, Hepatitis-C, or HIV with erbium laser resurfacing.

Smoke Evacuation

During the treatment with the erbium laser, a distinct dust and smoke formation must be expected due to the photoablation. The particles and aerosols being emitted are evacuated through the handpiece. Without a smoke evacuator, the optical part of the handpiece can be damaged due to the deposition of the particles.

Anesthesia

The local anesthesia should be varied according to the depth of treatment. There are several forms to choose from: surface anesthesia, applied topically and occlusively (EMLA) or infiltration anesthesia (aminoamides, aminoester) that is injected intradermally or subcutaneously. It is also possible to apply infiltration anesthesia topically after the ablation of epidermis.

Medication

Initiate levofloxacin 750 mg a day before the surgery and continue it for 5 days. In case there is a history of herpes labialis, famciclovir 250 mg TDS is also started.

Intraoperative

Principles

The goal of both CO_2 and erbium laser resurfacing is clean, char-free, layer-by-layer ablation of skin, resulting in the absolute or relative effacement of lesions, while avoiding the creation of dermal injury so deep that hypertrophic scarring or other untoward complications result. Penetration into the papillary or upper reticular dermis represents the end point of safe treatment. Several factors determine the actual treatment parameters for each laser system, including the anatomic location being resurfaced, the patient's skin type, individual tissue response to irradiation and prior treatments to the area.

In general, highly fibrotic areas, skin with more severe lesional involvement and facial regions with thicker skin—the cheeks, chin, perioral area and forehead—require higher fluences and a greater number of laser passes. However, thin or delicate skin, such as that in the periocular area, or skin with fewer adnexal structures as a result of prior treatment requires lower energies and/or fewer passes. Moreover, patients with darker skin phototypes (III and above) run an ever-greater risk of adverse pigmentary changes as the depth of ablation increases. Thus, the aggressiveness of treatment should always be case-specific.

Techniques

When performing resurfacing with the erbium:YAG laser, a homogeneous appearance must be obtained to produce an acceptable esthetic result. The laser tissue interaction produces ablative effects with "sharp" edges, as compared with the carbon dioxide laser and its Gaussian curve. To ensure a homogeneous appearance, significant (i.e. 30–50%) overlap of pulses is necessary. Smooth skin lesions can be ablated by applying overlapping laser spots to the area to be treated. The overlapping best adapted to the beam profile is 10–20% of the spot diameter. Of course, it is possible to work with a higher overlap but it has to be taken into consideration that energy may summate in the overlapped areas. Lower pulse energies have to be selected in this case. Overlap less than 10% is not recommended since ablation may be not as regular as usual. Uneven skin lesions can be treated by smoothing the entire treatment area and then flattening the edges of wrinkles or other lesions in a second pass. Three techniques are recommended for ablative lasers (Fig. 2.15).

Types of Resurfacing Techniques

Circular technique: In this, an overlap technique is used to flatten edges of lesion (e.g. acne scars) (Fig. 2.15).

Paintbrush technique: Paintbrush technique is used for extensive lesions (e.g. lentigines, Becker's nevi). After finishing one pass, the direction should be changed by 90°. If further passes are required, they should be given diagonally (Fig. 2.16). The ultimate aim is to avoid excessive thermal damage.

Single spot technique: This technique is for a single lesion (e.g. syringomas). The method that is used for layering passes is important (Fig. 2.15), as it ensures less overlap and consequentially minimal thermal damage.

End Points

Er:YAG: When resurfacing with the Erbium:YAG laser, clear visualization of the end points makes the procedure extremely accurate. Using magnifying glasses/Dermaview helps in assessing the end point. Because little necrotic tissue remains after erbium laser impact, wiping the skin between passes is *not* typically necessary, as it is after CO_2 irradiation.

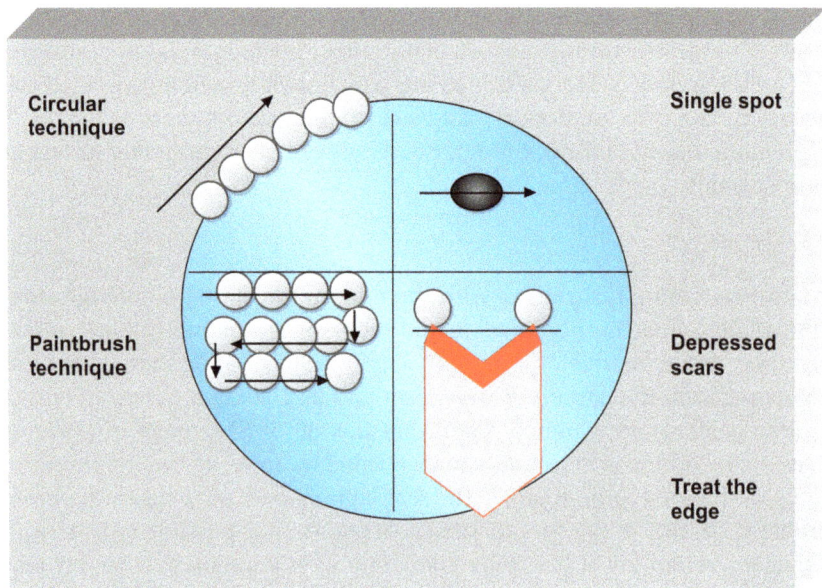

Fig. 2.15: Standard techniques employed while using ablative lasers.

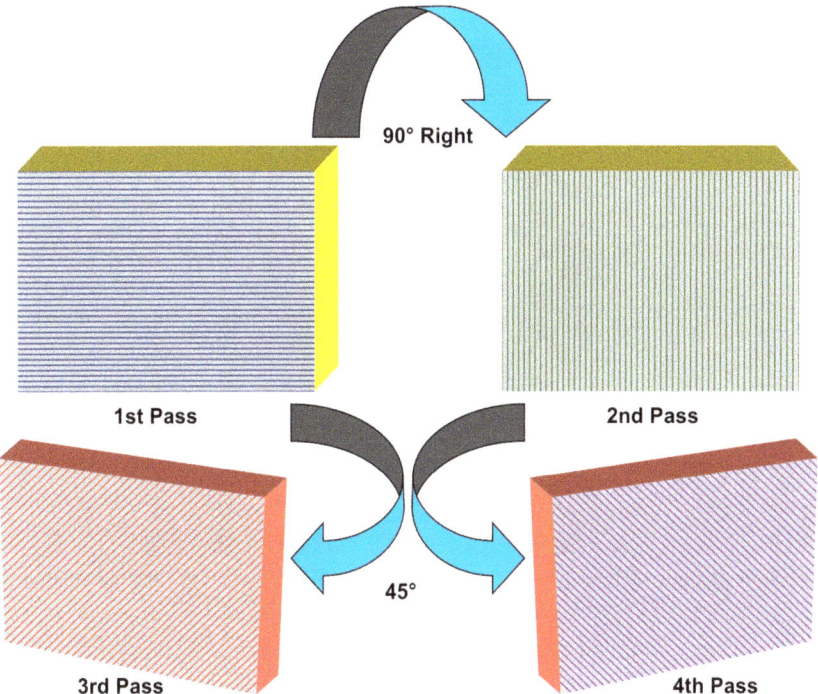

Fig. 2.16: Method of layering of passes with ablative lasers with the aim of avoiding excessive thermal damage.

Epidermis: Resurfacing within the epidermis produces a yellowish-brown appearance on the epidermis. This is preceded by a transient whitening of the skin.

Epidermal-dermal junction: Once the epidermis has been removed, the pinkish appearance of the upper papillary dermis will be readily appreciated (Fig. 2.17). The follicle openings look small and regular, like a fine sponge.

Lower papillary dermis: As resurfacing proceeds into the papillary dermis, pinpoint bleeding and a transudate develops, indicating injury to the small capillaries that are present in the papillary dermis. If local anesthesia with epinephrine is used, bleeding and transudation may be greatly reduced (Fig. 2.18). Follicle openings become wider and begin to stand out from the surrounding dermis.

Upper reticular dermis: When the upper reticular dermis is reached, bleeding may become splotchy, and the transudate becomes more profuse. Follicle openings become much wider and the collagen bundles become coarser and more haphazard in orientation. At this point, it is generally best to proceed no further.

Although the end points are clear, especially with the help of magnification, they may take several seconds or minutes to become evident.

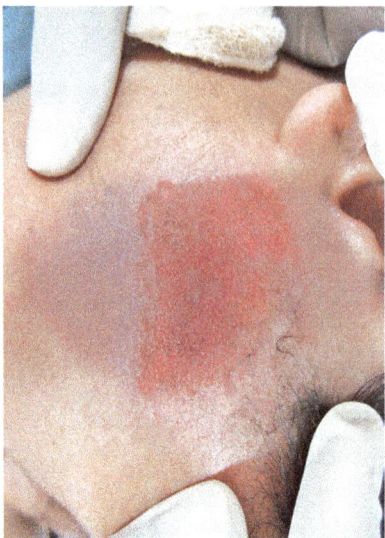

Fig. 2.17: A case of Becker's nevi treated with Er:YAG resurfacing, the pinkish hue of "papillary dermis" is the end point (Er:YAG, Ascepelion; 10 J/cm^2; 4 Hz).

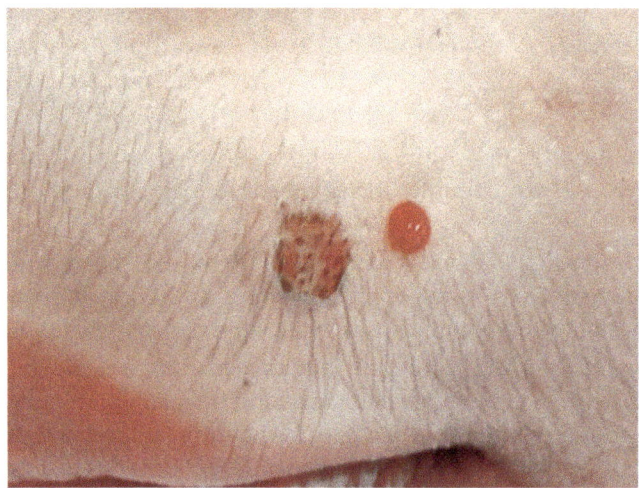

Fig. 2.18: A case of junctional nevus with pin point bleeding and the end point of prominent follicular openings (Er:YAG 7 J/cm^2; 4 Hz; level: lower papillary dermis).

Carbon Dioxide Laser

- Extensive prepping of the skin prior to laser treatment is unnecessary because the heat of the laser sterilizes the skin.
- The surgeon should use energy densities equal to or exceeding the critical irradiance threshold (5 J/cm^2) for tissue ablation. Lower irradiances on the contrary heat the tissue too slowly, thereby permitting greater heat

conduction into surrounding tissues. Excessively deep thermal injury, or even charring, can result.
- After each pass of the laser, the desiccated white debris must be wiped away with saline soaked gauze before the next pass because this debris acts as a heat sink and CO_2 laser energy delivered to this layer will result in excessive thermal injury and possible scarring. The wet gauze also serves to rehydrate the desiccated tissue. Dry gauze should be used to remove any remaining water and exudates prior to another pass because this surface water would absorb the energy and prevent further tissue ablation.
- Additional laser passes are used until the desired depth of vaporization is reached or until the treated lesion(s) are removed.
- One should not continue ablation once the distinctive yellowish color of the desiccated reticular dermis has been reached.
  Bleeding is not usually encountered with CO_2 laser ablation except when treating very thick lesions such as rhinophyma or vascular lesions such as warts.
- The desired treatment end point is visible removal of the target lesion and a smooth, even surface.

The first pass with a CO_2 laser will vaporize all or most of the epidermis. Because CO_2 ablation is primarily thermal, each pass will leave behind a detritus of coagulated necrotic tissue. This whitish debris must be thoroughly removed with saline-soaked gauze; if allowed to remain, it can act as a heat sink and promote excessive thermal damage with successive laser passes. Moreover, the removal of necrotic tissue allows better visualization of the surgical field. After the debris left by the first pass has been removed, the smooth, pink surface of the papillary dermis is apparent. With each subsequent pass, subtle color changes signal deeper dermal penetration. Collagen fibers appear as white, cotton-like threads. A change to a distinctly yellowish color, apparent when the surgeon reaches the upper reticular dermis, which signals the end point of treatment, even when lesions have not been fully effaced. As discussed above these end points are not always reliably seen.

Continued ablation and possibly greater residual thermal injury, could substantially injure the adnexal follicular structures essential for reepithelialization. In general, the thin skin of the periorbital region can sustain one to two passes with the CO_2 laser, whereas the thicker skin of other facial regions can tolerate three or four passes. More than four passes do not seem to improve clinical results and are not advised because tissue vaporization is reduced and progressive desiccation of the dermis occurs, which may cause excessive residual thermal injury.

Dosage and Settings

A rough guide to dosages is given in the *Appendix* but a useful method is to understand the end points to be achieved which are detailed above.

Wound Care

Dressings

In the area of resurfacing, occlusive dressings were used to absorb the exudate produced by the procedure. In spot therapy, we prefer an open wound care with topical fucidin ointment applied thrice a day till the crust falls off. Oral levofloxacin 750 mg HS for 5 days is routinely given to prevent bacterial infections.

Post Wound Care

A mild depigmenting agent, ideally HQ/Tretinoin free, is preferred (Melacare™) can be given after the crust has fallen off to avoid PIH. Sun avoidance is advisable for 10 days after the procedure.

LIMITATIONS OF ABLATIVE LASERS

Er:YAG

On impact, the erbium laser beam forcibly ejects desiccated tissue at supersonic speeds, hence, the distinctive skin popping during ablation and the superficially whitened area left behind quickly fades into inconspicuousness, offering the surgeon less guidance when treating large adjacent areas of the dermis than does the coagulated tissue remaining after CO_2 irradiation.

The Erbium:YAG laser is absorbed superficially in the skin due to its high water absorption. Higher fluences and multiple passes are necessary to obtain improvement in deeper wrinkles and acne scars, making the procedure slower than with the carbon dioxide laser. To overcome this problem, large scan patterns and higher fluence erbium machines have been developed.

Bleeding: When deeper resurfacing is being performed, dermal bleeding will occur, making the procedure more cumbersome and messy. Modulated lasers can help in increasing the coagulative potential of the lasers.

Noise level: Because the erbium laser tissue interaction is strong and explosive, the noise level in the operating room can become oppressive; ear muffs are recommended.

Plume: Because significant tissue ablation occurs with the Erbium:YAG laser, a large amount of plume containing live tissue is released. A powerful smoke evacuation system is needed to cope with the plume. Live viruses are a potential problem for operating room staff.

CO_2 Lasers

The major issues are due to the large degree of thermal damage that is caused by the systems. This can lead to postoperative erythema, scarring and pigmentary alterations especially in pigmented skins.

Conclusion

The use of modulated Er:YAG lasers (*see* Table 2.3) has tried to bridge the gap between ablative/coagulative potential of CO_2 and the fine ablation with less coagulative potential of Er:YAG. In most dermatological indications, we feel that, the less thermal damage and fine ablation makes the Er:YAG a better technology. The added advantage of less side effects (PIH) makes it useful in Indian skin.

APPENDIX

Treatment guidelines for pulsed CO_2 and Er:YAG laser have been detailed in Tables 2.5 and 2.6.

Table 2.5: Treatment guidelines for pulsed CO_2.

Indications	Energy	Diameter (mm)	Exposure time	Comments
Spot vaporization • Benign skin tumors • Condylomata acuminate • Epithelial dysplasia • Verrucae vulgaris	8–10-(20) Watt	0.5–2-(3) mm	0.1–0.2 s	This is the superpulse mode which has a higher thermal damage than the UltraPulse mode. Usually a controlled single pulse is given ranging from 0.01–0.09 sec
Large area vaporization • Condylomata acuminate • Epithelial dysplasia • Verrucae	5–10 Watt	0.5–1.5 mm	0.1 s	Either the superpulse mode or the repeat mode can be selected with a 0.4 s interval
UltraPulse mode • BCC • Flat benign • Scars • SCC • Skin ablation • Skin tumors	10–20 Watt	Fixed with scanner	<1 ms	The least thermal damage amongst all the modes of CO_2 lasers
Surgical resection	15–25 Watt	0.5–1 mm	Continuous wave	The ablation and thermal damage is the maximum

Table 2.6: Treatment guidelines for Er:YAG laser.

Indications	Diameter (mm)	Energy	Pattern	Comments
Acne scars	3–5 according to lesion size	4–5 J/cm^2	Circle	Plane acne scars edges with overlap technique
Becker nevi Café-au-lait Spots	3–5 according to lesion size	4–5 J/cm^2	Paintbrush	With darker skin types, transitory hypo-/hyperpigmentation possible (inform patient!) Continue the treatment until no more pigment is visible
Epidermal nevi (soft)	3–5 according to lesion size	4–5 J/cm^2	Paintbrush	Ablation down to the level of the skin or into the unaffected dermis (until whitish tissue of dermis becomes visible)
Exophytic scars (flat scars, no keloids)	3–5 according to lesion size	4–5 J/cm^2	Paintbrush	Ablation of exophytic portion
Lentigines spilus	3–6 according to lesion size	4–5 J/cm^2	Single spot (selective) Paintbrush (area)	The treatment is continued until no more pigment is visible
Stepped scars	3–6 according to lesion size	4–5 J/cm^2	Overlap	Plane the edge of the scar
Syringomas Xanthelasmas Adenoma Sebaceum	3–6 according to lesion size	4–5 J/cm^2	Single spot	Requires ablation of the complete lesion (trough-shaped depression)
Wrinkles	1–3 according to lesion size	4–5 J/cm^2	Overlap	Plane the shoulder of the wrinkle

BOOKS

1. Carcamo AS, Goldman MP. Skin resurfacing with ablative lasers. In: Goldman MP (Ed). Cutaneous and Cosmetic Laser Surgery, 2nd edition. USA: Mosby; 2009.
2. Willard RJ, Moody Br, Hruza GJ. Carbon dioxide and erbium:YAG laser ablation. In: Goldman MP (Ed). Cutaneous and Cosmetic Laser Surgery, 2nd edition. USA: Mosby; 2009.

BIBLIOGRAPHY

1. Alster TS. Cutaneous resurfacing with CO_2 and Erbium:YAG laser. Plast Reconstr Surg. 1999;103:619-32.

2. Alster TS, Nanni CA, Williams CM. Comparison of four carbon dioxide resurfacing lasers. A clinical and histopathologic evaluation. Dermatol Surg. 1999;25(3):153-8.
3. Alster TS. Clinical and histologic evaluation of 6 erbium: YAG lasers for cutaneous resurfacing. Lasers Surg Med. 1999;24:87-92.
4. Fitzpatrick RE, Tope WD, Goldman MP, et al. Pulsed carbon dioxide laser, trichloroacetic acid, Baker Gordon phenol, and dermabrasion: A comparative clinical and histologic study of cutaneous resurfacing in a porcine model. Arch Dermatol. 1996;132:469-71.
5. Jaisn ME. Achieving Er:YAG superior resurfacing results with the Er:YAG lasers. Arch Facial Plastic Surg. 2002;4:262-6.
6. Kauvar AN, Waldorf HA, Geronemus RG. A histopathological comparison of "char-free" carbon dioxide lasers. Dermatol Surg. 1996;22(4):343-8.
7. Kim S. Treatment of acne scars in Asian patients using a 2,790-nm fractional yttrium scandium gallium garnet laser. Dermatol Surg. 2011;37(10):1464-9.
8. Ross EV, Swann M, Soon S, et al. Full-face treatment with the 2790-nm erbium:YSGG laser system. J Drugs Dermatol. 2009;8:248-52.
9. Weinstein C. Carbon dioxide laser resurfacing. Long-term follow-up in 2123 patients. Clin Plast Surg. 1998;25(1):109-30.

ABLATIVE LASER TREATMENT OF COMMON CONDITIONS

INTRODUCTION

Even with the advent of novel laser systems, the popularity of Er:YAG and CO_2 has not waned, even though in terms of publications not much has been published in recent times. This reflects a bias as the laser industry sponsors newer technology, but older conventional lasers are still excellent tools.

The use of ablative lasers and its widespread appeal lies in the fact the water is the chromophore, and thus almost every skin lesion is a potential target. The clinicians must choose indications based on the **shallower tissue effects** due to higher water absorption of **Er:YAG** and the **deeper** effects of **CO_2**.

The basic principle guiding the use of CO_2 lasers is that its use is based on the dimensions of tolerability of the skin for scarring and dyspigmentation. As long as everything within the block of tissue vaporized or heated can be sacrificed without adverse side effects, the CO_2 laser is an attractive "*what you see is what you get laser.*" Once the CO_2 laser light impacts on the skin, there is immediate absorption, so that the injury is always *top to bottom* unless one irradiates the skin from the undersurface, which is a technique used by some physicians. For this reason, the CO_2 laser demands a high level of operator practice and skill to achieve reliable results. It follows that with greater use, one finds that the laser is as good or nearly as good as some of the pigment selective or vascular selective lasers for particular lesions.

It is our opinion that for most epidermal and dermal disorders, Er:YAG is superior as it has less thermal damage and a predictable depth, with easy to discern end points. Those who prefer the CO_2 laser should be adept at using the tool to minimize thermal damage.

Practice Points

- A useful **thumb** rule is, that when *fine ablation, cosmesis* and *fast healing* is the goal, **Er:YAG** is preferred. For deeper lesions, vascular lesions, lymphatic tumors CO_2 laser is preferred.

    Though variable pulse Er:YAG can mimic the coagulative effects of CO_2, those who do not use this laser prefer the controlled effect of carbon dioxide laser.

    Both the lasers can be used for numerous indications though as a **thumb** rule *deep dermal, vascular and lymphatic conditions* respond best to pulsed **CO_2 lasers** (Table 2.7).
- Where one needs *selective single spot damage* a *low fluence* and *pulse duration* should be used and where there is a need for *coagulation or ablation* the *pulse duration* and *dose* should be *increased*.
- The indications range from the A to Z of dermatology with almost one condition for each alphabet! But before attempting any laser procedure three questions must be asked.
    1. Is there a *need* for a laser ablation?
    2. What are the chances of *recurrences*?
    3. *How* should the laser be used?

    Though we will largely focus on the last aspect there are numerous indications where lasers are of little use and are best left alone as the ultimate cosmetic results may be worse than the initial appearance.
- A useful guide to indications is given in Table 2.8. Obviously just because water is the chromophore does not preclude to its use in all indications listed!

Table 2.7: Indications of ablative lasers.

	Focal treatment	*Resurfacing mode*
Epidermal disorders	• Actinic cheilitis • BXO (balanitis xerotica obliterans) • Epidermal nevi • Epidermal tumors • Lichen sclerosus • Melasma • Seborrheic keratoses • Verruca • Zoons balanitis	Wrinkles
Dermal disorders	• Benign dermal tumors • Lymphangiomas • Scars • Vascular growths	

Table 2.8: Indications of ablative lasers.

Ablative lasers as the potential treatment of choice	Ablative lasers offer distinct advantages	Ablative lasers where no specific advantages exists
Actinic cheilitis	Veruccae	Superficial BCC
Epidermal nevi	Condyloma accuminata	Bowen's disease
Rhinophyma	Various benign dermal tumors (e.g. adenoma sebaceum, trichoepitheliomas, syringomas)	Squamous cell carcinoma
Eyeliner tattoos	Erythroplasia of Queyrat Actinic keratoses Seborrheic keratoses Red tattoo reactions Xanthelasma Burn debridement Neurofibromas Other superficial lesions (balanitis xerotica obliterans, lichen sclerosus, Zoon's balanitis, etc)	Cherry angiomas Solar lentigines Granuloma faciale Angiokeratomas

INDICATIONS

Skin Tumors

Epidermal lesions (e.g. junctional nevi, trichoepithelioma, solar keratoses, seborrheic keratoses, and sebaceous hyperplasia) respond extremely well to the erbium:YAG laser. Dermal lesions (e.g. compound nevi, dermal nevi, syringoma, xanthelasmas) can be modified and the exophytic component removed, producing an improved cosmetic appearance, with both the lasers. However, where there is a deeper dermal component, these lesions will inevitably recur. Pulsed CO_2 lasers may be used in dermal disorders. In certain disorders where sensitive and thin areas of skin are involved, like in Zoon's balanitis, Er:YAG is probably an ideal tool to use.

Scars

The atrophic scars, most responsive to resurfacing, are those that are relatively shallow, soft and distensible. Extremely deep scars or pits bound with highly fibrotic tissue are far less responsive to either type of resurfacing.

i) Acne

Both the pulsed CO_2 and the erbium:YAG laser are useful for treating acne scars, but results with any resurfacing procedure alone are moderate at best. A combined approach to acne scar improvement produces the best results.

TCA cross can somewhat help in ice-pick scars and deep boxcar scars. Dermarollers help the rolling scars and superficial boxcar scars the results of which are probably similar to the results of fractional lasers (*see* **Chapters 4 and 12**).

ii) Chickenpox Scars

Modest improvement of mild-to-moderate acne scarring can be achieved with the short pulsed Er:YAG laser resurfacing. Deep acne scars have a better chance of improvement when resurfaced with a modulated Er:YAG laser. However, even with the modulated Er:YAG lasers, the reported improvement has been moderate at best. Adjunctive treatment with other modalities (e.g. subcision, punch excision, fillers, grafts) is usually required to achieve significant correction of this difficult-to-treat condition.

Though fractional lasers are used in acne scars for localized scars like chickenpox scars ablative lasers are superior to most fractional lasers.

The basic principle being, reducing the depth of the scar borders and stimulating neocollagenesis to fill in the depressions.

Step-by-step Approach
Spot laser resurfacing (Fig. 2.19A)
1. First the area ***around*** and **over** the scar is vaporized with one laser pass de-epithelialization typically requires one pass with the CO_2 laser at 300 mJ and two to three passes with the Er:YAG laser at 5 J/cm^2.
2. Additional passes are made along the ***edge*** of the scar.

    The purpose is to sculpt the scar edges or "shoulders" with additional vaporizing laser passes to bring the edge to approximate the level of the base. This is followed by 1–2 passes in the center of the scar. Aggressive passes over the center can cause a deeper scar. Partially desiccated tissue should be completely removed with saline- or water-soaked gauze after each laser pass in an effort to prevent charring.

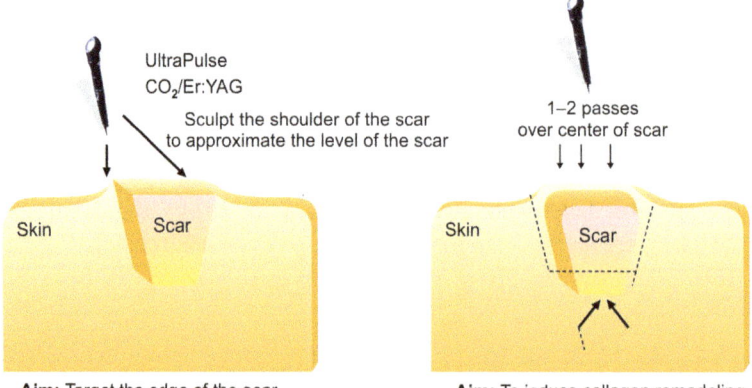

Fig. 2.19A: A figurative depiction of laser treatment of atrophic chickenpox scar.

3. *End point*: Effacement of the scar or bringing the surrounding skin to the level of the depth of the scar.

Weinstein et al. first flattened the shoulders of the scars by single spots at 8 J/cm^2, two to five passes, followed by treatment of the entire anatomical unit with the computerized scanner at 15 J/cm^2 and 30% pulse overlap with two to three passes. For deeper acne scars, she used the CO$_2$ laser (SilkTouch scanning device, 30-40 J/cm^2) for the shoulders followed by the Er:YAG laser as described before. Using this technique, she achieved, seven good (70-90% improvement), and three fair results (50-70% improvement).

A depiction of a case of chickenpox scar treated by Er:YAG laser is given in Figures 2.19B(i) and (ii).

Pearls/Pitfalls:
- Never ablate an atrophic scar "in toto" as it invariably leads to a deeper scar.
- Vary the spot size to adjust the beam to target the edge of the scar.
- Nonablative resurfacing and fractional lasers do not help substantially in chickenpox/smallpox scars.
- Subcision is usually of **no use** as these scars are "tissue defects" and not tethered unlike rolling scars of acne.

Level of Difficulty: High.

iii) Post-traumatic Scars

Post-traumatic and surgical scars may be modified by the Erbium:YAG/CO$_2$ laser if resurfacing is performed during the phase of collagen remodeling (i.e. within 90 days of the original trauma or surgery). Linear facial scars respond best. Extrafacial scars respond poorly. Raised scars can be planed down to the level of the surrounding skin (Fig. 2.20A). Most depressed scars require a sculpting approach where the edges are ablated till they are leveled with the

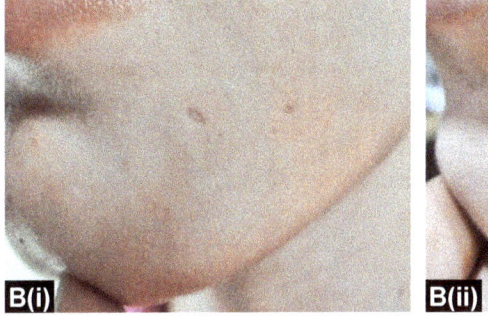
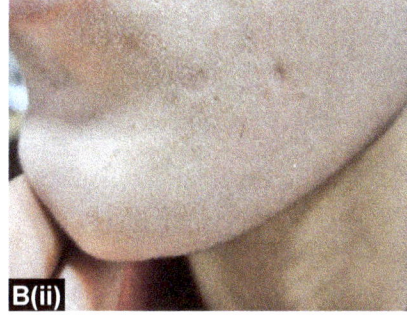

Figs. 2.19B(i) and (ii): B(i) A case of chickenpox scar, the "medial" scar was treated with an Er:YAG laser; B(ii) After 6 months marked improvement is seen in the treated scar as compared to the control (lateral) scar.

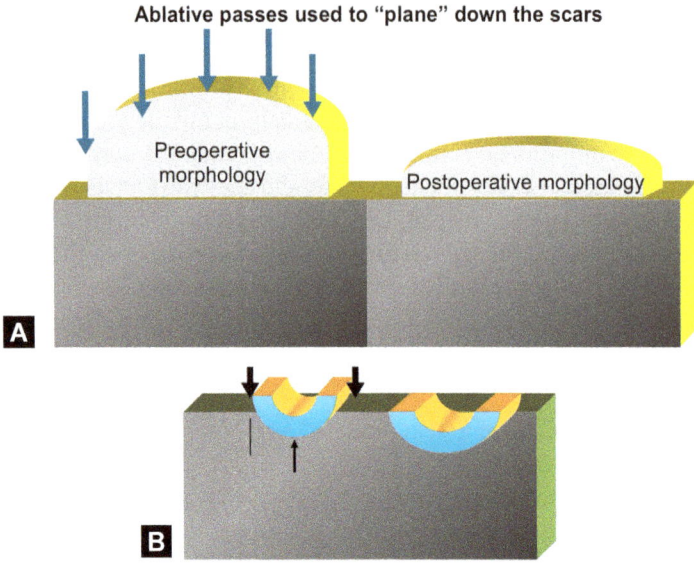

Figs. 2.20A and B: (A) Ablative lasers can ablate the elevated surface of hypertrophic scars; (B) Ablative lasers use in depressed scars. The elevated edges are planed down to the level of the adjacent epidermis skin.

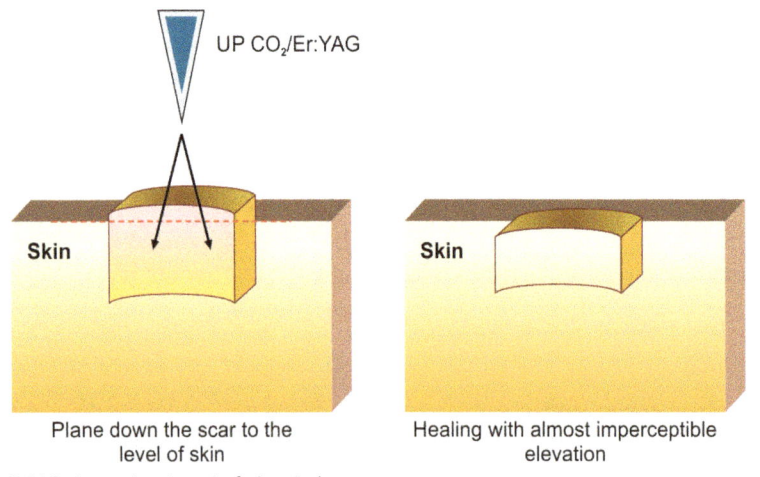

Fig. 2.20C: Laser treatment of elevated scar.

surrounding skin (Fig. 2.20B). A pass over the center of the scar can help to stimulate collagen to lift up the scar.

Step-by-step Approach
Spot laser resurfacing (Fig. 2.20C)
1. An elevated scar can simply be sculpted down to the level of the surrounding skin.
2. A few passes over the center of the scars can depress it further.

Combination approach
1. Initial sessions can be done with a PDL in the erythematous stage, this tends to cut off the vascular supply.
2. Concomitant topical agents can be used.
3. Treat a scar early.

Level of Difficulty: Easy.

Acne Keloidalis Nuchae

There are two approaches to treat this condition. One is to target the hair growth and second is to ablate the lesion. The former is slow and is rarely successful in our experience. Ablating with the CO_2 laser leads to better results. Recurrences ensue unless the lesions are vaporized down to the fat and the hair follicles are destroyed. But, the larger vessels (>0.5 mm) lead to profuse bleeding that requires coagulation by electrosurgery.

Kantor et al. treated eight patients with the CO_2 laser and found that as long as the lesions were excised to the **level of the fat**, there were no recurrences. Lesions were allowed to heal by **secondary intention**.

The primary advantage of the use of CO_2 laser in acne keloidalis nuchae is hemostasis versus the lack of the same in cold steel surgery.

Level of Difficulty: High.

BIBLIOGRAPHY

1. Dragoni F, Bassi A, Cannarozzo G, et al. Successful treatment of acne keloidalis nuchae resistant to conventional therapy with 1064-nm ND:YAG laser. G Ital Dermatol Venereol. 2013;148(2):231-2.
2. Esmat SM, Abdel Hay RM, Abu Zeid OM, et al. The efficacy of laser-assisted hair removal in the treatment of acne keloidalis nuchae; a pilot study. Eur J Dermatol. 2012;22(5):645-50.
3. Kantor GR, Ratz JL, Wheeland RG. Treatment of acne keloidalis nuchae with carbon dioxide laser. J Am Acad Dermatol. 1986;14(2 Pt 1):263-7.

Actinic Cheilitis

Though both the UltraPulse and the Cw laser have been used, we feel that an adequately gated Cw laser can give results comparable to the UltraPulse lasers.

Step-by-step Approach (Figs. 2.21A to C)

1. Cw mode of CO_2 power 3–8 W using defocused, 2–4 mm beams is used.
2. *End point*: After the first pass in Cw mode white bubbling of the surface (opalescence) is seen. This can be wiped away with either saline-soaked gauze or hydrogen peroxide. If there is a mildly damaged area, a bright pink papillary dermis is exposed. However, in areas where there is severe actinic damage, one sees a yellow-gray surface.

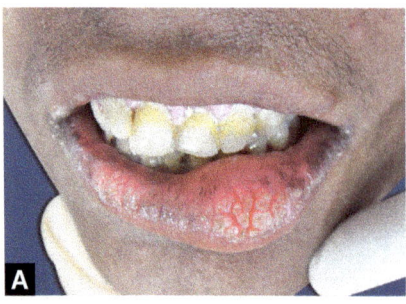
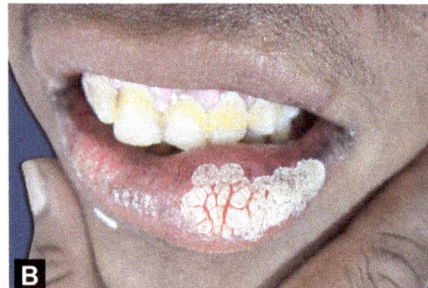
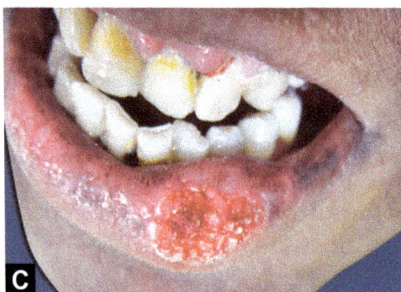

Figs. 2.21A to C: (A) A case of Actinic Cheilitis. Plan: Ablation of the epidermis with Er:YAG and coagulation of the dermal vessels with pulsed CO_2; (B) Note the whitening due to the tissue effects of Er:YAG; (C) 3–4 passes lead to bleeding, the desired end point.

Some authors have described **three colors** as end points namely, pink, white/gray, and white coarse. It was believed that the first two levels are desirable. But it is now believed that the whiter areas are those focal areas with the greatest clinical damage prior to treatment and may also be needed to be removed. The lack of surface pinkness is not only due to deeper treatment, but also due to preexisting fibrosis in these areas, as well as increased acanthosis and interdigitations between the lesion and the underlying dermis.

3. An additional pass is performed in this area with a very low power of about 2 W for 0.5–1 s.
4. The importance of moving the handpiece in a rapid brushing manner cannot be overstated. This in the case of Cw mode, the hand becomes a scanner, limiting the dwell time in a somewhat primitive manner, but one that becomes increasingly precise and reliable with practice.

Level of Difficulty

High.

Rhinophyma

Background

This consequence of rosacea is characterized by sebaceous hyperplasia of sebum and keratinous debris. Variable amounts of dermal fibroplasia and connective tissue increase may also occur.

Principle of Surgery/Lasers Used

The goal of surgical management of rhinophyma is to debulk the hypertrophied tissue and leave an adequate glandular reserve to allow scarless re-epithelization. Many patients request treatment, not for cosmetic considerations, but to improve air movement.

Many techniques have been used to treat rhinophyma, including dermabrasion, cold steel surgical sculpting, cryosurgery, electrosurgery, CO_2 laser ablation, and Er:YAG laser ablation. Dermabrasion may result in incomplete ablation of rhinophymatous tissue due to technical difficulties. Cryosurgery often results in uneven ablation because it is difficult to achieve a uniform depth of freezing. Electrosurgical sculpting allows easy tissue removal but heat conduction to deeper tissues may result in scarring. Lack of hemostasis with cold-steel surgery for rhinophyma makes this a suboptimal treatment modality.

Carbon dioxide continuous wave laser ablation allows for precision in nasal shaping. Hemostasis during the procedure allows visualization of the treated areas and greater control over contouring. The use of prerhinophymatous photographs helps to prevent oversculpting. Care must be taken, especially at the ala, not to overtreat, which can lead to scarring and nasal flaring. Consideration of the residual 1-2 mm of thermally denatured tissue with the Cw CO_2 laser should be taken into account. There is a definite risk of scarring when ablating to a deep plane. One must be aware of the extent of ablation by recognizing sebaceous gland structures as deeper layers of tissue are removed. During vaporization, the dermis contracts and sebum is visibly expressed from the sebaceous glands, indicating that scarring is unlikely at this depth. Re-epithelialization occurs by approximately 3-4 weeks with Cw CO_2 lasers.

A resurfacing CO_2 laser or variable pulsed Er:YAG laser can be used to treat mild-to-moderate rhinophyma. Re-epithelialization is complete in approximately 2-3 weeks. The risk of scarring with resurfacing lasers is very low. Some hypopigmentation is often seen and a reduced number of more prominent pores can also occur. Frank scarring is seen more often when using Cw lasers.

Step-by-step Approach

1. **Outline** the entire nose with additional markings of the rhinophymatous tissue.
2. Perform a **nasal "ring" block** by infiltrating local anesthetic along the nose cheek junction to anesthetize the infratrochlear, supratrochlear and infraorbital nerve branches. Infiltrate local anesthetic at the base of the collumella and finally inject anesthetic at the nasal bone and cartilage junction to the left and right of midline to anesthetize the anterior

ethmoidal nerves. This should provide complete nasal skin anesthesia and obviate the need for extensive painful injections into the often stiff rhinophymatous tissue.
3. Wrap the nose with wet towels and cover the patient's eyes with wet eye patches.
4. Ablate the rhinophymatous tissue until the nose shape approximates that of its prerhinophymatous state (compare with the "before" photographs). With resurfacing lasers, maximal energy fluences and pulse rates, along with pulse stacking, will be needed to achieve sufficient ablation. Although it has been advocated that, for severe rhinophyma, it may be advantageous to first use the Cw CO_2 laser with a small spot size to excise and debulk large phymatous areas followed by the use of a larger spot size for vaporization and fine contouring. It is advised not to cut away the rhinophyma nodules with the laser in the focused mode as we have found that areas so treated heal with scarring.
5. Ablation should stop while still in the sebaceous tissue plane. Once large vessels have been encountered or there is no more sebaceous tissue noted ablation has proceeded too deeply and those areas will be at increased risk for scarring.
6. It is better to err on the side of **undertreatment** rather than overtreatment.
7. Consider the anticipated postlaser treatment coagulated tissue slough and tissue contraction due to posttreatment fibrosis.
8. Special care should be taken at the nasal ala groove where too deep an ablation can result in unattractive nasal flaring.
9. Feather the treatment area by ablating into the papillary dermis the rest of the nose.

Pitfalls/Pearls

Hemostasis is achieved with lidocaine with epinephrine soaked gauze. Larger vessels that cannot be coagulated with the laser are sealed with spot electrocoagulation.

In Indian skin the high level of PIH makes such procedures uncommon. A modulated Er:YAG is a better tool in our opinion in Indian skin.

Level of Difficulty

High.

Nevi (Epidermal and Dermal)

Almost all types of epidermal and dermal nevi can be treated and thus we will discuss a few representative conditions in detail. As a general rule deeper the lesions, poorer are the results.

a) Epidermal Nevi/Nevus Comedonicus

Background: Epidermal nevi are developmental abnormalities resulting in excess keratinocytes. Lesions usually manifest early in life and have a predilection for the neck, trunk and extremities. While tumors, such as basal cell carcinoma and squamous cell carcinoma, have been reported to arise within these lesions, this is a rare occurrence and removal is primarily of a cosmetic nature in such nevi.

Laser Used: Excision is usually not an option due to the large size of many epidermal nevi. Laser ablation with CO_2 or Er:YAG lasers can successfully remove these lesions.

The Er:YAG can be used but the dermal bleeding is an issue even with the novel modulated lasers. The CO_2 laser may be combined with pigment targeting lasers to decrease the risk of scarring. The CO_2 laser is used to first ablate the clinically visible epidermal nevus followed by treatment with the frequency doubled Q-switched Nd:YAG laser at 3.5-4.0 J/cm^2. A combination with fractional CO_2 has been published recently. The same principles can be used to treat nevus comedonicus (Figs. 2.22A to C) and PEODN.

Though other lasers like PDL, Nd:YAG and argon have been tried we do not use them as the results do not match the results of the ablative lasers.

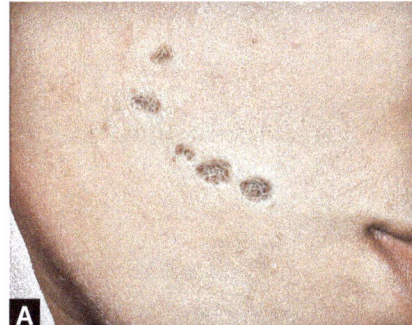
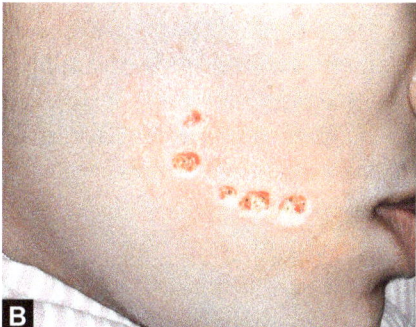
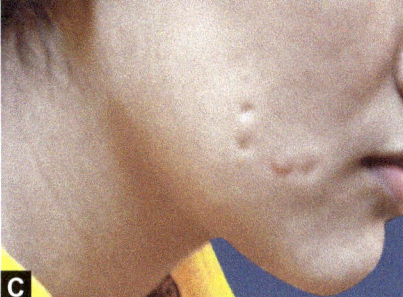

Figs. 2.22A to C: (A) A case of Nevus Comedonicus; (B) UltraPulse CO_2 laser (260 mJ), after three passes there is a clean ablation of the epidermis with partial ablation of the follicular plugs, "glistening" papillary dermis being the end point; (C) Complete removal of the follicular plugs.

Step-by-step Approach: Care must be taken to balance efficacy versus scarring. Epidermal ablation only will allow for recurrence of the abnormal keratinization. Excessive ablation will lead to scarring. The **ideal depth** of ablation is to the **papillary dermis**.

1. UltraPulse laser with the 3 mm handpiece and a pulse energy of 450–500 mJ. If using one of the SPCO$_2$ lasers, 5 J/cm^2; 2 ms pulse duration and a pulse interval of 20 ms can be used.
2. This results in epidermal ablation at the center of the spot, and after carefully heating the epidermis, the denatured epithelium can be wiped away (Fig. 2.23A).
3. Use a dermaview to see the altered dermis. Fine papillomatosis can be seen where the epidermal nevus remains.
4. These lesions require a reduction of the spot size to a 1-mm handpiece, which is then used to ablate the remaining areas with pulse energies ranging from 150 mJ to 250 mJ. The handpiece can be focused or defocused to either heat or ablate the remnant tissue. As the handpiece is moved closer to the lesion, one increases the fluence and a louder pop is heard. After a few passes, the papillomatosis disappears and the area is smooth (Fig. 2.23B).

End point: Yellowing of the dermis and loss of papillations.

Pitfalls/Pearls:
1. Do **not** try to achieve **complete** removal of the lesions as the residual thermal damage is usually sufficient to obtain long-term remissions without significant scaring or pigmentation changes.
2. If properly used a Cw CO$_2$ can achieve results as good as UltraPulse CO$_2$ lasers.

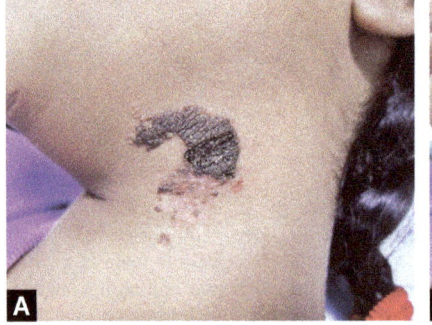 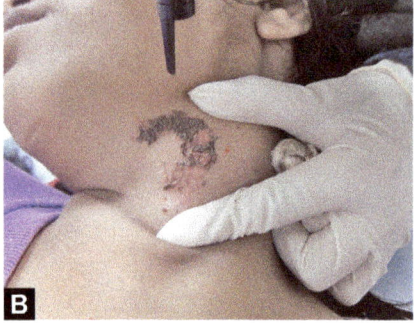

Figs. 2.23A and B: (A) An epidermal nevus being treated with the pulsed CO$_2$. Note the thermal necrosis on the surface; (B) The debris is wiped off leaving behind the remnant lesions subsequently the spot size is reduced to target the remaining tissue.

3. A soft nevi will respond better than the hard verrucous nevi.
4. A combination of CO_2 and Er:YAG can lead to excellent results (Fig. 2.27). A series of cases are depicted in Figures 2.24 to 2.28.

Level of Difficulty: Moderate to high. In Indian skin post-inflammatory hypopigmentation (Fig. 2.24) is a complication and hence a test spot should be attempted.

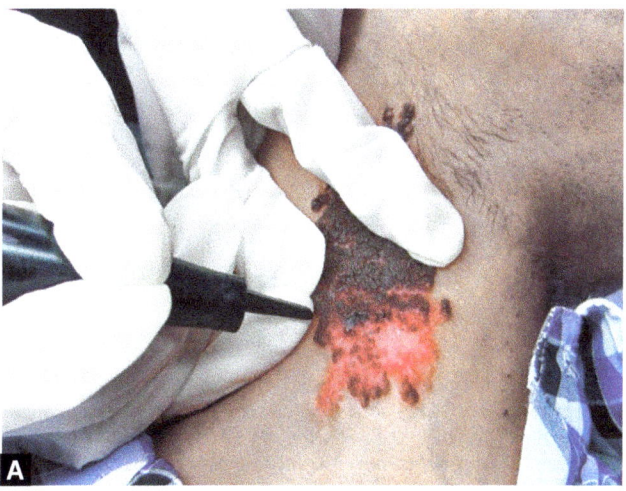

Fig. 2.24A: Intraoperative procedure using the "paintbrush technique" with the Up CO_2 lasers (350 mJ; 5 J/cm^2; <1 ms). Note the almost bloodless field due to the coagulative effect of the laser.

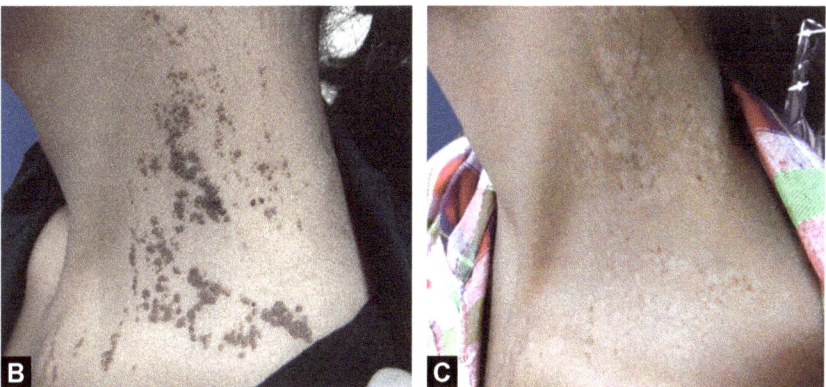

Figs. 2.24B and C: A case of "soft" epidermal nevi: The Er:YAG was attempted but there was rapid recurrence. An $SPCO_2$ at a setting of 2–3 J/cm^2 was used with a pulse duration of 0.08 seconds, staged sessions, at 6 weekly interval, excellent results, but the pigmentary sequelae is an issue with CO_2 lasers.

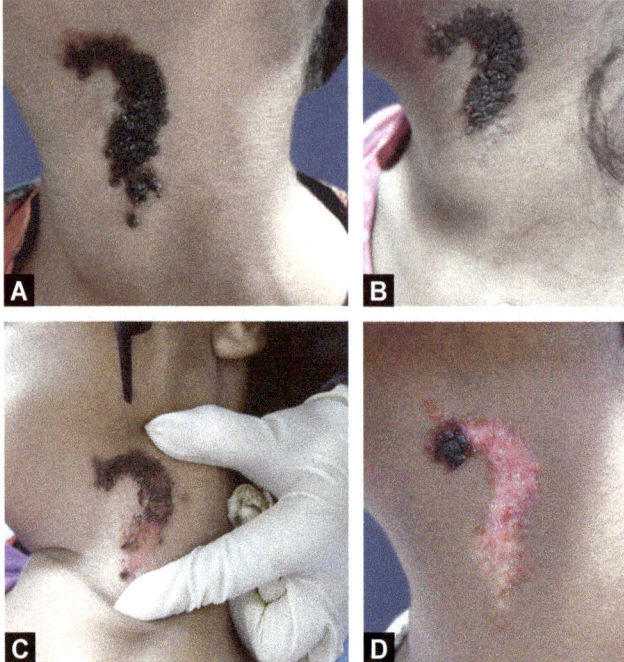

Figs. 2.25A to D: A case of soft epidermal nevi, treated over 6 months with staged SPCO$_2$ laser. The last photograph shows a reasonably good result but with pigmentary alteration and recurrence. The depth of CO$_2$ makes it better than Er:YAG but as is obvious here, lasers are not always the solution for epidermal nevi and recurrences are possible. The deeper you go more is the scarring while superficial ablation leads to recurrence.

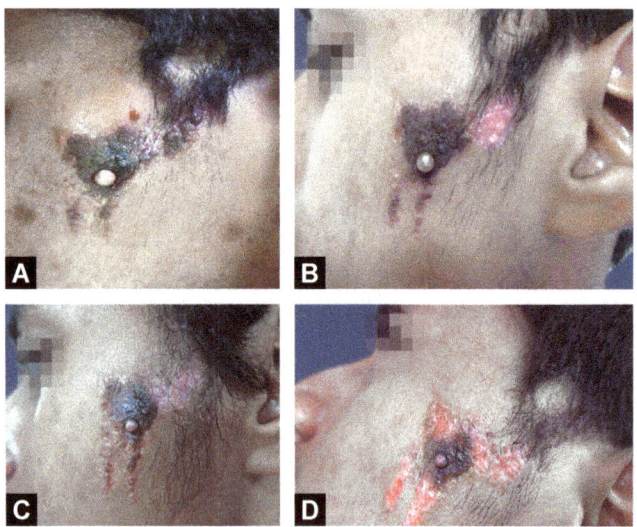

Figs. 2.26A to D: A case of "hard "epidermal nevi. Staged ablation with CO$_2$ laser in SP mode, note that the removal is far from perfect. It is my observation over so many years, that hard nevi rarely have satisfactory results.

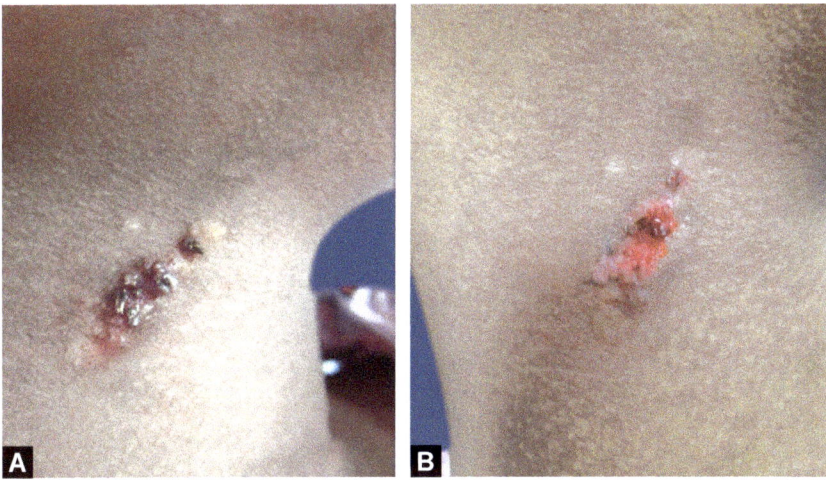

Figs. 2.27A and B: A case of epidermal nevi. Ablation with SPCO$_2$ (3 J/cm^2) followed by Er:YAG ablation till bleeding occurred which indicates the level of the papillary dermis. A combination of CO$_2$ followed by Er:YAG prevents excessive thermal damage caused by CO$_2$ and achieves the best of both lasers, the "ablative" advantage of CO$_2$ and the "precision" of Er:YAG.

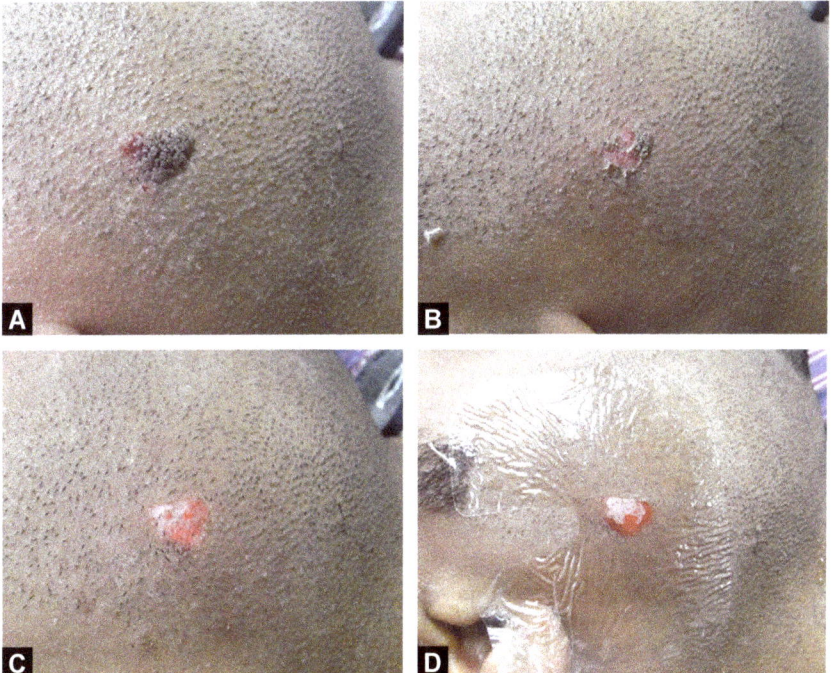

Figs. 2.28A to D: A soft epidermal nevi. This is an ideal case for Er:YAG laser, note the clean base following ablation, the bleeding indicates a level of papillary dermis which is a good point to reevaluate the depth and "feel" the tumor, here there was complete ablation, a Tegaderm dressing helps in excellent healing.

BIBLIOGRAPHY

1. Conti R, Bruscino N, Campolmi P, et al. Inflammatory linear verrucous epidermal nevus: why a combined laser therapy. J Cosmet Laser Ther. 2013;15(4):242-5.
2. Hammami GH, Lacour JP, Passeron T. Treatment of inflammatory linear verrucous epidermal nevus with 2940 nm erbium fractional laser. J Eur Acad Dermatol Venereol. 2013.
3. Jain S, Sardana K, Garg VK. Ultrapulse carbon dioxide laser treatment of porokeratotic eccrine ostial and dermal duct nevus. Pediatr Dermatol. 2013;30(2):264-6.
4. Sardana K, Garg VK. Successful treatment of nevus comedonicus with ultrapulse CO_2 laser. Indian J Dermatol Venereol Leprol. 2009;75(5):534-5.

b) Nevus Sebaceous

Principles: The concept and method is largely similar to that of epidermal nevi, but in our view these lesions are difficult to remove with incomplete removal.

Step-by-step Approach:
1. The plaques are vaporized with many passes to achieve a level where most of the yellow papules embedded in the lesion are removed.
2. As there is concomitant bleeding on reaching the dermis a CO_2 laser is ideal for the lesions.
3. The final end point to be achieved is a smooth pink surface. Healing is by secondary intention.

Pearls/Pitfalls: Like epidermal nevi, attempts to ablate the lesion down to the reticular dermis will result in longer remission but also in a greater likelihood of scarring.

Thus, it is better to use the laser in the defocused mode and remove only the exophytic portion, as aggressive therapy results in extensive scarring.

Level of Difficulty: High.

c) Melanocytic Nevi

This condition has been discussed at length in the following **Chapter 3**. It has been our experience that the use of ablative lasers achieved excellent results. Our approach is to use lasers depending on the type of the nevi.

Junctional nevi: Er:YAG laser, end point being complete ablation of the pigmented lesions.

Compound nevi: Initially an Er:YAG can be used to accurately remove the visible pigmented nevi. This can be followed by a 1-2 passes of a CO_2 in a single pulse mode to coagulate the vessels in the papillary dermis. Another option is to first use an Er:YAG laser followed by a Qs Nd:YAG to destroy the nevus cells.

Dermal nevi: Either an Er:YAG or a pulsed CO_2 can be used.

A representative depiction is given in Figures 2.29 to 2.33 while a detailed discussion follows in the next chapter.

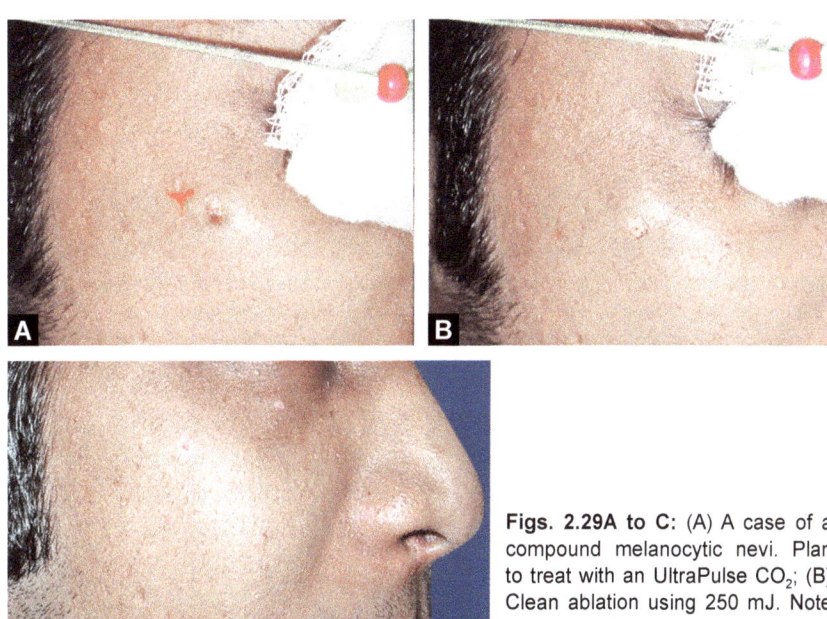

Figs. 2.29A to C: (A) A case of a compound melanocytic nevi. Plan to treat with an UltraPulse CO_2; (B) Clean ablation using 250 mJ. Note the lack of thermal damage; (C) Postoperative appearance after 7 days.

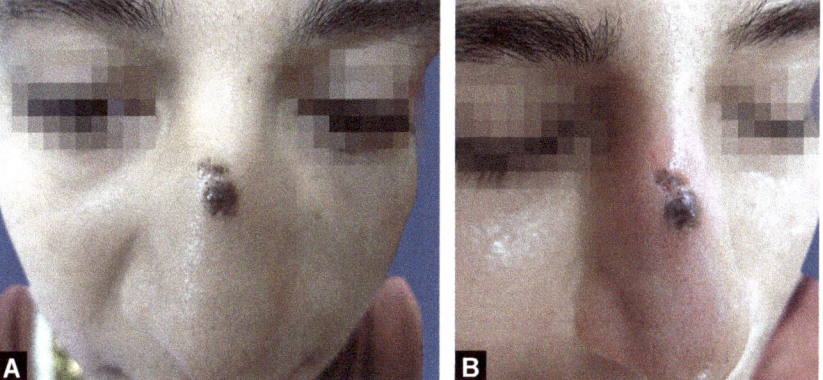

Figs. 2.30A and B: Melanoytic nevi: The smaller lesion was treated with CO_2 laser (superPulsed mode), after this lesion healed the second nevi was attempted with the CO_2 laser.

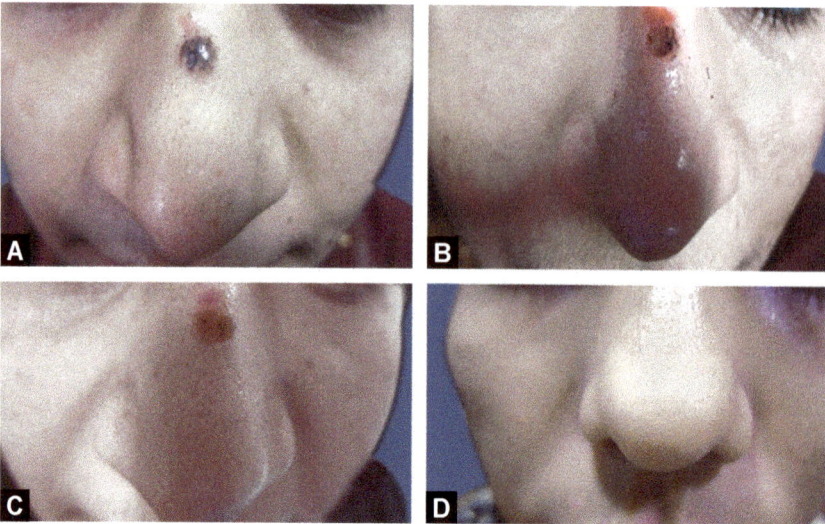

Figs. 2.31A to D: After the first compound nevi, healed, the second lesion was treated again with the Sp CO_2, note the healing after 4 weeks with a slight depression.

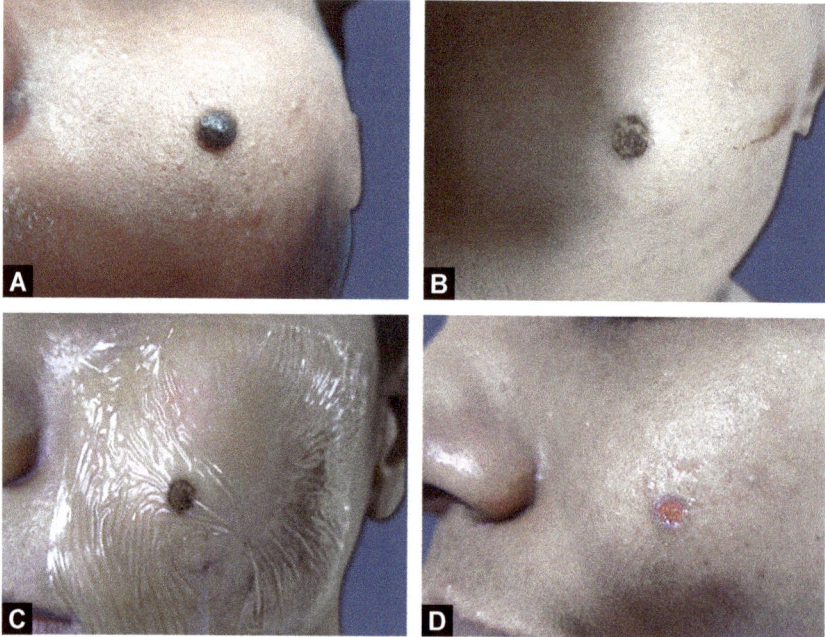

Figs. 2.32A to D: A case of compound nevi, ablated using Sp CO_2 laser, note the carbonization, which leads to minimal bleeding. It is a good idea to wipe the debris by a wet gauze and look for ablation of the nevi. Note the follicular pigment which is consequent to the hair follicles. A simple "trick" to enable good healing is to cover it with a Tegaderm dressing which also enables visualization of the wound.

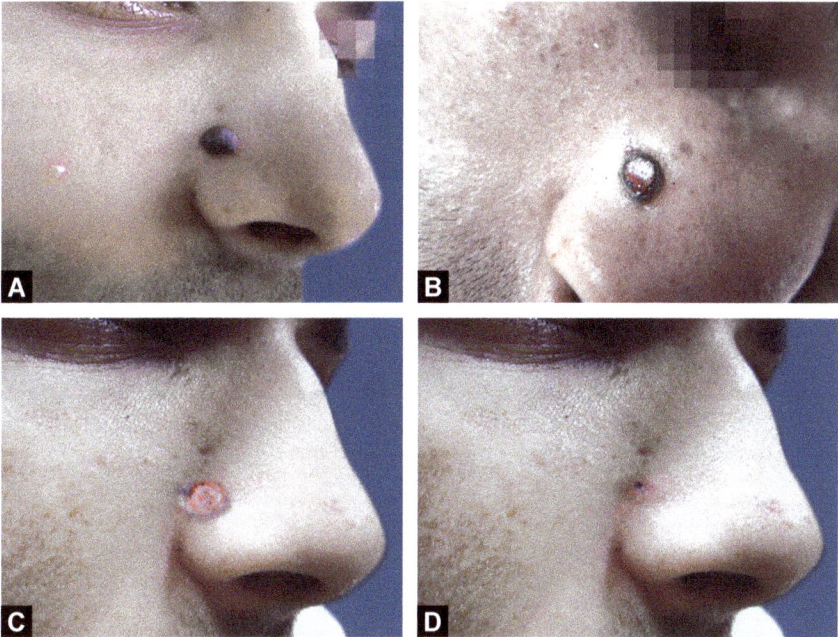

Figs. 2.33A to D: A large compound nevi treated with CO_2 followed by Er:YAG. The second picture (Fig. B) shows the ablation using Sp CO_2 laser. Note the lack of bleeding but a rim of carbonized tissue. The nevi are leveled with the surrounding skin. This is followed by a few passes of Er:YAG (1.5 J/cm^2) for a clean base. Complete healing after 4 weeks.

Pearls/Pitfalls: The problem of removing moles is that the end point of disappearance of pigment is masked by the carbonization of the CO_2 lasers. Thus, the trick is to keep the pulse duration low ideally less than 2 milliseconds. This ensures a clean base. Another option is to use the Er:YAG which does not cause carbonization. An ideal combination of Er:YAG followed by CO_2 is the best as then the ER:YAG ablates the nevi and after achieving the end point a pass of CO_2 suffices. Compound nevi have the maximum recurrence rates. In case of recurrences RF is an option (Figs. 2.34A and B).

BIBLIOGRAPHY

1. Sardana K, Chakravarty P, Goel K. Optimal management of common acquired melanocytic nevi (moles): current perspectives. Clin Cosmet Investig Dermatol. 2014;7:89-103.
2. Sardana K. The science, reality, and ethics of treating common acquired melanocytic nevi (moles) with lasers. J Cutan Aesthet Surg. 2013;6(1):27-9.

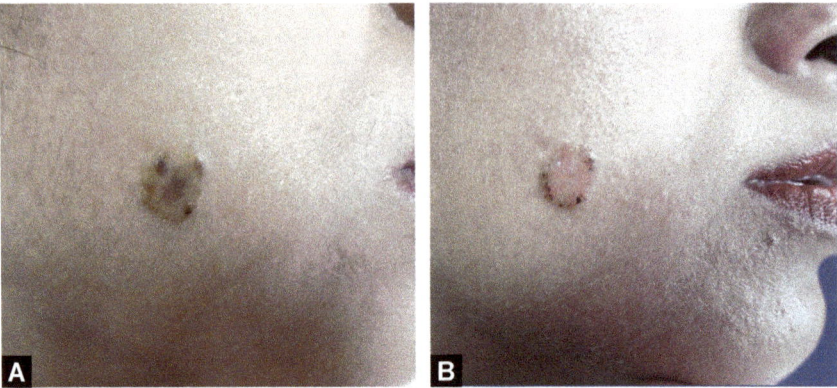

Figs. 2.34A and B: A case of recurrent nevi. After two sessions of Up and Sp CO_2 laser the patient had a recurrence. This is an ideal case for an Ellman RF!

Benign Tumors

Carbon dioxide lasers can be employed to treat a number of dermal growths. Adenoma sebaceum, trichoepitheliomas, syringomas, hidrocystomas, neurofibromas, myxoid cysts, sebaceous hyperplasia, syringocystadenoma papilliferum, and xanthelasma have all been treated with laser ablation. Though the lesions that are discussed below may seem to be disparate conditions with various etiologies including eccrine, pilar, sebaceous tumors, cysts and cholesterol deposition disorders, they are discussed here as they are essentially benign, acquired and largely dermal in nature.

Principles

1. For individual lesions, the growth is vaporized by using relatively low-power settings in the 3- to 5-W range with a spot size that *"matches the size of the lesion"*.
2. Though the approach depends upon the depth of the lesion being treated, the entire lesion should *not* be destroyed. Ablation should be carried out but to the level of the dermis since residual thermal damage will extend 0.5– 1 mm beyond the level of ablation. Thus, one should *not try to remove the entire lesion.*
3. If there is deep extension of the lesion recurrence may occur.
4. A useful end point is a smooth cutaneous contour matching the surrounding skin.

1) Adenoma Sebaceum

Er:YAG and Cw and UltraPulse CO_2 lasers have been used to treat these lesions, though the latter two are better in our opinion.

A study (Fioramonti P) has also used sequentially 3 lasers. The Er:YAG laser reduced lesion thickness (in the first and second sessions), whereas the dye laser attenuated the blush because of its efficacy on the vascular component. The sessions were repeated at 3 monthly intervals. Finally, a full face resurfacing was done by the CO_2 laser. Such a aggressive therapy is not advised in skin of color patients.

Settings: One can use the CO_2 laser with a low power of 2-3 W and 1-2 mm spot size with short application times of 0.25-0.5 s to gently vaporize/heat the papules so that they shrink over the subsequent few weeks. Though the PDL has been used, the CO_2 laser shows superior cosmetic results.

With the use of sirolimus and rapamycin, probably lasers may not be required.

2) Neurofibromas

As this condition has a dermal component, the CO_2 is preferred (Figs. 2.35A and B).

Step-by-step Approach:
1. UltraPulse laser, 1-3 mm spots with pulse energies ranging from 200 mJ to 500 mJ, can be used.
2. After reaching dermis, the tumor, which has a rubbery consistency, can be manually expelled by gentle pressure around the wound.
3. This is followed by additional passes of the laser to destroy the base.
4. Another approach is by using the cutting mode CW CO_2 laser. A 2-mm beam and power of 4-6 W can be used rapidly to treat patients with multiple pedunculated and sessile lesions.

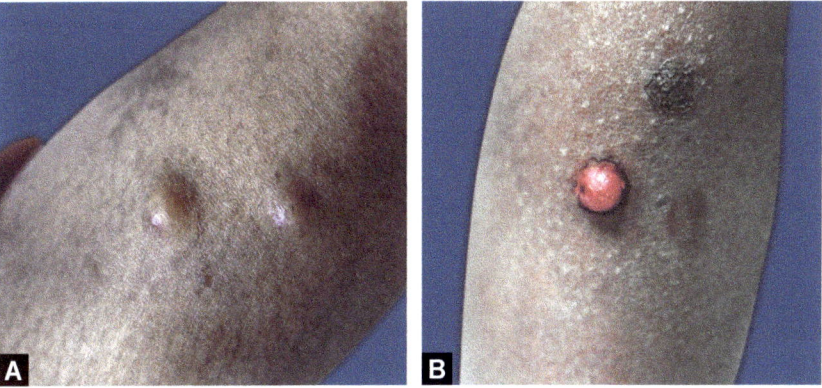

Figs. 2.35A and B: A case of neurofibroma. Settings: Cw CO_2, 2 J/cm^2, 0.5 second. The tumor was incised and the tumor popped out which was excised using the laser, the base was then cauterized using a lower fluence.

First the 0.2 mm spot can be used to excise the stalks in the *pedunculated* lesions, and a defocused beam at 35–60 W CW while squeezing the rubber nodule outward to remove the *sessile lesions*.

3) Pearly Penile Papules

An ablative pulsed or repeat mode CO_2 is a very useful technique as it can help minimize the bleeding.

A setting of 1–3 W, 0.25–0.5 s exposures in the repeat mode or a 5 W, 0.1 s burst is a useful method of achieving satisfactory results.

4) Syringoma

Treating syringoma is tricky as the depth has to be ideal to remove the pathology but should be controlled to avoid thermal damage.

The commonly used technique is the **pinhole technique or the multiple-drilling method** (Lee SJ) in which the normal tissue between each hole is used for wound healing; however, in plaque-type syringomas, there is no normal tissue between each hole.

Another technique is the ovoid technique (Kitano Y) where oval areas are removed by the Er:YAG to achieve better results for the larger, agminated variants of syringoma.

Step-by-step Approach: Surgical plan—*end point* is the ablation of syringoma to a depth just beneath the surrounding uninvolved skin surface. A conservative end point is removing about *half to two-thirds* of the lesion. This results in a depression the skin that heals with minimal hypopigmentation and scarring (Figs. 2.36A and B).

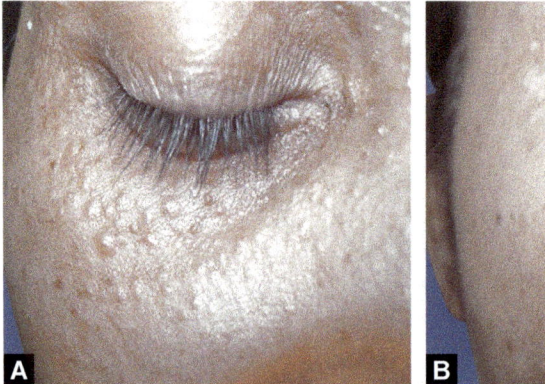
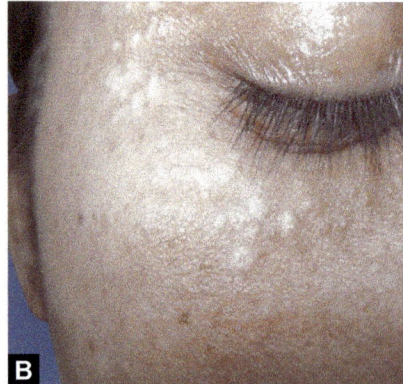

Figs. 2.36A and B: Syringoma are eccrine gland tumors. Ideal laser is Er:YAG due to its better side effect profile in pigmented skin especially on the face; (B) Post-treatment with Er:YAG (5 J/cm^2; 2 Hz; single spot technique) healing with pigmentary alteration, which is an inevitable but reversible sequelae.

1. Demarcate the syringoma with a surgical marking pen.
2. Infiltration anesthesia is required.
3. Place normal saline or sterile water soaked sponges and drapes around the treatment area. This is primarily as the ablative lasers are absorbed by water and this can minimize damage to the surrounding skin in case of inadvertent laser impaction.
4. Either the Er:YAG or CO_2 can be used.
   - CO_2 power 15 W, (repeat continuous, pulsed or scanned beam at 0.1–0.2 s), spot size (defocused beam with spot size of 2–3 mm at skin surface). The **spot size** may be adjusted manually with the **diameter** of the lesion.
   - UltraPulse mode is a remarkably more elegant tool in that one can ablate the lesions by 100–200 µm increments. Our typical end point is removing about *half to two-thirds* of the whitish lesion. This results in a *small dell* in the skin that heals with minimal hypopigmentation and scarring.
   - Er:YAG: 5 J/cm^2, two or three passes. A recent study used an ovoid ablation of 2-4 mm using the Er:YAG, with conservative settings (1 mm, an irradiation intensity of 9 J/cm^2, and a pulse-width of 250 sec.)
5. Vaporization—direct the shuttered beam to the lesion with one or two pulses. Debride the treated area with a normal saline or sterile water soaked sponge. Repeat vaporization and debridement, as necessary to reach desired end point.

Pearls/Pitfalls:
1. Dark-skinned patients should be warned that there will usually be some hyperpigmentation starting about 3 weeks after the procedure. This usually resolves within 2–3 months with or without bleaching creams.
2. Patients with **infraorbital pigmentation** should **not** be treated as the pigmentary consequences are disastrous.
3. *Always* do a test site with one or two lesions prior to treating an entire area.

5) Seborrheic Keratoses

Again the Er:YAG is superior to the CO_2 laser as it has a minimal thermal damage and almost perfect epidermal ablation (Figs. 2.37 and 2.38).

Settings: *Er:YAG (2–5 J/cm^2)*: End point is an epidermal ablation. A whitish hue is achieved by a single pass, this can be wiped off till a faint erythema appears which indicates the papillary dermis.

CO_2: Either a "single spot" Cw or UltraPulse modes can be used.

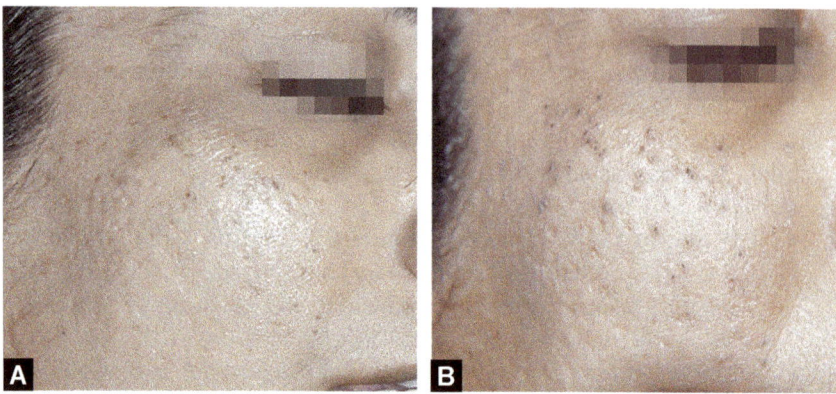

Figs. 2.37A and B: (A) Multiple seborrheic keratosis on the face; (B) Single spot technique using Up CO_2 (350 mJ; 5 J/cm^2; <1 ms). End point is mild crusting.

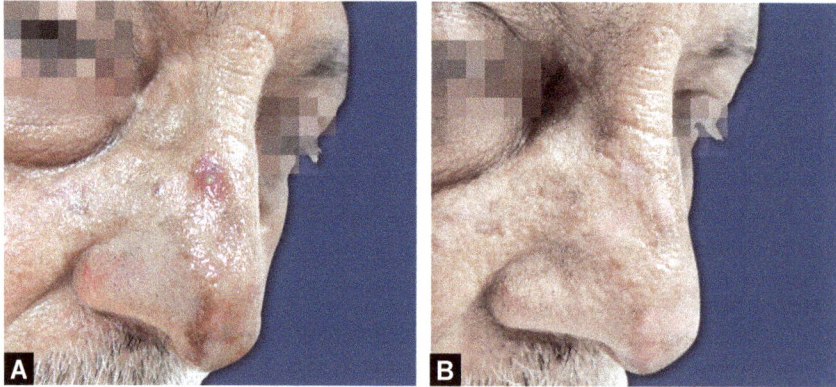

Figs. 2.38A and B: (A) Seborrheic keratosis on the face. Plan to treat with Er:YAG; (B) Postoperative view after 7 days, note the clean surface with little sign of PIH.

Pearls/Pitfalls: Care should be taken once the base of the lesion is reached so that unnecessary heating and subsequent pigmentation changes and scarring do not occur. This almost never occurs with the Er:YAG laser, which is a reason for our preference for using this system.

For cases of recurrent and progressive cases look for carcinomas the patient in Figures 2.38A and B underwent three repeat settings when he was diagnosed with pancreatic carcinoma followed by an unfortunate demise of the patient.

6) Sebaceous Hyperplasia

This is one of the most rewarding and easy tumors to treat. It is our opinion that for these the Er:YAG is an excellent tool and we prefer it over CO_2 laser.

Settings: Er:YAG (2-3 mm spot; 4-5 J/cm^2). CO_2 (1 mm handpiece; pulse energy of 200 mJ), the distance between the skin and handpiece tip is varied to accommodate the size of the lesion.

Step-by-step Approach:
1. A few overlapping passes are made to expose the yellow fatty nodules.
2. Once exposed, these punctate 0.5 mm lobules are treated with additional pulses until they are either extruded are heated.
3. The final result is a slight depression that resolves in 1-3 months.

7) Steatocystomas

The principle is to treat the *lining* of the cysts otherwise rapid recurrence is the rule.

Step-by-step Approach:
1. First pierce the central portion with the 1 mm spot in the pulsed mode (Repeat pulse).
   (CW CO_2; 1 mm spot and 5 W, 100 ms gated pulse)
2. Apply gentle pressure to the lesion to extrude the contents.
3. Apply a defocused laser passes to the lining.
4. Another alternative if the lesions are small, it is to vaporize the lesions with subsequent passes.
5. The wounds are allowed to heal by secondary intention.

Recently the fractional CO_2 laser has been sued in a single case using settings of 70 mJ, 70% coverage, 8 passes (Kassira S). A simpler technique without laser can be used , wherein a small incison can be made in the center and the contents taken out after dissecting the cyst out of the wall (Lin KP).

8) Trichoepitheliomas

Er:YAG and Cw and UltraPulse lasers have been used to treat these lesions.

End point: An ablation to a level **just below** the adjacent skin surface should be the goal. Deeper ablation results in scarring and more superficial ablation results in early recurrence.

Settings: The typical laser settings in Cw mode include 1-3 mm spot sizes and powers of 2-5 W. If an UltraPulse mode is used, 200-250 mJ energy is used. It is our experience that results with most lasers the results are not good (Fig. 2.39) as the depth of the lesion is not sufficiently targeted in most cases. A recent study used the ActiveFx scanning handpiece with a fluence of 100-125 mJ depending on anatomic area and thickness of individual lesions and noted good results (Sinha K).

9) Xanthelasma

This common condition has been treated by multiple modalities including surgery, TCA and lasers. Clinically the flat, papular, plaque and nodular

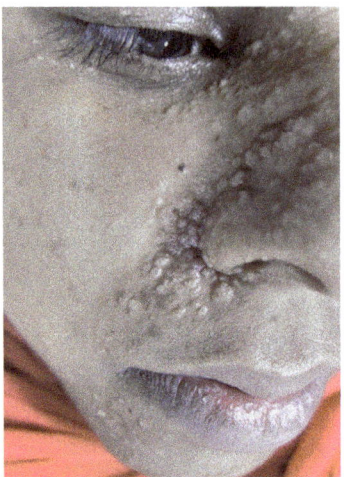

Fig. 2.39: A case of trichoepithelioma proposed to be treated by CO_2 laser. The patient underwent a test session, but the results were not satisfactory and hence further sessions were aborted. A test spot is advisable in case of dermal tumors and perfect ablation is not always met, hence the "good" results in studies usually means a reduction in size, which may mean little to the patient.

variants have been described. The importance being that for the last two variants the depth of infiltration makes them unresponsive to most methods except surgery **(Also *see* Chapter 12)**.

1. *Surgery*: There are various techniques that can be used but in spite of them recurrences are commonly seen. Moreover, it is impractical to employ surgical means for recurrences, which are seen in the deeper variants. We recommend surgery for a few, large lesions (plaques/nodular) with an appreciable depth.
2. *TCA*: There are two important principles that determine the use of TCA. First the concentration that should be used is at least 30–70% and secondly it is to be used in small lesions, with little depth. Moreover, a minimum of 3–5 sessions are required for most lesions.
3. *Laser*: Though various lasers have been used, the ablative lasers are superior to Nd:YAG, PDL, ruby and fractional lasers. Both CO_2 and Er:YAG can be used though the latter has a problem with the lack of coagulation that leads to a decrease in the achievable depth and that may lead to recurrences. As shown in **Figure 2.40** coagulative effect of CO_2 is ideal though in deeper lesions a residual lesion can still remain.

Step-by-step Approach (Figs. 2.41 and 2.42):
1. Our approach is to use the 1–2 mm handpiece with either the UltraPulse or Er:YAG laser.
2. A defocused beam is used to initially ablate the epidermis.

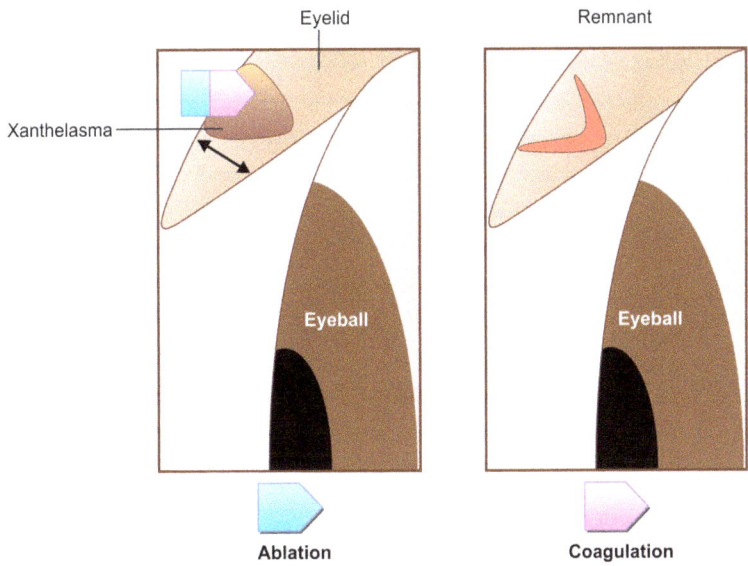

Fig. 2.40: A figurative depiction of the effect of CO_2 laser in xanthelasma. Note that for a deeper lesion, recurrence can occur even though there is a coagulative component of the pulsed CO_2 laser.

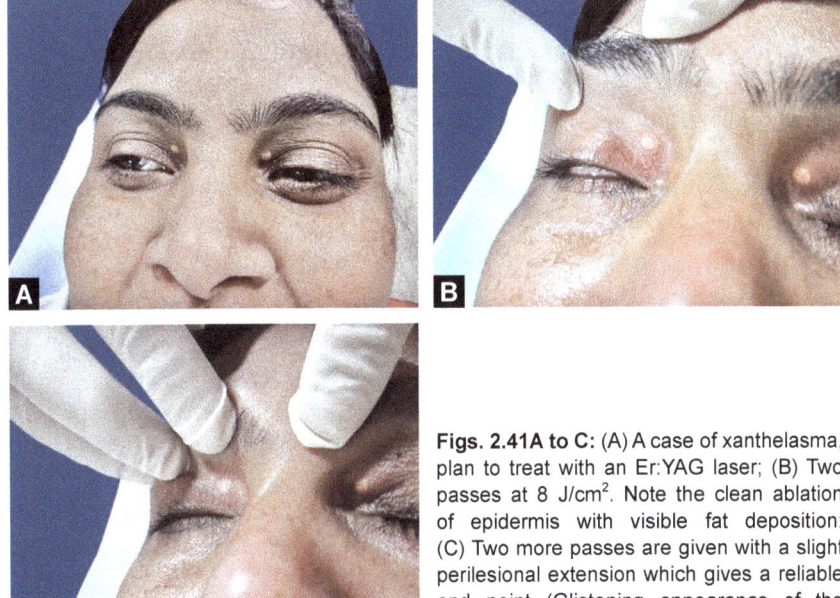

Figs. 2.41A to C: (A) A case of xanthelasma, plan to treat with an Er:YAG laser; (B) Two passes at 8 J/cm². Note the clean ablation of epidermis with visible fat deposition; (C) Two more passes are given with a slight perilesional extension which gives a reliable end point (Glistening appearance of the papillary dermis).

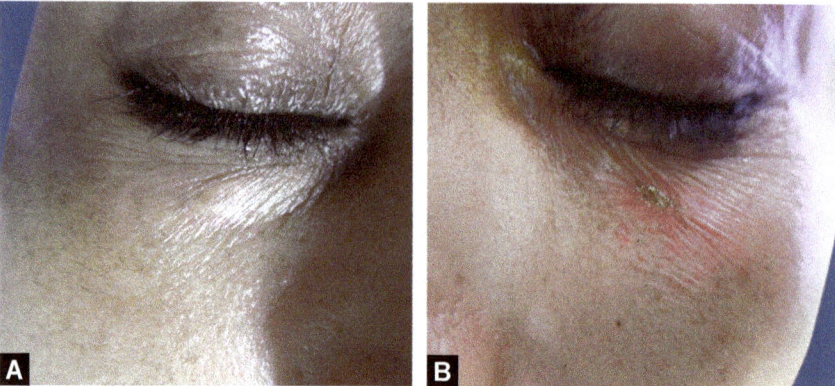

Figs. 2.42A and B: Xanthelasma. The Ideal laser is the Up CO_2 laser. Here the Sp CO_2 was used (0.8 W, 0.05 seconds). As the condition has fat tissue till the papillary dermis the end point is not removal of fat tissue. After every pass, it is best to feel the tumor and ablate till it is flat. A few more passes will be sufficient. Note that complete ablation is neither needed nor desirable as the zone of coagulation which lies below the zone of ablation helps to remove the fat tissue. Shrinkage of the tissue seen here is a sufficient end point to stop more passes.

3. This reveals the "fat" tissue. As the normal dermis is replaced by the fat tissue the normal signs that determine the depth are not readily visible.
4. With the Er:YAG it is a good "trick" to ablate the surrounding epidermis to give an idea about the depth achieved.
5. After ablating the epidermis, about 1–3 passes using a fluence of 10 J/cm^2 with the Er:YAG is enough. Even if visible tissue remains the procedure should be stopped. With the CO_2 (5 J/cm^2) again three passes are enough to cause sufficient ablation of the fat tissue. The residual "invisible" coagulation that extends deeper than the ablation is sufficient to help in the ultimate removal of the lesion.

Pearls/Pitfalls:
1. Even when some "fat tissue" is visible grossly, the coagulation and fibrosis helps to remove the lesion. Excessive treatment can lead to complications, thus it is better to undertreat than to overtreat.
2. After healing, at the next visit the residual lesion should be treated by TCA and not by the laser as the tissue depth required may be less and lead to overtreatment.

Our approach is to use the laser as a tool for both small and large lesions. For the former a single session suffices while for the latter lesion, after the initial session TCA can be used for residual lesions. If that fails surgical excision is the only option (Flowchart 2.1). A surgeon, though, may adopt a different approach.

Level of Difficulty: Variable.

Flowchart 2.1: A flowchart for management of xanthelasma with various modalities.

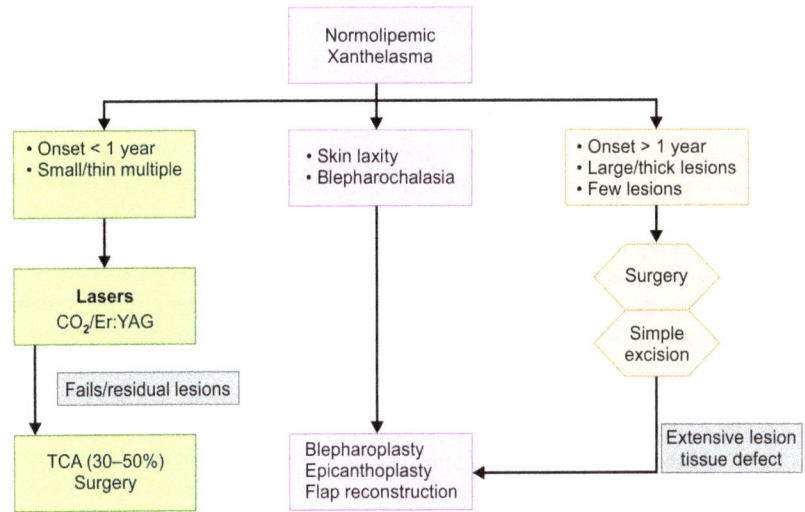

BIBLIOGRAPHY

1. Blickenstaff RD, Roenigk RK, Peters MS, et al. Recurrent pyogenic granuloma with satellitosis. J Am Acad Dermatol. 1989;21(6):1241-4.
2. Fioramonti P, De Santo L, Ruggieri M, et al. Erratum to: Co(2)/Erbium:YAG/Dye laser combination: An effective and successful treatment for angiofibromas in tuberous sclerosis. Aesthetic Plast Surg. 2017;41(3):760.
3. Goel K, Sardana K, Garg VK. A prospective study comparing ultrapulse CO_2 laser and trichloroacetic acid in treatment of Xanthelasma palpebrarum. J Cosmet Dermatol. 2015;14(2):130-9.
4. Janniger CK, Goldberg DJ. Angiofibromas in tuberous sclerosis: comparison of treatment by carbon dioxide and argon laser. J Dermatol Surg Oncol. 1990;16(4):317-20.
5. Karim A, Streitmann M. Excision of rhinophyma with the carbon dioxide laser: a ten-year experience. Ann Otol Rhinol Laryngol. 1997;106(11):952-5.
6. Kassira S, Korta DZ, de Feraudy S, et al. Fractionated ablative carbon dioxide laser treatment of steatocystoma multiplex. J Cosmet Laser Ther. 2016;18(7):364-6.
7. Kitano Y. Erbium YAG laser treatment of periorbital syringomas by using the multiple ovoid-shape ablation method. J Cosmet Laser Ther. 2016;18(5):280-5.
8. Lee CT, Tham SN, Tan T. Initial experience with CO_2 laser in treating dermatological conditions. Ann Acad Med Sing. 1987;16(4):713-5.
9. Lee SJ, Goo B, Choi MJ, et al. Treatment of periorbital syringoma by the pinhole method using a carbon dioxide laser in 29 Asian patients. J Cosmet Laser Ther. 2015;17(5):273-6.

10. Lin KP, Chang ME, Ho WT. Treatment of steatocystoma multiplex on axillae using keyhole approach technique. J Cosmet Laser Ther. 2018. p. 1.
11. Modica LA. Pyogenic granuloma of the tongue treated by carbon dioxide laser. J Am Geriatr Soc. 1988;36(11):1036-8.
12. Negosanti F, Tengattini V, Gurioli C, Neri I. Facial angiofibromas treated by rapamycin 0.05% ointment and a combined laser therapy. J Cosmet Dermatol. 2018;17(5):762-5.
13. Ries WR, Speyer MT. Cutaneous applications of lasers. Otolaryngol Clin North Am. 1996;29(6):915-29.
14. Robinson JK. Actinic cheilitis. A prospective study comparing four treatment methods. Arch Otolaryngol Head Neck Surg. 1989;115(7):848-52.
15. Rosenbach A, Alster TS. Multiple trichoepitheliomas successfully treated with a high-energy, pulsed carbon dioxide laser. Dermatol Surg. 1997;23(8):708-10.
16. Sinclair RJ, Sinclair PJ. Carbon dioxide laser in the treatment of cutaneous disorders. Australas J Dermatol. 1991;32(3):165-71.
17. Sinha K, Mallipeddi R, Sheth N, Al-Niaimi F. Carbon dioxide laser ablation for trichoepitheliomas: The largest reported series. J Cosmet Laser Ther. 2018;20(1): 9-11.
18. Stanley R, Roenigk R. Actinic cheilitis: treatment with the carbon dioxide laser. Mayo Clin Proc. 1988;63(3):230-5.
19. Wataya-Kaneda M, Ohno Y, Fujita Y, et al. Sirolimus gel treatment vs placebo for facial angiofibromas in patients with tuberous sclerosis complex: A randomized clinical trial. JAMA Dermatol. 2018;154(7):781-8.
20. Wheeland R, Bailin PL, Ratz JL. Combined carbon dioxide laser excision and vaporization in the treatment of rhinophyma. J Dermatol Surg Oncol. 1987;13(2): 172-7.
21. Zelickson B, Roenigk R. Actinic cheilitis. Treatment with the carbon dioxide laser. Cancer. 1990;65(6):1307-11.

10) Histiocytoma/Xanthoma Disseminatum

The ideal laser is the UP CO_2 though the SP CO_2 can also be used. This handpiece can be focused or defocused depending on the size of the lesion. Once the epidermis is removed, the yellow base of the lesions is seen. At this point, the smaller spot is used to ablate the remaining lesion. This will leave a depression if the lesion is completely removed. Leaving about 20% of the lesion at the base results in a very nice cosmetic result without recurrences.

11) Hailey-Hailey and Darier's Disease

Though various lasers have been used including the erbium:YAG laser and CO_2, the ideal laser would be the CO_2 in a defocused mode (2 mm spot, 10 W) to vaporize to a level without apparent disease, usually after two passes. The key is to remove the papillary dermis for long-term remission.

Warts

Lasers Used

Development of human papilloma virus induced verrucae is a common cutaneous disease process. The use of continuous wave or pulsed lasers has been shown to have an efficacy in the range of 56-81%. The use of ablative lasers is only for warts that have been *refractory* to less invasive and less costly measures. It has been noted that 80% of primary warts responded to laser therapy, whereas only 48% of refractory lesions responded. Warts that are particularly difficult to eradicate include those occurring in a periungual area.

The Er:YAG laser has also been used successfully and has a better safety profile. Most likely, the laser, like other destructive techniques, reduces the viral load and allows for innate immunity to control the remainder wart tissue. This should be the guiding principle of therapy with lasers.

Step-by-step Approach (Plantar Wart)

1. Surgical plan—*end point* is the ablation of the plantar wart and 5-10 mm of surrounding uninvolved epidermis.
2. Treatment margins are outlined with a surgical marking pen.
3. Manually **remove thickened hyperkeratotic debris**. This tissue has low water content and tends to act as a heat sink with laser impact, creating excessive thermal diffusion.
4. Anesthesia—local infiltration of 1% lidocaine with epinephrine into the treatment area. Regional block may also be useful.
5. Use normal saline or sterile water soaked sponges and drapes around treatment area.
6. Set *laser parameters*—power output 15-25 W, waveform (continuous wave, pulsed or scanned), spot size (defocused beam with spot size of 3-5 mm at skin surface).
7. *Vaporization*—move handpiece with air brush-like movements over wart and surrounding epidermis to margins. Sweep the laser over the verrucae 1-3 times. A cleavage plan at the dermoepidermal junction will be created allowing the keratotic epidermis to be curetted away. Vaporize any apparent wart tissue remaining. Coagulate the papillary dermis to seal blood vessels.
8. *Remove* large pieces of desiccated wart from surface. Wipe treated area with a normal saline or sterile water soaked sponge then blot with dry sponge.
9. Repeat vaporization and debridement as necessary until normal dermis is identified.
10. A 2-mm area around the wart should also be removed.

Dressing—bactroban ointment/fucidin which is covered by a sterile nonadherent dressing. We prefer using a Dynaplast instead of a routine bandage.

Step-by-step Approach (Common Wart)

1. If a wart is very exophytic, a higher energy of 15–20 W and a 2-mm spot size is used in the vaporization mode to ablate the surface of the lesion.
2. Residual debris is wiped away with moist gauze.
3. A curette can be used to separate the denatured tissue from the dermis. If the heating plane at the dermal-epidermal (DE) junction is sufficient, the wart will separate without much difficulty and the underlying dermal base will be only slightly heated. If one undertreats, the unheated remaining epidermis will still be attached to and interdigitated with the underlying dermis.
4. Once the denatured wart is separated, the base is heated gently with a lower power of 3–5 W. A rim 2–5 mm from the clinically obvious wart should be heated. The underlying dermis can be identified by the appearance of skin lines or the observation of slight tissue shrinkage.

Step-by-step Approach (Periungual Wart)

1. A tourniquet greatly aids in hemostasis.
2. An aggressive therapy is required with curettage.
3. As the "hard" wart tissue in the nailfold can be mistaken for the normal dermis, a simple measure is to remove the surface till a smooth surface is achieved.
4. If **focal fatty globules** are visible **stop** the treatment.

Step-by-step Approach (Condylomata Acuminata)

1. Patients with perianal lesions may benefit from anoscopic examination to evaluate for the presence of internal lesions.
2. Consider acetowhitening to help delineate subtle lesions.
3. Insert a moistened gauze into the anal sphincter or urethral orifice.
4. Used a pulsed laser or Er:YAG to treat the lesion until ablation of the lesion is achieved (Figs. 2.43A and B).
5. *Wound care*: Re-epitheliazation takes 3–4 weeks.
    a. Sitz baths with saltwater solution should be performed three or four times daily
    b. Use a hair dryer instead of wiping
    c. Consider the use of stool softeners
    d. Refrain from sexual intercourse, douching or the application of topical creams.

Pitfalls/Pearls

1. As most recurrences develop at the peripheral margin of a treated wart, laser ablation should incorporate a zone of 3–5 mm of clinically normal appearing tissue around the verruca.

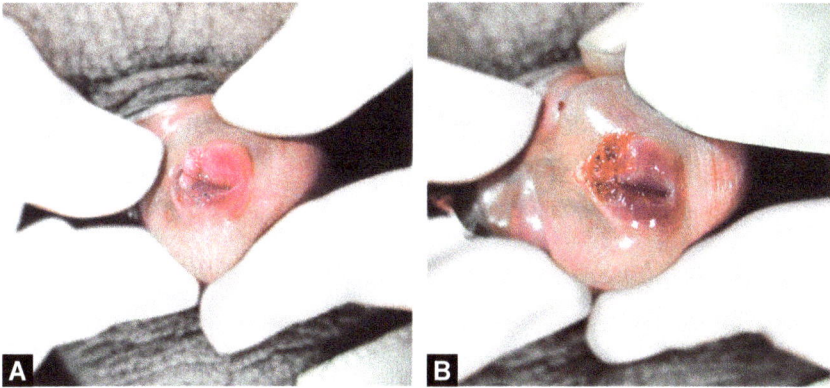

Figs. 2.43A and B: (A) An intraurethral wart. The location dictated the use of an Er:YAG laser as the CO_2 can cause marked thermal damage and lead to a stricture; (B) A modulated Er:YAG was used to ablate and coagulate the vessels.

2. Wart tissue "bubbles" upon treatment whereas normal epidermis exhibits dermatoglyphics that appear to contract with laser contact. Thus, a useful end point is *contraction* of tissue which indicates adequate ablation of the wart.
3. For periungual warts, vaporization of the nail plate to gain access to subungual extension of verrucae is not only helpful, but it eliminates the need for nail plate avulsion.
4. When treating virally mediated diseases with ablation, special safety considerations are warranted. Viable viral particles have been demonstrated in the smoke plume generated from the treatment of verrucae. Plantar warts (HPV type 1) are the richest in viral particles. Because HPV-6 and -11 cause both respiratory papillomatosis and genital warts, a major risk of inhalational HPV infection exists when treating condyloma accuminata. Although viral transmission to the laser surgeon has not been convincingly demonstrated, personal safety precautions are recommended. Intact and viable HIV particles have been identified in CO_2 laser plumes when HIV-infected tissue was treated. No transmission of HIV through laser plumes has been reported to date. Because of these factors, high efficacy smoke evacuators have to be employed and the evacuation tube opening should be within 1 cm of the laser plume. All personnel should don high-filtration laser masks with a particle filtration threshold of 0.1 micrometer.

BIBLIOGRAPHY

1. Baggish MS. Improved laser techniques for the elimination of genital and extragenital warts. Am J Obstet Gynecol. 1985;153(5):545-50.
2. Bellina JH. The use of the carbon dioxide laser in the management of condyloma acuminatum with eight-year follow-up. Am J Obstet Gynecol. 1983;147(4):375-8.

3. Ferenczy A. Laser therapy of genital condylomata acuminata. Obstet Gynecol. 1984;63(5):703-7.
4. Hahn GA. Carbon dioxide laser surgery in treatment of condyloma. Am J Obstet Gynecol. 1981;141(8):1000-8.
5. Kryger-Baggesen N, Falck-Larson J, Hjortkjaer Pederson P. CO_2-laser treatment of condylo mata acuminata. Acta Obstet Gynecol Scand. 1984;63(4):341-3.
6. Lassus J, Happonen HP, Niemi KM, et al. Carbon dioxide (CO_2)-laser therapy cures macroscopic lesions, but viral genome is not eradicated in men with therapy-resistant HPV infection. Sex Transm Dis. 1994;21(6):297-302.

Excisional Surgery/Debridement

Excisions performed on infected issue may best be performed using a CO_2 laser as the heat that is generated sterilizes the surgical field. Debridement of decubitus ulcers, exuberant granulation tissue, and various cutaneous infections such as botryomycosis and cutaneous leishmaniasis as well as ablation of dermatophyte-infected nails have been effectively carried out with a CO_2 laser. Treatment of hidradenitis suppurativa, acne keloidalis nuchae, and dissecting folliculitis of the scalp has also been reported. In case of *Hailey–Hailey* disease as the depth to be achieved is less we feel that the erbium:YAG laser is the ideal ablative lasers.

Nail Matrixectomy

Ingrowing Toe Nail: Ingrowing toe nail is classified in three stages. Stage 1 is characterized by erythema, slight edema and pain on pressure. In stage 2, the symptoms increase with local infection and discharge. In stage 3, granulation tissue and lateral wall hypertrophy are seen.

Anesthesia: Proximal or distal digital block.

Tools:
- Tourniquet
- Nail avulsion tray
- Curette 3 mm.

Step-by-step Approach (Figs. 2.44A to D):
1. A tourniquet is placed to ensure a complete bloodless field.
2. The roof of the PNF is retracted with a hook or a thread allowing the lateral matrix horn to be vaporized with the CO_2 laser. Usually, a continuous wave mode with about 4 W and a spot size of 1 mm is used; however, this may be varied according to personal experience and the machine used.
3. Extend the laser excision from the distal end to a point 5 mm medial to a point at the intersection of proximal and lateral nail fold and a further 1 cm proximally.
4. Then extend this further laterally as a wedge excision of the hypertrophied soft tissue.

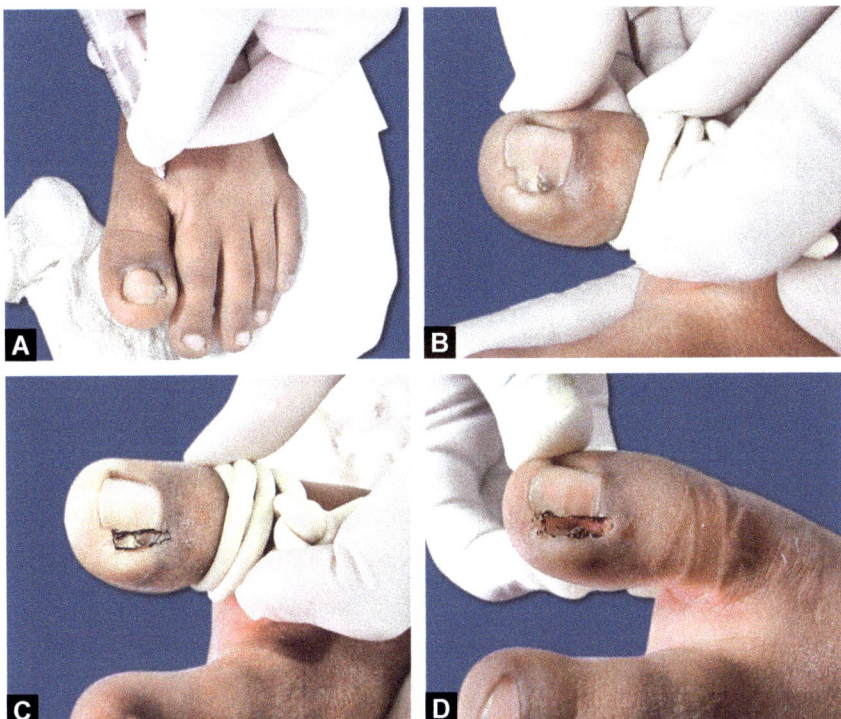

Figs. 2.44A to D: Steps of surgery (A) Nail block (proximal nail block); (B) Application of tourniquet; (C) Lateral excision of nail and nail fold up to the matrix; (D) Immediate postoperative; note the complete absence of bleeding (CO_2 laser, Cw TW, 1 mm spot size).

5. 1–2 passes are given on the edge of the incision.
6. This is followed by visualization of the cavity. If a white glistening fiber is seen, they indicate the matrix and this should again be ablated.

Pearls/Pitfalls: Some authors prefer to open the PNF over the lateral matrix horn to see more clearly the extension of laser vaporization.

The speed and the excellent hemostasis are unique advantages of the CO_2 laser which is used in preference to the Er:YAG laser.

The most important advantage of the CO_2 laser is that the coagulation zone tends to take care of the remnant matrix tissue.

BIBLIOGRAPHY

1. Farley-Sakevich T, Grady JF, Zager E, et al. Onychoplasty with carbon dioxide laser matrixectomy for treatment of ingrown toe nails. J Am Podiatr Med Assoc. 2005;95(2):175-9.
2. Karpen M. The CO_2 laser used for matrixectomy. J Clin Laser Med Surg. 1992;10(6):454-6.

Keloids

Earlobe Keloids

Earlobe keloids are particularly well suited to treatment with the CO_2 laser. As long as most of the keloid is vaporized and care is taken in the postoperative period, a low rate of recurrence and a high degree of patient satisfaction can be achieved.

Step-by-step Approach:
1. A 3-mm handpiece with the UltraPulse laser with maximum pulse energy and a high repetition rate of 20–40 Hz is used the Cw CO_2 with a setting of 5–6 J/cm², 0.09 sec can also be used.
2. Vaporize the lesion down to a point where one *feels* and *sees* very little keloid at the base. This requires many passes.
3. Use the thumb to push the keloidal tissue toward the laser handpiece. After many passes, one will begin to feel mild heating on the finger as the keloidal tissue is vaporized.

Pearls/Pitfalls:
1. The pulsed mode allows for a relatively char-free tissue removal.
2. Even though a substantial amount of tissue may be removed, the contour of the lower earlobe is unaffected.
3. Combination with interferons, imiquimod and IL steroid can also be used.

Larger Keloids and Nonearlobe Keloids

The evidence does ***not*** favor the use of laser for other keloids and the CO_2 laser probably offers little advantage over excisional surgery of keloids.

Hair Transplants

In hair transplantation, Er:YAG lasers may be used to "drill" holes for recipient sites. Even in scarring alopecia, modern Er:YAG lasers with high pulse energy can drill holes for hair transplants efficiently, with less bleeding than with punches, and with less tissue damage as with CO_2 lasers, which is important for graft uptake.

Pyogenic Granuloma

These lesions respond very well to CO_2 laser vaporization, provided that the level of destruction is adequate. This includes cases that have recurred after electrodesiccation and curettage (ED&C) and cryotherapy. This is probably as the coagulative capacity of the CO_2 laser helps to effectively seal the vessels. **(Also *see* Chapter 12).**

Step-by-step Approach *(Figs. 2.45A and B):*
1. The lesion is vaporized with 3–5 W power and a 2–4 mm spot size.
2. End point is to make the lesion **flush** with the surrounding skin.
3. This is followed by removal of the denatured friable surface using a curette.
4. Use a dermaview to visualize the central feeder vessel which is surrounded by dermis or fibrofatty tissue.
5. Change the spot size of the laser and vaporize the bleeder using a defocused beam with a long pulse duration. The spot size should be just large enough to accommodate the diameter of the vessel and the surrounding tissue is lightly grayed with a defocused beam.

Pearls/Pitfalls

A postoperative application of TCA 90% with an adhesive dressing like "Dynaplast" helps in healing of the lesion. GO DEEP is the key principle. The key to effective one-time treatment is the depth of destruction. Patients who have been referred after treatment failure have invariably noted that the initial treatment had been more superficial.

Lymphangioma Circumscriptum

As CO_2 has an ability to seal lymphatics this is the ideal **laser to** treat lymphatic tumors. The ideal end point is lack of visible lymphatic drainage. Mild hypertrophic scarring can occur (Figs. 2.46A to C). Because of the deep nature of the lesions, lesions usually recur regardless of the treatment modality.

There are many other modalities tried including the fractional lasers, Er:YAG, RF and bleomycin, sirolimus and isotretinoin.

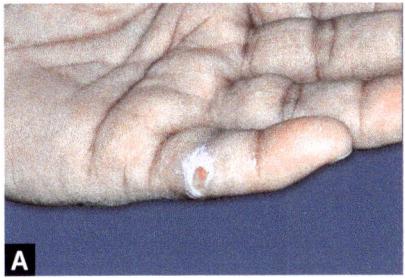 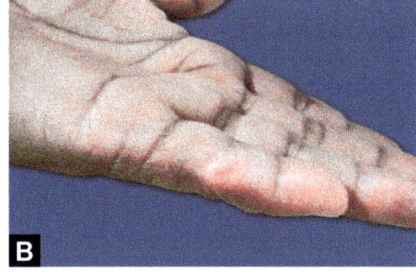

Figs. 2.45A and B: (A) Pyogenic granuloma on the medial border of the hand. Plan to treat with a Cw CO_2 laser; (B) Healing after 3 weeks with a scar, which is consequent to the thermal damage induced by the CO_2 laser, which is useful in vascular indications.

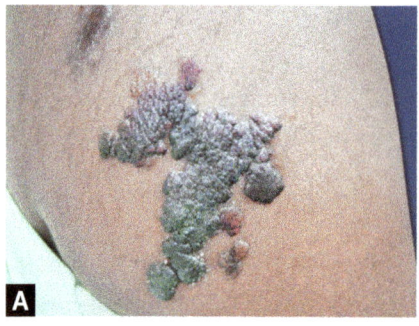
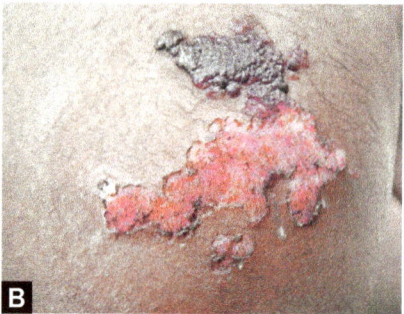
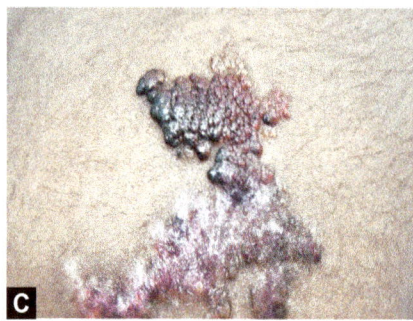

Figs. 2.46A to C: A preoperative photograph of lympho (hemangioma) circumscriptum: Intraoperative use of CO_2 (superpulsed mode; paintbrush technique) which is the ideal laser for coagulation of lymphatic vessels. Healing with hypertrophy of the skin due to the concomitant thermal tissue effect of the CO_2 laser can be appreciated.

BIBLIOGRAPHY

1. Ayhan E. Lymphangioma circumscriptum: Good clinical response to isotretinoin therapy. Pediatr Dermatol. 2016;33(3):e208-9.
2. Bailin PL, Kantor GR, Wheeland RG. Carbon dioxide laser vaporization of lymphangioma circumscriptum. J Am Acad Dermatol. 1986;14(2, Pt 1):257-62.
3. Haas AF, Narurkar VA. Recalcitrant breast lymphangioma circumscriptum treated by Ultra-Pulse carbon dioxide laser. Dermatol Surg. 1998;24(8):893-5.
4. Khurana A, Gupta A, Ahuja A, et al. Lymphangioma circumscriptum treated with combination of bleomycin sclerotherapy and Radiofrequency ablation. J Cosmet Laser Ther. 2018. pp. 1-4.
5. Makdisi J, de Feraudy S, Zachary CB. Vulvar lymphangioma circumscriptum treated with fractional ablative erbium: yttrium aluminium garnet laser. Dermatol Surg. 2018;44(8):1149-51.
6. Saluja S, Petersen M, Summers E. Fractional carbon dioxide laser ablation for the treatment of microcystic lymphatic malformations (lymphangioma circumscriptum) in an adult patient with Klippel-Trenaunay syndrome. Lasers Surg Med. 2015;47(7):539-41.

Vitiligo Surgery

Er:YAG has also been used for vitiligo surgery for preparation of the lesional site for autologous melanocyte transfer, though not all believe it adds substantially to the ultimate clinical results (Figs. 2.47A and B).

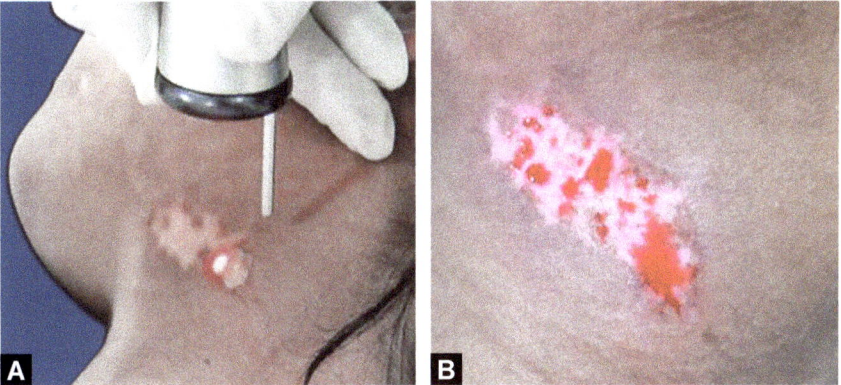

Figs. 2.47A and B: (A) A vitiligo patch prepared with Er:YAG (5 J/cm^2); (B) End point is mild bleeding, indicating the papillary dermis which is the desired end point.
Source: Dr Sumit Gupta, MD, Delhi.

The Er:YAG laser with its exact ablation and no residual thermal damage is ideal for preparing transplantation beds in bizarre and geometrically complicated lesions and sites, like the nose, lips, ear and folds of skin.

Tattoo Removal

Laser tattoo removal has primarily fallen within the domain of Q-switched lasers. However, in selected circumstances, CO_2 or Er:YAG laser ablation can be considered.

1. In patients with allergic reactions to tattoo ink, the use of a Q-switched laser can lead to systemic reactions. In these cases, ablation of the tattoo can be considered.
2. Additionally, patients who desire tattoo removal without the multiple treatment sessions required with Q-switched lasers may benefit from laser ablation, which can usually achieve tattoo removal in a single treatment session. To diminish scarring, the entire depth of the tattoo is not ablated. Approximately 30–50% of the ink is removed via laser. This technique is known as the *RTR technique* (rapid tattoo removal technique) and is depicted in the Figure 2.48.

   This method involves ablation of the epidermis overlying the tattoo to gain better access to the pigment for Q-switched laser therapy in the same treatment session. Epidermal ablation results in less beam scattering for the Q-switched laser. This technique may reduce the number of treatment sessions with a Q-switched laser by 50% without significantly increasing the risk of scarring.

   We have found the short-pulse Er:YAG laser and CO_2 laser to be particularly useful for tattoo ablation as there is no need for thermal tissue coagulation. The ultimate cosmetic outcome is superior if the entire region of the tattoo is ablated, rather than simply tracing the outline of

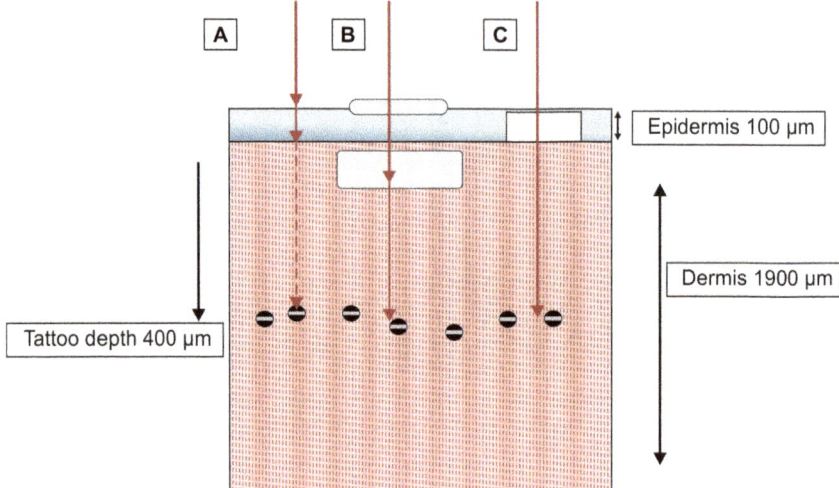

Fig. 2.48: A schematic diagram highlighting techniques to enhance tattoo removal. (A) The laser beam gets attenuated by the epidermis and the dermis due to epidermal and dermal scattering; (B) Topically applied clearing agents can help in reducing the dermal scatter and enhance results. They can be placed either on the skin or intradermally; (C) Epidermal ablation is another effective tool for enhancing results by eliminating epidermal scatter.
Source: Sardana K, Ranjan R, Ghunawat. Optimising laser tattoo removal. J Cutan Aesthet Surg. 2015;8(1):16-24.

the tattoo. The latter approach can lead to a ghost of the tattoo remaining. Ultimately, the treated area resembles a superficial burn scar.

3. Some patients may require a second "touch-up" treatment to remove any residual visible tattoo ink 6 months after the initial ablative treatment.
4. For tattoos that have been treated with Q-switched lasers, certain pigments (skin-colored, white, brown, some red pigments) that contain iron or titanium oxides undergo a reduction reaction that converts the treated pigment into a black color. Additional Q-switched laser therapy is not an option for this black pigment, but it can be efficiently ablated with a resurfacing laser.

BIBLIOGRAPHY

1. Sardana K, Ranjan R, Ghunawat S. Optimising laser tattoo removal. J Cutan Aesthet Surg. 2015;8(1):16-24.
2. Sardana K, Ranjan R, Kochhar AM, et al. A rapid tattoo removal technique using a combination of pulsed Er:YAG and Q-Switched Nd:YAG in a split lesion protocol. J Cosmet Laser Ther. 2015;17(4):177-83.
3. Sardana K, Garg VK, Bansal S, et al. A promising split-lesion technique for rapid tattoo removal using a novel sequential approach of a single sitting of pulsed CO_2 followed by Q-switched Nd: YAG laser (1064 nm). J Cosmet Dermatol. 2013;12(4):296-305.

Miscellaneous Conditions

Various lesions in difficult surgical locations may be addressed advantageously using ablative lasers. A number of inflammatory conditions have been reported to respond to ablation with the CO_2 laser. The experience with treating these conditions is limited to small numbers and large scale clinical trial data are not available.

Some of these conditions include balanitis xerotica obliterans, Zoon's balanitis, kraurosis vulvae, lichen sclerosis et atrophicus, porokeratosis, keratoderma, chondrodermatitis nodularis helices, granuloma faciale, genital lichen planus, oral florid papillomatosis, psoriasis, and lupus erythematosus (*See* Chapter 12).

Dyspigmentation

Pigmentation of the skin due to sun damage or chloasma can respond to the Erbium:YAG laser. The so-called "Erbium peel" is effective in fair skinned and Southeast Asian skin types. Chloasma does tend to recur, so the use of long-term bleaching preparations and ultraviolet A light-blocking sunscreens is mandatory.

Wrinkles

Although the Erbium:YAG laser has been specifically promoted for the treatment of superficial wrinkles, it can successfully remove both superficial and deeper wrinkles with great accuracy. Treating deeper wrinkles leads to dermal bleeding, which makes the procedure slightly cumbersome and messy. CO_2 and Er:YAG are not effective in effacing movement-associated rhytides in the glabellar region and the nasolabial folds. Thus, wrinkles caused by excessive ultraviolet light exposure are primarily indicated for resurfacing with either laser, those associated with movement are secondarily indicated.

STEP BY STEP APPROACH

CO_2 LASER

Preoperative Considerations

Ideal patient: The ideal patient for treatment, regardless of disease, is either very dark or very light-skinned, as patients tend to return to their constitutive color after CO_2 laser surgery.

Bronzed patients with Types II and III skin are at high risk for permanent hypopigmentation with increasing depth of injury.

Any patient with *decreased* adnexal structures from previous radiation therapy or even laser hair removal or electrolysis should probably receive at least a test site. This advice is controversial for laser hair reduction, as there are no reports of compromised healing in CO_2 laser induced areas previously treated with hair reduction lasers.

The recommended minimum time interval between isotretinoin treatment and resurfacing (and vice versa) ranges from 6 months to 2 years.

Preoperative Regimen

For adnexal tumors, test sites, and small-scar abrasions, no systemic or topical medications are prescribed. We have found that topical retinoids and bleaching preparations do *not* appear to alter the postoperative course.

Intraoperative

Technique

Defocused mode is ideal for vaporization while focused mode is used for cutting. For most dermatological indications a pulsed laser is ideal. For patients where a deeper ablation is required a superpulsed mode or a Cw (interrupted pulse) can be used. Prolonging the pulse duration in a superpulsed mode is another method of increasing the energy.

1. *Modes (shuttered continuous wave, pulsed or scanned beam at 0.1–0.2 s)*: Most CO_2 lasers have Cw (continuous wave), repeat, single, Sp (super pulse) and Up (UltraPulse) modes. The repeat and single are basically CW modes.

   As a **thumb rule** for small, appendageal tumors (e.g. milia) the single pulse mode is ideal. For a larger lesion (xanthelasma), the repeat mode in appropriate settings (see below) should be used.
2. Spot size (defocused beam) with spot size of 2–3 mm at skin surface.
3. The power density may be varied by changing the power output, beam configuration, spot size, movement speed of handpiece, or shuttering the laser beam. These changes may be done either by hand or with the use of a mechanical scanning device (details are given in the preceding chapters).

Steps

1. After setting the power (at least 5 J/cm^2) one pass is given.
   Method: Air brush-like movements with the defocused laser beam of the continuous wave carbon dioxide laser or discrete pulses of the pulsed or rapidly scanned carbon dioxide laser create visible vaporization and/or coagulation.
2. The surgeon should rely on visual inspection of the treatment site after each pass of the laser and wiping the site with wet and dry sponges in order to determine the extent of the lesion and surrounding tissue damage.
   First pass: Vaporization of skin results in a *white* and slightly scaly surface. Once the treated area is gently wiped with a wet sponge, the epidermis

may still be visible if the treated lesion is particularly thick or the power density was very low and the speed of movement was very fast. If the epidermis is thin and a greater power density is delivered, the superficial dermis is seen with normal dermatoglyphic markings.

Dermis: When the dermis is heated or vaporized, visible *collagen contraction* is noted. If coarse and woven collagen bundles are seen, the tissue has been ablated into the deep dermis.

Subcutaneous: If ablation is continued further, subcutaneous fat will be obvious.

If charring is seen, there has been slow tissue burning at very high temperatures resulting in heat diffusion to surrounding tissues rather than tissue ablation. Charring is therefore not desired.

Postoperative Care

1. With the exception of excised wounds, in which sutures should be left in 3–5 days longer than in scalpel wounds, wounds are left to heal by secondary intention and will heal optimally when kept moist and clean. Dressings will speed healing if they are changed (at least every 2 days).
2. We have used a combination of fucidin cream (less sensitizing than neomycin) with application of aloe vera gel (J Alokem 75) till the crusting falls off. We routinely recommend an antibiotic, starting 1 day prior to 4 days after the surgery (Levofloxacin 750 mg HS) with an anti-inflammatory drug for 2 days (Zymoflam-D).
3. To avoid PIH a combination of sunscreen and non-HQ/steroid based creams is given. A physical block sunscreen is advisable.
4. More disturbing than the almost always temporary, especially on the face, postinflammatory hyperpigmentation is the delayed onset of hypopigmentation after the CO_2 laser in some cases. Thus, as far as possible Cw CO_2 should be restricted to small areas of the face.

Pitfalls/Pearls

1. Optimal use of the carbon dioxide as an ablative instrument includes many steps.
2. The most important is to determine the desired clinical **end point** which *varies* depending on the lesion treated.
    a. *Actinic cheilitis*: End point is coagulation or white discoloration of the entire external lower mucosal lip is seen.
    b. *Epidermal nevus*: Evidence of some coagulation in the dermis under the ablated area.
    c. *Plantar wart*: The presence of normal dermis under the visible wart as well as 5–10 mm surrounding it.
    d. *Appendageal tumors*: The clinical end point for the treatment of small appendageal tumors of the face includes vaporization of epidermis and dermis to a depth just beneath the surrounding uninvolved skin.

ERBIUM:YAG

Though most of the aspects mentioned under CO_2 laser surgery are common some unique aspects apply to the Er:YAG laser.
1. Wherever full face resurfacing is needed modulated Er:YAG is superior to CO_2 laser.
2. Although the superficial ablation and minimal collateral thermal damage achieved with the Er:YAG laser allow physicians to treat patients with more confidence, careful patient selection is still essential.
3. For most dermatological indications except vascular and lymphatic disorders Er:YAG is the ideal laser.

Patient Selection

Absolute contraindications to laser resurfacing include active bacterial or viral infections, impaired immune system, use of isotretinoin in the past year, and history of poor healing, especially hypertrophic scars or keloids in the treatment area. Skin that has received extensive radiation therapy or patients with scleroderma show decreased amounts of adnexal structures and should not be resurfaced because of risks of poor healing. Patients with unrealistic expectations should not be resurfaced.

Pregnant patients are also not treated due to the unknown risk of anesthesia on the fetus.

Relative contraindications include history of prior skin dyspigmentation, skin types V and VI, and koebnerizing diseases such as vitiligo or labile psoriasis. Patients who had a prior blepharoplasty or who have significant eyelid laxity should be approached cautiously, since the tightening achieved during laser resurfacing may result in ectropion formation.

Pretreatment Regimen

All patients undergoing laser resurfacing of the face are typically prophylactically given either acyclovir 400 mg PO tds, valacyclovir 500 mg PO bid, or famciclovir 250 mg PO bid. The antiviral is started 2 days prior to the procedure and continued for 10 days after the procedure. We, though, do not follow this as a rule and if there is no elicitable history of herpes labialis there is no need to administer antivirals.

Prophylactic use of systemic antibiotics, such as dicloxacillin, cephalexin, or azithromycin in penicillin allergic patients, should be given 2 days prior and continuing until the skin has re-epithelialized, to diminish the incidence of postoperative infection. We prefer levofloxacin 750 mg HS.

A moist, warm wound environment also promotes candidal infections. Occasionally, a single dose of fluconazole may be given on the day of surgery to patients, especially those with a significant history of recurrent vaginal discharge.

Intraoperative

Anesthesia: Infiltration anesthesia.

Treatment Technique

The basics have been described in the text and today resurfacing is not the primary indication. For almost all ablative indications except vascular and lymphatic, Er:YAG is better than CO_2 laser. This is especially true of the new variable pulse lasers where the pulse duration can be increased to match the coagulative effects of CO_2 laser.

Method

1. Erbium:YAG resurfacing can be performed either freehand or with a scanner. If the freehand method is used, it is important to ensure that overlapping of pulses is moderate, but not great. Significant overlapping and stacking of pulses will increase the depth of ablation and collateral thermal damage.
2. The number of passes necessary to vaporize the epidermis depends on the fluence and spot size used. In general, a fluence of 5–7 J/cm^2 will ablate the epidermis in two to four passes and a fluence of 8–15 J/cm^2 will do so in one or two passes. Subsequent passes will ablate between 5 mm and 40 mm of tissue depending on the energy fluence used. This is based on a rough estimation of an ablation of 5 µm of the skin per J/cm^2 of energy.
3. To minimize thermal damage subsequent passes should be oriented perpendicular or at an angle to the preceding passes to further enhance the uniformity of the ablation.
4. The margins of the treatment areas can be blended into the untreated skin by using pulses of lower fluence or by defocusing the handpiece or scanner (which, in effect decreases the fluence).
5. A quick wipe between passes with moistened gauze is recommended to remove the fine tissue debris, to rehydrate the skin, and to allow better visualization of the plane being treated. This process only takes a few seconds and does not require the time and effort associated with wiping between CO_2 passes.

Dose/Depth

With a of 5 J/cm^2, the following ablation depths are usually achieved: one pass, 20–40 µm or down to the granular layer of the epidermis; two passes, up to 60 µm or down to the basal cell layer; three to four passes, 80–120 µm or down to the papillary dermis, and deeper into the papillary and superficial reticular dermis after five to six passes (Alster, Perez).

Weinstein (1997) described the following ablation depths using a scanner of 20 Hz and 30% pulse overlap: 5 J/cm^2, superficial epidermal injury (30–40 µm) with negligible thermal necrosis; 10 J/cm^2, epidermal injury to the level of the basal layer (50 µm) with minimal thermal necrosis (5 mm); 15 J/cm^2, full-thickness epidermal injury through the basement membrane, minimal ablation of the papillary dermis (20 µm), and a narrow band of thermal necrosis (10–15 µm). These schematic histological ablation depths provide an approximation of the real ablation depth achievable with different fluences and numbers of passes.

End Point

The visual *end point* for treatment with the Er:YAG laser differs from that of the CO_2 laser. The chamois yellow color seen with CO_2 resurfacing, which indicates that the deep papillary dermis or superficial reticular dermis is reached, is not seen with Er:YAG laser resurfacing.

Epidermis: Resurfacing within the epidermis produces a *yellowish brown* appearance on the epidermis.

Epidermo-dermal junction: Once the epidermis is removed, a *pinkish* appearance of the upper papillary dermis will be readily appreciated. The follicle openings look small and regular like a fine sponge.

Lower papillary dermis: When proceeding into the papillary dermis, *pinpoint bleeding* and a *transudate* develops, indicating injury to the small capillaries. The follicle openings become wider and begin to stand out from the surrounding dermis.

Upper reticular dermis: When the upper reticular dermis is reached, bleeding increases and the transudate becomes more profuse. Follicle openings become much *wider* and the *collagen bands become coarser* and more haphazard in orientation. At this point it is generally best not to proceed no further.

Therefore, the physician must be mindful of the estimated depth of ablation associated with each pass of the laser at the fluence being used, and compare that with the average depth of the epidermis and dermis of the area being treated. As the collateral thermal injury induced by the Er:YAG laser is insufficient to coagulate medium-sized vessels, a common visual clue indicating that ablation has reached the mid-dermis is *pinpoint bleeding*. This bleeding will often inhibit further treatment beyond a certain level.

Thus, if the rhytides, acne scars, or other lesions are adequately effaced before the bleeding and exudate limit further treatment, then one or two additional passes are done to compensate for the impact edema. If oozing is remarkable, gauze soaked with 1% lidocaine with epinephrine can be placed over the resurfaced area at the end of the procedure.

Postoperative Care

For small lesions, we recommend topical antibiotic ointments or ointments specifically designed to accelerate wound healing (e.g. fucidin). This should be used until complete re-epithelialization has occurred and prevents the formation of irritating crusts.

For extensive lesions as in skin resurfacing, either the open technique (application of ointments several times a day, following irrigation with water or vinegar solutions) or the closed technique (application of various kinds of occlusive dressings for several days) can be used.

Pearls/Pitfalls

To complement the effect of Er:YAG and CO_2, a **combination** approach is a useful concept. This helps to balance out the advantage of fine ablation of Er:YAG and coagulation of CO_2.

An often asked question is whether this may lead to accentuated thermal damage. This has been answered by the histological examinations of Utley et al., who found the following residual thermal damage zones after ablation with an Er:YAG and a pulsed CO_2 laser (at 4.7 J/cm^2 each).

- CO_2 alone (four passes) 89 μm, Er:YAG (four passes) and CO_2 (two passes) 97 μm.
- Er:YAG alone (eight passes) 43 μm, and CO_2 (two passes) and Er:YAG (four passes) 56 μm.

Thus, a simple protocol is to combine Er:YAG initially followed by CO_2 for deep pathologies while Er:YAG suffices for most superficial indications.

This helps to maximize results by using the almost predictable ablation of Er:YAG with coagulation of CO_2 lasers.

BIBLIOGRAPHY

1. Alster TS. Clinical and histologic evaluation of six erbium:YAG lasers for cutaneous resurfacing. Lasers Surg Med. 1999;24:87-92.
2. Hohenleutner U, Landthaler M. Er:YAG Lasers. In: Kauvar AN, Hruza GJ (Eds). Principles and Practices in Cutaneous Laser Surgery. Abingdon: Taylor and Francis; 2005.
3. Perez MI, Bank DE, Silvers D. Skin resurfacing of the face with the erbium:YAG laser. Dermatol Surg. 1998;24:653-9.
4. Ross EV. Continuous wave and pulsed CO_2 lasers. In: Kauvar AN, Hruza GJ (Eds). Principles and Practices in Cutaneous Laser Surgery. Abingdon: Taylor and Francis; 2005.
5. Tse Y, Manuskiatti W, Detwiler SP, et al. Tissue effects of the erbium:YAG laser with varying passes, energy and pulse overlap. Lasers Surg Med. 1998;22(suppl 10):70.
6. Utley DS, Koch RJ, Egbert BM. Histologic analysis of the thermal effect on epidermal and dermal structures following treatment with the superpulsed CO_2 laser and the erbium:YAG laser: an in vivo study. Lasers Surg Med. 1999;24:93-102.
7. Weinstein C. Computerized scanning erbium:YAG laser for skin resurfacing. Dermatol Surg. 1998;24:83-9.
8. Weinstein C. Erbium laser resurfacing: current concepts. Plast Reconstr Surg. 1999;103:602-16.

CHAPTER 3

Pigmented Lesions and Tattoos

Kabir Sardana, Seema Rani, Pooja Arora Mrig

INTRODUCTION

Arguably, after ablative lasers and to some extent ablative fractional lasers one of the most *happening* and clinically *satisfying* indications of lasers are pigmented disorders. Lasers were first used in the treatment of pigmented lesions by Leon Goldman in the 1960s when he used the ruby laser (694 nm) to treat nevi and tattoos. The focus then shifted to the use of continuous wave modalities such as the carbon dioxide laser (10,600 nm) and the argon laser (418 nm, 514 nm). These continuous-wave lasers were used to treat pigmented lesions via nonselective destruction. Due to the lack of selectivity, the results were often unpredictable, with frequent complications such as scarring and pigmentary changes. Though out of vogue in the West in India Er:YAG is still used at low fluences of 1.4 J/cm^2 to treat epidermal pigmented disorders. The Q second technology has now been supplanted by the picosecond technology but this has not consistently proved to be superior to the Q-switched technology.

LASER-TISSUE INTERACTIONS IN PIGMENTED SKIN

Selective photothermolysis was originally applied to the treatment of vascular lesions with oxyhemoglobin as the target chromophore. Thereafter, selective photothermolysis was applied to pigmented lesions by targeting endogenous melanin and exogenous carbon particles as target chromophores.

Selective destruction of human epidermis with lasers using melanin as the target chromophore was first demonstrated in the early 1960s using a normal-mode ruby laser (wave-length 694 nm, pulse width 500 ms). Subsequent studies with the Q-switched ruby laser using a 50-ns pulse width showed the threshold radiant exposure to be 10–100 times lower, suggesting a more selective effect of the shorter pulse width (Goldman L). For the next 20 years, this work was largely overlooked, until the emergence of Anderson and Parrish's theory of selective photothermolysis (Andreson RR).

As a target chromophore, melanin has a broad absorption spectrum within the ultraviolet, visible and near-infrared light range (Fig. 3.1). Thus, while most lasers can be used for treating pigmented disorders, the light absorption in melanin decreases steadily with increasing wavelength. Also, as there are competing chromophores especially in pigmented skin, thus the *window of opportunity* is between the wavelengths of **630–1100 nm** where the melanin absorption exceeds that of Hb. But as the absorption of melanin falls with a higher wavelength, a higher fluence is needed.

The melanin containing melanosomes are 0.5 µm in diameter and are predicted to have a thermal relaxation time between 50 ns and 500 ns. Thus, ideally Q-switched lasers would be effective in treating the disorders. As stated previously, with increasing wavelengths, melanin absorption decreases but the required threshold laser exposure dose increases. This is relevant (Fig. 3.1) as the lasers that is used in India QS Nd:YAG (1,064 nm) would require a *higher* fluence than the other lasers. This can lead to postinflammatory hyperpigmentation (PIH), which is a decidedly common feature. More importantly is the sequelae of dyspigmentation and thus the authors do **not** (Sardana K, 2014) recommend using this laser for melasma in Indian skin.

When treating pigmented lesions, Q-switched lasers generate an immediate ash-white color at the site of impact (Figs. 3.2A and B). The cause of this tissue response is due to heat-induced steam cavities in melanosomes,

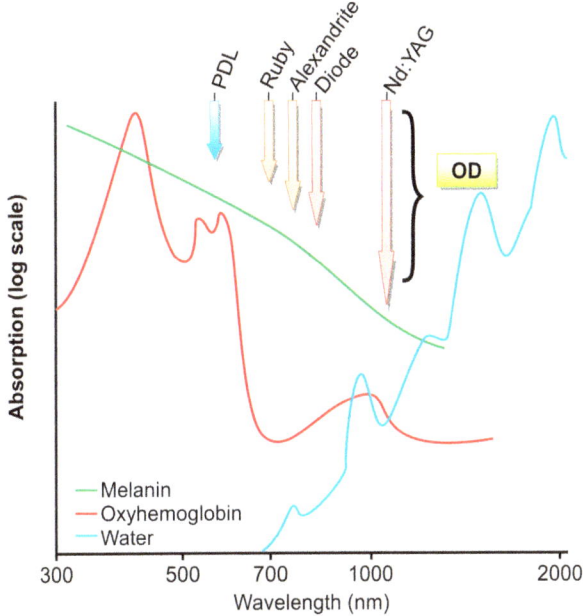

Fig. 3.1: Absorption coefficient of melanin in relation to the common lasers used for pigmented lesions
(OD: optical depth)

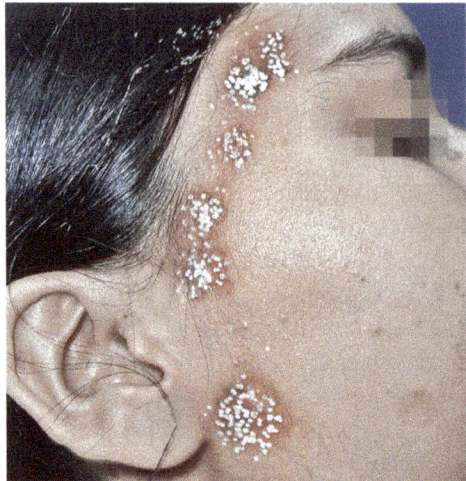

Fig. 3.2A: A 'white' end point is the ideal dose level for a QSw Nd:YAG laser for epidermal disorders.

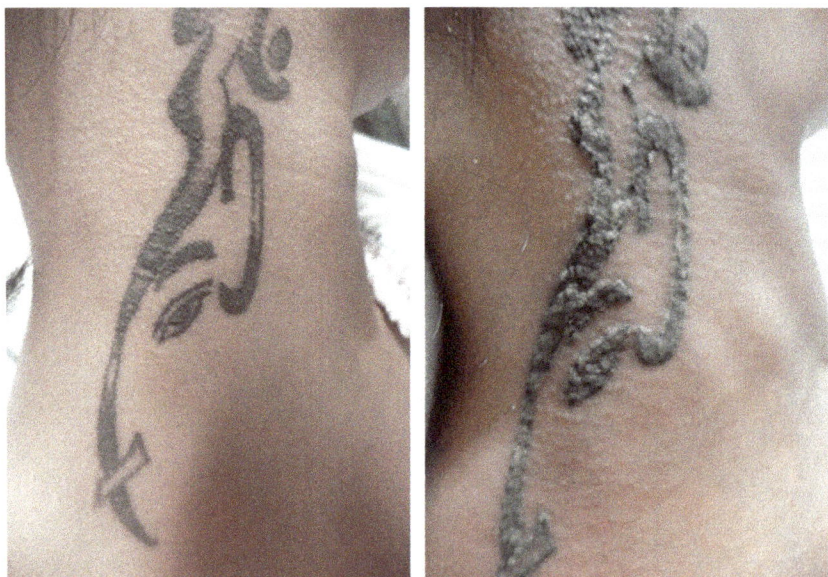

Fig. 3.2B: A black tattoo on the neck, note the whitening and edema after a pass of QS Nd:YAG 1064.

which cause a scattering of visible light, producing a white color. The adequate laser exposure dose for melanosome damage correlates well with the clinical threshold for immediate skin whitening. In other words, if the clinical ash-white color is not visible, the laser exposure dose is not sufficient. *Darker skin has a* **lower threshold** *for whitening due to a higher epidermal melanin* *content, thus a lower dosage than recommended for fairer skin types should be used.* Also remember for dermal disorders this end point is not consistently seen.

There are certain *variables* that determine the efficacy of lasers in pigmented lesions. Also endpoints depend on *multiple factors*, including
- Laser wavelength
- Pulse width
- Target organelle
- Fluence
- Skin type.

If an endpoint is not achieved, increasing the fluence may *not* be the solution-always look carefully for warning endpoints. With Q-switched lasers increasing the *diameter* may be a better option *(see* **Chapter 1: Laser-Tissue Interactions and its Clinical Correlates)**. Achieving a therapeutic endpoint does not guarantee the absence of side effects. Q-switched lasers cause immediate whitening while long pulsed lasers and light sources cause subtle darkening that will take several minutes to appear.

Wavelength selectivity limits absorption to a specific target chromophore. Thermal damage is then confined to that target by limiting the *pulse width* to less than or equal to the thermal relaxation time of the target chromophore. Once the pulse width is determined, energy levels can be optimized to achieve a desired effect. As a generic rule, melanocytes or melanin-containing keratinocytes are best targeted with a Q-switched laser in the nanosecond (ns) domain, whereas longer pulse is used in lasers for hair removal better target clumped melanin. In both cases, when appropriate settings are used for the risk of dyspigmentation and scarring is rare.

It must be understood that the *increased melanin content and sometimes unpredictable reactions of the Asian skin increase the risk of complications when using higher energies.* The larger, more melanized melanosomes in darker skin types absorb and scatter more energy, providing higher photo protection. Conversely, the melanocytes and mesenchyme in darker skin seem to be more vulnerable to trauma and inflammatory conditions. The Q-switched laser is a high impact laser and its use should be marked by judicious caution lest side effects occur.

Wavelengths

The various lasers used include the pulsed tunable dye laser (wavelength 435–750 nm, pulse width 300–750 ns), Q-switched ruby laser (wavelength 694 nm, pulse width 40 ns) and the QS Nd:YAG laser (wavelength 355, 532 and 1,064 nm; pulse width 10–12 ns). While shorter wavelengths, such as 351 nm are better at absorbing melanin, longer wavelengths penetrate deeper into the skin, increasing their ability to reach deeper melanosomes (Fig. 3.3). This principle accounts for the use of Qsw Nd:YAG 532/1064 nm in dermal disorders.

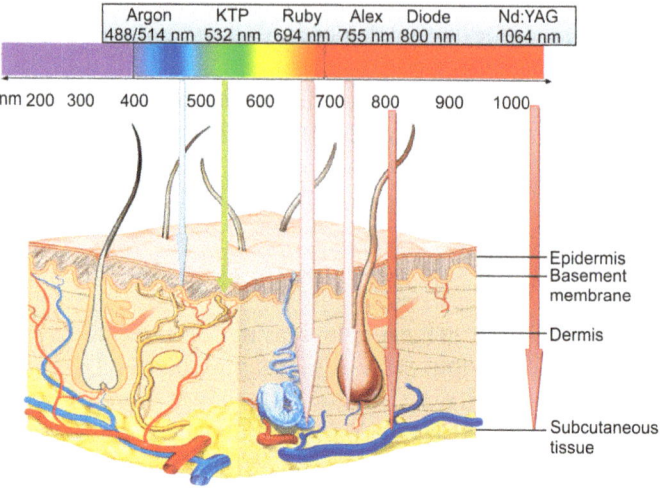

Fig. 3.3: Common lasers used for pigmented lesions with their penetration depth.

Lasers Used

The laser used varies, but in accordance with the principles of selective photothermolysis, ideally pigment selective lasers should be used. Other systems have also been used and are enumerated in Table 3.1. The lasers used include:
- Pigment nonselective
- Highly pigment selective (Qsw lasers) and picosecond lasers
- Less pigment selective lasers.

Pigment Nonselective Lasers/Fractional Lasers

The carbon dioxide (10,600 nm), Erbium-YAG (2,940 nm) and the yttrium-scandium-gallium-garnet (YSGG) (2,790 nm) lasers are pigment nonselective lasers that remove epidermal pigment because of their ability to target water and ablate the entire epidermis, including melanocytes and melanized keratinocytes. They are useful only if used in a dose settings within the thermal relaxation time of the skin (<1 ms). If it is beyond that then thermal damage will ensue that would lead to more side effects. They are though very useful in removing acquired melanocytic nevus.

The fractionated CO_2 and fractionated Erbium:YAG lasers work in the same manner as their nonfractionated counterparts but deliver the light in many small columns. Because only fractions of the pigmented epidermis are affected, a series of treatments is necessary to achieve the desired result and at least some of the original pigmented epidermal lesion would remain even after a series of treatments resulting in incomplete lesion removal. We are not proponents of using this technology except the fractional Q-switched

Table 3.1: A summary of the various lasers used for pigmented conditions (Med-lite C6, Hoya Con Bio Inc., Fremont, CA, USA, Q-Switched Nd:YAG laser machine use in Dr RMLH, PGIMER).

Device (manufacturer)	Laser type	Wavelength (nm)	Pulse duration	Spot size (mm)	Hz	Comments
Alex TriVantage (Candela)	QS FD Nd:YAG QS Alexandrite QS Nd:YAG	532 755 1,064	50 ns	2, 3, 5 2, 3, 4	5 5	
AlexLAZR (Candela)	QS Alexandrite	755	50 ns	2, 3, 4	5	Fiberoptic delivery system
EpiTouch (Lumenis)	QS Ruby	694	25 ns	5	0.8	Long pulse mode available for hair removal
Medlite C6 HOYA (ConBio)	QS FD Nd:YAG QS Nd:YAG	532 1,064	5–20 ns	2, 3, 4, 6 3, 4, 6, 8	10	Handpiece converts wavelength to 585 nm and 650 nm
ProTMQ-1064/532 (Protocadmus)	QS Nd:YAG	1,064 532	6 ns	1–4	2–5	
SkinClear (Sybaritic)	QS FD Nd:YAG QS Nd:YAG	532 1,064	10 ns 10 ns	1, 2, 3 1, 2, 3		
Spectrum RD-1200 (Palomar)	QS Ruby	694	28 ns	5, 6.5	0.8	Large spot size promotes deeper penetration
Tattoo Star Q-switched laser (Ascepelion)	Q-switched Nd:YAG laser Q-switched ruby laser Fractional ruby	1,064 and 532 694	8 ns 40 ns	2–4.5	10 2	First fractional, Qsw ruby laser
Versa Pulse VPC (Lumenis)	FD Nd:YAG	532	2–50 ms	2–10	6	Four lasers within one

versions (Tattoo star Fr:QS Ruby) for pigmented lesions (Table 3.1). This is simply as the quantum of improvement is *miniscule* compared to the amount of melanin removed by the fractional lasers (*see* **Chapter 12D**).

Highly Pigment Selective Lasers

There are three short-pulsed, pigment selective lasers that are widely used today: (1) The Q-switched ruby laser (QSRL) (694 nm), (2) the Q-switched alexandrite laser (755 nm), and (3) the Q-switched neodymium:YAG (Nd:YAG and KTP) laser (1,064, 532 nm).

These lasers selectively target melanin by delivering high-intensity, short-pulsed radiation at varying wavelengths (Fig. 3.3). The QSRL emits light at a wavelength of 694 nm and a pulse duration of 28–40 ns. The Q-switched alexandrite laser has a near infrared wavelength of 755 nm, pulse duration of 50–100 ns, spot size of 2–4 mm, and a repetition rate up to 10 Hz. The Q-switched Nd:YAG laser emits infrared light at 1,064 nm. The wavelength can be halved by placing a frequency-doubling KTP (potassium-titanyl-phosphate) crystal in the laser beam's path. Dye-impregnated handpieces can convert the 532 nm wavelength to either 585 nm (yellow) or 650 nm (red). An articulated arm delivers pulses with a spot size to 1.5–8 mm, a pulse duration of 5–10 ns, and a repetition rate up to 10 Hz (Fig. 3.4A). The difference between non-FDA approved lasers and the FDA approved devices is in the beam profile. Most lasers in these classes have a Gaussian beam profile, thus requiring overlap and thus leading to more thermal damage. In pigmented lesions, this can have a detrimental effect. This is depicted in Figure 3.4B.

The 1064-nm Q-switched Nd:YAG laser should be used when treating darker skin types, because it greatly reduces the risk of epidermal injury and pigmentary alteration. Some basic caveats in procuring a good QSw Nd:YAG are in Box 3.1.

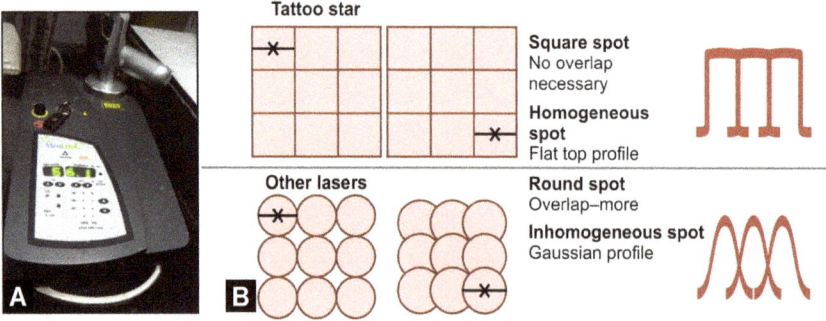

Figs. 3.4A and B: (A) Q-switched Nd:YAG laser machine used in Dr RMLH, PGIMER (Medlite C6, Hoya Con Bio Inc., Fremont, CA, USA); (B) A comparison of the beam profile of QS laser (Asclepion Laser Technologies, GmbH).

Box 3.1: Ideal check for buying a good QSw 1064 nm laser

- 1064 nm is the main wavelength
- This is converted to 532, 650-585 nm
- The ideal energy dose per pulse of 1064 nm—2000 mJ
- Dose per pulse of 532 nm–900 mJ
- Dose per pulse for other wavelengths 600–700 mJ

Picosecond

Picosecond Lasers: The Q-switched nanosecond technology was based on the possibility of being able to move from purely thermal heating of melanin and tattoo ink to a photomechanical process with the creation of pressure waves in targeted tissue with nanosecond pulses (Fig. 3.4C). Lowering the pulse duration is presumed to be superior as the very short pulse duration, causes both photomechanical and photothermal effects in the tissue and produces greater tensile strength than when using nanosecond lasers (Saedi N). Thus, the superiority of the picosecond laser is based on the premise that high-energy picosecond energy generates an intense shock wave that leads to fragmentation of targets via a photomechanical, rather than photothermolytic effect.

The picosecond laser is characterized by the concept of Stress lock-in (Stress relaxation time theory). Here when a certain particle is heated, thermal expansion of the particle occurs with consequent expansion of the vibration and is called stress diffusion (Fig. 3.4D). When the pulse duration is very short, the stress generated within the particle does not have enough time to diffuse and stress lock-in is achieved. The stress relaxation time (SRT), for tattoo pigments, is thought to be slightly shorter than 1 ns. Therefore, a ps-laser is ideal here. The major action involves the photoacoustic destruction of the particle, with a minor photothermal component.

The first pico laser with a pulse duration less than 1 ns (1.0 ns = 10^{-9} s) was studied in the late 1990s with an experimental laboratory-based ps-laser. This was not deemed to be commercially viable and after 15 years again a spate of such lasers have been launched. This includes the PicoSure (755 nm/750 ps) by Cynosure Inc., enLIGHTen (1064 nm, 532 nm/750 ps) by Cutera Inc. and PicoWay (1064 nm, 532 nm/450 ps, 375ps) by Syneron Candela Inc. It must be emphasized that the picosecond lasers were made primarily for tattoo removal where it may be better than the ns lasers, for certain difficult to treat tattoos (see next section). The spate of articles on its use in other disorders should be read with caution unless they are compared with the existing standard of care lasers and found to be superior.

A comparison of existing picosecond lasers

Wavelength (nm)	532/1064	755	532/1064	532/585/650/1064
Energy per pulse (mJ)	200/400	165–200	300/600	250/500
Pulse duration	375 ps	500–750 ps	750 ps, 2 ns	600 ps, 2 ns, 8 ns
Peak power	0/53 GW	0.36 GW	0.40/0.80 GW	0.80 GW
Spot size (mm)	2–10 mm	1,2,5,10 mm	2–8 mm	2–15

*This is calculated using the highest energy per pulse with the lowest spot size and lowest pulse duration

QS laser simplified operation

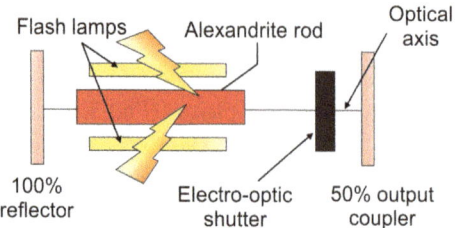

1. Flash lamps store energy in the laser rod while the shutter blocks the resonator
2. The shutter is opened and a nanosecond short pulse is emitted

Picosure simplified operation

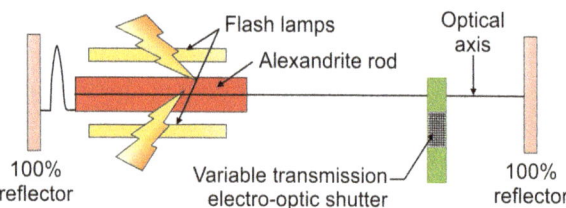

1. Flash lamps store energy in the laser rod while the shutter blocks the resonator
2. A single short seed pulse is established by the variable transmission shutter
3. The pulse is amplified in a low loss resonator configuration
4. The pulse is extracted from the resonator and delivered to the patient

Fig. 3.4C: A depiction of the Q-switched and picosecond laser operation.

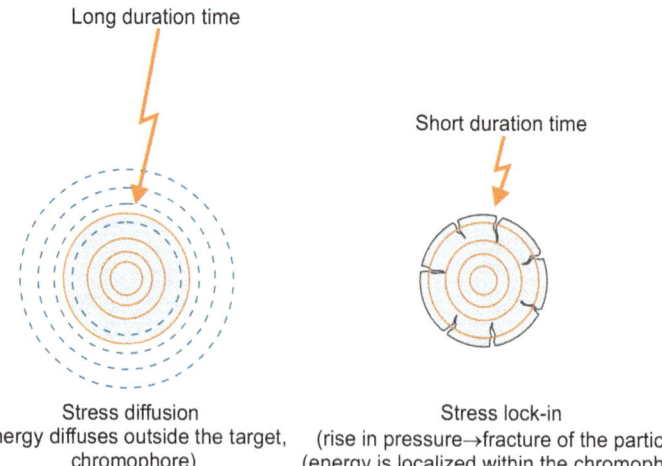

Fig. 3.4D: A depiction of the concept of stress lock-in phenomenon.

Picosecond Lasers and its Real life Applicability: Before we extoll the virtues of this laser remember that one has to understand that it is early days for this technology and we need to see if it is really superior to Q-switched lasers. Also one has to examine comparative trials and most importantly there are many variables that determine the end results not just the pulse duration. The concept of reducing the pulse duration is not so important as long as pulse widths are below the estimated thermal relaxation time of melanosomes. Studies have shown that there is no added advantage of picosecond or femtosecond pulse duration for targeting melanosomes (Watanabe S).

The main advantage of the pico lasers is that the peak power is undeniably high. But it must be noted that this is when we take into consideration, the smallest spot size. In actual practice as the spot size increases the energy per pulse would decrease as the penetration depth increases with increase in spot size. This would lead to extremely low pulse energies than described. Also remember that the Qs laser can have very high peak energy levels. Like the maximum energy, settings of a 1064 nm laser can be 250 J/cm^2, which is higher than most ps lasers.

In real life scenarios, like say melasma a higher spot size would be needed. With the 755 nm lasers, an ideal setting would be to keep the pulse duration as low as possible. Keeping the same pulse duration mode, the fluence decreases while the spot size increases. But the end points need to be achieved and hence for melasma a 650 pulse duration is preferred. The actual energy levels would of course then depend on the spot size. Thus in real life, the high energy levels are rarely achieved as the pulse duration needs to be changed to suit the end points.

Also one must understand that a true pico laser is one that is as close to 1 ps (Fig. 3.4E). What we have are lasers that are in actual terms close to 1 ns laser as their pulse duration are >500 ps (0.5 ns). Most importantly, for pigmented skin the 1064 nm Q-second lasers are ideal as they are not absorbed by competing pigment in the epidermis, but what we have is a spate of articles on the 755 nm which is not ideal for skin of color.

Hence, it must be appreciated that the pico laser, is definitely superior for certain tattoo colors, it is by no means superior for other conditions, unless comparative studies are done with maximum doses of the Qs lasers in a comparative trial.

Salient Studies: Though numerous studies have been done and are referenced in further sections a few studies are listed here to give a practical view of the technology.
- The picosecond laser was used for tattoo removal where Brauer and colleagues demonstrated the successful treatment of green and/or blue tattoos using the picosecond 755 nm alexandrite laser with a 75% clearance of pigment after 1–2 treatments. These promising results have been attributed to more rapid heating and greater fragmentation

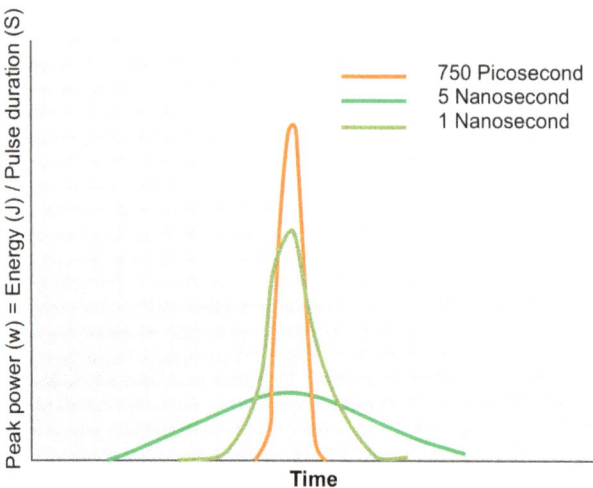

Fig. 3.4E: A comparison of picosecond and nanosecond pulse.

achieved by the ultra-short picosecond pulses. Here it must be noted that the picolaser is not superior to the Qs laser for the common black tattoos. This has been discussed in the next section on tattoos.

- A retrospective chart and photographic review to evaluate the efficacy and safety profile of various lasers used for the treatment of pigmentary disorders in SOC (skin of color) patients, including the current standard-of-care treatment with the Q-switched ruby and Nd:YAG lasers and the newer alexandrite picosecond laser was examined in an important study (Levin MK, 2016). The most common pigmentary disorder treated was Nevus of Ota (38.1%), followed by solar lentigines (23.8%). Other pigmentary disorders included PIH, congenital nevus, café-au-lait macule, dermal melanocytosis, Nevus of Ito, and Becker's nevus. Eighty four percent of subjects receiving Q-switched nanosecond laser treatments and 50% of the subjects receiving alexandrite 755 nm picosecond laser treatments felt satisfied with the therapy. Side effects observed in subjects treated with the alexandrite 755 nm picosecond laser, were similar to those commonly observed and reported with the nanosecond Q-switched technology. Importantly the 755 nm alexandrite picosecond, 694 nm ruby, 532 nm, and 1064 nm neodymium:YAG nanosecond lasers appear to be safe and *equally effective* modalities for removal of pigmentary disorders in skin of color patients with no long-term complications if used appropriately. Thus, the key message is that the 755 nm is *not* superior to the existing standard of care lasers in pigmented disorders studied.
- The short pulse durations of Q switched lasers allow for optimal, targeted photothermal damage to melanosomes, which has a thermal relaxation time of between 50 and 250 ns. The existing Qs lasers have a pulse duration

ranging from 1 ns to 5 ns and is already less than the melanosomes and hence it does not seem that the ps laser would benefit in pigmentary disorders.

Most importantly the ideal laser wavelength for skin of color in the 1064 nm hence, except for tattoos, we should look at the comparative studies of the 1064 nm pico versus the Qs 1064 nm.

An overview of the advantages and lacunae are depicted in Table 3.2 and the reader is advised to take a balanced view of the technology.

Table 3.2: Overview of picosecond technology.

Advantages	Disadvantages
• Useful for facial lesions and tattoos • Causes less peripheral damage • Less postinflammatory hyperpigmentation • Causes less peripheral damage (Thermal confinement) • Lower pulse duration • Lower pulse energy is needed • Worth the cost if multicolored tattoos are the major source of revenue in practice	• May not be useful or superior for dermal pigmented lesions located on the extremities or trunk • Similar wavelengths have not been compared with adequate settings (example-1064 nm Q-switched vs picosecond of 1064 nm) • Not superior for Nevus of Ota/Congenital nevi/other dermal pigmented lesions • Not tested in type VI skin type subjects • Very costly laser

Less Pigment Selective

The Q-switched ruby, alexandrite and Nd:YAG lasers also have long-pulsed counterparts with the same wavelengths that operate in a normal (non-Q-switched) mode. These normal mode lasers are often used for laser hair removal because their higher fluences and longer pulse durations target large pigmented structures such as hair follicles or nests of cells rather than individual melanosomes or pigmented cells (Ueda et al.).

Normal mode lasers have been shown to be effective in the removal of epidermal pigmented lesions but are not ideal because damage may be imparted on surrounding tissue. Long-pulsed (millisecond rather than nanosecond domain) 532 nm (KTP) Nd:YAG lasers and 595 nm pulsed-dye lasers, which are traditionally used to treat vascular lesions, can also be used to treat superficial pigmented lesions. The millisecond (ms) pulse width more closely matches the thermal relaxation time of nested melanocytes, and collateral thermal damage provides a lethal injury to melanocytes that are adjacent to the target area but that might not actually contain melanin at the time of treatment. In fact the pulse width of these lasers closely matches the thermal relaxation time of the entire epidermis (about 10 ms) and therefore, does not allow for selective damage to melanosomes. Because of their longer pulse width, millisecond domain lasers produce a purely thermal effect on their target, unlike the photomechanical effect of Q-switched lasers.

Regardless, these longer pulse duration devices, just like intense pulsed light devices are highly effective in removing unwanted epidermal pigment. These lasers are not suitable for treating dermal pigmented lesions because of the limited penetration depth (Kono et al.).

Intense Pulsed Light

The noncoherent, broadband, intense pulsed light (IPL) source has also demonstrated efficacy in the treatment of pigmented lesions. IPL is particularly effective in the treatment of epidermal pigmented lesions, such as lentigines. This modality can also be safely used on darker skin types when used in a double or triple pulsed mode that allows the epidermis to cool between light pulses as well as its low risk of PIH.

INDICATIONS

Pigment lasers can be used for various indications and are conveniently divided into epidermal and dermal disorders (Fig. 3.5). As a **thumb rule**, the efficacy of lasers results depends on the site of pigment epidermal > dermal > mixed. Another practical method of classifying the conditions are static conditions (Nevocellular nevus) and dynamic conditions like melasma, the latter consistently have inconsistent results (Table 3.3).

Pigment Location and Lasers Used

Epidermal: Pigmented lesions include lentigo, café-au-lait macule, ephelide, junctional nevus, nevus spilus, and seborrheic keratosis.

Dermal: Pigmented lesions include blue nevus and nevus of Ota or Ito. Some pigmented lesions, such as melasma, Becker nevus, and compound nevus, have both an epidermal and a dermal component.

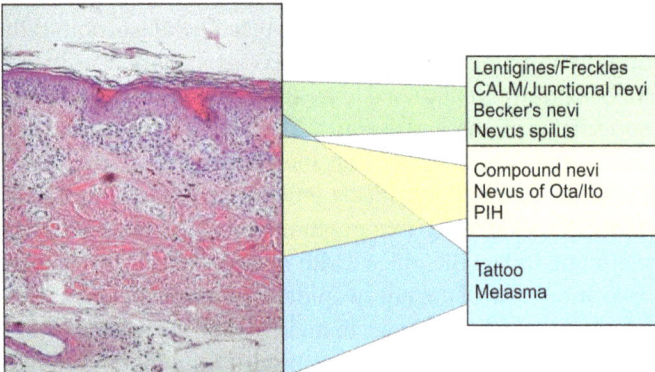

Fig. 3.5: Summary of the salient conditions amenable to treatment by pigmented lasers. Remember the cardinal rule, "dynamic" disorders should not be treated with pigment lasers.

Table 3.3: A summary of laser treatment for selected disorders.

Pathology	Condition	Laser	Results
Epidermal/ Dermal	Acquired melanocytic nevi (Moles)*	QS ruby laser (694 nm) QS Alex (755 nm) QS Nd:YAG (1,064 nm) Normal–mode ruby laser (NMRL) Long Pulse Alex Er:YAG Up CO_2	Recurrence is a distinct possibility Lighter nevi respond best to shorter wavelengths while darker nevi typically respond to any wavelength within the melanin absorption spectrum Compound nevi have the maximum recurrence We prefer the Er:YAG/ Up CO_2 laser over the pigment specific lasers
	Becker's nevus	Er:YAG lasers QS 1,064 nm Nd:YAG Long-pulse 755 nm Alex laser	Incomplete results with most lasers In resistant cases Er:YAG ablation is an option *Combination of two lasers* a. Hair removal laser appropriate for skin and hair type b. Pigment-specific laser such as QS ruby, alexandrite, or Nd:YAG
	Melasma	Resurfacing lasers Fractional lasers Fractional ruby Pigment lasers/IPL Q-switched lasers Laser toning (low-fluence, QS 1,064 nm Nd:YAG laser, setting (6–8 mm spot size, 1.6–2.3 J/cm^2) Vascular lasers	In Indian skin, the results are erratic and transient with all lasers
	Lichen planus (LP) pigmentosus	QS 1,064 nm Nd:YAG laser (low fluence) (Kim JE et al.) IPL (Harmony, with a wavelength of 570 nm, exposure time 12 ms, fluence 15 J/cm^2) (Meire Brasil Parada et al.)	

Contd...

Contd...

Pathology	Condition	Laser	Results
Epidermal	Café-au-lait patches	QS 694 nm ruby laser QS 532 nm Nd:YAG NMRL or LP Alex Er:YAG	Inconsistent and incomplete results *Long Pulse Alex* has been used as its tends to decrease recurrence and the number of sittings The **principle** is that the longer pulse allows for collateral damage to nonpigment containing melanocytes
	Freckles and lentigines	Almost all Qsw lasers can be used. Ideal is QS-532 nm Long pulse lasers have also been tried	Easy to treat with consistent results (1–3 sittings)
	Nevus spilus	QS ruby QS Alex QS 532 nm Nd:YAG laser Combination of carbon	The darker nevocellular nevus clears but the background pigment persists
Dermal	Drug-induced pigmentation	Q-switched 532 nm/ 1,064 nm Q-switched Alexandrite	Useful for minocycline induced pigmentation
	Infraorbital hyperpigmentation	QS Ruby lasers QS Alex lasers	Effective only in cases with deposition of dermal melanin
	Congenital nevus	None are reliably effective	Laser treatment should be undertaken with caution
	** Nevus of Ota	QS Nd:YAG-1064/532 nm QS Alexandrite (Alex)- 755 nm	The number of treatment session varies and depends on age, color and size of the lesion A study gives a realistic view of results based on the color** of the lesion (Felton SJ et al.)
	Blue nevus	QS ruby (694 nm) QS alexandrite (755 nm) QS Nd:YAG (1064 nm)	Variable results

*Congenital nevus are difficult to treat and require a ablative laser in combination with a pigment specific laser ** blue-colored lesions improved with all modalities, brown with QS Nd:YAG-532 nm/QS Alex-755 nm, blue-gray with QS Alex-755 nm/QS Nd:YAG-1064 nm while gray lesions are the most resistant. Type V skin were the most resistant to therapy (Felton SJ et al.).

For some pigmented lesions, the target is melanosomes in *keratinocytes*, whereas in most cases it is melanosomes in *melanocytes* or the whole melanocyte. In some cases, the spread of thermal damage from pigment containing melanocytes may be advantageous in targeting adjacent melanocytes lacking significant melanin content (i.e. dermal nevi or compound melanocytic nevi).

The success of the Q-switched lasers in the realm of pigmented lesions is based on the ability of these lasers to selectively target melanosomes situated within melanocytes and keratinocytes. The melanosome-specific damage is due to the absorption of high-energy, nanosecond, laser pulses. Long pulsed lasers in the millisecond domain were developed to target pigmented hair. These lasers can also be used to target epidermal and dermal pigment found in larger clumps such as those in nested melanocytes or confluent melanin in the epidermis (Kurban K). The picosecond laser has also been used but the results do not seem to be superior to the Q second lasers.

Epidermal Pigmented Lesions

The common indications include: ephelides, lentigines, café-au-lait macules, seborrheic keratoses, nevus spilus and Becker's nevi. Since pigment in epidermal lesions is found superficially, shorter-wavelength devices can be used successfully despite their limited penetration depth (Fig. 3.3). The 510 nm wavelength of the pigmented lesion pulsed dye laser and 532 nm pulsed lasers are highly absorbed by melanin but penetrates to a depth 250 μm into the skin (Anderson et al.). The Q-switched ruby and alexandrite lasers effectively treat both epidermal and dermal pigmented lesions since their wavelengths are still within the melanin absorption spectrum and they penetrate deeply into the dermis. The Nd:YAG (1,064 nm) laser penetrates deeply but is poorly absorbed by melanin, making the 532 nm wavelength preferable for epidermal lesions.

When using the 510 nm and 532 nm wavelengths, hemoglobin competes with melanin for absorption of light. Nanosecond pulses at these wavelengths causes rupture of superficial blood vessels, which may manifest clinically as purpura. A variable spot size that covers the epidermal lesion should be used and the lesions treated with single pass with minimal overlap.

Dermal Pigmented Lesions

The conditions amenable to treatment include: melanocytic nevi (acquired and congenital), nevus of Ota, tattoos and melasma. Other dermal pigmented lesions where laser can be used in combination with medical therapy like lichen planus (LP) pigmentosus, PIH, fixed drug eruption and persisted Mongolian spots. The Q-switched ruby, alexandrite and 1,064 nm Nd:YAG are the most commonly used lasers. All of these lasers are still within the absorption spectrum of melanin yet also have wavelengths that are long enough to penetrate into the dermis (Fig. 3.3). A list of common disorders with the modes of treatment is listed in Table 3.3 while details are listed in the following section.

BOOKS

1. Goldberg, Dover JS, Alam M. Procedures in cosmetic dermatology series: Lasers and Lights: Part1/2; 2006.
2. Hruza GJ, Avram M. Lasers and Lights: Procedures in Cosmetic Dermatology Series (Expert Consult - Online and Print), 3rd ed., 2012.
3. Laser dermatology: Pearls and problems by Goldberg DJ, 2011.
4. Lasers in dermatology and medicine. Nouri K (Ed); 2011.
5. Sanjeev Aurangabad. Laser for pigmented lesions and tattoos. In: Mysore V (Ed). ACSI Textbook on Cutaneous and Aesthetic Surgery. New Delhi: Jaypee Brothers Publishing; 2013.pp.797-13.

BIBLIOGRAPHY

1. Anderson RR, Parrish JA. Selective photothermolysis: precise microsurgery by selective absorption of pulsed irradiation. Science. 1983;220:524.
2. Anderson RR, Parrish JA. The optics of human skin. J Invest Dermatol. 1981;77:13-9.
3. Brauer JA, Reddy KK, Anolik R, et al. Successful and rapid treatment of blue and green tattoo pigment with a novel picosecond laser. Arch Dermatol. 2012;148:820-3.
4. Felton SJ, Al-Niaimi F, Ferguson JE, Madan V. Our perspective of the treatment of naevus of Ota with 1,064-, 755- and 532-nm wavelength lasers. Lasers in medical science, 2013.
5. Goldman L. Optical radiation hazards to the skin. In: Sliney D, Wolbarsht M (Eds.). Safety with Lasers and Other Optical Sources: A Comprehensive Handbook. New York: Plenum; 1983.
6. Kim JE, Won CH, Chang S, et al. Linear lichen planus pigmentosus of the forehead treated by neodymium: Yttrium-aluminum-garnet laser and topical tacrolimus. J Dermatol. 2012;39:189-91.
7. Kono T, Manstein D, Chan HH. Q-switched ruby versus long-pulsed dye laser delivered with compression for treatment of facial lentigines in Asians. Lasers Surg Med. 2006;38(2):94-7.
8. Kurban AK, Morrison PR, Trainor S, et al. Pulse duration effects on cutaneous pigment. Lasers Surg Med. 1992;12:282.
9. Levin MK, Ng E, Bae YS, et al. Treatment of pigmentary disorders in patients with skin of color with a novel 755 nm picosecond, Q-switched ruby, and Q-switched Nd:YAG nanosecond lasers: A retrospective photographic review. Lasers Surg Med. 2016;48(2):181-7.
10. Parada MB, Yarak S, Michalany NS. Treatment of lichen planus pigmentosus. Surgical & Cosmetic Dermatology. 2009;1(4):192-4.
11. Molly Wanner, Fernanda HS, Mathew MA, et al. Immediate skin responses to laser and light treatment therapeutic endpoints: How to obtain efficacy. J Am Acad Dermatol. 2016;74(5):30-42.
12. Olson RL, Gaylor J, Everett MA. Skin color, melanin, and erythema. Arch Dermatology. 1988;124:869.
13. Saedi N, Metelitsa A, Petrell K, et al. Treatment of tattoos with a picosecond alexandrite laser: A prospective trial. Arch Dermatol. 2012;148(12):1360-3.

14. Sanjeev Aurangabad. Laser for pigmented lesions and tattoos. In: Mysore V (Ed). ACSI Textbook on Cutaneous and Aesthetic Surgery. New Delhi: Jaypee Brothers Publishing; 2013.pp.797-13.
15. Sardana K, Chugh S, Garg V. Are Q-switched lasers for nevus of Ota really effective in pigmented skin? Indian J Dermatol Venereol Leprol. 2012;78(2):187-9.
16. Sardana K, Chugh S, Garg VK. Which therapy works for melasma in pigmented skin: lasers, peels, or triple combination creams? Indian J Dermatol Venereol Leprol. 2013;79(3):420-2.
17. Sardana K, Garg VK. Lasers are not effective for melasma in darkly pigmented skin. J Cutan Aesthet Surg. 2014;7(1):57-60.
18. Sardana K. The science, reality, and ethics of treating common acquired melanocytic nevi (moles) with lasers. J Cutan Aesthet Surg. 2013;6(1):27-9.
19. Ueda S, Imayama S. Normal-mode ruby laser for treating congenital nevi. Arch Dermatol. 1997;133:355-9.
20. Watanabe S, Anderson RR, Brorson S, et al. Comparative studies of femtosecond to microsecond laser pulses on selective pigmented cell injury in skin. Photochem Photobiol. 1991;53(6):757-62.

LASER TREATMENT OF COMMON PIGMENTED CONDITIONS

Some basic **principles** about lasers should be understood before attempting pigmented lesions specially in pigmented skin:

- *Dynamic conditions do not respond as well as static lesions:* This principle explains why conditions like lentigines and nevus of Ota tend to respond better than say melasma, a classic dynamic lesion.
- *Low contrast lesions respond to lasers:* In pigmented skin, melasma is not a *low contrast* lesion, while in a fair skin type, it might be the case. Thus, the results of most procedures are disappointing in melasma.
- *Dermal disorders are poorly responsive in pigmented skin:* The rapid and predictable response of lentigines as compared to the slow, variable response of nevus of Ota is explained by the effect of the competing pigmented epidermis, which alters the laser physics dynamics.

LASERS USED

Pigment in epidermal lesions is located superficially, so shorter wavelength devices can be used effectively despite their limited penetration depth. For example, the 510 nm wavelength of the pulsed dye laser penetrates only 250 μm into the skin but is highly absorbed by melanin. The Q-switched ruby and alexandrite lasers effectively treat both epidermal and dermal lesions since their wavelengths are well absorbed by melanin and penetrate deeply into the dermis. The 1,064 nm wavelength of the Nd:YAG laser penetrates deeply but is poorly absorbed by melanin, making the 532 nm wavelength a better choice when treating epidermal lesions. At the 510 nm and 532 nm (green) wavelengths, hemoglobin competes with melanin for absorption of light. Ultrashort (nanosecond range) pulses at these wavelengths cause rupture of superficial blood vessels, which is evident clinically as purpura.

The efficacy and side effect profile of QS ruby and QS Nd:YAG (1,064 nm, 532 nm) lasers have been compared in the treatment of cutaneous pigmented lesions, including lentigines, café-au-lait macule (CALM), nevus of Ota, nevus spilus, Becker's nevus, PIH, and melasma. With the exception of melasma for which poor results are reported the QS ruby laser produced good-to-excellent results (50–95% clearing), as opposed to fair-to-good (25–75% clearing) results for the QS Nd:YAG for all remaining conditions.

EPIDERMAL DISORDERS

Lentigines

Lentigines are extremely common hyperpigmented macules that are most often due to chronic sun exposure and are then referred to as solar lentigines. On pathology, lentigines display increased single melanocytes along the basal layer with elongation of club-shaped rete ridges.

Lasers Used

Q-switched devices: All three Q-switched lasers are highly effective for treating all types of lentigines. If properly performed, 1–2 sessions are sufficient. With one treatment using a Q-switched laser, at least 50% clearing of lentigines is expected. Treatment with Q-switched lasers is more effective than with other modalities such as liquid nitrogen, 35% trichloroacetic acid and glycolic acid peels (Jiang et al.) and (Chan HH et al.) (Fig. 3.3).

Picosecond lasers: Apart from the 755 nm, for skin of color the 532 and 1064 nm is more relevant. A study by Kung KY et al. used the 532 and 1064 nm pico which delivers pulse energy up to 400 mJ, and pulse duration of 450 ps. They found excellent results, better than the 755 nm picolaser.

Millisecond devices: Although less selective, non-Q-switched (millisecond domain) KTP, 595 nm pulsed-dye, ruby, alexandrite, and diode lasers may also be used to treat lentigines. Pulsed dye laser delivered with firm diascopy through a transparent window can also be used to treat lentigines without concomitant damage to blood vessels (Kono et al.). The advantages are **less** PIH. The logic is that long pulse lasers have a longer millisecond pulse width, which result in more absorption by target melanin and less absorption by competing chromophores such as oxyhemoglobin, and surrounding pigmented skin. Also these lasers target melanin by photothermolysis only.

Long pulsed lasers are associated with a lower risk of PIH than the use of Q-switched laser in Asian patients (Kono et al.). In contrast, QS lasers emit high-energy, nanosecond radiation, causing both photothermal and photomechanical effects. This paradoxically stimulates the surrounding melanin and oxyhemoglobins are causing PIH.

Intense pulsed light (IPL): Though this has been tried, but in our experience, multiple treatments are required and the large spot size, leads to complications in Indian skin. In fact, IPL suffer from the classical "catch 22" situation as if a low energy is used, the results are poor while a high energy leads to risk of injury to surrounding normal skin.

If a targeted IPL treatment is envisaged, a wavelength between 500 and 635 nm with contact cooling is the ideal parameter.

Pearls/Pitfalls

Always use a **test spot** to determine the optimal energy level. This is as in our skin type hypopigmentation is an eventual result. Use the **lowest fluence** that causes mild whitening as Q-switched lasers have narrow therapeutic window. Lower fluence may incompletely eradicate lesions, whereas higher fluence can result in pigmentary alteration especially when treating dark complexioned skin. Also consistent SPF 30 sunscreen is advisable as a tanned skin leads to a high test spot dose.

Level of Difficulty

Easy to trust and the results are predictable and good with occasional cases of dyspigmentation. Recurrence occurs but late (Figs. 3.6A to E).

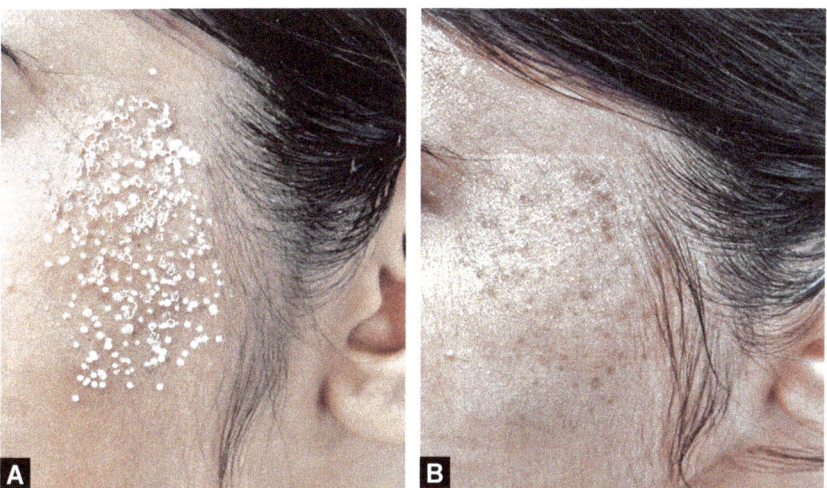

Figs. 3.6A and B: (A) A case of segmental lentiginosis. Plan: Qsw Nd:YAG (532 nm, 2 Hz 2.5 J/cm^2). "Single spot" technique (B) Immediate postoperative view using the protocadamus Qsw Nd:YAG. Note the end point of whitening and slight bleeding.

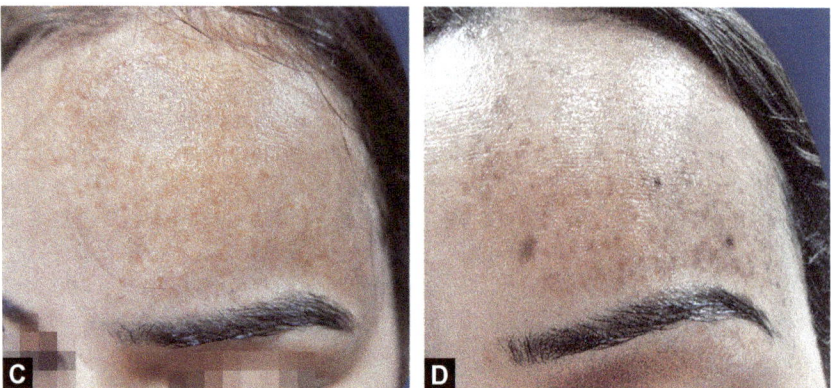

Figs. 3.6C and D: (C) A female patient with segmental lentigines; (D) Same patient after 4 sessions with a Qsw Nd:YAG (532 nm, 3 Hz).

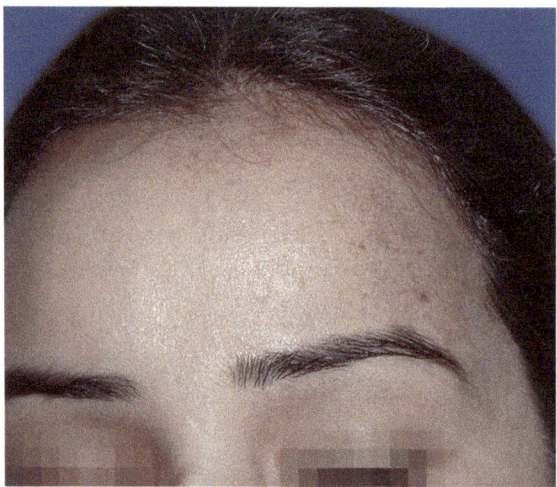

Fig. 3.6E: After 5 sessions and at 6 months follow-up, there is marked improvement of the lesion.

BIBLIOGRAPHY

1. Chan HH, Fung WK, Ying SY, et al. An in vivo trial comparing the use of different types of 532 nm Nd:YAG lases in the treatment facial lentigines in oriental patients. Dermatol Surg. 2000;26:743-9.
2. Jiang SB, Levine V, Ashinoff R. The treatment of solar lentigines with Diode (Diolite532nm) and the Q-switched ruby laser: a comparative study. Laser Surg Med Suppl. 2000;12:55.
3. Kilmer SL, Wheeland RG, Goldberg DJ, et al. Treatment of epidermal pigmented lesions with the frequency-doubled Q-switched Nd:YAG laser. A controlled, single-impact, dose-response, multicenter trial. Arch Dermatol. 1994;130(12):1515-9.

4. Kono T, Manstein D, Chan HH, et al. Q-switched ruby versus long-pulsed dye laser delivered with compression for treatment of facial lentigines in Asians. Laser Surg Med. 2006;38:94-7.
5. Kung KY, Shek SY, Yeung CK, Chan HH. Evaluation of the safety and efficacy of the dual wavelength picosecond laser for the treatment of benign pigmented lesions in Asians. Lasers Surg Med. 2018 Oct 25. doi: 10.1002/lsm.23028.
6. Tse Y, Levine VJ, McClain SA, et al. The removal of cutaneous pigmented lesions with the Q-switched ruby laser and the Q-switched neodymium:yttrium aluminum-garnet laser. A comparative study. J Dermatol Surg Oncol. 1994; 20(12):795-800.

Labial Melanotic Macules

Melanotic macules on the lip vermilion are a feature of several entities including physiological racial pigmentation, Laugier-Hunziker syndrome, and Peutz-Jeghers syndrome.

Laser Used

These can be treated using the QS ruby or QS alexandrite or frequency-doubled QS Nd:YAG lasers. In the case of the syndromes, patients should be made aware that new macules will develop over time. Partial or complete clearance has been reported with use of Q-switched lasers, long-pulsed lasers and IPL (Grevelink et al., Abecassis et al.) (Figs. 3.7A and B).

Level of Difficulty

Easy.

Nevus Spilus

A nevus spilus (speckled lentiginous nevus) consists of a background CALM and scattered nests of nevi cells. Successful clearing of the darker nevocellular component has been reported with the QSRL, but the CALM component tends to recur. Partial or complete clearance has been reported with use of Q-switched lasers, long-pulsed lasers and IPL (Grevelink et al., Abecassis et al.).

A recent paper (Mingjun Tang et al.) describes the *combination* of a fractional CO_2 laser and a Qs laser. The settings used were ActiveFX™ mode (energy 90–125 mJ/cm^2) to scan the nevi to the level of normal skin, ensuring that the depth of treatment did not exceed the superficial layer of the dermis. This was followed by the MedLite C6 laser (wavelength 1064 nm, energy 4.0 J/cm^2, beam 3 mm, frequency 10 Hz) and the wavelength 532 nm (energy 1.2 J/cm^2, beam 2 mm, frequency 10 Hz). The only issue as always is that excessive use of a fractional CO_2 in this case may cause PIH.

Level of Difficulty

Easy for the nevocellular component but the background pigmentation persists (Figs. 3.8 and 3.9).

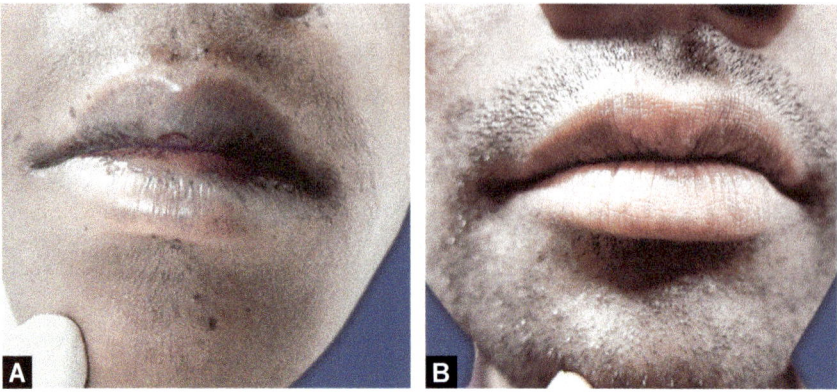

Figs. 3.7A and B: A case of labial melanotic macule treated with two sessions of 532 QS Nd:YAG.

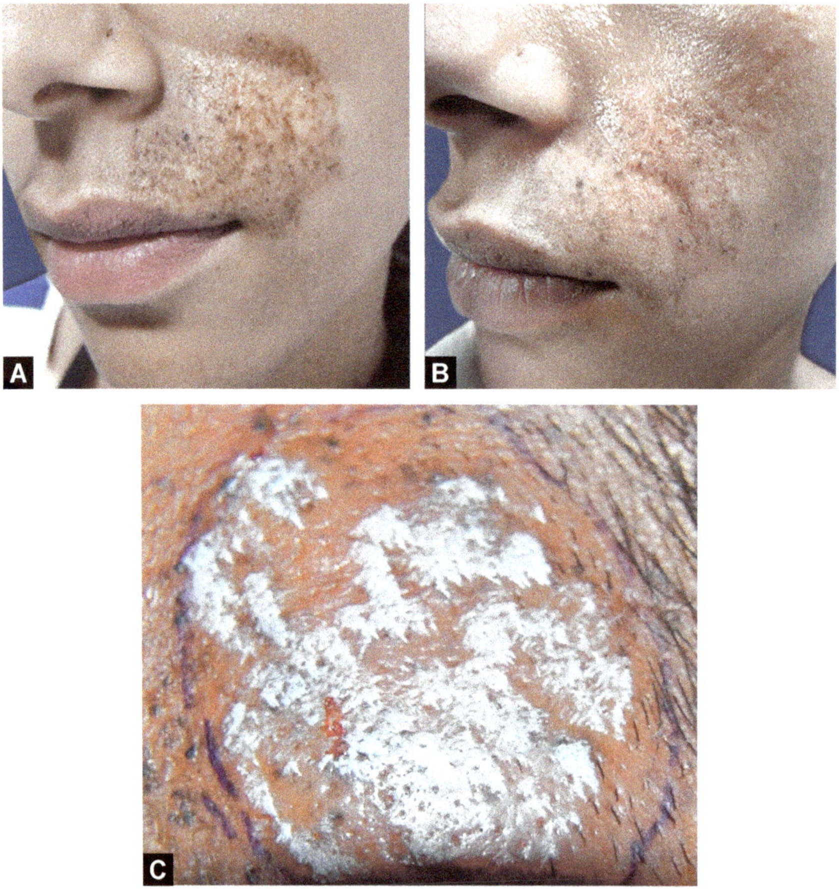

Figs. 3.8A to C: (A and B) Nevus spilus: After 6 sessions of 532 nm QS Nd:YAG. An appreciable but not complete improvement; (C) *Note* the diffuse whitening due to the Qsw 532 nm in a case of nevus spilus (2.5 J/cm^2 Protocadamus, device).

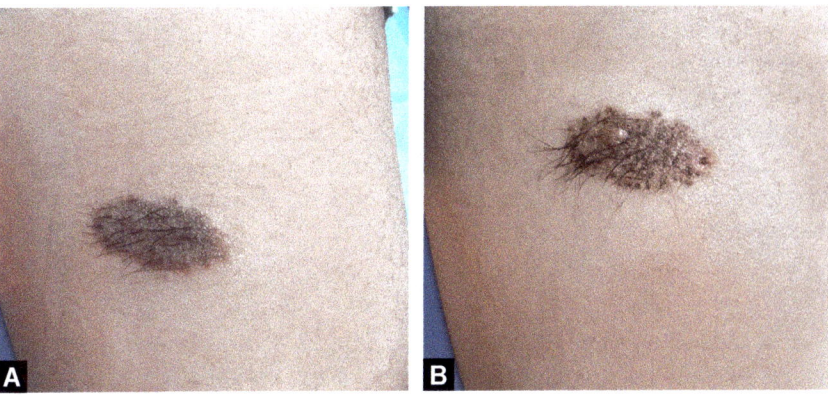

Figs. 3.9A and B: (A) Nevus spilus before treatment with Q-switched Nd:YAG; (B) During treatment with Q-switched Nd:YAG laser (532 nm).

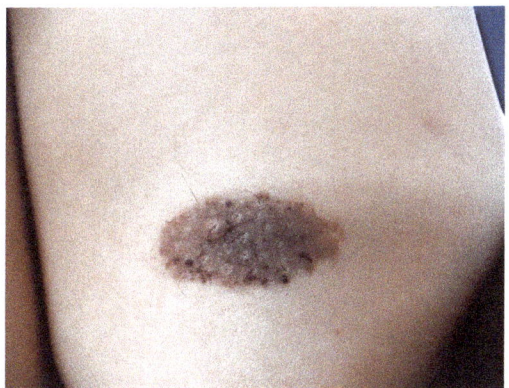

Fig. 3.9C: Post-treatment (after six sittings) improvement in the form of reduced pigmentations and smoothening of overlying skin, improvement of nevocellular component but persistence of CALM.

BIBLIOGRAPHY

1. Abecassis S, Spatz A, Cazeneuve C, et al. Melanoma within naevus spilus: 5 cases. Ann Dermatol Venereol. 2006;133:323-8.
2. Grevelink JM, Gonzalez S, Bonoan R, et al. Treatment of nevus spilus with the Q-switched Ruby laser. Dermatol Surg. 1997;23:365-9.
3. Tang M, Cheng Y, Yang C, et al. Nevus spilus: treatment with fractional CO_2 laser in combination with MedLite C6 laser: a preliminary study. Lasers Med Sci. 2017;32(7):1659-62.

Café-au-lait Macules

The lesions are easy to diagnose but remarkably difficult to treat. The pathology shows giant melanin granules. Laser modalities comprise the most widely used method to eradicate CALMs, and they include the use of pulsed dye, copper vapor, Q-switched, and erbium-doped YAG garnet lasers. The most widely used laser modality for the removal of CALMs is the QSNd:YAG (1064 nm) laser.

Although it is considered as being the most effective modality, only one-third of the reported cases demonstrated complete or nearly complete clearance, and a 24% recurrence at 4 months (on average) after laser treatment, has been reported as well.

Lasers Used

Q-switched lasers: QS Nd:YAG, QS ruby, and QS alexandrite lasers—Treatment of CALMs with lasers is minimally successful and often unpredictable (Figs. 3.10A to C). Temporary lightening or clearing can be achieved after multiple treatments. They frequently recur which is seen in up to 50% of lesions even

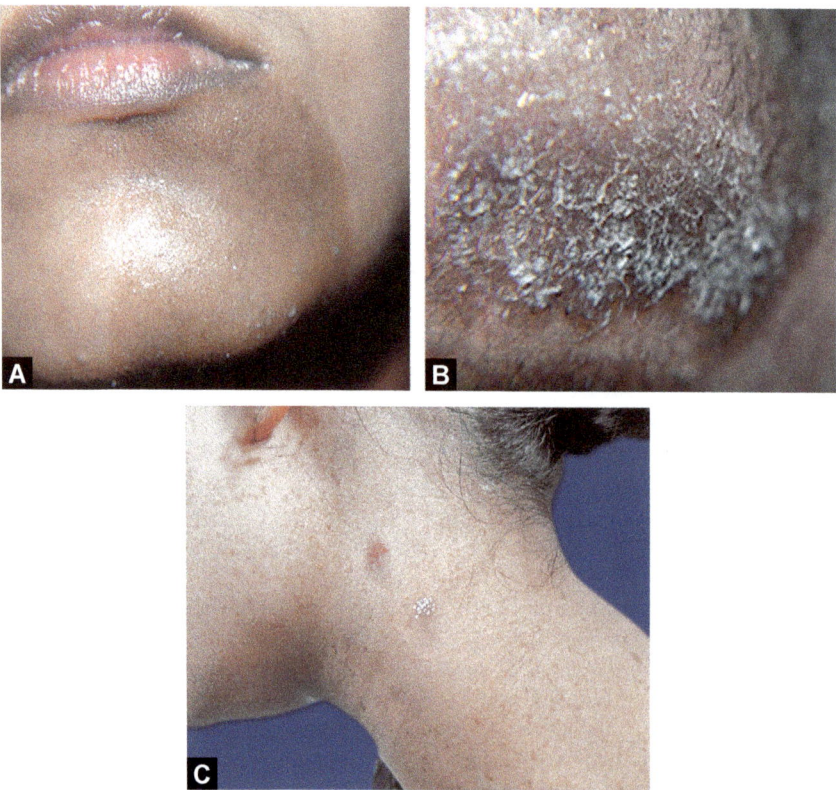

Figs. 3.10A to C: (A and B) Test spot for a CALM using an Nd:YAG 1064 nm. Note the whitening. A close-up reveals that the hair have also turned white. Thus shaving the area before attempting lasers intervention is a good idea to avoid competing laser absorption by the hair of the lesion; (C) A case of CALM, an initial test spot is given with the Qsw 1,064 nm for the upper part and 532 nm for the lower part of the lesion. The post laser sequelae will dictate the ideal laser (wavelength) to be used (2.5 J/cm^2).

when clearing is initially achieved. Treatment sessions are spaced at least 8 weeks apart and clearance requires at least 2–4 treatment sessions.

Among all lasers, Q-switched lasers yielded the most *variable* results with *high recurrence* rates, and paradoxical darkening has also been reported. In a study using a Q-switched 694 nm ruby laser and a Q-switched 532 nm Nd:YAG laser, it was found that the degree of clearance was highly variable. This is possibly as the QS lasers failed to remove the *follicular melanocytic* component of the café-au-lait macules (Grossman).

Picosecond laser: A recent study (Artzi O) used the picosecond 532 nm laser for CALM. Most patients experienced significant improvement and were highly satisfied with the results. They all reported excellent tolerance to the device and minimal pain, discomfort, and swelling which subsided shortly after treatment. The PS 532 laser demonstrated a higher clearance rate, a lower recurrence rate, and fewer and less severe side effects. These advantages might be related to the combined photoacoustic and photothermic effects of the PS laser. Its disadvantages are its relatively high cost.

Long pulse lasers: Longer pulsed alexandrite lasers have been used recently in hopes of decreasing the recurrence rate and also decreasing the number of treatment sessions required. It is possible that the longer pulse width allows for collateral thermal damage to nonpigment containing melanocytes.

Ablative lasers: Er:YAG can be used but as can fractional lasers, but again the results are disappointing.

Pearls/Pitfalls

1. Light-skinned patients are the ideal candidates for CALM removal, but recurrences, residual hyperpigmentation, and incomplete pigment removal are common.
2. CALMs may recur weeks to months after laser treatment, but are often responsive to retreatment; in other cases, they can recur years later or can be very resistant to treatment. The variable behavior of CALMs implies a subset of lesions with unique biologic behavior. Repigmentation may occur from normal melanocytes in the normal surrounding skin or from melanocytes that were inactive at the time of treatment.
3. Because the response of these lesions to laser treatment is unpredictable, it is advisable that a test spot be performed prior to treating the entire lesion.
4. One current approach is to use an LP pigment laser, such as normal mode ruby lasers (NMRL) or long pulse (LP) Alex laser without cooling, to target not only the epidermal melanocytes but also the *follicular melanocytes*. In doing so, the recurrence rate can be reduced.
5. The results with the picosecond may be better but an interesting observation is that the results may depend on the morphology of the lesion.

A study by Belkin DA used various lasers, including Q-switched ruby laser, Q-switched alexandrite and Nd:YAG. Only 1 lesion in each group was treated with a picosecond device alone. In a few cases, more than 1 type of laser was used.

Irregular bordered lesions were far more likely to achieve good or excellent clearance than smooth-bordered coast of California lesions. Furthermore, there was a trend toward higher risk of hypopigmentation in smooth-bordered lesions.

This study has implications beyond the morphology of CALM as this study used conventional Qs laser and found them to be as good as the pico laser.

In Indian skin, the results are disappointing. A combination of Er:YAG with a pigmented laser may be tried. The most important pearl is not to unnecessarily intervene and to forewarn the patient about the largely dismal response rate.

Level of Difficulty

Difficult.

BIBLIOGRAPHY

1. Artzi O, Mehrabi JN, Koren A, Niv R, Lapidoth M, Levi A. Picosecond 532-nm neodymium-doped yttrium aluminium garnet laser-a novel and promising modality for the treatment of café-au-lait macules. Lasers Med Sci; 2017.
2. Alora MB, Arndt KA. Successful treatment of a café-au-lait macule with the erbium:YAG laser. J Am Acad Dermatol. 2001;45(4):566-8.
3. Belkin DA, Neckman JP, Jeon H, et al. Response to Laser Treatment of Café au Lait Macules Based on Morphologic Features. JAMA Dermatol. 2017;153(11): 1158-61.
4. Grossman MC, Anderson RR, Farinelli W, et al. Treatment of cafe au lait macules with lasers. A clinicopathologic correlation. Arch Dermatol. 1995;131:1416-20.
5. Levy JL, Mordon S, Pizzi-Anselme M. Treatment of individual café au lait macules with the Q-switched Nd:YAG: a clinicopathologic correlation. J Cutan Laser Ther. 1999;1(4):217-23.
6. Polder KD, Landau JM, Vergilis-Kalner IJ, et al. Laser eradication of pigmented lesions: A review. Dermatol Surg. 2011;37(5):572-95. doi: 10.1111/j.1524-4725.2011.01971.x.
7. Shah S, Alster TS. Laser treatment of dark skin: An updated review. Am J Clin Dermatol. 2010;11(6):389-97.

Ephelides (Freckles)

These are hyperpigmented small macules located on sun-exposed skin and become darker in the summer and lighter in the winter. There is no increase in the number of melanocytes on pathology, but there is an increase in melanin.

Lasers Used

Ephelides respond well to Q-switched laser treatment (Figs. 3.11A to C).

Level of Difficulty

Easy.

Seborrheic Keratoses

These respond better to pulsed CO_2 lasers and Er:YAG as the results are much faster than Q-switched lasers and a single session is enough in most cases.

In general, thinner seborrheic keratoses respond better to laser treatment than thick lesions with Q-switched lasers.

Level of Difficulty

Easy.

Becker's Nevus

Becker's nevus is a hyperpigmented, hair-bearing plaque that most commonly occurs on the upper trunk or shoulder of males. These lesions may also be associated with a dermal smooth muscle hamartoma.

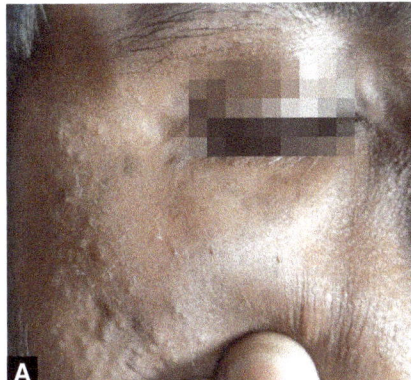
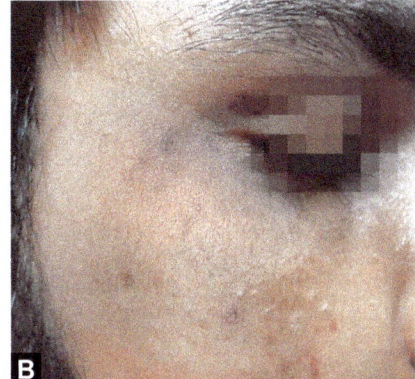
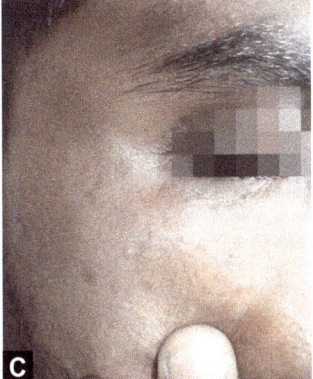

Figs. 3.11A to C: (A) Freckles near the outer canthus before Q-switched Nd:YAG; (B) During treatment with 532 nm Q-Switched Nd:YAG; (C) Post-treatment with near total clearance with Q-switched Nd:YAG.

Lasers Used

As the lesion has **three** components: the hair, the pigmented cells and a dermal component, three lasers are ideally used in *sequence* (Figs. 3.12A to E). Treatment sessions should be spaced 8–12 weeks apart and 3–5 treatment sessions are usually necessary.

Principle: The chromophore that must be targeted in its treatment is melanin. The fine clumping of melanin granules in the epidermis requires shorter pulse widths (nanosecond domain), than the larger hair follicles, which typically respond best to the millisecond pulse widths used in hair removal lasers.

Hypertrichotic BN treated with only pigment-specific QS lasers have demonstrated unsatisfactory long-term remission likely due to follicle-

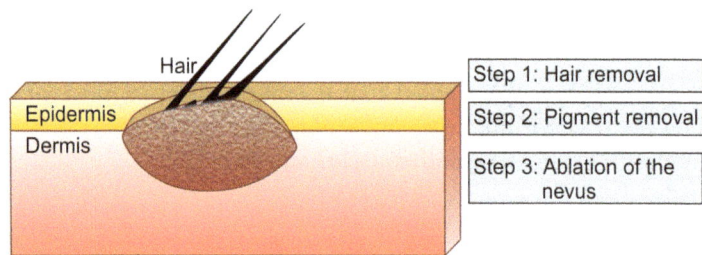

Fig. 3.12A: Steps involved in treatment of Becker's nevi. A figurative depiction of Becker's nevus and the combination of lasers needed for optimal therapy.

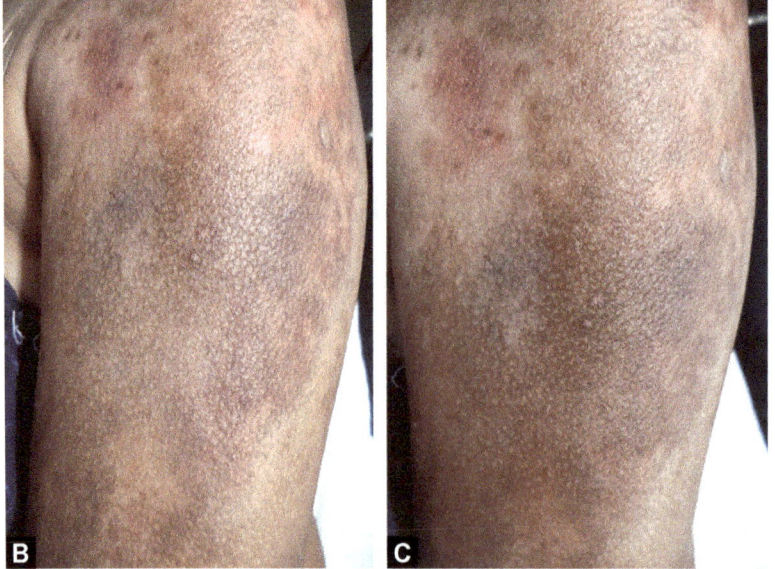

Figs. 3.12B and C: Becker's nevus. Little response after multiple sessions of Q Sw Nd:YAG 1064 nm.

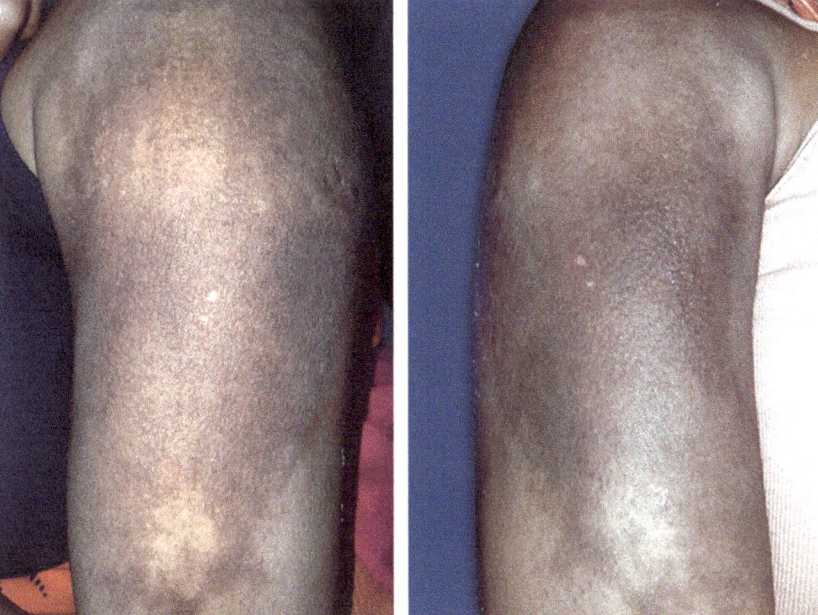

Fig. 3.12D: Becker's nevus after 8 sittings with Q-switched Nd:YAG (532 nm), incomplete removal.

derived repigmentation. Several studies have also demonstrated variable efficacy with monotherapy laser hair removal using LP alexandrite (LPAL), normal-mode ruby laser (NMRL), and diode lasers which is likely due to inadequate evacuation of dermal and epidermal pigment.

Studies evaluating QS lasers for the treatment of BN have produced variable results and high recurrence rates.

1. Q-switched ruby, Q-switched Nd: YAG, and 1,550 nm fractional erbium-doped fiber laser. Of the QS lasers, the ruby is slightly more effective than the Nd: YAG. The hyperpigmented component of Becker's nevi respond similarly to laser treatment for CALMs. Our experience though is not as heartening (Figs. 3.12B to D) and frequent recurrences (within 6–12 months) and PIH is seen.
2. The terminal hairs can be removed with the hair removal lasers. This can be followed by a Q-switched or fractional laser.
3. Often a Er:YAG laser is used, which though is not specific for the pigment can remove or reduce the extent of the lesion. Clinical evaluation at 2 years after treatment with the Er:YAG laser showed complete clearance (100%) in 54% of the patients (n = 6) and clearance of more than 50% in 100% of the subjects and was superior to Q-switched lasers (Trelles M). We have used the Er:YAG with satisfactory results (Fig. 3.12E).

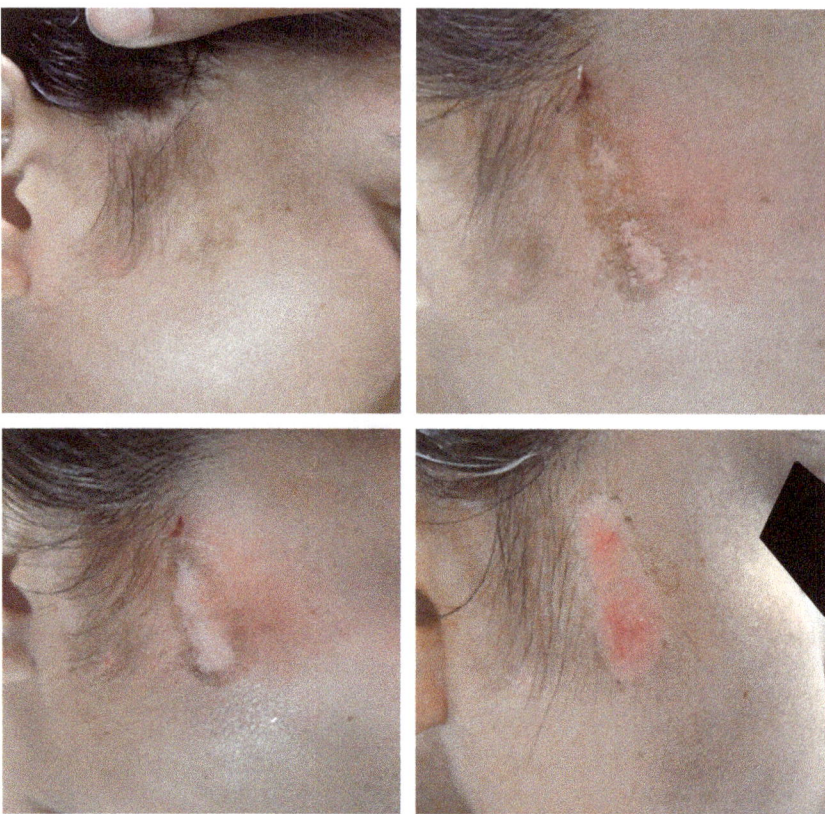

Fig. 3.12E: Becker's nevi (nonhypertrichotic): This case was treated with Er:YAG laser as here fine and accurate ablation is the requirement with minimal thermal damage. The almost "butter knife" like ablation seen in the second photo (top right) is followed by a complete and clean removal of the epidermis. The third photograph (lower left) reveals the papillary dermis. A good healing at 3 weeks.

4. Two male patients with Becker's nevi were treated with the 1,550 nm wavelength erbium-doped fiber laser 6–10 mJ at 4 weeks intervals with 5–6 treatment sessions. More than 75% of the pigment had faded by 1 month in both patients. There was no improvement in hypertrichosis (Glaich AS).

Pearls/Pitfalls

It should be understood that a combination of lasers is useful and even after this also a complete response may not be seen. This author (Kabir Sardana) routinely uses a combination of fine ablation with Er:YAG (5 J/cm^2, 2 passes) followed by Q-switched Nd:YAG (1,064 nm).

The long pulsed alexandrite laser offers the best possibility for more permanent clearing of both the pigmentation and the increased hair growth. Settings are similar to CALM for the surrounding pigment and the hair removal lasers are used at their appropriate settings for hair color and shaft size (Nanni CA).

But the treatment of ethnic patients with Q-switched lasers, LPAL, NMRL, and ablative lasers may further induce undesired scarring, and hypo- or hyperpigmentation.

As a thumb rule, *hypetrichotic BN are the most difficult to treat* (**Also *see* Chapter 4: Fractional Photothermolysis**).

Level of Difficulty

Difficult. Monotherapy with Q-switched laser has disheartening results in most cases.

BIBLIOGRAPHY

1. Glaich AS, Goldberg LH, Dai T, et al. Fractional resurfacing: a new therapeutic modality for Becker's nevus. Arch Dermatol. 2007;143:1488-9.
2. Lapidoth M, Adatto M, Cohen S, et al. Hypertrichosis in Becker's nevus: effective low-fluence laser hair removal. Lasers Med Sci. 2014;29(1):191-3.
3. Nanni CA, Alster TS. Treatment of a Becker's nevus using a 694-nm long-pulsed ruby laser. Dermatol Surg. 1998;24:1032-4.
4. Trelles MA, Allones I, Moreno-Arias GA, et al. Becker's naevus: a comparative study between erbium: YAG and Q-switched neodymium:YAG; clinical and histopathological findings. Br J Dermatol. 2005;152(2):308-13.

DERMAL DISORDERS

Q-switched lasers have revolutionized the treatment of dermal pigmented lesions including: melanocytic nevi, nevus of Ota, and melasma. But it must be appreciated that as a *thumb rule*, **deeper the pathology, slower the results**.

The Q-switched ruby, alexandrite and 1,064 nm Nd:YAG are the most commonly used lasers. All of these lasers are still within the absorption spectrum of melanin yet also have wavelengths that are long enough to penetrate into the dermis. Broadband light sources (such as IPL) lack wavelength specificity and have longer (ms range rather than nanosecond range) pulse durations, making them unsuitable for treating dermal pigmented lesions.

We have developed a simple tool to modify the lasers used in accordance with the condition. Thus, if the target particle is large, a millisecond or microsecond laser can be used with equally good results. This principle is used in in removing the acquired melanocyte nevus, where a Er:YAG or pulsed CO_2 can have excellent results if used properly.

Acquired Melanocytic Nevi (Moles)

These are classified into junctional, dermal and compound types depending on the site of nevus cells. The acquired melanocytic nevi (AMN) is a useful condition to understand the principle of combination of lasers, thus we will dwell on it in detail.

Lasers Used

The lasers used for CAMN range from pigment-selective lasers to ablative lasers. The use of lasers in CAMN (moles) is complicated by many practical issues and scenarios which have to be properly understood before attempting this mode of therapy (Fig. 3.13).

Principles of Therapy

Like any other indication, the use of lasers in pigmented lesions begins at the helm of laser physics and depends on the absorption spectra of the target chromophore, which is believed to be the melanocyte (melanosome). The spectrum of laser wavelength used ranges from the green lasers [(pulsed dye, Q-switched)], and neodymium (Nd):yttrium aluminum garnet (Nd:YAG) 532) to the far-infrared lasers [(CO_2 10,600 nm and erbium (Er):YAG 2,940 nm)]. Except for the ablative lasers, the rest are strongly absorbed by melanin.

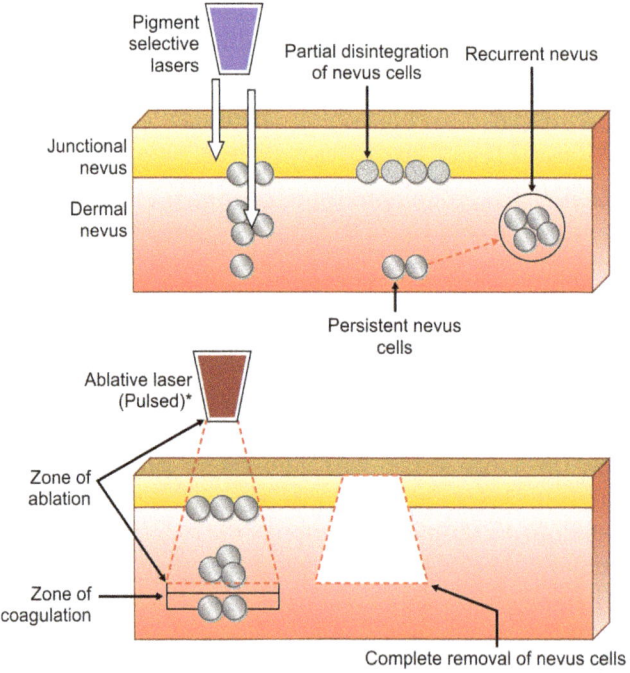

*Er:YAG (200–300 μs, pulse duration)/ultrapulse CO_2 (<1 ms, pulse duration)

Fig. 3.13: Effect of pigment selective and ablative lasers in removal and recurrence of melanocytic nevi. A properly used ablative lasers may achieve excellent results with minimal recurrence.
Source: Sardana K, et al. Optimal management of common acquired melanocytic nevi (moles): current perspectives. Clin Cosmet Investig Dermatol. 2014;7:89-103.

The second important proviso is to minimize heat damage, which requires optimal setting of the pulse duration of the laser. A laser with a pulse duration less or equal to the thermal relaxation time (TRT) of the target tissue should be employed. This, in turn, depends on the size of the target tissue which dictates TRT. This ranges from 0.25 μs to 1.00 μs for the melanosome to 0.1 ms (100 μs) for the melanocyte. Although the nanosecond lasers (Qsw) have been conventionally used to treat pigmented lesions, the same principle cannot apply to CAMN. The geometry (and therefore, the microscopic characteristics) of the lesion is important, and as the nevus is composed of melanocytes in aggregates (collectively of a size of 100 μm in diameter) this corresponds to a TRT of about 10 ms, thus accounting for the use of normal mode (ms) and far-infrared lasers to treat CAMN.

The third requirement is to achieve an adequate depth to target the chromophore for which the red (ruby 694 nm, alexandrite 755 nm) (and near-infrared Qsw Nd:YAG 1,064 nm) lasers (approximately 600–1,100 nm) are ideal.

Based on these three principles, the devices useful for treating melanocytic lesions are of **two basic classes**: infrared skin resurfacing lasers and pulsed lasers/IPL lasers (Fig. 3.14).

The pulsed lasers are further divided into long-pulse (ms) devices, which tend to target relatively large pigmented structures such as hair follicles and "nests" of nevus cells, and short-pulse (Qsw ns lasers) devices, which are capable of targeting individual pigmented cells.

Histologically, CAMN have both isolated nevomelanocyte cells, and "nests," or clusters, of cells. Thus, a mixture of lasers targeting both should ideally be used, with the use of short (ns) pulses and long (ms) pulses. This is the reason why melanocytic nevi are better treated with a combination of lasers or just ablative lasers.

Clinical Experience and Principles

A side-by-side comparison of QS alexandrite (755 nm, 100 ns, 3 mm, and 6.0 J/cm^2) and the Nd:YAG (1,064 nm, 10 ns, 3 mm, 6.0 J/cm^2) lasers for treatment of benign acquired melanocytic nevi with a fluence of 6.0 J/cm^2 and a 3 mm spot size was done to opposite halves of a large (1.5 cm) or to two small (0.7 mm) adjacent nevi (Rosenbach A). After one treatment, 10% lightening was noted for both lasers whereas after three treatments, more lightening was observed after alexandrite (60%) than after Nd:YAG (30%) laser treatment possibly explained by the more superficial location of the target melanosomes (i.e. at the dermal–epidermal junction) in common-acquired melanocytic nevi, as compared to nevus of Ota, which respond better to the longer and deeper penetrating wavelength of the QS Nd:YAG (1,064 nm) laser.

Thus, some basic principles can be used to treat acquired melanocytic nevi:
1. Lighter nevi respond best to shorter wavelengths that maximize melanin absorption, while darker nevi typically respond to any wavelength within the melanin absorption spectrum. Multiple treatments are frequently necessary for optimal lightening. Clinical lightening is also associated

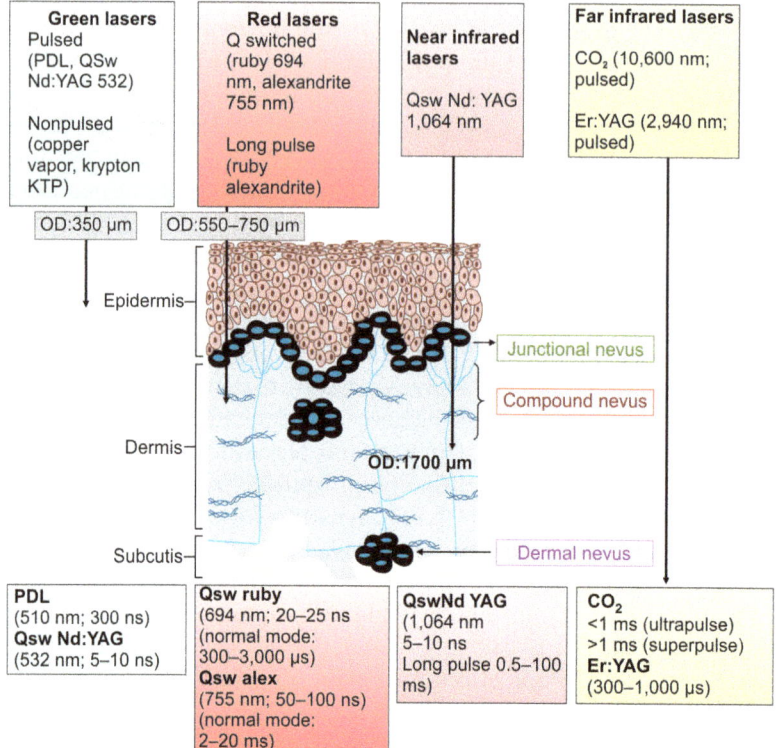

Fig. 3.14: An overview of different lasers used for moles and their parameters and depth of penetration.

with the development of a subtle microscopic scar up to 1 mm thick that obscures residual nevus cells.
2. The goal of complete resolution is difficult in most cases and recurrence after laser treatment is common. This is as there may be persistence of nevus cells containing little pigment located in the deeper dermis that are shielded from laser radiation by the more pigmented superficial cells.
3. Long pulsed lasers (alexandrite, diode) have been shown to more effectively eradicate these nevi in fewer treatment sessions, using fluences of 40–60J/cm^2, and 8- to 12-mm spot sizes.
4. Deep dermal nevi and thick moles do not respond to the Q-switched laser. The short pulsed Er:YAG laser is useful in such cases (5.2–14 J/cm^2) (Baba M).
5. Ablative lasers are an useful tool and more effective (*see* **Chapter 2: Ablative Lasers**).

Protocol Used (Flowchart 3.1)

As shown in the Figure 3.14, there is little advantage in using conventional nanosecond lasers as there is a high chance of recurrence. But if employed,

Flowchart 3.1: An algorithm depicting the role of various lasers in the treatment of acquired benign melanocytic nevi (Sardana K, 2014).

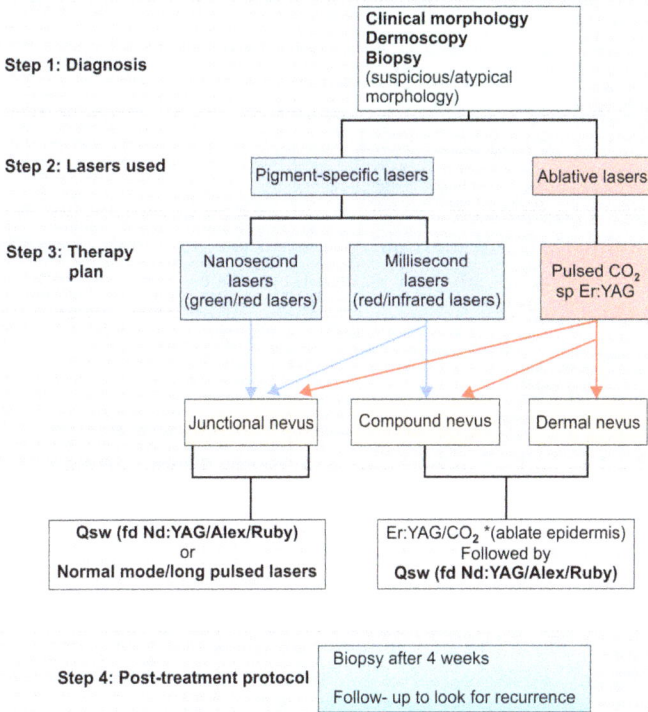

the chance of recurrence is to be expected. Good pulsed laser due to the added coagulative effect has better results.

1. The logic employed in the use of combination lasers (normal mode and Q-switched ruby laser, CO_2 and Q-switched alexandrite, CO_2 and Q-switched frequency-doubled Nd:YAG laser, CO_2 and Q-switched ruby laser) is to expose the otherwise unaffected, deep-sited nevomelanocytes to the pigment-specific laser.
2. Nevus cells in the superficial dermis are additionally removed by the CO_2 laser.
3. Alternatively, for a smaller "mole" (1.5 cm), a short-pulsed Er:YAG would be an ideal tool, as apart from the pulse duration (300–1,000 µs) the Er:YAG laser has a predictable depth (5 µm/J/cm^2), minimal thermal damage (20–30 µm), and a high absorption coefficient of water (Er:YAG 12,800 cm^{-1}; CO_2 800 cm^{-1}), and is thus capable of a far finer and safer superficial ablation, with minimal sequelae. A comparison of various modalities at our center revealed that the combined or pulsed ablative method is better than using the Q-switched lasers for CAMN.

Pearls/Pitfalls

1. The use of a laser is to be reserved for benign nevomelanocytic lesions exhibiting little to no atypia. If any doubt exists about the clinical diagnosis, a biopsy should be performed prior to laser treatment.
2. Use a laser depending on the pathology. In our experience, pigment specific laser requires more sessions while an ablative laser requires 1–2 sessions.
3. A biopsy is useful in case of recurrence or atypia.
4. Compound and intradermal nevi are best treated by radiofrequency, ablative lasers or surgical excision whereas in junctional nevi, the response is variable.

BIBLIOGRAPHY

1. Baba M, Bal N. Efficacy and safety of the short-pulse erbium:YAG laser in the treatment of acquired melanocytic nevi. Dermatol Surg. 2006;32:256-60.
2. Duke D, Byers R, Sober AJ, et al. Treatment of benign and atypical nevi with the normal-mode ruby laser and the Q-switched ruby laser: Clinical improvement but failure to completely eliminate nevomelanocytes. Arch Dermatol. 1999;135:290-6.
3. Rosenbach A, Williams CM, Alster TS. Comparison of the Q-switched alexandrite (755 nm) and Q-switched Nd:YAG (1064 nm) lasers in the treatment of benign melanocytic nevi. Dermatol Surg. 1997;23:239-45.
4: Sardana K, Chakravarty P, Goel K. Optimal management of common acquired melanocytic nevi (moles): Current perspectives. Clin Cosmet Investig Dermatol. 2014;7:89-103. eCollection 2014. Review.
5. Vibhagool C, Byers R, Grevelink JM. Treatment of small nevomelanocytic nevi with a Q-switched ruby laser. J Am Acad Dermatol. 1997;36:738-41.

Congenital Melanocytic Nevi

The variable depth of the nevus cells, concomitant presence of hair in a majority of cases and epidermal changes makes the results of lasers erratic and unpredictable.

Although Q-switched lasers may effectively lighten congenital nevi, there is frequently *repigmentation* due to persistence of nevus cells within the deeper reticular dermis and within adnexae (Grevelink JM). There is a greater clearance with a Q-switched and normal-mode ruby laser (NMRL) than in NMRL alone. In theory, *millisecond-domain* pulses are more appropriate than Q-switched pulses for treating thick lesions such as congenital nevi because they produce less selective thermal damage, destroying entire nests of cells rather than individual pigmented cells.

Lasers Used

Although Q-switched lasers may effectively lighten congenital nevi, there is frequently repigmentation due to persistence of nevus cells within the deeper reticular dermis and within adnexae.

Combination of Lasers

Pigment laser: The use of a Q-switched ruby laser followed immediately, or 2 weeks later, by a normal-mode ruby laser (NMRL) can lead to a 52% visible decrease in pigment without complete histologic clearance (Duke et al.). The short- and long-term histologic findings of congenital nevi that have been treated with an NMRL indicate that subtle microscopic scars reaching 1 mm in diameter are frequent which cover the underlying nevus cells, leading to cosmetic improvement (Imaya S).

Better cosmetic result has been reported by first using an NMRL to remove the epidermis, followed immediately by multiple passes with a Q-switched ruby laser (Kono). This approach for allows the effective removal of the epidermis and enables a greater degree of penetration by the QS ruby, of which multiple passes further enhance the clinical efficacy.

Ablative lasers with pigment lasers: Combinations of pulsed CO_2 and Er:YAG or with Q-switched lasers have been used. The principle being that the ablative laser removes the bulk of the tissue, but being nonspecific for the pigment, the pigment specific laser is then used to target the nevus cells. Compared with macular congenital melanocytic nevi (CMN), mammillated CMN show a marginally better response to laser treatment. Also CMN on the limbs respond poorly (August PJ).

Surgical excision followed by Er:YAG: The basic principle is a surgical/shave excision followed by Er:YAG. This method is "blind" as the Er:YAG has affinity for water and not the pigmented nevus cells.

Pearls/Pitfalls

As congenital nevi have the potential to transform into malignant melanoma, and residual nevus cells persist in the dermis after laser treatment, cautious long-term follow-up of nevi treated with lasers is required. A recent study has examined the comparison of lasers versus surgical excision and found that surgical excision gives better results for small to medium CMN (Lim JM). When choosing a treatment option, location seemed to be an important factor, possibly because better cosmetic results are more important to the patient when the lesion is located on easily exposed areas. Excision followed by pigment-specific laser was likely to be chosen for females, smaller lesions, and lesions on the face. Just monotherapy with laser leads to incomplete removal and recurrences.

Thus, lasers should be restricted small and medium-sized CMN (Figs. 3.15 and 3.16). But as there are very few RCT in literature and the complexities of surgical excision does not eliminate the nevus cells or the risk of melanoma, a close regular follow-up should be the aim.

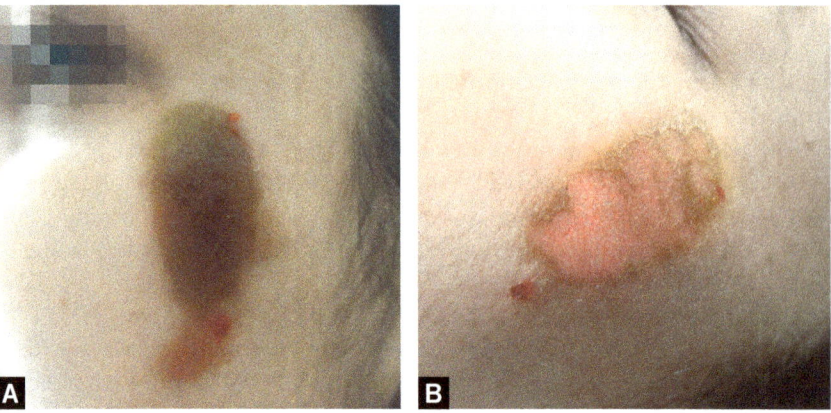

Figs. 3.15A and B: A case of CMN on the face: Ablation with Er:YAG laser (3.5 J/cm^2) the end point being fine bleeding that indicates level of papillary dermis.

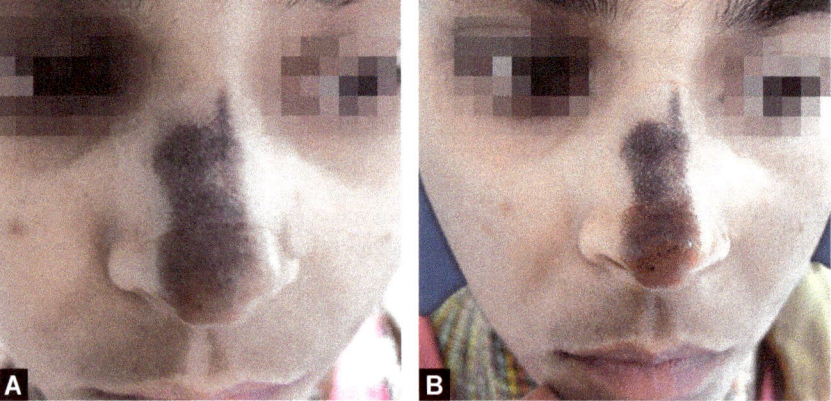

Figs. 3.16A and B: A case of CMN. A test spot was attempted in the distal aspect of the lesion, there was prompt recurrence and the procedure was aborted (Er:YAG), highlighting the importance of a test spot.

BIBLIOGRAPHY

1. Al-Hadithy N, Al-Nakib K, Quaba A. Outcomes of 52 patients with congenital melanocytic naevi treated with UltraPulse carbon dioxide and frequency doubled Q-Switched Nd-YAG laser. J Plast Reconstr Aesthet Surg. 2012;65(8):1019-28.
2. August PJ, Ferguson JE, Madan V. A study of the efficacy of carbon dioxide and pigment-specific lasers in the treatment of medium-sized congenital melanocytic naevi. Br J Dermatol. 2011;164(5):1037-42.
3. Duke D, Byers HR, Sober AJ, et al. Treatment of benign and atypical nevi with the normal-mode ruby laser and the Q-switched ruby laser: Clinical improvement but failure to completely eliminate nevomelanocytes. Arch Dermatol. 1999;135:290-6.

4. Grevelink JM, van Leeuwen RL, Anderson RR, et al. Clinical and histological responses of congenital melanocytic nevi after single treatment with Q-switched lasers. Arch Dermatol. 1997;133:349-53.
5. Imayama S, Ueda S. Long- and short-term histological observations of congenital nevi treated with the normal-mode ruby laser. Arch Dermatol. 1999;135:1211-8.
6. Kono T, Nozaki M, Chan HH, et al. Combined use of normal mode and Q-switched ruby lasers in the treatment of congenital melanocytic naevi. Br J Plast Surg. 2001;54:640-3.
7. Lim JM, Oh Y, Lee SH, et al. Comparison of treatment options for small to medium congenital melanocytic nevi: A retrospective review of 119 cases. Lasers Surg Med. 2018 Oct 30. doi: 10.1002/lsm.23030.
8. Lim JY, Jeong Y, Whang KK. A combination of dual-mode 2,940 nm Er:YAG laser. Ann Dermatol. 2009;21(2):120-4.

Melasma

It is said that "a medical condition with no cure, has many treatments". While in medicine, common cold is a classic example, in dermatology, this honor can be safely bestowed upon, melasma. Every possible intervention from triple combination (TC) creams, peels to lasers have been tried, but as is the universal experience, probably, TC creams with form the mainstay of therapy. Even with TC creams, transient results have been seen for the epidermal subtype, but dermal melasma and the mixed type which constitute the majority of patients in pigmented skin are difficult to treat.

Two recent reviews aptly summarize the present evidence on melasma. The use of lasers for the treatment of melasma cannot be recommended, due to unpredictable safety and efficacy, time-limited clinical improvement, and no clear benefit over conventional treatments. Thus, probably melasma is nature's way to compensate for the high ambient UV flux in tropical countries and any method to remove it would probably lead to indifferent results and rapid recurrence. Though we have no experience in treating fair skin types, in darkly pigmented skin melasma should **not** be a favored indication for laser therapy.

Lasers Used

Pigment specific and pico lasers: "Laser toning" involves the use of large spot size, and a low-fluence, Q-switched 1,064-nm Nd:YAG laser (6–8 mm spot size, 1.6–2.3 J/cm^2). The results, without any additional therapy, are variable even in fairer skin types, with a large number of cases, reporting mottled depigmentation. In our patients, a high degree of disconcerting hyperpigmentation has been noted (Figs. 3.17 to 3.19).

Here it must be emphasized that laser toning is a complex concept and if the correct machine and settings are done, good results have been seen (See section on Laser Toning). But it is relevant to point out that a study from Korea (Won KH) where a split face comparison was made between fractional

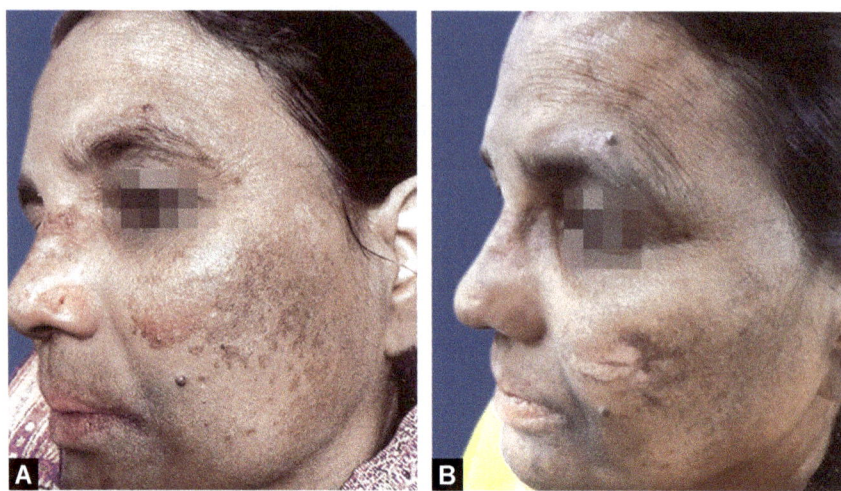

Figs. 3.17A and B: Perils of laser toning, depigmentation following therapy in melasma. *Courtesy:* Dr Shilpa Garg, New Delhi.

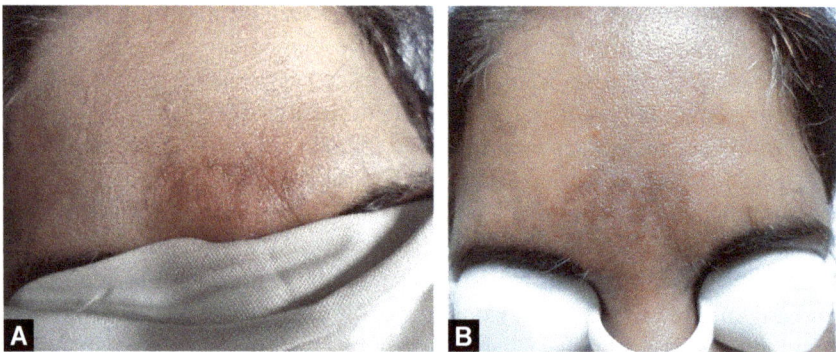

Figs. 3.18A and B: (A) Melasma before treatment; (B) Six sitting after laser toning with Q-switched Nd:YAG (1064 nm).

Nd:YAG 1064 nm versus conventional setting found EQUAL results on both sides. Here please note Korean skin is much "fairer" than our skin. The settings used were laser toning in three passes with a fluence of 1.5 J/cm^2 for fractional 1064-nm QSNY and a fluence of 2.0 J/cm^2 for conventional 1064-nm QSNY to obtain a total energy of approximately 750 mJ per pulse.

Fractional lasers: The principles of laser therapy involve a pertinent target (melanocytes in melasma), appropriate wavelength and the right pulse duration. The fractional lasers are selective for water and their pulse duration is in milliseconds unlike the microsecond TRT of melanocyte making them intrinsically inappropriate in melasma. This coupled with the fact that only a

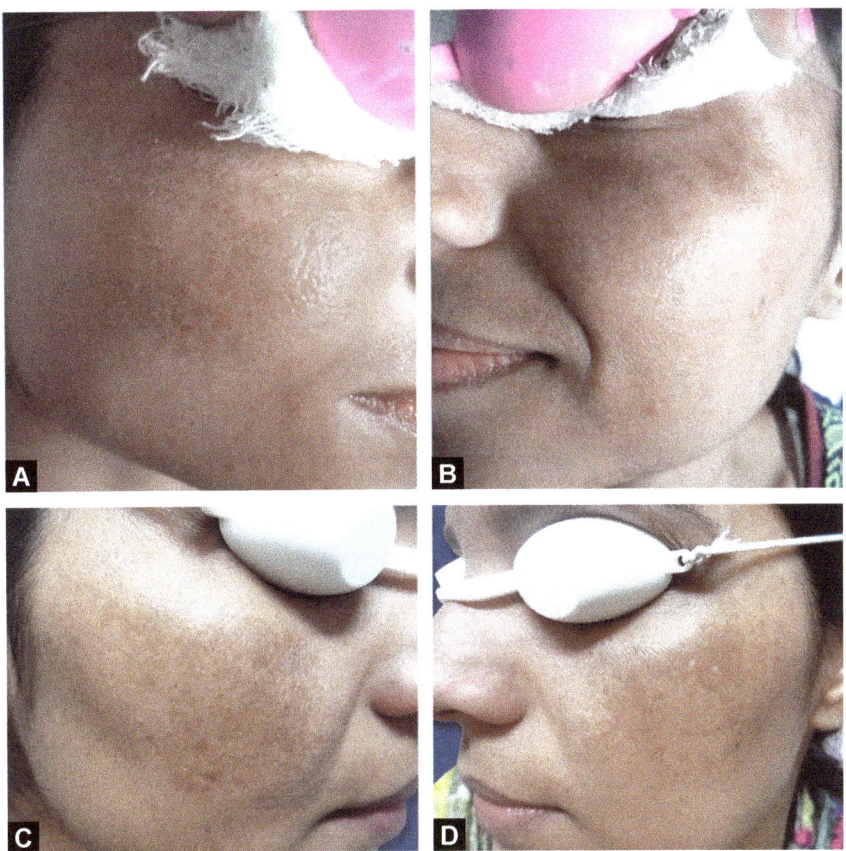

Figs. 3.19A to D: (A and B) Melasma before treatment with Q-switched ND:YAG; (C and D) After 12 sittings with laser toning (1064 nm, at 2 weeks interval).

"fraction" of the skin is damaged, makes the technology inherently ineffective for melasma (Fig. 3.20). Fractionated laser treatment may work by expelling columns of microscopic epidermal debris that contains melanin but is probably insufficient to make a clinical difference. The data suggests a high rate of repigmentation and sometimes even an increase in pigmentation after the treatment makes it a risky option in a pigmented skin.

On the contrary, if a fractional, pigment specific laser is used the results are better, as seen by the results of the fractional *ruby* laser (Figs. 3.21A to F) and probably the fractional *thulium* laser.

Intense pulsed light: In our opinion, there is little practical use in using this technology for melasma.

Er:YAG: A low fluence (1-2 J/cm^2) Erbium peel has been tried but again is inadvisable in pigmented skin. We have used it with unfavorable results.

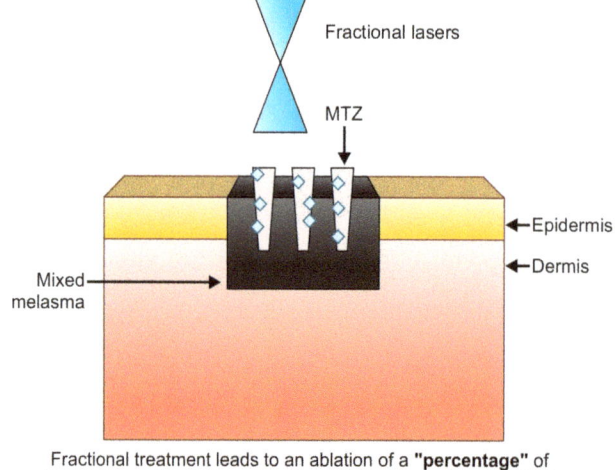
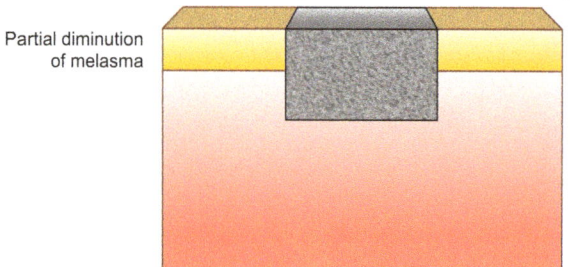

Fig. 3.20: The mode of action of fractional lasers in melasma.
Source: Sardana K, Garg VK. Lasers are not effective for melasma in darkly pigmented skin. J Cutan Aesthet Surg. 2014;7(1):57-60.

Literature Review

An overview of the literature (Table 3.4) reveals certain salient facts that should have a sobering effect on the unbridled enthusiasm of laser practitioners who use this therapy for melasma specially in pigmented skin.

1. *Evaluation (Objective versus subjective)*: It must be emphasized that melasma area and severity index (MASI) is a highly subjective tool and the use of this and the often used percentile scoring is never of any practical use as the improvement does not mirror the actual clinical results.
2. The pigment in the epidermis alters the laser physics dynamics especially in pigmented skin accounting for the variable results. Also the pigment in melasma is not homogeneous either in distribution or depth and studies have to be structured to account for a similar type of melasma (epidermal/dermal or mixed).

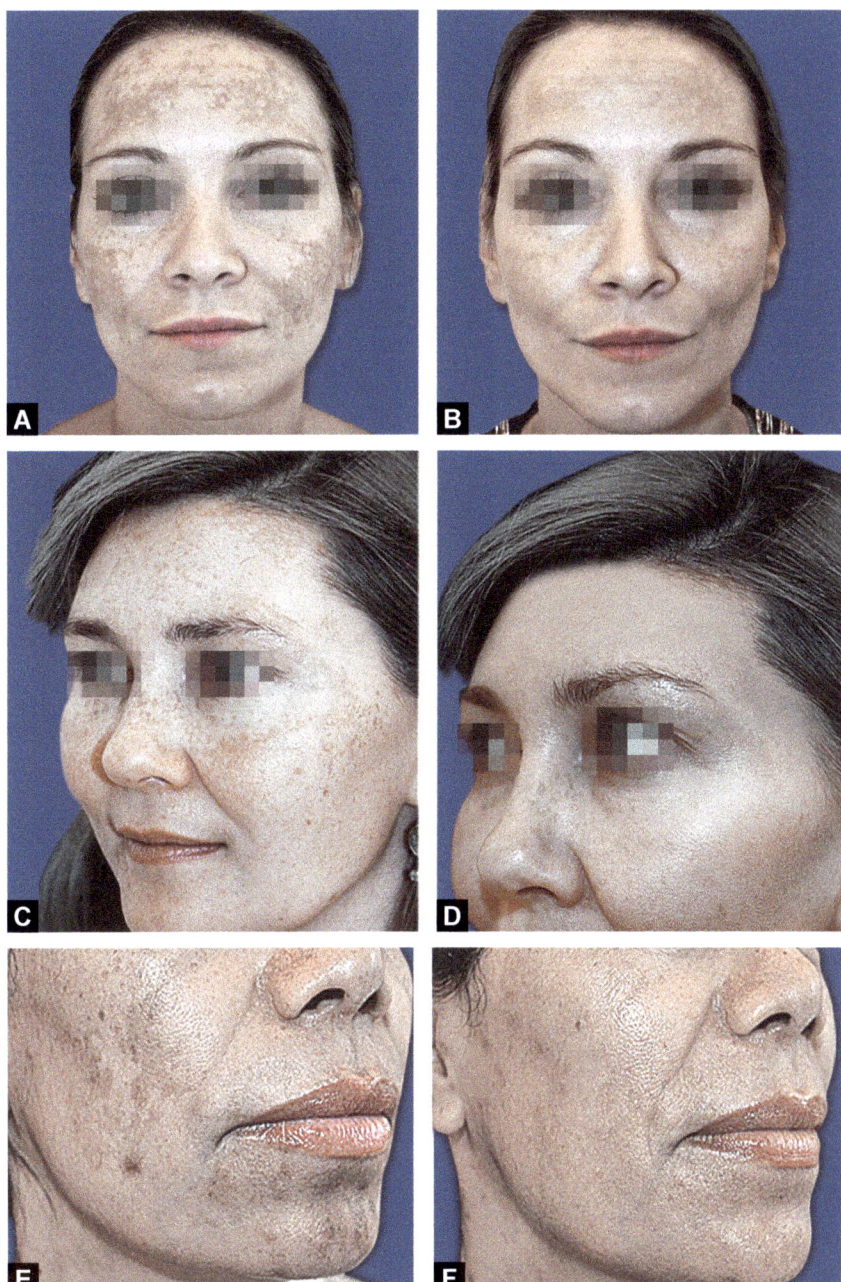

Figs. 3.21A to F: A series of patients treated by the fractional mode Q-switched ruby laser tattoo star for melasma.
Courtesy: Asclepion laser technologies GmbH.

Table 3.4: Chronological summary of the salient work on lasers and their combinations in melasma.

Author	Therapy	Demography	Trial	Dosages	Assess	Results
Monotherapy						
Polder KD et al., 2012	Fractional thulium laser (1,927 nm)	14 patients	O	10–20 mJ, 6–8 passes, 3–4 sessions/4 weekly	Blinded physician and patient assessment (subjective)	51% decrease in MASI at 1 month follow-up ($p < 0.05$)
Zhou X et al., 2011	Qsw Nd:YAG 1,064 nm	50 patients FP IV-VI	O	2.5–3.4 J/cm², Spot size: 6 mm, 9 sessions/weekly	MASI, Melanin Index	Mean decrease in MI by 35.8% ($p < 0.001$) MASI decreased by 61.3% ($p < 0.001$) 70% had >50% clearance
Jang WS et al., 2011	Fractional Qsw 694 nm ruby laser	15 Korean patients Dermal/mixed melasma	O	6 sessions at 2 weeks interval	MASI, skin reflectance	Mean decrease in MASI 15.1 to 10.6. Skin reflectance increase from 56.6 to 59.9
Suh KS et al., 2011	Low dose Nd:YAG 1,064 nm	23 Korean patients FP III-V	O	2–4 J/cm², Spot size: 4,6,8 mm, 10 sessions (once/week)	MASI satisfaction index	Mean MASI decreased significantly even at 3 month f/u visit
Chan NP et al., 2010	Low fluence Qsw Nd:YAG (1,064 nm)	5 Asian patients	CS	1.6–3.5 J/cm², Spot size: 6–8 mm, 6–50 sessions (22.67)	UV photographic images	All patients failed to show improvement in melasma
Choi M et al., 2010	Low dose 1 Qsw Nd:YAG (1,064 nm)	20 patients FP-III-IV	O	2.0–3.5 J/cm², Spot size: 6 mm, 5 sessions at weekly interval	Mexameter, cutometer, chromameter, corneometer, visiometer	L value increased and melanin index decreased

Contd...

Contd...

Author	Therapy	Demography	Trial	Dosages	Assess	Results
Sardana K* et al.	IPL Er:YAG AFR (Er:YAG) NAFR (Er:Glass) Qsw Nd:YAG	3 IPL 2 Er:YAG 7 AFR 1 NAFR 2 Nd:YAG	O	22 J/cm^2 5 J/cm^2 90 J/cm^2 70 mJ/mb 5–6 J/cm^2	MASI percentile score	The results with AFR, NAFR and IPL were disappointing with Er:YAG and Qsw Nd:YAG temporary
Combination therapy						
Kauvar AN, 2012	Microderm abrasion with Qsw Nd:YAG with HQ and sunscreens	27 female patients FP II-IV Mixed resistant melasma	O	1.6–2.0 J/cm^2/4 weeks Average no. of sessions–2.6.	Blinded comparison of digital photographs using quartile system (Subjective)	40% patients achieved >95% clearance 81% patients achieved >75% clearance Remission lasted 6 months
Park KY et al, 2011	1,064 nm Qsw Nd:YAG Laser with 30% GA peels Vs laser monotherapy	16 patients Mixed melasma	RCT SF	Laser: 2.0–2.3 J/cm^2, 6 mm spotsize 6 sessions (once/week) GA peels: 3 sessions (once/2 weeks)	Mexameter mMASI	Combined therapy 32.6% improvement with mexameter and 37.4% in mMASI Vs 22% and 16.7%, respectively by laser alone ($p < 0.05$)
Wattanakrai P et al., 2010	Qsw Nd:YAG with 2% HQ vs 2% HQ	22 patients Dermal/mixed melasma/ FP II–IV	RCT SF	3.0–3.8 J/cm^2 Spot size: 6 mm 5 sessions at weekly intervals	Colorimetric (objective) and mMASI (subjective)	73% patients in the combination group had excellent results

Contd...

Contd...

Author	Therapy	Demography	Trial	Dosages	Assess	Results
Angsuwarangsee S et al., 2003	Up CO_2 laser and Qsw alexandrite laser (QSAL) vs QSAL alone	6 Thai patients FP II–V refractory melasma	SF	CO_2: 300 mJ; Power: 5W; Spotsize: 3 mm QSAL: 5–7 J/cm^2 Spot size: 3 mm	mMASI and the Melanin index score	Combination treatment had a statistically significant reduction compared to QSAL side
Combination therapy with TC creams						
Goldman MP et al., 2011	IPL with TC (4% HQ) cream vs IPL with control cream	56 patients Symmetrical melasma	RCT SF	2 IPL treatments at 2 and 6 weeks	MASI	Significant improvement in melasma severity in the combination group vs IPL alone
Passerson T et al., 2011	PDL and TC vs TC cream	17 patients FP II–III	RCT SF	7–10 J/cm^2 Pulse duration: 1.5 ms 3 sessions at 3 weekly interval	MASI, Satisfaction index	Greater patient satisfaction in combination group
Trelles MA et al., 2010	TC alone vs AFR (CO_2) vs combination therapy	30 females FP II–IV	O	High power fixed pulse width, low frequency	MASI, satisfaction index	100% improvement in all 3 groups, results were maintained, however, only in combination group at 12 months

Contd...

Contd...

Author	Therapy	Demography	Trial	Dosages	Assess	Results
Wind BS et al., 2010	NAFR 1,550 nm vs TC (5% HQ)	29 patients	RCT SF	15 mJ/mb, 2000–2500 MTZ/cm^2 4–5 sessions vs TC for 15 weeks	(PGA), patient's satisfaction, (PhGA), Melanin index, and lightness (L-value)	Mean PGA and satisfaction index were significantly lower for laser treated site. PhGA, Melanin index, and L-value showed a significant worsening of hyperpigmentation at the laser side. At 6 months follow-up, most patients preferred TC
Jeong SY et al., 2010	Low dose Qsw Nd:YAG 1,064 nm with pre- and post-TC cream	13 patients FP III–IV	RCT SF cross-over	3.0–3.8 J/cm^2 6 mm spot size 5 sessions (once/week)	Lightness index/ Colorimetry	Mean MASI decreased significantly on laser side

HQ: hydroquinone; FP: fitzpatrick type; AFR: ablative fractional laser; NAFR: non-ablative fractional laser; O: observational therapy; RCT: randomized control trial; SF: split face trial; CS: case series; mMASI: modified melasma area and severity index score; PGA: patient's global assessment; PhGA: physician's global assessment; Combinations with microdermabrasion, Up CO_2, AFR, HQ, Peels and QSw Alex.; * Data of the laser clinic (2008–12)

3. All the lasers tried for melasma, including the pigment specific lasers (Q-switched, long-pulsed lasers and IPL), ablative lasers (Er:YAG), and fractional lasers have had indifferent results (Table 3.4). Transient results have been seen for the epidermal subtype, but dermal melasma and the mixed type which constitute the majority of patients in pigmented skin are difficult to treat.
4. Though peels have been touted as an useful intervention, it is a universal "practical" experience that without TC creams (triple combination creams) the results are not great, especially in pigmented skin. This is probably as deep peels (papillary dermis level) which are useful in the common mixed dermal melasma cases, are difficult to use in pigmented skin due to their potential for PIH. Hurley in their study pointed out that a TC cream would have superior results to the chemical peel, which is the 'real-life' scenario, though few authors admit this upfront.
5. A combination of TC creams/peels plus laser (Table 3.4) is an admission of the fact that probably-assisted therapy is better which puts a question mark on the role of lasers per se.
6. Fractional laser do not target melanin but target water so their use in melasma make little logical sense. While the theory that they can "shuttle" out the pigment is elegant, it ignores the fact that the pigment reverts back rapidly, sometimes making it worse than before! In fact, with the fractional lasers, a rebound hyperpigmentation has been noted in our analysis which is similar to the results noted by Karsai S et al.
7. Melasma is a **dynamic** disorder and in active stages of melasma, laser intervention is a cardinal mistake. Pigment lasers are effective for static disorders and not dynamic disorders. Laser toning has now largely fallen out of use as its results are not commensurate with the "hype" around its use.

The experience of Dr Kwang Hee Won is explicit and I quote "In our experience, laser toning or intense pulsed light (IPL) is either *ineffective* against or in fact often *aggravates* (rebound) this type of estrogen-dependent melasma. Because the subtypes of melasma are heterogeneous, the evidence for improvement results following laser therapy has been mixed to date with evidence of a significant potential for worsening." In fact, the study goes to state that, "the other subtype of melasma can be categorized into photoaging-associated mottled pigmentary (PMP) lesions." The main target of laser toning should be PMP lesions because 1064 nm QSNY is intended to rejuvenate the skin and PMP is the most common and earliest sign of photoaging in Asian women.

Pearls/Pitfalls

If after all the disheartening data (Table 3.4), lasers are attempted, scrupulous sunscreen use (preferably a physical block) with the use of a midpotent steroid for a week should be used. After that till 21 days, which is believed to be the time by which PIH appears in the majority of cases, a non-HQ/tretinoin based cream should be used.

BIBLIOGRAPHY

1. Angsuwarangsee S, Polnikorn N. Combined ultrapulse CO_2 laser and Q-switched alexandrite laser compared with Q-switched alexandrite laser alone for refractory melasma: split-face design. Dermatol Surg. 2003;29:59-64.
2. Chan HHL. Pigmentation and hypopigmentation: Benign pigmented lesions. In: Raulin C, Karsai S (Eds). Laser and IPL Technology in Dermatology and Aesthetic Medicine, Ist edition. London: Springer-Verlag Berlin Heidelberg; 2011.pp.151-3.
3. Chan NP, Ho SG, Shek SY, et al. A case series of facial depigmentation associated with low fluence Q-switched 1,064 nm Nd:YAG laser for skin rejuvenation and melasma. Lasers Surg Med. 2010;42:712-9.
4. Choi M, Choi JW, Lee SY, et al. Low-dose 1064-nm Q-switched Nd:YAG laser for the treatment of melasma. J Dermatolog Treat. 2010;21:224-8.
5. Goldberg DJ. Pigmented Lesions, Tattoos, and Disorders of Hypopigmentation. In:Laser Dermatology Pearls and Problems, Ist edition. Massachusetts: Blackwell Publishing; 2008. pp. 91-3.
6. Halachmi S, Haedersdal M, Lapidoth M. Melasma and laser treatment: an evidenced-based analysis. Lasers Med Sci. 2014;29:589-98.
7. Jang WS, Lee CK, Kim BJ, Kim MN. Efficacy of 694-nm Q-switched ruby fractional laser treatment of melasma in female Korean patients. Dermatol Surg. 2011;37:1133-40.
8. Kar HK, Gupta L, Chauhan A. A comparative study on efficacy of high and low fluence Q-switched Nd:YAG laser and glycolic acid peel in melasma. Indian J Dermatol Venereol Leprol. 2012;78(2):165-71.
9. Karsai S, Raulin C. Fractional photothermolysis: a new option for treating melasma? Hautarzt. 2008;59(2):92-100.
10. Kauvar AN. Successful treatment of melasma using a combination of microdermabrasion and Q-switched Nd:YAG lasers. Lasers Surg Med. 2012;44:117-24.
11. Lee HI, Lim YY, Kim BJ, et al. Clinicopathologic efficacy of copper bromide plus/yellow laser (578 nm with 511 nm) for treatment of melasma in Asian patients. Dermatol Surg. 2010;36:885-93.
12. Passeron T, Fontas E, Kang HY, et al. Melasma treatment with pulsed-dye laser and triple combination cream: a prospective, randomized, single-blind, split-face study. Arch Dermatol. 2011;147(9):1106-8.
13. Polder KD, Bruce S. Treatment of melasma using a novel 1,927-nm fractional thulium fiber laser: a pilot study. Dermatol Surg. 2012;38:199-206.
14. Polnikorn N. Treatment of refractory melasma with the MedLite C6 Q-switched Nd:YAG laser and alpha arbutin: a prospective study. J Cosmet Laser Ther. 2010;12:126-31.
15. Rivas S, Pandya AG. Treatment of melasma with topical agents, peels and lasers: an evidence-based review. Am J Clin Dermatol. 2013;14(5):359-76.
16. Sardana K, Chugh S, Garg VK. Which therapy works for melasma in pigmented skin: lasers, peels, or triple combination creams? Indian J Dermatol Venereol Leprol. 2013;79(3):420-2.

17. Suh KS, Sung JY, Roh HJ, et al. Efficacy of the 1064-nm Q-switched Nd:YAG laser in melasma. J Dermatolog Treat. 2011;22:233-8.
18. Trelles MA, Velez M, Gold MH. The treatment of melasma with topical creamsalone, CO_2 fractional ablative resurfacing alone, or a combination of the two: a comparative study. J Drugs Dermatol. 2010;9:315-22.
19. Wattanakrai P, Mornchan R, Eimpunth S. Low-fluence Q-switched neodymium-doped yttrium aluminum garnet (1,064 nm) laser for the treatment of facial melasma in Asians. Dermatol Surg. 2010;36:76-87.
20. Won KH, Lee SH, Lee MH, et al. A prospective, split-face, double-blinded, randomized study of the efficacy and safety of a fractional 1064-nm Q-switched Nd:YAG laser for photoaging-associated mottled pigmentation in Asian skin. J Cosmet Laser Ther. 2016;18(7):381-6.
21. Zhou X, Gold MH, Lu Z, Li Y. Efficacy and safety of Q-switched 1,064-nm neodymium-doped yttrium aluminum garnet laser treatment of melasma. Dermatol Surg. 2011;37:962-70.

Postinflammatory Hyperpigmentation

Postinflammatory hyperpigmentation occurs due to hemosiderin and/or melanin deposition. Because this condition arises due to inflammation, it is important to use low fluences and ensure that the patient does not develop significant post-treatment erythema to provoke additional PIH. For this reason, test spots are encouraged prior to treating large areas.

Lasers Used

Pigmented lasers: Though a variety of QS and Pico lasers have been used, close reading shows that they were combined with topical measures. Also PIH responds to many nonlaser modalities.

Vascular lasers: Vascular lasers, such as the 595 nm LPDL, target mainly oxyhemoglobin, and can be used to treat the vascular component of the inflammatory process.

Fractional lasers: The laser system currently used most often for PIH is the fractional photothermolysis system, even though treatment with this laser has been reported to induce PIH itself. The fractional Er:YAG and possibly the thulium laser may prove to be useful in this regard.

Pearls/Pitfalls

Prevention is a better option, which can be achieved by effective sun protection pre- and postprocedure, the use of long-pulsed lasers, cooling, diascopy, and lower fluences.

A study that is relevant here, compared three groups, treated with topical agents, 595 nm long pulsed dye laser and/or 1064 nm Q-switched Nd:YAG, or combination topical and laser treatments. Topical treatment, laser therapy, and combination topical and laser treatments all appeared to be effective management strategies for acne PIH in Fitzpatrick types III and IV skin with little complications. Hence, there is little rationale in the use of lasers in PIH.

We prefer administering hydroquinone-free products include compounds such as kojic acid, and arbutin to prevent PIH. Postlaser tretinoin-based compounds may cause irritation and aggravate PIH.

Nevus of Ota/Ito

Nevus of Ota (also known as oculodermal melanoma or nevus fuscoceruleus ophthalmomaxillaris) is a mottled, blue-gray macule that is usually located unilaterally within the distribution of the first and second branches of the trigeminal nerve. The clinical appearance resembles a powder blast, with poorly demarcated macules and patches blending readily with the normal surrounding skin. Lesions vary in color from brown to darker shades such as blue, gray, and purple.

Histologic examination of both lesions shows long, slender dermal melanocytes scattered largely in the upper half of the dermis. The normal dermal collagen architecture is well preserved. Although the epidermis is generally normal, focal basal hyperpigmentation may also be seen.

Lasers Used

It must be appreciated though, the Q-switched lasers are the mainstay, there are variations in the dose, fluence and sessions required depending on the depth, size and color of the lesion.

Q-switched Lasers: Q-switched lasers are extremely helpful in treating nevus of Ota. The degree of lightening is usually directly proportional to the number of treatments performed. Lightening of 70% or more has been reported in the majority of patients treated four or five times with the QSRL (Watanabe S).

A few basic principles that have emerged from the use of QS lasers are:
1. *Treat early:* QSRL treatment of nevus of Ota in children results in fewer required sessions and complications, but recurrence is still a concern.
2. *Multiple sessions:* Treatment sessions with QSRL increases response rate.
3. Q-switched Nd:YAG is superior to QS Alex in subjective assessments of lightening, but no statistical difference in efficacy has been shown.
4. Q-switched Alex treatment is efficacious and can be without side effects. Histologic evidence demonstrates laser-induced elimination of upper dermal pigmentation without epidermal disruption.

Picosecond Lasers: If pico lasers can treat nevus of Ota better than the Qs lasers, this will be a major boon for patients and a breakthrough as our experience in Indian skin has been dismal (Sardana K).

Though there is a study with the alexandrite 755-nm picosecond which was superior to the Qs 755 nm (Yu W), it still did not remove the lesion completely. In skin of color, a pico 1064 nm would have more relevance and we await such a comparative study.

Combination of Lasers

1. *Scanned CO_2 with Q-switched laser:* Mauskiatti et al. demonstrated greater clearing of bilateral nevus of Ota like macules with a combination of carbon dioxide (CO_2) and Q-switched ruby laser (QSRL) treatment than with QSRL alone.
2. *Fractional laser:* There are reports of the use of 1440 nm and 1550 nm fractional lasers, which ostensibly help in better penetration of the pigment specific laser. They are unlikely to appreciably improve the condition by itself.
3. *Combination of various lasers (Felton SJ):* It is well known that not all cases respond to the Qsw lasers. This is possibly as the lesion can have varying colors, which logically will respond to various wavelengths. Thus, a combination of QS Nd:YAG-1,064 nm, QS alexandrite 755 nm and QS Nd:YAG 532 nm lasers were used in accordance with the test patch results. Laser modality was switched following repeated test patches if there was no or no sustained improvement. Though most of the patients had ≥90% improvement compared to baseline photographs, the results were dependent on the color. Gray lesions and those on the forehead/temple were most *resistant.*

Literature Review

The analysis of the results of laser in nevus of Ota (Table 3.5), give some sobering facts of the actual efficacy which are important to understand before the treatment is attempted.

1. The *success rate* especially in pigmented skin is rarely 100%. The average results are 50% and this is also after multiple sittings.
2. Various *combinations* have been tried which is proof of the less reliability of monotherapy with a Q-switched laser. Conversely combination with fractional laser may look impressive in clinical reports, but the actual results may not be superior to monotherapy.
3. It is important to focus on the *color of the lesion* that predicts the response. A study by Ueda et al. found that the 22 brown lesions attained an excellent

Table 3.5: Overview of results with various lasers used for nevus of Ota.

Author	Clearing (%)	Laser used	Conclusions
Kono et al. 2003	100	QSRL	Early QSRL treatment of nevus of Ota in children results in fewer required sessions and complications, but *recurrence* is still a concern
Kono et al. 2001	75	QSRL	Side effects are pigmentary changes; mainly hypopigmentation that may be permanent. *Recurrence* is rare but important in childhood cases
Yang et al.	50	QSRL	QSRL treatment is efficacious and safe, without scarring. However, transient pigmentary changes, especially hyperpigmentation, are common
Suh et al.	7% patients with improvement	QS Alex	QS Alex is safe and effective, with better results after repeated treatments. Histologic evidence of laser-induced thermal damage of melanocytes demonstrated
Wang et al.	Variable	QS Alex	QS Alex treatment is safe and effective with few cases of transient hypopigmentation as the main side effect. Increased treatment sessions yielded better results
Kang et al.	75%	QS Alex	QS Alex treatment is safe and effective but limited by hyperpigmentation in darker skin types, delay in therapeutic effect, and lack of complete clearing. Histologic evidence of laser-induced selective destruction of melanocytes is demonstrated
Chan et al.	Alex: 10–26 YAG: 35–62	QS Alex QS Nd:YAG	QS Nd:YAG is superior to QS Alex in subjective assessments of lightening, but no statistical difference in efficacy was determined
Kar HK et al. 2011	8% had excellent efficacy	QS Nd:YAG	
Sardana K	25%	QS Nd:YAG	In our experience the efficacy is not as marked as with Western skin type
Sethuraman G	>50% pigment clearance	QS Nd:YAG	Though melanin index showed an improvement, clinical results were not as dramatic as revealed by the percentile improvement

(QS Nd:YAG: Q-switched neodymium-doped yttrium aluminum garnet)

Box 3.2: Factors that predict response of NOA to lasers.

- Laser wavelength
- Dose
- Spot size
- Pulse duration
- Interval between sessions
- Number of sessions
- Age of the patients
- Site
- Coloring nevus of Ota
- Skin type

(95–100%) or good (75–95%) cosmetic results (3 treatments). Of the other 42 brown-violet lesions, only 25 of the 29 had good or excellent results after four treatments, of the 81 violet-blue lesions, 54 of the 65 had good or excellent results after four treatments while the six blue-green lesions, had the poorest response.

Brown lesions can be cleared by 3 laser treatments, brown–violet lesions by 4 sessions, violet–blue lesions can be eliminated after 5 sessions, and blue–green lesions require at least 6 treatment sessions for complete clearance.

This concept was again proved by a study by Fulton et al. wherein only 20% of patients, was the QS-1,064 nm found to be efficacious. Also the number of treatments required varied significantly according to lesional color and site: gray lesions and those on the forehead/temple were most resistant.

Thus before we embark on the laser therapy, various aspects (Box 3.2) must be considered. Reporting of results in studies do not reflect actual patient improvements as they employ subjective methods of assessment, which invariably do not reflect actual improvement.

Pearls/Pitfalls

1. Lesion clearance is generally noted with fluences ranging from 6 to 10J/cm^2, after one to seven treatments. Start with a *larger spot size* at maximal fluence, then *decrease spot size* and retreat the area and maximal fluence available. (Figs. 3.22 and 3.23). More resistant lesions generally continue to demonstrate improvement with successive treatments, though more slowly. As PIH is a common complication in Indian skin a *low dose* of **2.5 j/cm^2** can be tried which has been shown to reduce the side effects.
2. Hori nevus is difficult to treat and the results are inferior to that of N of Ota.
3. The use of topical fusidic acid plus betamethasone valerate cream for 2 weeks after the session has been shown to reduce the pigmentation (Uaboonkul T). But excessive use can lead to hypopigmentation.
4. In pigmented skin, conservative fluencies are advisable as occasionally melasma like lesions may develop consequent to laser therapy (Lee WJ).

CHAPTER 3: Pigmented Lesions and Tattoos

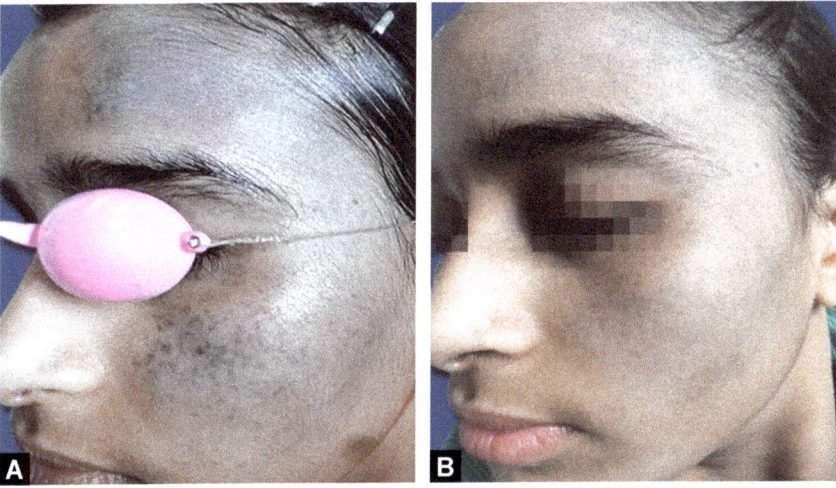

Figs. 3.22A and B: (A) Nevus of Ota before treatment; (B) Post-treatment with Q-switched Nd:YAG (1064 nm) after 7–8 sitting.

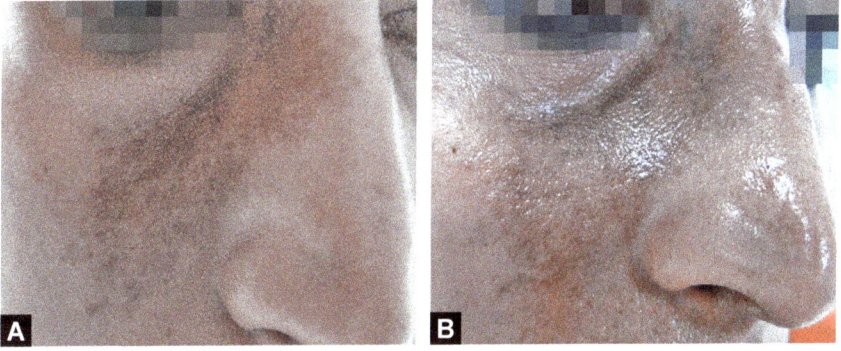

Figs. 3.23A and B: A brownish nevus of Ota in a female patient. Plan: Treat with Qsw Nd:YAG (1,064 nm). After 7 sessions there is a partial diminution in the lesion. A large probe size 3–4 mm is ideal for treating dermal disorders over a large area.

BIBLIOGRAPHY

1. Chan HH, Ying SY, Ho WS, et al. An in vivo trial comparing the Q-switched 1064 nm Nd:YAG lasers in the treatment of nevus of Ota. Dermatol Surg. 2000;26(10):919-22.
2. Felton SJ, Al-Niaimi F, Ferguson JE, et al. Our perspective of the treatment of naevus of Ota with 1,064, 755 and 532 nm wavelength lasers. Lasers Med Sci. 2014;29:1749-9.
3. Ho SG, Yeung CK, Chan NP, et al. A retrospective analysis of the management of acne post-inflammatory hyperpigmentation using topical treatment, laser treatment, or combination topical and laser treatments in oriental patients. Lasers Surg Med. 2011;43(1):1-7.
4. Kang W, Lee E, Choi GS. Treatment of Ota's nevus by Q-switched alexandrite laser: therapeutic outcome in relation to clinical and histopathological findings. Eur J Dermatol. 1999;9(8):639-43.

5. Kar HK, Gupta L. 1064 nm Q-switched Nd:YAG laser treatment of nevus of Ota: An Indian open label prospective study of 50 patients. Indian J Dermatol Venereol Leprol. 2011;77(5):565-70.
6. Kono T, Chan HH, Ercocen AR, et al. Use of Q-switched ruby laser in the treatment of nevus of Ota in different age groups. Lasers Surg Med. 2003;32(5):391-5.
7. Kono T, Nozaki M, Chan HH, Mikashima Y. A retrospective study looking at the long-term complications of Q-switched ruby laser in the treatment of nevus of Ota. Lasers Surg Med. 2001;29(2):156-9.
8. Lee WJ, Kim YJ, Noh TK, Chang SE. Formation of new melasma lesions in the periorbital area following high-fluence, 1064-nm, Q-switched Nd/YAG laser. J Cosmet Laser Ther. 2013;15(3):163-5.
9. Manuskiatte W, Sivayathorn A, Leelaudomlipi P, et al. Treatment of acquired bilateral nevus of Ota-like macules (Hori's nevus) using a combination of scanned carbon dioxide laser followed by Q-switched ruby laser. J Am Acad Dermatol. 2003;48(4):584-91.
10. Moody MN, Landau JM, Vergilis-Kalner IJ, et al. 1,064-nm Q-switched neodymium-doped yttrium aluminum garnet laser and 1,550 nm fractionated erbium-doped fiber laser for the treatment of nevus of Ota in Fitzpatrick skin type IV. Dermatol Surg. 2011;37(8):1163-7.
11. Sardana K, Chugh S, Garg V. Are Q-switched lasers for Nevus of Ota really effective in pigmented skin? Indian J Dermatol Venereol Leprol. 2012;78(2):187-9.
12. Sethuraman G, Sharma VK, Sreenivas V. Melanin index in assessing the treatment efficacy of 1064 nm Q Switched Nd-Yag laser in nevus of Ota. J Cutan Aesthet Surg. 2013;6(4):189-93.
13. Uaboonkul T, Nakakes A, Ayuthaya PK. A randomized control study of the prevention of hyperpigmentation post Q-switched Nd:YAG laser treatment of Horinevus using topical fusidic acid plus betamethasone valerate cream versus fusidic acid cream. J Cosmet Laser Ther. 2012;14(3):145-9.
14. Wang HW, Liu YH, Zhang GK, et al. Analysis of 602 Chinese cases of nevus of Ota and the treatment results treated by Q-switched alexandrite laser. Dermatol Surg. 2007;33(4):455-60.
15. Watanabe S, Takahashi H. Treatment of nevus of Ota with the Q-switched ruby laser. N Engl J Med. 1994;331:1745-50.
16. Yu W, Zhu J, Yu W, et al. A split-face, single-blinded, randomized controlled comparison of alexandrite 755-nm picosecond laser versus alexandrite 755-nm nanosecond laser in the treatment of acquired bilateral nevus of Ota-like macules. J Am Acad Dermatol. 2018;79(3):479-86.

Acquired Bilateral Nevus of Ota-like Macules (ABNOM or Hori's Macules)

Hori's macules are dermal hyperpigmentations commonly seen in Asian patients that affect approximately 0.8% of the population. Hori's macules present as bilateral blue-gray macules typically located over the malar region in a symmetrical pattern. The lateral temples, alae nasi, eyelids, and foreheads can also be involved. Histologically, dermal melanocytes are dispersed in the papillary and middle part of the dermis.

In contrast to nevus of Ota, the pigmentation of Hori's macules is acquired, has a late onset in adulthood, and does not affect the mucosa. Melasma and Hori's macules can coexist in some patients.

Lasers Used

Like nevus of Ota, QS lasers have been shown to be effective for treatment of Hori's macules. Combined laser therapy has also been found to be effective. One study indicated that a QS 532-nm Nd:YAG laser used in conjunction with a QS 1,064 nm Nd:YAG laser can achieve better results than laser on its own. Another option is to use an ablative laser to first remove the epidermis and to allow better penetration of the QS ruby laser (Figs. 3.24 and 3.25).

A recent study has compared a picosecond laser (755 nm Alex) with a Qs laser (755 nm) and found that former to be better with less PIH. When targeting pigmented chromophores, laser energy emitted by PSLs in the shorter picosecond domains is thought to generate a greater photomechanical effect, with tensile strength, which exceeds the tissue's ultimate tensile stress, leading

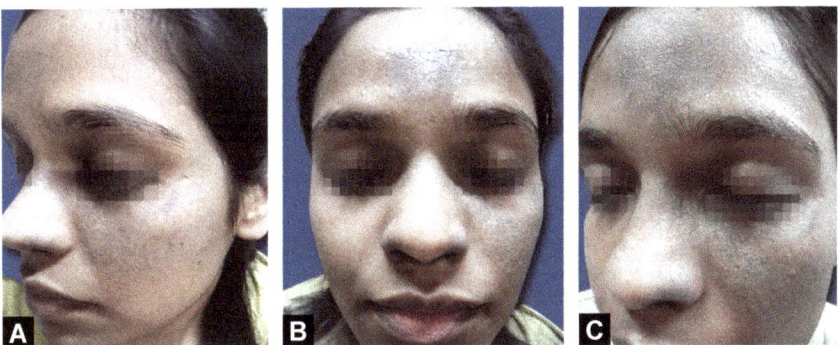

Figs. 3.24A to C: (A and B) Hori's nevus; (C) After 4–5 sittings with Q-switched Nd:YAG.

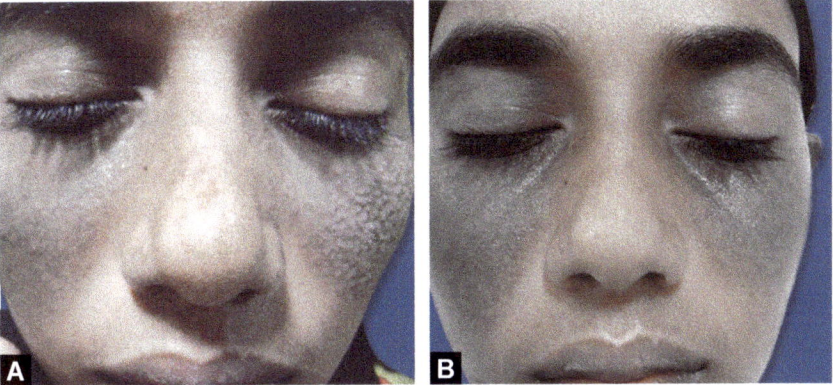

Figs. 3.25A and B: A case of Hori nevus extremely recalcitrant to therapy.

to tissue fracture and ablation. Theoretically, the additional photomechanical effect produced by the shorter pulse duration would translate into superior clinical efficacy compared to QSALs. Also the PIH in ABNOM is said to be consequent to perivascular melanocytes. The indirect vascular damage caused by nanosecond laser irradiation could induce inflammatory changes, as well as melanogenesis. Presumably since the pulse duration of the PSAL is far shorter than the thermal relaxation time of melanosomes, the laser energy absorbed is confined within the target chromophores, which results in minimal disruption to surrounding structures and vasculature.

A recent paper used the 1064 nm pico LIGHTen Picosecond Laser system (Cutera Inc) with the fractional lens with excellent results. ABNOM is difficult to treat and requires fluence up to 9.5 J/cm^2 and up to 11 sessions for clinical success. The low level of energies used (1.8–3.0 J/cm^2) makes this a great tool for Asian patients (Wong THS).

BIBLIOGRAPHY

1. Ee HL, Goh CL, Khoo LS, et al. Treatment of acquired bilateral nevus of Ota-like macules (Hori's nevus) with a combination of the 532 nm Q-Switched Nd:YAG laser followed by the 1,064 nm Q-switched Nd:YAG is more effective: prospective study. Dermatol Surg. 2006;32:34-40.
2. Manuskiatti W, Sivayathorn A, Leelaudomlipi P, et al. Treatment of acquired bilateral nevus of Ota-like macules (Hori's nevus) using a combination of scanned carbon dioxide laser followed by Q-switched ruby laser. J Am Acad Dermatol. 2003;48:584-91.
3. Wong THS. Picosecond laser treatment for acquired bilateral nevus of Ota-like macules. JAMA Dermatol. 2018;154(10):1226-8.
4. Yu W, Zhu J, Yu W, et al. A split-face, single-blinded, randomized controlled comparison of Alexandrite 755 nm picosecond laser vs. Alexandrite 755 nm nanosecond laser in the treatment of acquired bilateral nevus of Ota-like macules (ABNOM). J Am Acad Dermatol, 2017. pii: S0190-9622(17) 32893-1.

Congenital Dermal Melanocytosis

Mongolian spots are congenital and confluent hyperpigmented areas that are usually grayish blue in color. They are found most frequently in the sacral region in infants and typically disappear during childhood. Occasionally, they persist to adulthood.

Lasers

Q-switched alexandrite laser has been used though extrasacral lesions are more resistant to therapy. In adults, more frequent irradiation, longer intervals between treatment sessions and use of bleaching creams is required in the treatment of persistent sacral Mongolian spots in adults.

BIBLIOGRAPHY

1. Kagami S, Asahina A, Uwajima Y, et al. Treatment of persistent Mongolian spots with Q-switched alexandrite laser. Lasers Med Sci. 2012;27(6):1229-32.
2. Shirakawa M, Ozawa T, Ohasi N, et al. Comparison of regional efficacy and complications in the treatment of aberrant Mongolian spots with the Q-switched ruby laser. J Cosmet Laser Ther. 2010;12(3):138-42.

Infraorbital Hyperpigmentation (Dark Circles)

This may result from a variety of causes, including dermal melanin deposition, postinflammatory hyperpigmentation from atopic or allergic contact dermatitis, prominent superficial blood vessels, and shadowing from skin laxity and infraorbital swelling.

Thus, the therapy will require correction of the pigmentation, the skin laxity and the vascular accentuation.

Hyperpigmentation of the delicate under eye skin can be especially problematic to treat due to the potential for mixed pigmentation presentation (hemosiderin vs melanin) and the propensity toward postinflammatory hyperpigmentation especially in darker skin types.

Lasers Used

Lasers primarily work on the pigmentation, which in our experience responds as well to topical creams. Here it is important to understand that the Nd:YAG can achieve deeper penetrative energy levels and can potentially cause hyperpigmentation in Indian skin types.

Q-switched lasers: The QSRL has been reported to effectively treat infraorbital hyperpigmentation due to deposition of dermal melanin. The other Q-switched lasers, especially the Q-switched alexandrite laser, are also effective treatments in studies.

Picosecond: The dual wavelength picosecond Nd:YAG laser emits both 532 and 1,064 nm wavelengths and thus has the potential to target both superficial and deep components of the infraorbital dark circle pathophysiology. In several published studies, the picosecond 755 nm alexandrite laser has demonstrated efficacy in photorejuvenation and treatment of benign pigmented lesions. A recent study though found the 755 nm pico to be superior.

Another study compared the dual wavelength pico (1064/532 nm) with the 755 nm pico. There was an overall lack of improvement in hyperpigmentation and the high rate of post-inflammatory hyperpigmentation in the dual wavelength fractionated picosecond Nd:YAG trial even after on session reflecting the perils of using this wavelength. Though the 755 nm pico did not cause PIH, the objective improvement was mild. While optimization of settings was suggested, it is our view that in pigmented skin this may not be a successful therapy.

Ablative lasers: Improvement of this condition has also been reported following carbon dioxide laser resurfacing and the combination of carbon dioxide laser followed by Q-switched alexandrite laser.

Fractional lasers YSGG 2,790 nm: The 2,790 nm Er:YSGG wavelength has a lower water absorption coefficient than the 2,940 nm. Er:YAG, but a higher coefficient than the 10,600 nm CO_2 laser. This allows ablative resurfacing with mild thermal coagulation, which may increase clinical efficacy while reducing patient downtime. Two studies have been done with this laser, and we feel that the fractional Er:YAG would be a better option as this laser would penetrate even lesser than the YSSG laser, thus would be safer.

Other options: Blepharoplasty may be indicated when infraorbital darkening is due to excessive skin laxity. Soft tissue augmentation with fillers may be beneficial if there is shadowing due to a hollow in the tear trough.

Pearls/Pitfalls

A combination therapy will help to target the various causes of infraorbital darkening.

Probably the Thulium laser would be the safest of all the fractional lasers, though it has not been formally tried. Picosecond is the new "flavor" of the season but an objective look at results are not "earth shattering" in any respect.

BIBLIOGRAPHY

1. Ma G, Lin XX, Hu XJ, et al. Treatment of venous infraorbital dark circles using a long-pulsed 1,064-nm neodymium-doped yttrium aluminum garnet laser. Dermatol Surg. 2012;38(8):1277-82.
2. Park KY, Oh IY, Moon NJ, Seo SJ. Treatment of infraorbital dark circles in atopic dermatitis with a 2790-nm erbium: yttrium scandium gallium garnet laser: a pilot study. J Cosmet Laser Ther. 2013;15(2):102-6.
3. Vanaman Wilson MJ, Jones IT, Bolton J, et al. Prospective studies of the efficacy and safety of the picosecond 755, 1,064, and 532 nm lasers for the treatment of infraorbital dark circles. Lasers Surg Med. 2018;50(1):45-50.
4. Walgrave SE, Kist DA, Noyaner-Turley A, Zelickson BD. Minimally ablative resurfacing with the confluent 2,790 nm erbium:YSGG laser: a pilot study on safety and efficacy. Lasers Surg Med. 2012;44(2):103-11.

Drug-induced Hyperpigmentation

Minocycline, doxycycline, amiodarone, and azidothymidine (AZT, zidovudine) can cause hyperpigmentation of the skin that appears as gray-brown to brown. Despite the fact that the Q-switched Nd:YAG (1,064 nm) laser theoretically has a greater penetration depth, the present data does not allow any comparisons to be made between the various lasers.

Minocycline Pigmentation

The maximum experience regarding minocycline-induced hyperpigmentation is with the Q-switched ruby laser though in India primarily the Q-switched Nd:YAG laser at a wavelength of 1,064 nm is used and requires up to eight sessions for complete removal.

Type I is a blue/black pigment that occurs on the face, generally within acne scars. **Type II** is a blue/gray pigment found on the shins and forearms involving normal skin. **Type III** is photo-distributed muddy-brown discoloration. **Type I** minocycline-induced hyperpigmentation is responsive to Q-switched Nd:YAG laser **(1,064 nm)**. This is as the pigment is in the dermis. In particular, histological staining for type I minocycline pigmentation demonstrates iron and melanin, which exist extra-cellularly and within dermal macrophages.

In cases of **Type II** minocycline-induced hyperpigmentation (i.e. generalized hyperpigmentation along the basal membrane zone), the Q-switched ruby laser is more effective because the shorter wavelength **(694 nm)** is better absorbed by the pigment particle in the epidermis.

The mechanism by which Q-switched laser therapy removes the pigment associated with minocycline use is not fully elucidated, but is thought to result from fragmentation of the intracellular and extracellular pigmentation and resulting drainage through the lymphatic system. Case reports have detailed that complete resolution of pigmentation can take from two to nine treatment sessions.

Pearls/Pitfalls

Caution is advised when treating drug-induced dyschromia with Q-switched lasers, even despite the therapeutic successes noted in literature. Patients who take or have taken gold medication may experience mottled hyperpigmentation (laser-induced chrysiasis) after treatment with a Q-switched laser, regardless of the indication for laser therapy. The skin type and extent of tanning pose constraints on the efficacy of the pigment laser.

A recent report combined a Fractional nonablative 1550 nm fractional photothermolysis followed immediately by 755 nm Q-switched alexandrite laser in one treatment session (Vangipuram RK). The settings used were, (Fraxel 1DUAL; Solta, Inc., Hayward, California) using a 15 mm spot size and fluence of 60 J/cm^2 at treatment level 8 (23% coverage) with eight passes and a total kilojoule deliver of 0.53 kJ. Patient comfort was maintained with topical ice cooling and cold-air (Cryo 5: Zimmer Medizin Systems, Irvine, California). Immediately following the nonablative 1550 nm fractional photothermolysis, a 755-nm Q-switched alexandrite laser was used to treat the same areas with a 4 mm spot size, pulse width of 50 ms, and fluence of 5.5 J/cm^2.

The picosecond laser has been shown in a singular case that failed with Qs Nd:YAG 1064/532 nm over 6 sessions to respond completely within 4 sessions using a fluence of 0.7 J, 7 mm spot size, 755 nm (Barret T et al.). The proposed mechanism seems to be the shorter pulse duration that is less than the thermal relaxation time of the target chromophore melanin which is present in the basal layer of Type III minocycline pigmentation.

Level of Difficulty

Time consuming and prolonged. A combination of fractional laser plus Qs laser and the pico dual laser is promising (Barret T et al., Vangipuram RK).

BIBLIOGRAPHY

1. Argenyi ZB, Finelli L, Bergfeld WF, et al. Minocycline-related cutaneous hyperpigmentation as demonstrated by light microscopy, electron microscopy and X-ray energy spectroscopy. J Cutan Pathol. 1987;14:176-80.
2. Barrett T, de Zwaan S. Picosecond alexandrite laser is superior to Q-switched Nd:YAG laser in treatment of minocycline-induced hyperpigmentation: A case study and review of the literature. J Cosmet Laser Ther. 2018. pp. 1-4.
3. Vangipuram RK, DeLozier WL, Geddes E, et al. Complete resolution of minocycline pigmentation following a single treatment with non-ablative 1550-nm fractional resurfacing in combination with the 755-nm Q-switched alexandrite laser. Lasers Surg Med. 2016;48(3):234-7.

Lichen Planus Pigmentosus

Lichen planus pigmentosus (LPP) is a common pigmentary disorder seen in the Indian population, although it may be present in other racial groups. Clinically, it presents as oval or irregularly shaped gray-brown to brown macules and patches in sun-exposed areas, including the forehead, temples and neck, or intertriginous areas, typically asymptomatic, but sometimes associated with mild pruritus and/or burning. The etiology for LPP is unknown. Photo distribution suggests that UV radiation may play a pathogenic role. Also, topical application of mustard oil which contains a potential photosensitizer, allyl isothiocyanate, and also amla oil have been proposed as possible inciting agents (Kanwar AJ et al) wherein the most likely diagnosis possibly is pigmented contact dermatitis. The differential diagnosis includes lichen planus, erythema dyschromicus pigmentosus (EDP), melasma, lichenoid drug eruptions and postinflammatory hyperpigmentation. Of note, in contrast to EDP, an erythematous border of early lesions is not a feature of LPP. LPP is a chronic disorder with exacerbations and remissions.

Treatment of LPP can be challenging because the clinical course is variable. Some cases may spontaneously resolve within weeks; other cases may persist for years. A study done by AI Mutairi et al., lightening of the pigmentation occurred in 54% (seven of 13) of patients treated with topical tacrolimus for 12–16 weeks.

Laser

In a recent case report, a combination of low-fluence 1064 nm pulse Q-switched ND:YAG with topical tacrolimus was reported to be successful (Kim JE et al.). Long pulse Q-switched ND:YAG 1064 is required five to six sessions at 4–8 weeks interval in LPP showed favorable response (Aurangabadkar SJ). The disease need to be managed medically to stabilized before initiation of laser.

Our Experience

The results of Q-switched Nd:YAG ,given at low fluence (2–2.5 j/cm^2), large spot size, given at 4–6 week interval time, lead to a variable response.

Level of Difficulty

Easy to do but difficult to get results! (Figs. 3.26A to I)

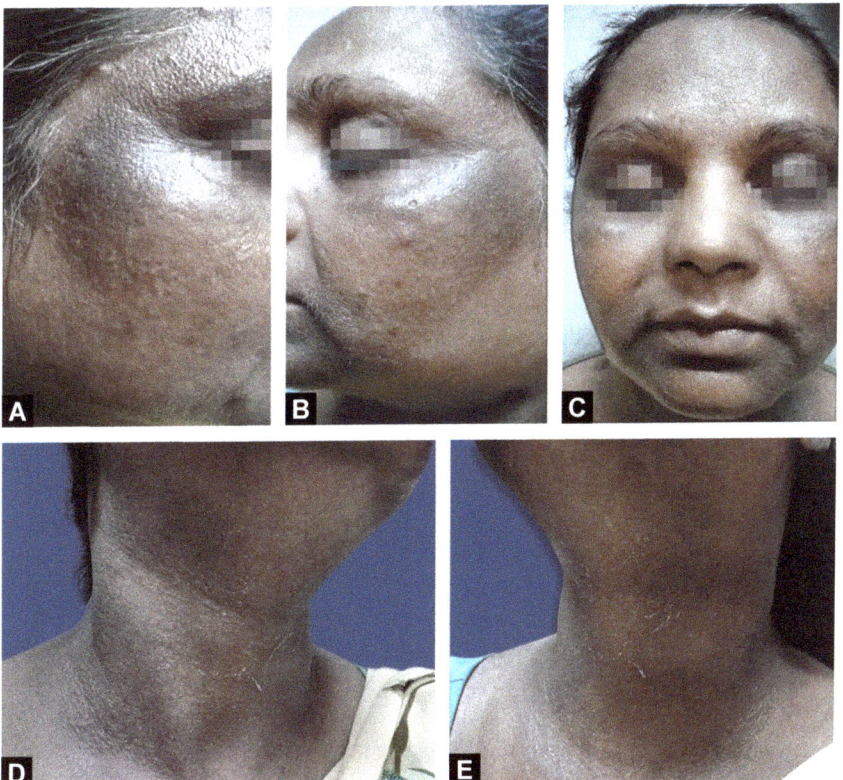

Figs. 3.26A to E: Lichen planus pigmentosus (LPP) before laser.

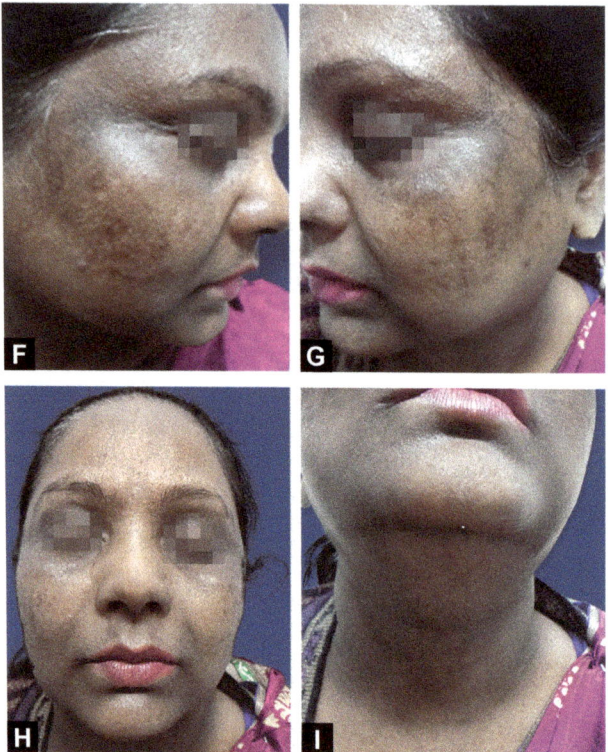

Figs. 3.26F to I: Postlaser toning with Q-switched ND:YAG (1064 nm).

BIBLIOGRAPHY

1. Al-Mutairi N, El-Khalawany M. Clinicopathological characteristics of lichen planus pigmentosus and its response to tacrolimus ointment: an open label, non-randomized, prospective study. J Eur Acad Dermatol Venereol. 2010;24:535-40.
2. Aurangabadkar SJ. Laser and light for pigmented lesion: opportunities and limitations. In: Kaushik Lahiri (Ed). Textbook of Laser in Dermatology. New Delhi: Jaypee Brothers Publishing; 2016.pp.87-8.
3. Kanwar AJ, Dogra S, Handa S, et al. A study of 124 Indian patients with lichen planus pigmentosus. Clin Exp Dermatol. 2003;28:481-5.
4. Kim JE, Won CH, Chang S, et al. Linear lichen planus pigmentosus of the forehead treated by neodymium:yttrium-aluminum-garnet laser and topical tacrolimus. J Dermatol. 2012;39:189-91.

Macular Amyloidosis

Macular amyloidosis is a form of cutaneous amyloidosis characterized by dusky-brown lace-like lesions usually located on the upper back between the shoulder blades, more infrequently, on the arms, chest and legs. Treatment of cutaneous amyloidoses usually yields disappointing results. Most cases can be treated with strong topical corticosteroids, normally for a short period. Calcipotriol or phototherapies are of limited use (Khoo, Jin et al.).

Lasers Used

Literature review shown encouraging results with the use of Q-switched Nd:YAG laser (1064–532 nm). Among the treatment modalities that has been used for amyloidosis, the pulsed dye laser has shown success in the treatment of nodular amyloidosis, and the Q-switched Nd:YAG laser has reduced the appearance of amyloid plaques in macular amyloidosis (Barsky M).

In a prospective, side-by-side, controlled, clinical trial study, Ostovari et al. used the Q-switched Nd:YAG laser (532 nm and 1064 nm) in 20 subjects with a clinical diagnosis and pathology confirmation of macular amyloidosis. Using colorimetric score assessment and digital photographs before laser therapy and 8 weeks after treatment, they concluded that the 2 lasers are effective in reducing the degree of macular amyloidosis pigmentation, with the 532 nm laser being more effective than the 1064 nm laser.

In an isolated case report in female of macular amyloidosis, resistant to all topical treatment has shown significant improvement after seven sessions of Q-switched Nd:YAG given at monthly interval (Nevil Khurana).

The fractional CO_2 has been used both in isolation and also in combination with topical agents wherein the laser helped in transdermal application of the drugs. AFR-assisted drug delivery is a promising tool for the future of dermatology.

In a recent study (Sobhi RM et al.), a combination of Fr CO_2 laser with topical steroids lead to a visible clinical and histological decrease in amyloid. The laser treatments were performed using fractional CO_2 laser (DEKA SmartXide DOT) with parameters of power 18 W, spacing 800 µm, dwell time 600 µs, and stacking 3.

BIBLIOGRAPHY

1. Barsky M, Buka RL. Pulsed dye laser for the treatment of macular amyloidosis: a case report. Cutis. 2014;93(4):189-92.
2. Jin AG, Por A, Wee LK, et al. Comparative study of phototherapy (UVB) vs photochemotherapy (PUVA) vs topical steroids in the treatment of primary cutaneous lichen amyloidosis. Photodermal Photoimmunol Photomed. 2001;17:42-3.
3. Khoo BP, Tay YK, Goh CL. Calcipotriol ointment vs. betamethasone 17-valerate ointment in the treatment of lichen amyloidosis. Int J Dermatol. 1999;38:539-41.
4. Nevil Khurana, Christine Urman. The Efficacy of Q-switched ND:YAG 1064 nm. LASer in recalcitrant macular amyloidosis: A case report. J Drugs Dermatol. 2016;15(11):1456-8.
5. Ostovari N, Mohtasham N, Oadras MS, et al. 532-nm and 1064-nm Q-switched Nd:YAG laser therapy for reduction of pigmentation in macular amyloidosis patches. J Eur Acad Dermatol Venereol. 2008;22:442-6.
6. Sobhi RM, Sharaoui I, El Nabarawy EA, et al. Comparative study of fractional CO(2) laser and fractional CO(2) laser-assisted drug delivery of topical steroid and topical vitamin C in macular amyloidosis. Lasers Med Sci. 2018;33(4):909-16.

TREATMENT APPROACH OF PIGMENTED LESIONS/TATTOO

Prerequisites

1. History of keloids, any bleeding diathesis, or history of infectious diseases, particularly hepatitis and HIV infection.
2. Patients with a recent history of isotretinoin use should be treated with caution.
3. A pretreatment biopsy should be performed if there is any possibility of atypia in a pigmented lesion or if the diagnosis is at all in question.
4. *Realistic goals:* Lasers are **NOT ERASERS**. This should be probably highlighted early on in the discussions with the patient. The patients of Becker's nevi, CALM and nevus spilus should be forewarned about the possibility of incomplete results. For tattoos, it can take 6–10 treatments or more to remove a tattoo and sometimes a "ghost" image of the tattoo may remain.
5. In some instances, the mixed nature of some lesions will require changes to the laser parameters or the use of multiple lasers.
6. Always take a pretreatment digital photographs and TEST SPOT the patient.

Pretreatment Preparation

The main competing chromophore during tattoo treatment is melanin pigment. The laser light has to traverse this to reach the tattoo. Thus, a bleaching agent such as alpha-hydroxy acid lotions combined with topical corticosteroids and/or hydroquinone may be used (2–4 weeks). It is the opinion of some authors (including us) that this does not markedly affect the final results.

Steps of Therapy

1. Topical EMLA is sufficient in most cases. In case of pain infiltration, anesthesia is an option.
2. Eye protection is a must and either eye shields or an eye cover should be provided.
3. A hydrocolloid dressing can be applied, as pieces of skin can often be aerosolized and blood can spatter during tattoo treatments with Q-switched lasers.
    This is because the rapid heating of the skin surface during the extremely short pulses delivered by Q-switching, causes a shock wave to be generated.
4. The laser handpiece should be held perpendicular to the skin with the attached plastic cone or guide resting on the skin to ensure that the laser beam is focused on the area to be treated. In some models, there is no

such guide, thus, the probe should be moved closer till the "popping sound" is heard.
5. Appropriate wavelength-specific safety goggles must be worn by all personnel in the treatment room. Retinal injury is the primary hazard of laser treatment for pigmented lesions.
6. Nonflammable, water-based lubricants may be used to protect eyebrows and other hair bearing areas from singeing.

Dose/Method

1. In general, **lower fluence** is used for dark lesions that contain larger amounts of absorbing chromophore.
2. One or two laser pulses should be fired at the lesion to ensure that a threshold response occurs, which is defined as immediate whitening of the lesion. The optimal tissue end point is uniform immediate whitening without epidermal disruption.
3. The *lowest* fluence required to invoke this response should be used. When the fluence is too low, the whitening will be barely noticeable. If the fluence is too high, whitening is a confluent bright white and epidermal damage with bleeding may occur. This may result in tissue sloughing, prolonged healing and also a greater likelihood of postinflammatory hyperpigmentation or hypopigmentation or textural changes.
4. It is advisable specially in pigmented skin that a test spot be done before deciding the final therapy regimen.
5. After the optimal fluence is determined, pulses can be delivered rapidly (up to 10 Hz, depending on the laser). As far as possible, overlapping should be avoided.

For Dermal Pigmented Lesions

1. Use anesthesia for larger lesions in the form of topical or local infiltration of lidocaine or regional nerve blocks.
2. For deeper lesions such as nevi of Ota and Ito, nerve blocks and supplemental infiltration of anesthesia can be used.
3. Larger spot sizes (4–6.5 mm), higher fluences, and longer wavelengths are required **than** for epidermal lesions to achieve deeper penetration.

Subsequent Sittings

They are performed 6 weeks after the original treatment. An increment of 1–2 J/cm^2 can be done, if needed. In nevus of OTA, a 3-month interval is ideal.

Number of Sittings

While some pigmented lesions (e.g. lentigines) may require only one to two treatments, other lesions (e.g. Café-au-lait macules) may need multiple treatments.

An overview of treatment and guide to dosimetry is given in Appendix 1, the details are discussed in chapter.

Appendix 1: A summary of standard dosimetry for select disorders.

Dermatoses	Wavelength	Diameter (mm)	Dose (initial)	Comments
Café-au-lait spot	532 nm	4	2 J/cm²	Treatment not successful in every case
Freckles	532 nm	4	2 J/cm²	The results are temporary with rapid recurrence
Amateur tattoo*	1,064 nm	1–4	3.5 J/cm²	On average 4–6 treatments
Professional tattoo,* very black	1,064 nm	1–4	3 J/cm²	On average 6–10, sometimes up to 20 treatments
Professional tattoo,* red	532 nm	1–4	2 J/cm²	On average 6–10, sometimes up to 20 treatments
Dirt tattoo*	1,064 nm	1–4	3.5 J/cm²	Dirt particles can shoot out

*See following section

Postoperative Course

The white tissue reaction that occurs immediately after Q-switched laser treatment fades within 20 minutes. An urticarial reaction, causing erythema, edema, itching, and stinging, may develop in and around the treated area.

In all patients, the treated lesions appear darker for several days then develop a thin crust that flakes off in 7-10 days. The risk of blistering is highest when shorter wavelength devices (e.g. QSRL) are used to treat patients with dark skin phototypes. Following treatment with the Q-switched 532 nm Nd:YAG, purpura usually develops after skin whitening has faded. This occurs because these wavelengths are well absorbed by both melanin and hemoglobin.

Patients should be instructed to gently wash the treated area with mild soap and apply an occlusive ointment (e.g. petrolatum) twice a day. We routinely advise a combination of aloe vera gel (40%) in the morning with Fucidin/colloidal silver cream at night. Any crusting should be allowed to slough spontaneously. To minimize the risk of hyperpigmentation and recurrence, patients should avoid excessive sun exposure and use a broad-spectrum sunscreen of SPF 30 or higher for several months after treatment.

TATTOO REMOVAL: VARIABLES AND MODIFICATIONS THAT PREDICT EFFICACY

Kabir Sardana, Pooja Arora Mrig

INTRODUCTION

Laser removal of tattoos is probably the most satisfying and at the same time the most challenging indication for pigment-specific lasers. Not all tattoos are cosmetic in nature and some are dictated by medical need to demarcate a radiation treatment field, or by traumatic embedment of foreign, pigmented matter in explosions, and other accidents. This results in a wide range of tattoo types (Table 3.6). The various types of tattoo pigments ranging from inorganic materials to azo dyes and their differing absorption spectrum makes the task of choosing the correct laser even more challenging (Box 3.1).

Table 3.6: Types of tattoo and their response to laser.

Tattoos	Pigment	Response	Side effects
Amateur	Most often black India ink, but also various other organic substances	Excellent: Complete clearance can be achieved with few treatment sessions	Rare
Professional	Diverse pigments, often inorganic metal salts	• Difficult as the pigment density is more and is deeply placed • Inorganic dyes and azo dyes are particularly difficult to treat	• Pigmentary changes and residual ink frequently seen • Allergic reactions possible
Cosmetic	• Often brown, white, or flesh tones • Enhanced with iron or titanium	• Difficult as the flesh-tone pigments poorly targetable by available wavelengths • Ablative lasers have to be used	Risk of paradoxical darkening
Medicinal	Most often blue-black India ink	Easily removed in 1–2 sessions	None
Iatrogenic	Metallic	Good response to QS Alex and QSRL	
Traumatic	Pigment from gunpowder, tar, and other particulate matter	Varies	May be combustible

(QS Alex: Q-switched alexandrite; QSRL: Q-switched ruby laser)

Box 3.1: Pigments used by tattoo artists.

Black:
- Carbon
- Iron oxide
- Logwood (extract from logwood tree).

Blue:
- Cobalt aluminate (azure blue).

Green:
- Chromium oxide (casalis green)
- Hydrated chromium sesquioxide (guignet green)
- Malachite green
- Lead chromate
- Ferrous ferricyanide
- Curcumin green
- Phthalocyanine dyes (copper salts with yellow coal tar dyes).

Red:
- Mercury sulfide (cinnabar)
- Cadmium selenide (cadmium red)
- Sienna (ochre: ferric hydrate and ferric sulfate).

Yellow:
- Cadmium sulfide (cadmium yellow)
- Ochre
- Curcumin yellow.

Brown:
- Ochre.

Violet:
- Manganese violet.

White:
- Titanium dioxide, zinc oxide.

Flesh:
- Iron oxides (variant of ochre).

CHOOSING THE CORRECT LASER

Though picoseconds lasers have emerged as a new option, the challenges that we face in tattoo removal are twofolds.

Firstly correctly interpreting the absorption spectrum of tattoos and then trying to ensure rapid tattoo removal (RTR) (Fig. 3.27). This figure may depict a simplistic view and the plethora of lasers used (Flowchart 3.2), reflects the difficult conundrum of tattoo removal, wherein numerous techniques are still being experimented with to arrive at a perfect technique for removal of the pigment.

The most important aspect is the *depth of the tattoo*, which may depend on the mode of placement, amateur or professional, the latter being more difficult to treat as the pigment is deeper. Thus, the focus of articles and research should be primarily the deeply placed professional tattoos.

From the perspective of the physician and laser operator, the pigment has to have a chemical composition that can be broken down with minimal

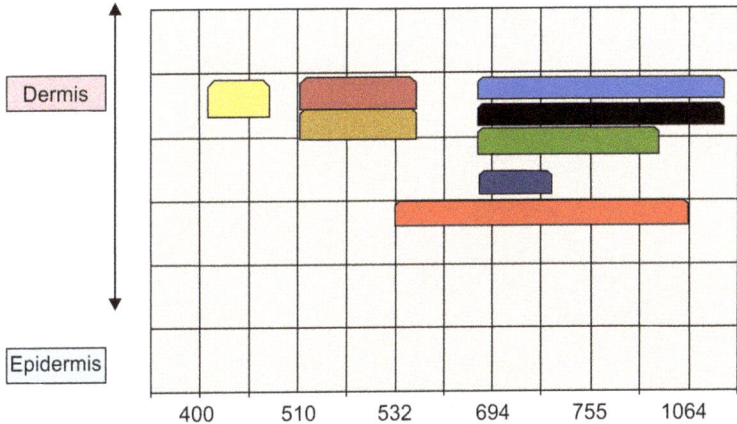

Fig. 3.27: The various pigment colors are depicted inset and correspond to the absorption spectrum of the wavelengths.
Source: Sardana K, Ranjan R, Ghunawat S. Optimising laser tattoo removal. J Cutan Aesthet Surg. 2015;8:16-24.

effort and without the formation of any toxic byproducts. To prevent such carcinogenic substances as much as possible, tattoo inks should be completely free of azo compounds; it is unlikely that an aromatic amine will occur as an impurity or be cleaved by a laser if no amines were used as starting substances in manufacturing the pigments. But without any guidelines on the same, this is unlikely to happen any day sooner.

PIGMENT-SPECIFIC LASERS AND TATTOO REMOVAL

For the selective removal of pigment, the laser light must penetrate far enough into the skin to reach the target pigment, and must be highly absorbed by the pigment relative to the surrounding skin. Different pigments, therefore, require different laser colors (Fig. 3.28). For example, red light is highly absorbed by green tattoo pigments. In current practice, numerous lasers can specifically target pigmented lesions, including red-light lasers (e.g. 694 nm ruby, 755 nm alexandrite), green-light lasers [e.g. 532 nm frequency-doubled neodymium-doped yttrium aluminum garnet (Nd:YAG)], and near-infrared lasers (e.g. 1,064 nm Nd:YAG). The wide range of lasers that can be used to treat pigment is a result of the broad absorption spectrum of melanin.

Though a detailed discussion on factors that determine laser tattoo removal will follow, the available evidence suggests that there is graded response of the various colored tattoos to the laser. Consequently, at least *three wavelengths* are needed to cover *most* of the pigments. Thus, possessing a 532 nm, 694 nm, and 1,064 nm laser, is a good starting point.

Flowchart 3.2: Overview of lasers used in tattoo removal (Sardana K, 2013).

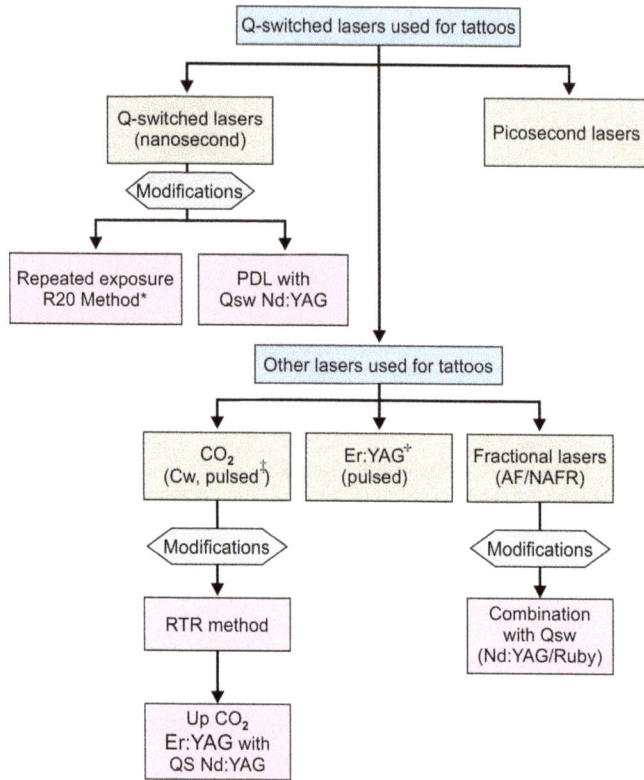

(CO_2: carbon dioxide; Er:YAG: erbium yttrium aluminum garnet; NAFR: nonablative fractional resurfacing; PDL: pulsed dye laser; QS Nd:YAG: Q-switched neodymium-doped yttrium aluminum garnet)
*Q-switched alexandrite laser (four passes with an interval of 20 minutes between passes), ‡used for cosmetic tattoo with multiple colors and flesh-colored iron oxide tattoo, and †used for traumatic tattoos and tattoo allergy, Q-switched ruby with AFR (10,600 nm)/NAFR (1,550 nm) or AFR (2,940 nm) with QS Nd:YAG.

As depicted here (Table 3.7 and Fig. 3.29) the basic principle is of complementary color absorption. Thus, a green tattoo will respond to a red laser while a red tattoo to a green laser. This simplistic observation is confounded by the use of other shades (Box 3.1) where an absorption spectrum analysis may be needed before arriving at the appropriate wavelength.

LASER-INDUCED RESOLUTION OF TATTOO PIGMENT

The laser works by impaction and dissolution of the tattoo pigment. A little researched topic is the course of events subsequent to this dissolution. Very little is known regarding the natural history of an intradermally placed

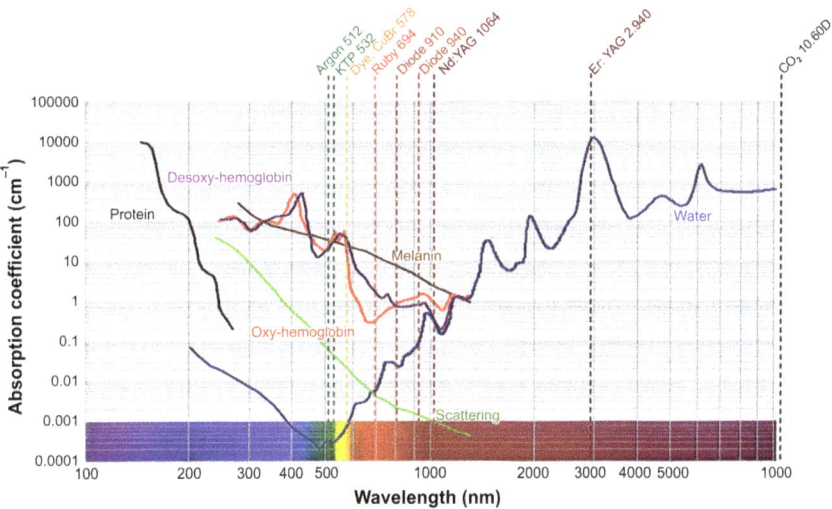

Fig. 3.28: Absorption spectrum of common lasers used for tattoo removal (Asclepion Laser Technologies, GmbH) (CO_2: carbon dioxide; Er:YAG: erbium:yttrium aluminum garnet; Nd:YAG: neodymium-doped yttrium aluminum garnet)

Table 3.7: Ideal laser for various tattoo pigments.

Color	QS Nd:YAG 532 nm	QSRL 694 nm	QS Alex 755 nm	QS Nd:YAG 1,064 nm	Pico 785 (Ti-Sapphire)	Ablative
Black	×	×	Ideal	Ideal	×	×
India ink	×	×	Ideal	×	×	×
Brown	×	×	×	Used*	×	×
Blue	×	×	Ideal	Ideal	Ideal	×
Green	×	Used*	Ideal	Used*	Ideal	×
Orange	Used*	×	×	×	×	×
Red	Ideal	×	×	×	×	×
Yellow	Ideal	×	×	×	×	×
Purple	×	Used*	×	×	Ideal	×
Flesh/White	×	×	×	×	×	Er:YAG/CO_2

(CO_2: carbon dioxide; Er:YAG: erbium:yttrium aluminum garnet; QS Alex: Q-switched alexandrite; QS Nd:YAG: Q-switched neodymium-doped yttrium aluminum garnet; QSRL: Q-switched ruby laser)
*Results are variable

tattoo. Initially, ink particles are found within large phagosomes in the cytoplasm of both keratinocytes and phagocytic cells, including fibroblasts, macrophages, and mast cells. The epidermis, epidermal–dermal junction, and papillary dermis appear homogenized immediately after tattoo

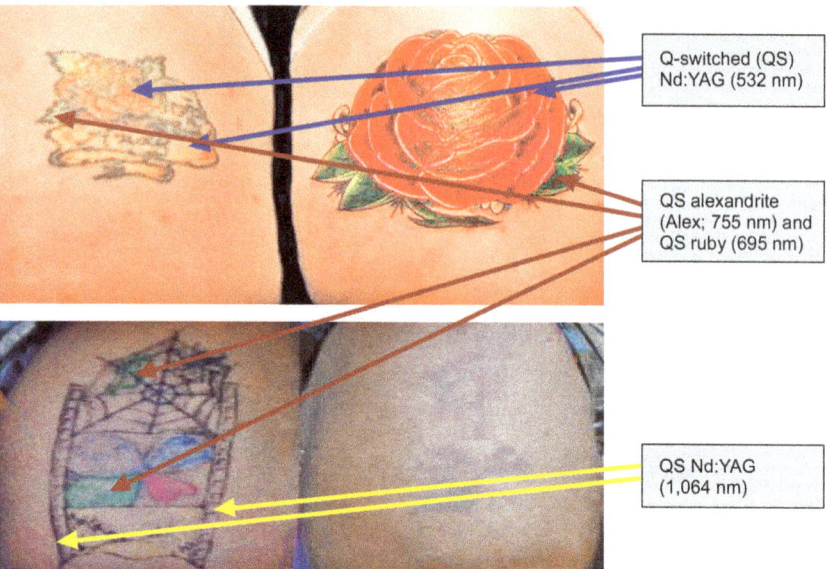

Fig. 3.29: A depiction of the various lasers used for multicolored tattoos. (QS Nd:YAG: Q-switched neodymium-doped yttrium aluminum garnet)

injection. At *1 month*, the basement membrane is reforming and aggregates of ink particles are present within basal cells. In the dermis, ink-containing phagocytic cells concentrate along the epidermal–dermal border below a layer of granulation tissue closely surrounded by collagen. At *1 month*, transepidermal elimination of ink particles through the epidermis is still in progress, with ink particles present in keratinocytes, macrophages, and fibroblasts. Reestablishment of an intact basement membrane prevents further transepidermal loss. In biopsies obtained at 2–3 months and 40 years, ink particles are found only in dermal fibroblasts, predominantly in a perivascular location beneath a layer of fibrosis, which had replaced the granulation tissue. Despite the diverse tattoo pigment, the light and electron microscopy of all pigments are remarkably similar.

It is common to observe that a tattoo becomes more indistinct, and blurred with time presumably as a consequence of ink particles moving deeper into the dermis. Indeed biopsies of older tattoos demonstrate pigment in the lower dermis.

The consequence of laser on the tattoo is twofold. Firstly some part of the tattoo ink is partially extruded through the scale crust that forms following epidermal injury. A greater proportion of the ink particles may be fragmented and released into the extracellular space and eliminated into the lymphatics or rephagocytosed as laser-altered residual tattoo particles, perhaps with altered optical properties. The last is important as in the R20R technique, the laser optics do not take into consideration the tissue effects of repeated shots of the laser.

VARIABLES AFFECTING TATTOO REMOVAL

A large study analyzed the variables that affect tattoo removal using the Q-switched neodymium-doped yttrium aluminum garnet (QS Nd:YAG) and alexandrite lasers. This study by Bencini et al. gives a realistic outcome of results with lasers. The cumulative rates of patients with successful tattoo removal were 47.2% after 10 sessions and 74.8% after 15 sessions.

Smoking, the presence of colors other than black and red, a tattoo larger than 30 cm^2, a tattoo located on the feet or legs or older than 36 months, high color density, treatment intervals of 8 weeks or less, and development of a darkening phenomenon were associated with a reduced clinical response to treatment. This highlights the numerous variables influencing response rates and the same should be considered when planning tattoo removal treatments. The Kirby-Desai scale is a useful index to predict the number of sittings required for tattoo removal (Fig. 3.30) but does *not* take into account the size depth and the duration of tattoo.

A recent review (Sardana K, 2015) has discussed this topic and a simple way to understand the variables involved is to focus on the steps involved in tattoo placement and eventual removal (Fig. 3.31). Three broad aspects are involved: (1) The laser(s) used, (2) The skin phenotype, and (3) Tattoo-dependent factors, which includes the type, depth, and size of tattoo (Fig. 3.27 and Table 3.8). A rarely appreciated aspect of tattoo removal is the role of the host immune response, which ultimately phagocytosis the tattoo particles and drains them away via the lymphatics. Thus, it is the inflammation consequent to the laser therapy and the concomitant stimulation of the host response that ultimately results in removal of tattoo ink via the lymphatics.

Patient-dependent Factors (Kirby et al.)

While a patient might believe that the laser treatment is the sole reason for tattoo ink reduction, the theory behind tattoo removal involves the patient's own immune system. It is hypothesized that these laser-altered residual particles are phagocytosed by the body's lymphatic system.

Patients suffering from short and long-term immunosuppression (i.e. via chemotherapy, drug-induced, or a medical condition) may experience poor healing, which can further lead to ink retention following laser treatments. Individuals presenting with underlying immunosuppression should be referred to the appropriate specialist for comprehensive care. Once the condition has stabilized or resolved, they should be considered appropriate candidates for laser tattoo removal treatment.

Tattoo-dependent Factors

Size of Tattoo Particle

The diameters of tattoo ink granules have been measured, and before irradiation, the granules within the dermis have a maximum diameter of **6 µm**. This mean diameter reduces after successive laser treatment. Since the

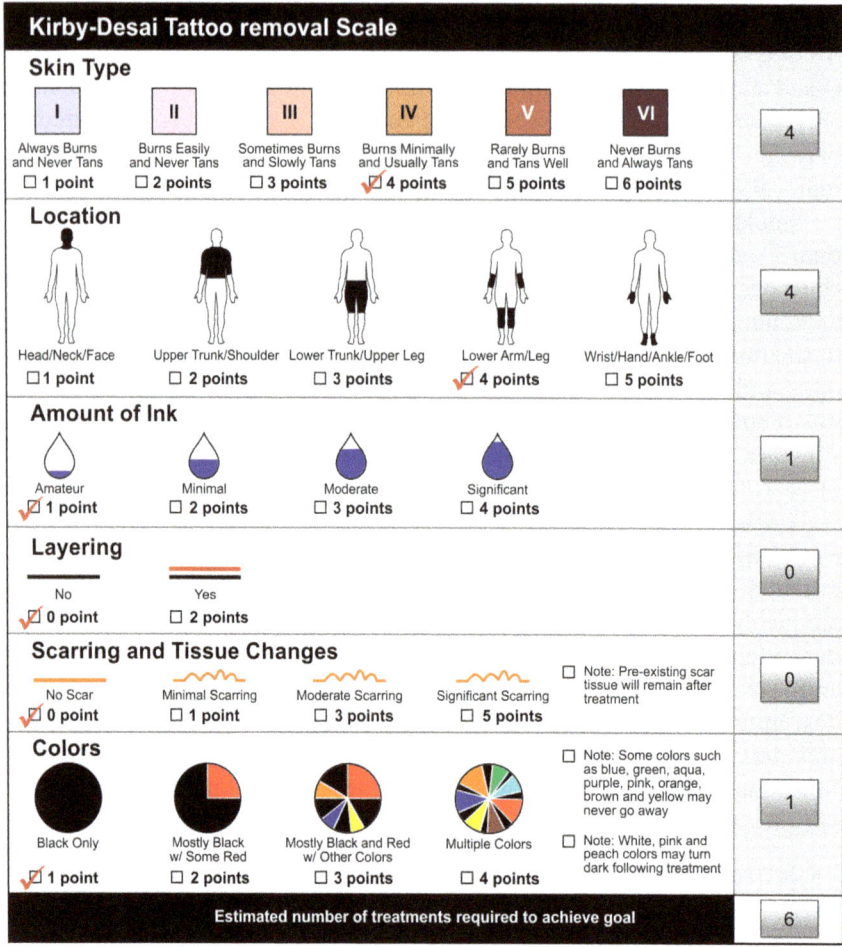

Fig. 3.30: Predicted number of sittings required for an amateur tattoo in an Indian patient using the Kirby-Desai scale.

maximum diameter of granule that can be absorbed by the lymphatic system is approximately 0.4 μm, any laser procedure that tries to fractionate them further is of little clinical use. This scientific concept goes against the concept of the R20R technique, as repeated thermal damage to the tattoo has little effect once the particle size of 0.4 μm is reached. Also as smaller granules absorb less energy, *larger* spot diameters and *higher* fluence settings are needed to reach the appropriate granule temperatures. Though this concept is generally true, it is also dependent on the color of the tattoo.

Depth of Tattoos

The granule depth remains uniform and is located at a depth of about 400 μm, as professional tattoos are generally located in the upper to mid-dermis

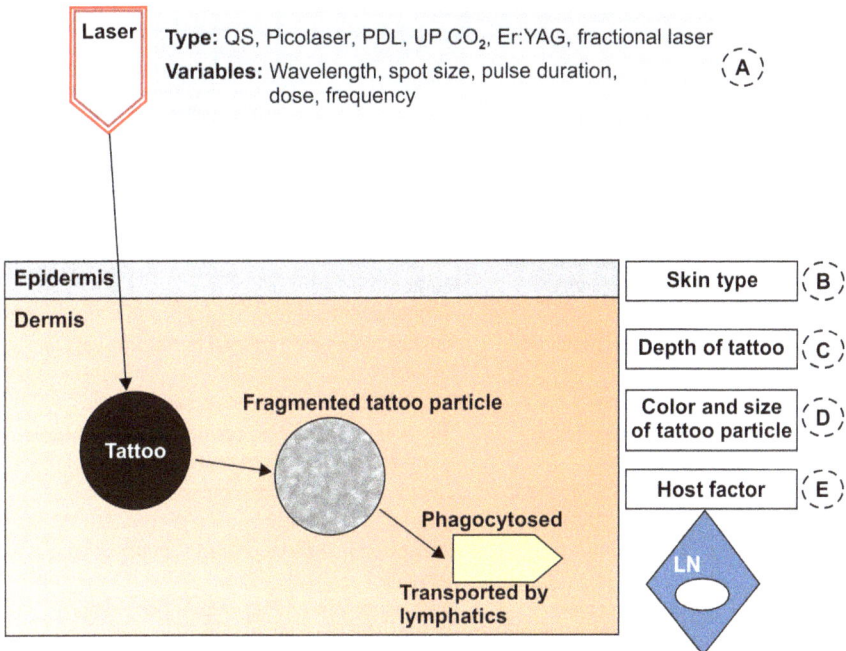

Fig. 3.31: Variables that affect tattoo removal. The normal process involves fragmentation followed by phagocytosis and transport via the lymphatics. Each step (A-E) plays a role and thus the variations in results are enormous. The color and mixture of tattoo color is probably the most important determinant in laser application for tattoo. (CO_2: carbon dioxide; Er:YAG: erbium:yttrium aluminum garnet; PDL: pulsed dye laser)

region (Fig. 3.32). This explains the difficulty in treating these tattoos as compared to amateur tattoos, which are superficially placed.

An *interesting* concept was proposed by Ho et al. who demonstrated that laser fluence attenuates rapidly in the dermis, thus a lower-intensity laser may used first for the removal of the top layer of the tattoo pigment. Subsequent sessions, with increasing fluence can help remove the pigment deep inside the dermis. This sequence can minimize the overall laser energy, and consequently reduce the collateral damage.

Professional versus Amateur

The number of sessions required varies though 5-10 sessions are standard for amateur tattoos and 15-20 for professional tattoos, even up to 25 sessions in some cases. The variable depth is a big problem as shown in Figure 3.33.

In professional tattoos, the particles may reach as far as the subcutis; depending on the location of the tattoo on the body, this can mean a depth of 5 mm or more. The penetration depth of the laser into the tissue is determined by the wavelength (the two factors correlate proportionally) and the spot size, which is usually limited to about 3-4 mm. The penetration depth of the

Table 3.8: Variables that affect laser response in tattoos.

Main variables	Characteristics	Variables
Tattoo	Type of tattoo	Professional/Amateur/Traumatic
	Duration	**Longer** the duration more difficult the removal as the size, depth and shape of the tattoo granules change
	Depth	**Deeper** the tattoo, more the sessions are required
	Volume surface area	A **larger** area requires more sessions
	Color of tattoo	**Multicolored** specially green tattoos are more difficult to remove
	Allergic reactions	Ablative lasers are required for removal of pigment
	Layering	**Double** tattoos require more sessions
	Cosmetic tattoo darkening	This is seen with **white** colored tattoos. Ablative lasers are required to remove the pigment
Laser	Type (Q switched/picoseconds)	It has been shown that a picosecond laser is superior to QS laser*
	Energy	Fluence should be increased with successive sessions
	Beam profile	Larger spot size enable deeper penetration
Host factors	Age	Poor response in **old age**
	Site	Poor response in **distal** anatomical regions
	Pigmented skin	Bleaching agents should be used before attempting tattoo removal
	Host removal of tattoo pigment	Depends on macrophages activity, which in turn depends on the host **immune response**

*Specially for older tattoos, purple, blue and green colors.

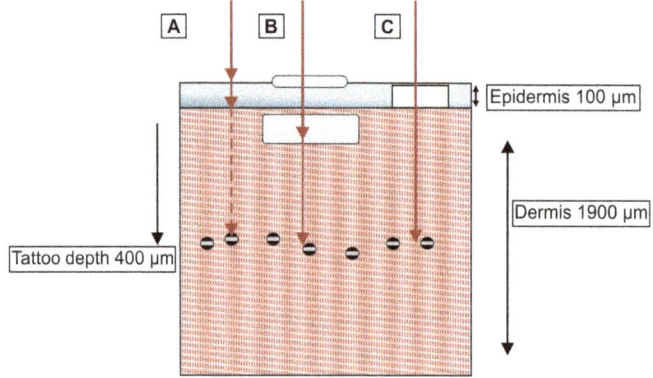

Fig. 3.32: A schematic diagram highlighting techniques to enhance tattoo removal. (A) The laser beam gets attenuated by the epidermis and the dermis due to epidermal and dermal scattering; (B) Topically applied clearing agents can help in reducing the dermal scatter and enhance results. They can be placed either on the skin or intradermally; and (C) Epidermal ablation is another effective tool for enhancing results by eliminating epidermal scatter.

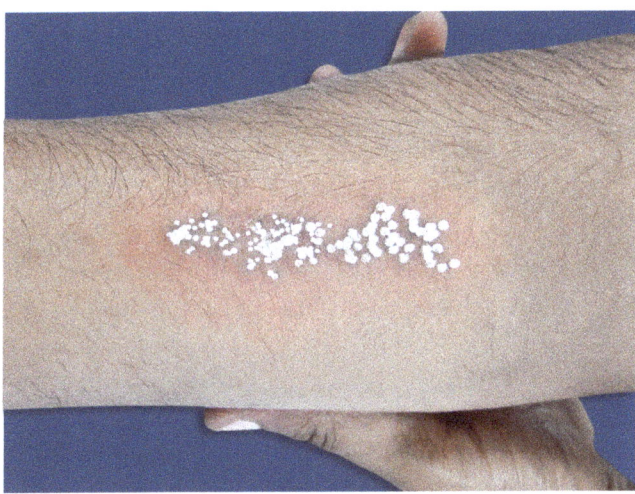

Fig. 3.33: Laser treatment of an amateur tattoo showing the variable whitening which indicates the variation in depth of the tattoo pigment leading to erratic removal of pigment.

laser can be optimized by using the largest spot size possible (4 mm) and a homogeneous beam profile (Karsai et al.).

Color

In clinical practice, all laser systems (ruby, 1,064 nm Nd:YAG, and alexandrite lasers) have proven effective in treating black, black-blue, blue, and brown inks. Red and orange tattoos only absorb light from the Q-switched frequency-doubled Nd:YAG lasers (532 nm) and pulsed dye lasers (510 nm). Green tattoos respond best to treatment with Q-switched ruby or alexandrite lasers, purple, yellow, white, and flesh-tone dyes do not yield satisfactory results (Prinz Ross, 2001).

An example of the complexities involved in tattoo removal is depicted in Figure 3.29 and Table 3.9.

We have treated various colors and some like blue-green are partially responsive to the 1,064 nm Nd:YAG laser (Figs. 3.34A to D).

Composition of Tattoo Dye

Detailed knowledge with respect to the identity and dye composition of tattoo pigments would be beneficial not only with regard to photoallergic, granulomatous, and anaphylactic reactions but will also be useful in improving treatment planning and response prediction to laser therapy. Klitzman designed a permanent and more removable tattoo ink using insoluble and bioresorbable pigments (such as beta-carotene and iron oxide), which are stabilized through microencapsulation in transparent polymethylmethacrylate (PMMA) beads. The microspheres contain discrete

Table 3.9: A summary of lasers used for various tattoo pigments.

Laser used	Violet*	Blue	Green	Red/brown*/orange/yellow	Black
532 nm neodymium-doped yttrium aluminum garnet (Nd:YAG)	No	No	No	Yes/Yes/Yes/Yes	No
694 nm ruby	Yes	Yes	Yes	No/Yes/No/No	Yes
755 nm alexandrite	No	Yes	Yes	No/Yes/No/No	Yes
1,064 nm Nd:YAG	No	Yes	No	No/Yes/No/No	Yes
Pico 785 nm	Yes	Yes	Yes	No	Yes

*Poor response

pigment that can be targeted by specific laser wavelengths. Laser-based tattoo removal causes the capsule to break, exposing the pigment, which is then reabsorbed by the body. Thus, one laser treatment can effectively remove 80% of tattoo pigment, contrary to the 20% removal with conventional ink. Although these results appear promising, the safety and efficacy of microencapsulated tattoo ink in human skin needs to be investigated in further studies as no clinical data have yet been published.

Location

Experience shows that it takes longer to lighten tattoos in distal anatomical regions such as forearms and calves. This may be due to slower lymphatic transport, which in turn leads to delayed elimination of the color pigments.

Age

It is believed that older the tattoo, worse is the response as the macrophages tend to engulf the pigment. Also, the tattoo is deeper and thus a higher dose and larger number of sittings are required.

Skin Type

Pigmented skin has delayed response as the epidermal pigment competes with the light.

Scar/Granuloma

If the skin is palpably thickened because of tattoo-related permanent infiltrate or scarring, (Fig. 3.35), it is more difficult for the laser to penetrate the dermis, and the pigment particles' ability to absorb light will be affected.

Paradoxical Ink Darkening

Paradoxical darkening of tattoo ink can occur after Q-switched treatment and has been reported in multiple ink colors. Certain colors including *yellow, white, peach, or pink* may be susceptible to paradoxical ink darkening

CHAPTER 3: Pigmented Lesions and Tattoos **213**

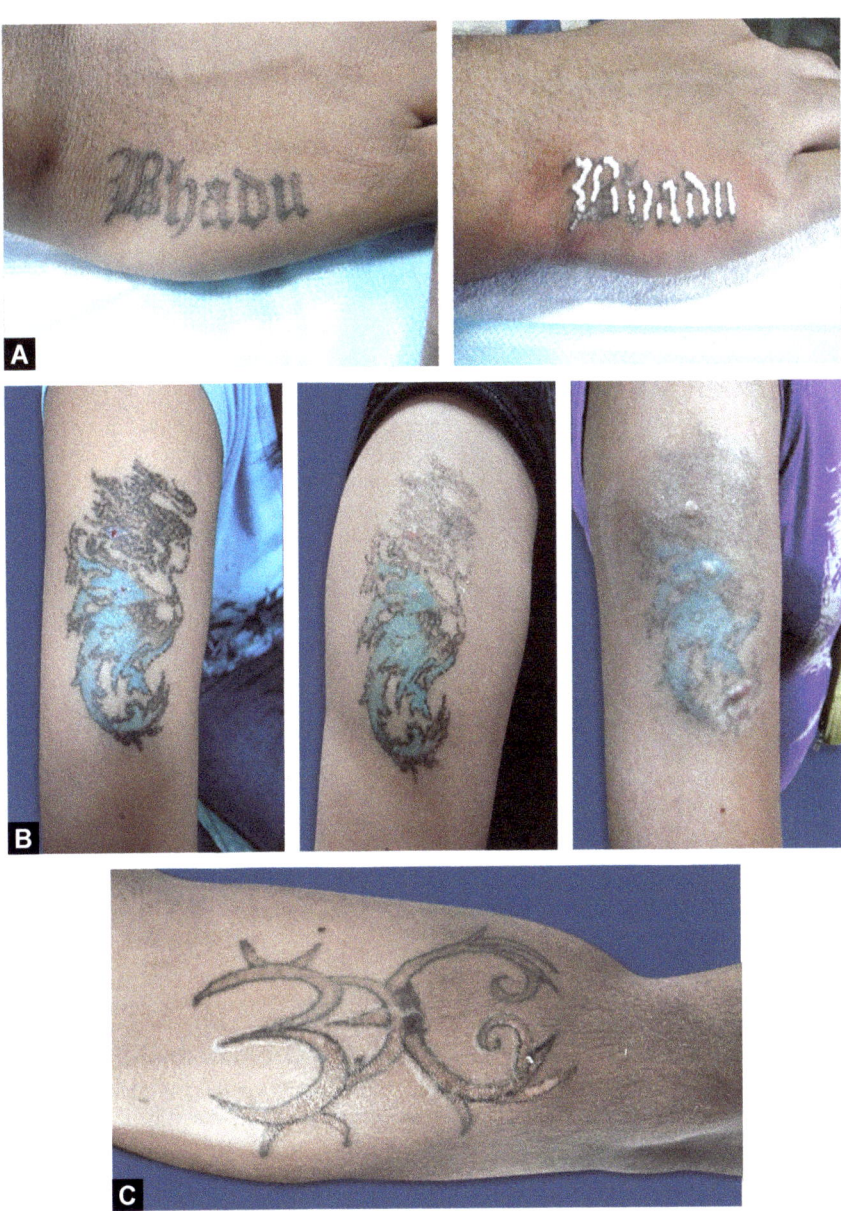

Figs. 3.34A to C: (A) Use of two different lasers for a black-red tattoo. The 532 nm was used for the red tattoo and the 1,064 nm for the blue-green tattoo; (B) A blue-black tattoo treated with 1,064 nm Q-switched neodymium-doped yttrium aluminum garnet (QS Nd:YAG). Though the same settings were used the black component was amenable to removal (six sessions) while the green/blue component faded only after 11 sessions; (C) A multicolored professional tattoo. Plan to treat the black tattoo with QS Nd:YAG 1,064 nm and red tattoo with QS Nd:YAG 532 nm.

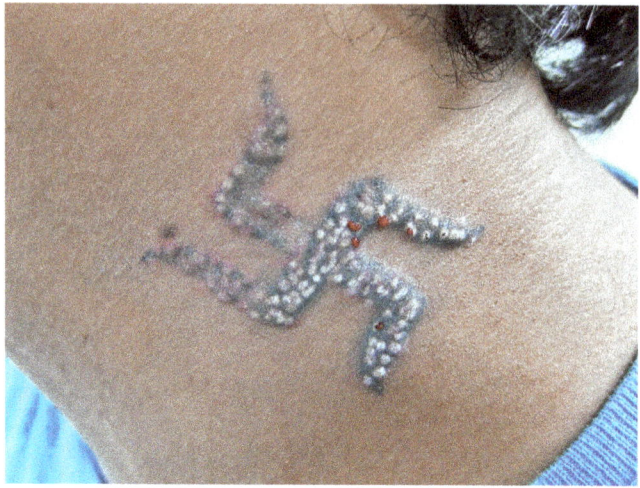

Fig. 3.34D: Professional black tattoo treated with QS Nd:YAG (1,064 nm; 5.1 J/cm^2).

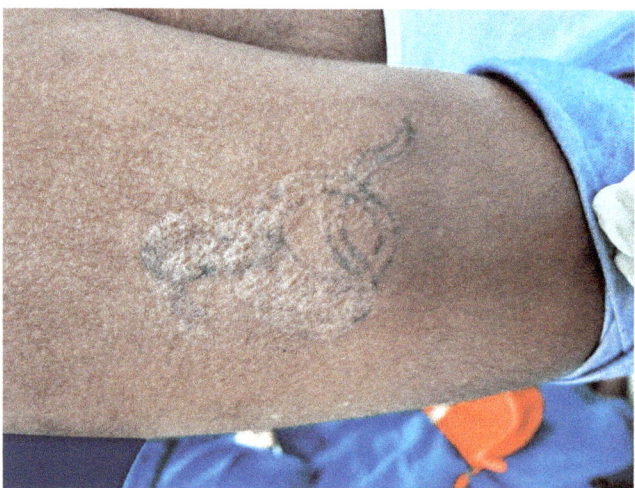

Fig. 3.35: A case of a tattoo with scarring noted before initiation of laser sessions. This has medicolegal implications and the patient should be told of the pre-existent scarring lest it becomes obvious after the sessions are over.

secondary to reduction of ferric oxide to ferrous oxide, which leads to a darkening of the ink. *Titanium* was found to be overrepresented in biopsy specimens analyzed in darkened tattoos after laser treatment. Titanium dioxide (TiO_2) is used to enhance the brilliance of tattoos and can be found in green, white, and flesh-colored tattoos, but can be seen in many other colors. *Mercury* was also reported to be seen in a red-colored tattoo that darkened after treatment with frequency-doubled Nd:YAG laser with fluences of 2–4 J/cm^2 and spot size of 2–3 mm.

Another possibility to explain paradoxical ink darkening may be the Tyndall effect, since tattoo pigments are found in the dermis and can cause a diffraction of incident light.

Tattoos that experience paradoxical darkening often require additional treatments to obtain complete ink resolution, but the newly darkened ink may also be an unfortunate permanent consequence. Paradoxical ink darkening can be a contributing factor to ink retention and patients who will likely experience this phenomenon should be forewarned of the possibility that ink retention is a possibility following paradoxical color changes with particular tattoo colors.

The 532 nm and 1,064 nm picosecond laser may be advantageous over the QS Nd:YAG laser for the treatment of paradoxical darkening as overall less energy is needed. Picosecond laser causes less heating, so that further darkening may be avoided and other heat-related side effects can be minimized. Furthermore, the greater mechanical disruption of pigment particles with picosecond pulses (breaking up particles into smaller parts that are more easily phagocytosed) may be an additional benefit of the picosecond laser.

Nonresponsive Tattoo Ink

Numerous tattoo ink formulations are now available. Although many inks respond to laser treatment as anticipated, some tattoo ink formulations are recalcitrant to treatment. The most common tattoo ink color is black and the wavelength of light used most frequently to treat this color is 1,064 nm. Tattoo artists will mix colors and ingredients and acknowledge that the formulations themselves are not uniform, frequently change, and are poorly regulated. In these cases, patients may experience ink retention and require more treatment sessions than originally anticipated. Clinicians may need to use more than one wavelength of light in these cases.

Undesired Pigmentary Alteration

Transient hyperpigmentation following Q-switched treatment is a well-established phenomenon upon complete resolution of tattoo ink following laser treatment. Patients and novice practitioners may occasionally confuse this hyperpigmentation with ink retention. Continued exposure to laser light may only prolong this transient hyperpigmentation and thus, treatments should cease once tattoo ink has resolved completely or at least improved significantly. Prolonging the intervals between treatments, topical hydroquinone, and sun avoidance measures should be considered for any patient that confuses undesired pigment alterations with ink retention.

Laser-dependent Factors

A summary of the seminal studies on lasers for tattoos is depicted here in Table 3.10 and the interpretations follow in the text.

Table 3.10: A list of seminal studies where QS lasers were employed for tattoo removal.

Authors	QS Nd:YAG 532	QSRL 694	AS Alex 755	QSNd:YAG 1064	Settings (J/cm²)	Session	Results
Taylor et al.	X	Yes	X	X	1.5–8	5	Clearance in 78% amateur and 23% professional tattoos
Kilmer et al.	X	X	X	Yes	6–12	4	> 75% in black tattoos >95% multicolored tattoos
Leuenberger et al.	X	Yes	Yes	Yes	4–10 (QSRU) 6–8 (QS Alex) 5–10 (QS ND:YAG)	4–6	QSRL was the best for black/blue tattoos but resulted in pigmentary changes
Ross et al.	X	X	X	Yes	0.6/35 picoseconds to 10 nanoseconds	4	12 out of 16 tattoos showed lightening with the picosecond laser
Ferguson and August	Yes	X	X	Yes	5–7 (532 nm) 10–4 (1064 nm)	1–5 (532 nm) 2–6 (1064 nm)	QS lasers are effective for black and red tattoos
Fitzpatrick and Goldman	X	X	Yes	X	4–8	8.9	95% clearance for black. Also effective for blue and green.

(QS Alex: Q-switched alexandrite; QS Nd:YAG: Q-switched neodymium-doped yttrium aluminum garnet; QSRL: Q-switched ruby laser)

Fluence

The fluence can be increased by the reduction of the laser beam to a smaller spot size area. However, this results in a longer treatment time. More importantly, the effective treatment of fluence is reduced at smaller spot sizes. As a beam propagates into the skin, light scattering by the skin spreads the beam radially outward on each side, which decreases the beam's effective fluence as it penetrates into the skin. This effect is more pronounced in smaller spot sizes where the spreading of the beam is relatively large compared to the incoming beam spot size (Fig. 3.36). This is why the effective fluence within the skin of, for example, a 2 mm incoming laser beam is approximately two times smaller than the effective fluence of an 8 mm laser beam. This results in approximately two times lower treatment efficacy when using a 2 mm spot size beam compared to an 8 mm spot size beam. When the incoming laser fluence is the same for both spot sizes, the resulting effective fluence is lower not only on the surface but also within the skin.

It must be remembered that the Q-switched laser is a high impact laser (Fig. 3.37A) and successive treatments with a laser result in fewer and smaller ink granules. Thus, if laser parameters are not altered to account for the progressive reduction in the size and number of the ink granules, greater number of treatment sessions may be required to reach a satisfactory clinical end point. As in vitro model (Humphries A), had predicted that the optimal absolute fluence for the *initial session* should be in the range of *7 J/cm^2*, while for the *latter session* it should be *11 J/cm^2* to achieve maximal ink fragmentation while maintaining only a small risk of thermal damage. This can be used as a rough guide for dose settings in clinical practice. A simple method to avoid "backspatter" of tissue and blood is to apply a hydrocolloid dressing while doing a tattoo (Fig. 3.37B).

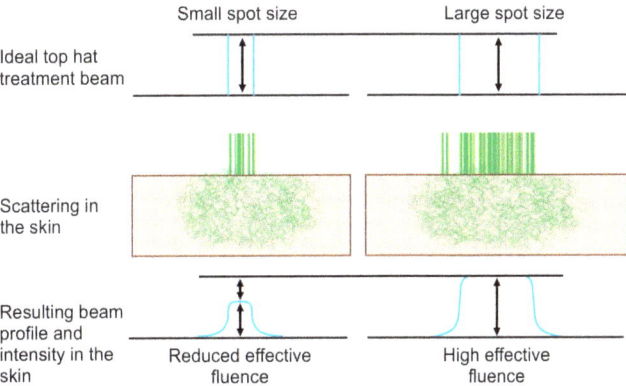

Fig. 3.36: Effect of spot size in Q-switched laser. The scattering of light is more when the spot size is small, thus it is useful to increase the diameter in case of recalcitrant lesion.

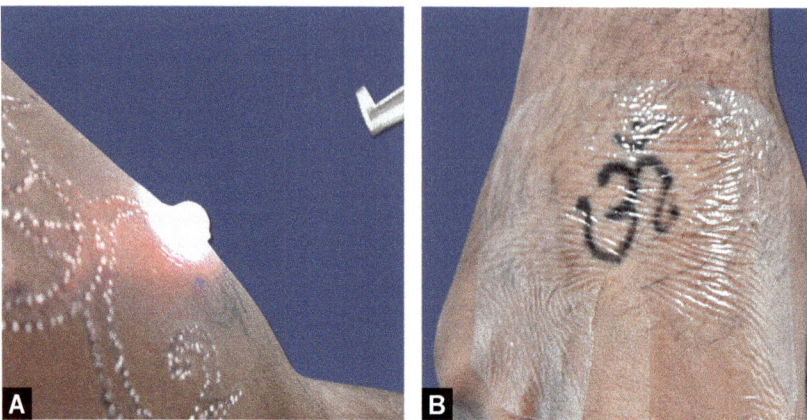

Figs. 3.37A and B: (A) Intense photothermal effect of a 1,064 nm neodymium-doped yttrium aluminum garnet (Nd:YAG) in Q-switched mode in a case of tattoo; (B) Hydrocolloid dressings are useful in cases of tattoos where higher fluences are needed and tissue splattering occurs.

Spot Size

Based on the earlier concept (Fig. 3.36), *larger spot sizes* enable deeper penetration and more effective treatment of pigment. Better beam profiles also minimize epidermal damage and decrease bleeding, tissue splatter, and transient textural changes. Of course, the practitioner can treat pigments with smaller beam spot sizes if the laser fluence is adjusted accordingly. For example, if the incoming fluence of a 2 mm laser beam is increased by a factor of two, the penetration and the treatment efficacy resulting from 2 mm and 8 mm laser beams become similar. This technique is successfully employed for variable square pulse (VSP) skin rejuvenation and hair removal treatments since VSP lasers are capable of generating sufficiently high laser pulse energies in the millisecond pulse duration range. However, this is often not a viable strategy for Q-switched lasers where high laser energies within extremely short, nanosecond pulses are difficult to obtain.

Extremely high laser powers may damage laser optics and cause optical breakdown in the air. For this reason, some commercially available devices use a rapid sequence of two or more lower power laser pulses, instead of a single giant pulse, to increase the total delivered laser fluence to the treated tissue. Others have modified it as the "R20R" technique. But this has a singular problem, as tissue characteristics change following the irradiation with a laser pulse. This may reduce the pigment removal efficacy of subsequent laser pulses.

A novel concept is of a *dynamic spot size*. Because tattoo ink fades with each treatment, increasing fluences are necessary to achieve optimal tattoo removal with each subsequent treatment. If too high fluence is used, especially during the initial treatment sessions when the tattoo is darkest, injury to the skin with scarring can occur. A dynamic spot diameter would progressively get smaller as the fluence gets higher thus avoiding unnecessary thermal injury. This is contrary to most Q-switched lasers where a 2–3 mm diameter spot size is used to achieve fluences as high as 12 J/cm^2 at 1,064 nm, which can cause more thermal damage.

Ideal Interval

Appropriate treatment interval has been rarely studied. It was initially hoped that a condensed protocol of three sessions within a 7–10 days period, followed by adequate time for macrophage activity (3 months), would result in an RTR with fewer total treatments but this was not found to help. Treatment intervals of 1 month interval could interfere with macrophage activity, because the pigment containing macrophages are laser targets as well as the stationary pigment-laden macrophages. Thus, extending the interval to *2–3 months* was ideal and lead to a 50% improvement after three sessions.

Sessions

It is difficult to predict the number of treatment sessions necessary for tattoo removal. Frequently the initial treatment session produces a more dramatic response than subsequent sessions. Very definite sites of clearing, corresponding to laser impacts, are often visible. Other tattoos are strongly unresponsive during early treatment phases, even though biopsies reveal fragmentation of tattoo granules. The explanation of these differences in response from one patient to another is likely to involve the efficiency of mobile macrophages in removal of fragmented tattoo pigment debris, as well as the density and amount of tattoo pigment present. The speed of the macrophage response, as well as the maximum amount of pigment removed per session, likely varies from patient to patient and to some extent from treatment to treatment.

A few general *assumptions* can be safely made, larger and deeper the tattoo more the sessions required. As a *general rule*, new tattoos treated with Q-switched alexandrite lasers cleared faster, possibly because of the more superficial location of a new tattoo.

As a rule with exceptions, 5–10 sessions are standard for amateur tattoos and 15–20 for professional tattoos, even up to 25 sessions in rare cases (Figs. 3.37C and D). More recently placed tattoos with deeply located pigment on a distal site are harder to remove due to the reduced lymphatic distribution, which helps in removing residual ink particles.

Pulse Duration

Recently, Saedi N et al. have used a picosecond alexandrite laser for removing tattoos. Most tattoo pigments have a particle size of 30–300 nm,

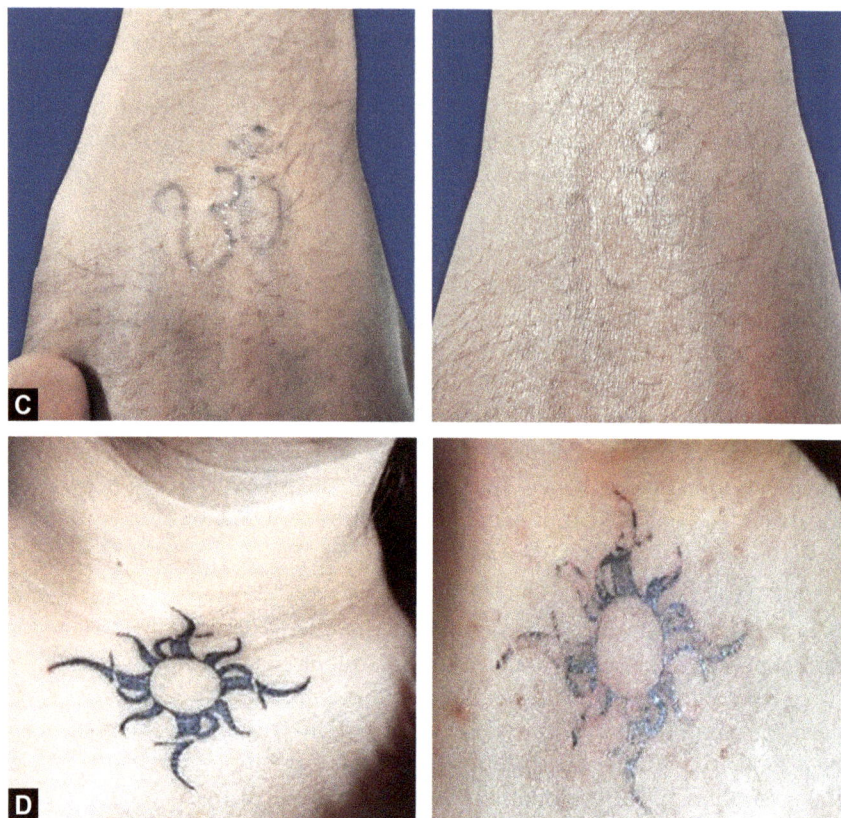

Figs. 3.37C and D: (C) A simple black amateur tattoo. Plan: Q-switched neodymium-doped yttrium aluminum garnet (QS Nd:YAG) 1,064 nm. Such tattoos respond to Q-switched laser. Complete removal after three sessions; (D) Baseline photograph of a patient with professional tattoo. Response after six sittings with ND:YAG laser (1,064 nm).

corresponding to a thermal relaxation time of less than 10 ns. Thus, an ideal laser should have a pulse duration in nanoseconds, which is the logic of using Q-switched lasers (10^{-9} s). Newer laser technologies shorten than pulse time to picoseconds (10^{-12} s), are promising but should be invested after understanding the myriad variables as detailed here.

Ideal Technique

A "Polka-dot" technique is employed. This means, gaps between consecutive shots. These gaps then have to be treated with an additional treatment. This technique reduces side effects related to the high absorption in very black professional tattoos.

NOVEL LASER THERAPY AND MODIFICATIONS FOR TATTOO REMOVAL

Is Picosecond the Latest Hype or are they Really Superior to Q-Switched Lasers?

In spite of this novel technology, there are certain contrarian views on the picoseconds laser which are listed below and the reader can take a informed decision of the technology:

- There are fundamental arguments against the concept of reduced pulse width that are achieved by the picolasers. Humphries et al. had elegantly demonstrated that variations in the pulse width had little influence on the fragmentation response. Also experimental data on the effect of laser-fluences on skin whitening for a wide range of tested pulse durations, has shown that the plasma formation threshold changed only slightly, even though the pulse duration varied by a factor of 25 (from 2–50 ns). It is thus highly unlikely that shortening of the pulse duration by another factor of 2.5 (to obtain subnanosecond pulses) would result in any further significant change. The plasma formation in highly absorbing tissues is insensitive to pulse duration and thus reducing the pulse duration into the sub-nanosecond range will not contribute significantly to the thermal mechanisms involved in tattoo removal.
- The predominant mechanism with sub-nanosecond pulses is the fracturing of tattoo particles under increased mechanical stress. However, as has been shown, tattoo particle fragmentation does not occur even when 20-times shorter (e.g. 35 ps) pulses are used.
- Though the first study published in 1998 and performed in 16 patients with a Q-switched Nd:YAG laser delivering 35 ps pulses was shown to be more efficient in clearing cosmetic tattoos than a Q-switched Nd:YAG laser delivering 10-nanosecond pulses, the present pico lasers are at best sub-nanosecond lasers, as they have a pulse duration of 300 and 750 ps and do not seem to be vastly superior to the nanosecond lasers (Ross v, 1998). Here it is important to note that Ross et al. had shown that temperature-induced changes, rather than particle fragmentation, are responsible for tattoo clearing. It is also worth noting that picosecond pulses of a sufficiently high fluence are difficult to generate, and thus picosecond lasers are capable of delivering fluences above plasma formation threshold only at small spot sizes. These small spot sizes result not only in procedures being slow, but also result in unacceptable scattering losses, so that the tissue penetration and treatment efficacy are compromised. Moreover, as is the need after the first few sessions, the spot size needs to be increased to target deep tattoo particles which would translate into a lower pulse energy, which is a issue as the effective pulse energy of the Pico systems are already low!

- Exact comparisons of these devices are needed to compare maximally tolerated fluences for each color within a given tattoo [Bernstein et al. 2013]. While there are many articles attesting to the efficacy of picosecond lasers, few actually compare nanosecond and picosecond lasers with equivalent spot sizes, fluences, and wavelengths. Most of the studies that extol the virtues of picosecond technology are based on treating resistant tattoos and then applying picosecond pulses, or the studies are simply a stand-alone assessment of picosecond lasers in treating various tattoos. The study by Pinto et al. that compared clearance after two treatments with picosecond and nanosecond lasers, essentially showing equivalence between the two pulse durations but the maximum fluences were not used.
- The use of the present "pseudo-picosecond lasers" is based on the premise that they are useful when the tattoo particles are small, but the smallest of these particles (< 0.5 μm) cannot be identified with light microscopy due to the resolution limit. Thus, there is no demonstrable histological proof that these pico lasers actually achieve the results based on "back of the envelope" calculations.
- A recent study compared in a split lesion protocol (Lorgeou A) two picosecond lasers, the Picoway© (Syneron Candela Corp, Wayland, MA, USA) with a pulse duration of 450 ps at 1064 nm and 375 ps at 532 nm and the Enlighten© (Cutera, Brisbane, CA, USA) with a pulse duration of 750 ps at 1064 and 532 nm. The nanosecond lasers used was the VersaPulse VP Cosmetic© (Coherent, Santa Clara, CA, USA), with a pulse duration of 5 ns at 1064 and 532 nm. A reduction of 75% or more of the color intensity was obtained for 33% of the tattoos treated with the picosecond lasers compared to 14% with the nanosecond laser. More importantly, the Picosecond lasers were superior to the nanosecond laser for professional tattoos, but this was not true for the amateur and cosmetic tattoos. Significantly for polychromatic tattoos the two were similarly effective. Thus, it is important to understand if the major cost difference justifies the pico lasers in routine tattoo practice, as they were equally effective for multicolored tattoos.
- We have treated countless professional multicolored tattoos with a modification of the standard tattoo techniques (RTR technique—Sardana K, 2015) and we do not share the unbridled enthusiasm of the picosecond lasers. At the end of the day, it is the host immune response that matters as it effects the removal of the tattoo particles and the laser used does not impact on that crucial process markedly (Fig. 3.38A).

Though there are many issues and debatable advantages that have now been considered as some as marketing gimmicks, there is no doubt that for certain colored tattoos, the pico has an advantage over the nanosecond lasers. A marked and unmistakable difference is in the ability to remove yellow tattoo inks in a few treatments with picosecond-domain devices [Alabdulrazzaq H,

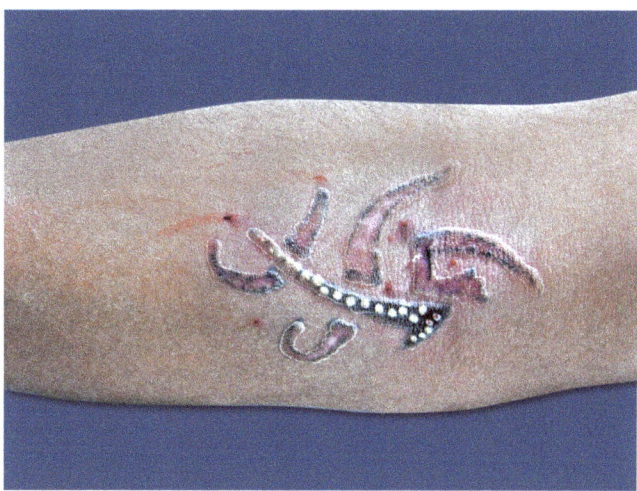

Fig. 3.38A: A tattoo being treated by the modified two step technique. First the epidermis is ablated using the erbium:yttrium aluminum garnet (Er:YAG) laser, is then followed by the Q-switched neodymium-doped yttrium aluminum garnet (QS Nd:YAG) laser. *Note:* The polka-dot pattern, wherein in the first pass, a gap is ensured between consecutive laser shots, which are then covered subsequently.
Source: Sardana K, Garg VK, Bansal S, et al. A promising split-lesion technique for rapid tattoo removal using a novel sequential approach of a single sitting of pulsed CO(2) followed by Q-switched Nd: YAG laser (1064 nm). J Cosmet Dermatol. 2013;12:296-305.

Bernstein EF, 2015]. A recent study (Bernstein et al. 2018) used a novel 785 nm, titanium:sapphire (Ti:sapphire) laser for removing multicolored tattoos, specially targeted at purple, blue and green and found it to improve 85%, 81%, and 74%, of these colored tattoos after four treatments (Fig. 3.38B). The 1064 nm and 532 nm are able to effectively treat the commonly seen black, red and yellow tattoos (Fig. 3.38B).

Here it is important to understand that this additional wavelength (785 nm) is useful as a quarter of tattoos (Bencini et al.) contain green, purple, or blue ink that has traditionally been targeted by the 755 nm alexandrite laser and is not always effective. This can also account for the relative failure of the conventionally used Qs lasers as they do not cater for this color combination.

Thus, there are certain scenarios where the picolasers may have an edge over the nanosecond laser.

1. The case of certain green-blue tattoos, where 750 ps red-light lasers (alexandrite) are able to clear tattoos better than a 50 ns alexandrite laser, even where higher fluences are applied in the nanosecond case. The recently studied 785 nm is another notable addition to the ps Alex lasers.
2. Possibly certain yellow tattoos, where there is evidence that they respond particularly well to low-energy picosecond green-light pulses.
3. Partially treated tattoos (where presumably the tattoo particles are smaller than pretreatment), in which case picosecond lasers are likely to clear tattoos faster.

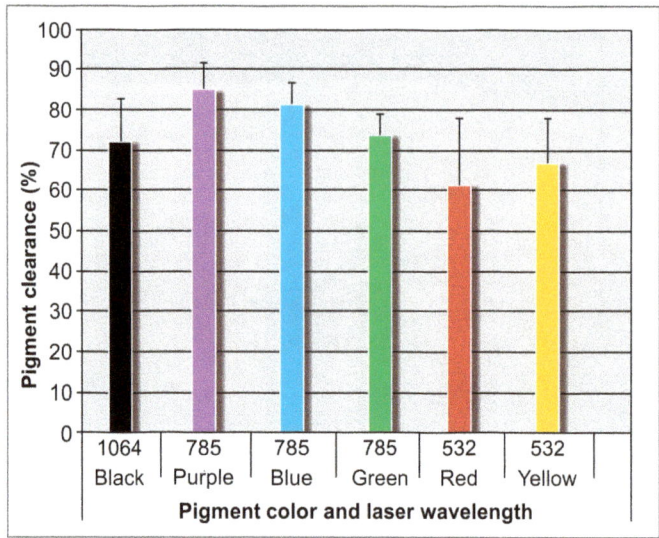

Fig. 3.38B: A comparison of the efficacy of different wavelengths for various colored tattoos (Bernstein et al. 2018).

In conclusion, the relationship between pulse-duration, tattoo ink composition, age of tattoo, and the biology of individual patients needs to be further explored to arrive at a definitive conclusion regarding the comparative superiority of the picosecond laser over the nanosecond laser.

BIBLIOGRAPHY

1. Alabdulrazzaq H, Brauer JA, Bae YS, Geronemus RG. Clearance of yellow tattoo ink with a novel 532-nm picosecond laser. Lasers Surg Med. 2015;47(4):285-8.
2. Bencini PL, Cazzaniga S, Tourlaki A, Glaimberti MG. Removal of tattoos by Q-switched laser: variables influencing outcome and sequelae in a large cohort of treated patients. Arch Dermatol. 2012;148:1364-9.
3. Bernstein EF, Bhawalkar J, Schomacker KT. A novel titanium sapphire picosecond-domain laser safely and effectively removes purple, blue, and green tattoo inks. Lasers Surg Med. 2018 May 20.
4. Bernstein EF, Civiok JM. A continuously variable beamdiameter, high fluence, Q-switched Nd:YAG laser for tattoo removal: comparison of the maximum beam diameter to a standard 4-mm diameter treatment beam. Lasers Surg Med. 2013;45:621-7.
5. Bernstein EF, Schomacker KT, Basilavecchio LD, et al. A novel dual-wavelength, Nd:YAG, picosecond-domain laser safely and effectively removes multicolor tattoos. Lasers Surg Med. 2015;47:542-8.
6. Lorgeou A, Perrillat Y, Gral N, et al. Comparison of two picosecond lasers to a nanosecond laser for treating tattoos: a prospective randomized study on 49 patients. J Eur Acad Dermatol Venereol. 2018;32(2):265-70.

7. Ross V, Naseef G, Lin G, et al. Comparison of responses of tattoos to picosecond and nanosecond Q-switched neodymium: YAG lasers. Arch Dermatol. 1998;134:167-71.
8. Sardana K, Ranjan R, Kochhar AM, et al. A rapid tattoo removal technique using a combination of pulsed Er:YAG and Q-Switched Nd:YAG in a split lesion protocol. J Cosmet Laser Ther. 2015;17(4):177-83.

Combination of Lasers (RTR Technique)

- A novel concept that was first propounded by Goldman MP and Fitzpatrick RE was based on ablation of the epidermis which helped to target the dermal tattoo pigment with less beam scattering and faster results (Fig. 3.32). This technique fell out of favor as conventional ablative lasers lead to scarring that is consequent to the use of doses and settings that exceed the thermal relaxation time of the skin. But pulsed lasers like erbium:yttrium aluminum garnet (Er:YAG) and the ultrapulsed carbon dioxide (CO_2) lasers can be used to precisely remove epidermal layers (Sardana K, 2013, 2015).

    This was studied initially using a combination of ultrapulse CO_2 laser followed by QS Nd:YAG, in a split lesion design which led to a significant reduction in the number of sessions with negligible side effects (Fig. 3.32). This has been further modified using the Er:YAG followed by the QS Nd:YAG with better results and has been christened the **RTR technique**. An example of this is depicted in Figure 3.38B. This was expanded later and a host of various tattoos have been treated including *professional and colored* (Figs. 3.39 to 3.42) and *amateur* (Figs. 3.43 and 3.44) tattoos. If a combination procedure is to be used, an Er:YAG is much safer, predictable, and has a perfect tissue ablation potential.

    Another study from Delhi conducted by Vanarase et al. in 60 patients with black tattoo, randomized patient into two groups, and treated with QS Nd:YAG laser (1,064 nm) alone and its combination with ultrapulse CO_2 laser. The sessions were repeated at interval of 4 weeks for a maximum of six sittings. The response was evaluated using visual analog scale (VAS) and tattoo ink lightening (TIL) scores. The authors found that combination laser showed statistically significant improvement in mean VAS and TIL scores. This was especially true for professional tattoos. The authors concluded that combination of ultrapulse CO_2 laser and QS Nd:YAG laser is superior to pigment-specific laser alone, especially for the treatment of refractory professional tattoos (Figs. 3.44A and B).

- Another option is to use a combination of fractional ablative laser and Q-switched laser, though in our experience this is not as effective as using a pulsed ablative laser. This technique creates microablation zones, through which the Q-switched lasers are presumed to penetrate more effectively into the dermis. This needs a spot diameter that corresponds

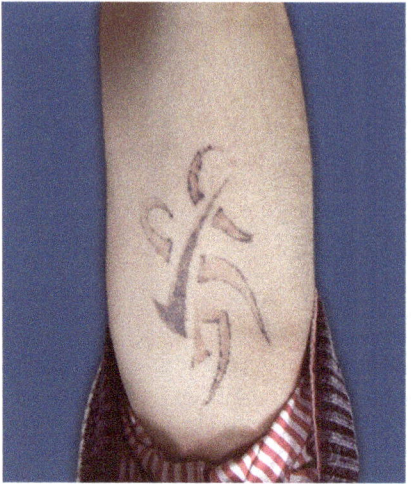
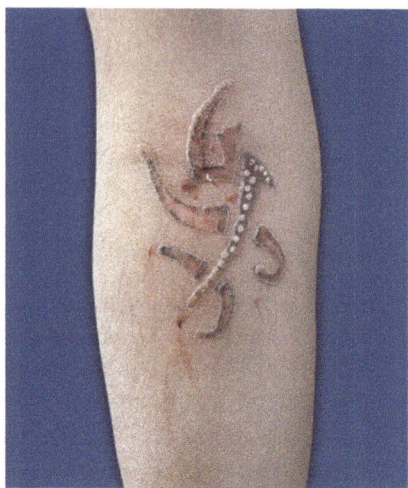

Fig. 3.39A: RTR technique: Er:YAG/Up CO_2 followed by QS Nd:YAG laser: Multicolored tattoo. In the first session ablate the epidermis till signs of a papillary bleed. The settings used were 4 J/cm^2 of the Er:YAG. At that point wipe off the debris and give a pass of the appropriate QS Nd:YAG. In this case 532 nm for the red tattoo and 1,064 nm for the black tattoo. (CO_2: carbon dioxide; Er:YAG: erbium:yttrium aluminum garnet; RTR: rapid tattoo removal; QS Nd:YAG: Q-switched neodymium-doped yttrium aluminum garnet)

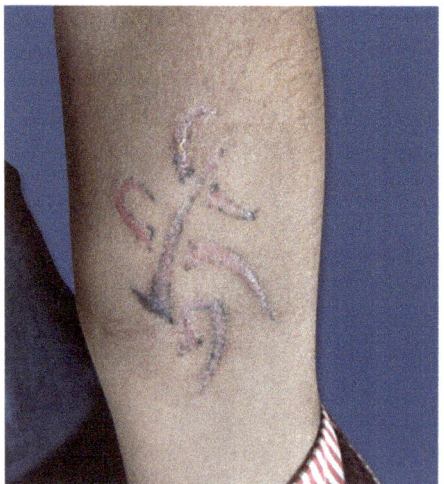
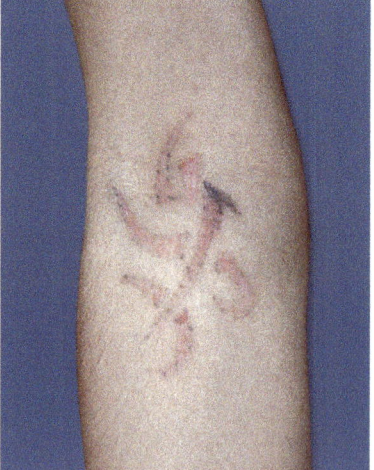

Fig. 3.39B: In the subsequent sessions do not ablate the epidermis. In 3–5 sessions most tattoos fade. Sessions at 3 months intervals.

to the microablation zones created by the fractional laser. Probably an accurate and complete ablation of the epidermis followed by Q-switched laser is a more appropriate method when emergent tattoo removal is required. And our extensive experience on this (Figs. 3.39 to 3.44) finds this to be a superior method than using the fractional laser.

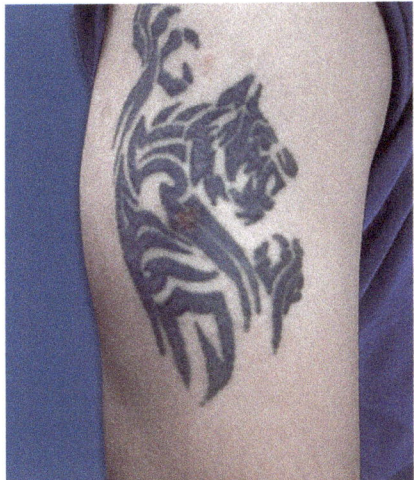 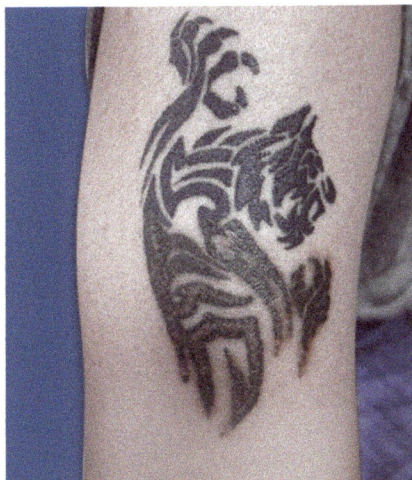

Fig. 3.40A: RTR technique: Er:YAG/Up CO_2 followed by QS Nd:YAG laser: A split lesion tattoo removal: Upper end QS 1,064 nm/lower part Er:YAG f/b Nd:YAG. (CO_2: carbon dioxide; Er:YAG: erbium:yttrium aluminum garnet; RTR: rapid tattoo removal; QS Nd:YAG: Q-switched neodymium-doped yttrium aluminum garnet)

Manipulation of the Laser Tissue Interface

An elegant concept that can be used to improve results is by manipulating the interface between the laser and the tattoo. This will effectively lead to reduced scatter and attenuation of the laser energy, thus resulting in enhanced results (Fig. 3.32). This can be achieved by various means:
- Epidermal injury can be reduced by topical application of hyperosmotic solutions prior to laser therapy, such as sucrose, glycerol, and water-soluble gels (e.g. surgilube) that have a refractive index matching closely to that of stratum corneum, i.e. 1.4 which will in effect reduce the surface scatter from incident light. The problem being that such solutions are highly hydrophilic and penetrate intact skin very poorly when applied topically.

  Khan et al. used clearing agents such as polypropylene glycol (PPG) and polyethylene glycol (PEG) which allowed more photons to reach the target apart from reducing the scattered light. The scattering coefficient of epidermis and superficial papillary dermis (upper 200–300 μm thickness) reduced from 0.4 mm^{-1} to 0.2–0.1 mm^{-1} after the application of these clearing agents. The resulting heat source term profiles showed a 40% decrease at the dermoepidermal junction (DEJ) due to reduced epidermal scattering, thus predicting a safer tissue impact profile.
- Another option is to reduce dermal scatter by using a transdermal application of a clearing agent (glycerol) which has been shown to improve treatment outcomes in tattoos (Fig. 3.32).

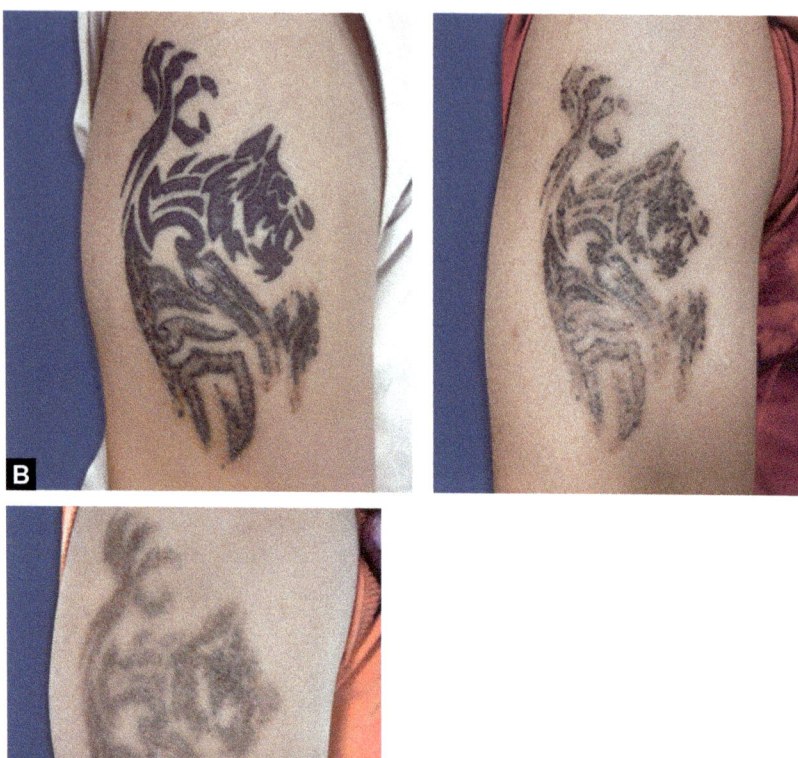

Figs. 3.40B and C: (B) A marked difference in the combination side [rapid tattoo removal (RTR) technique]; (C) At the end of six sessions. The "shadow" of the tattoo remains.

- A third modification has been described earlier, (*RTR* method) wherein a pulsed laser can be used to remove the epidermis, which eliminates the epidermal diffraction and scatter and this has been shown to reduce the number of sessions markedly.

R20 Method

This method is based on the observation that the "whitening" that occurs after most Q-switched lasers can prevent successive laser pulses to penetrate into the dermis. To obviate this repeated sessions after an interval of 20 minutes between pulses can help to dissipate this phenomenon and thus multiple passes can be achieved in a single session.

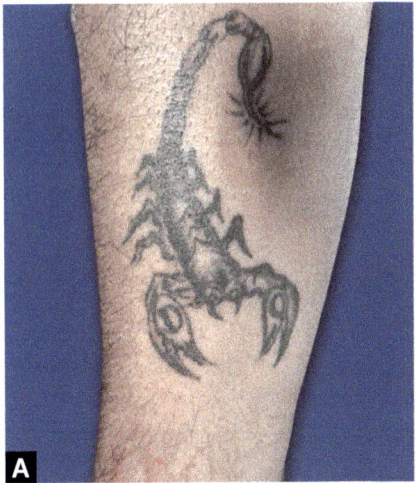 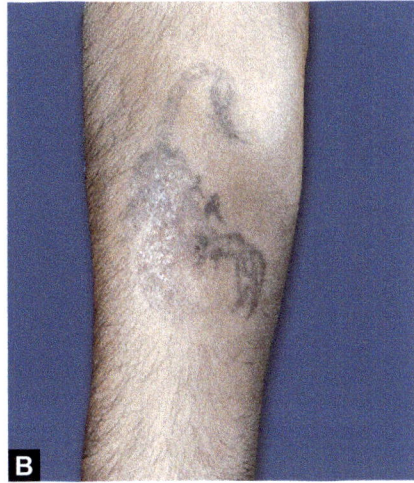

Figs. 3.41A and B: RTR technique: Er:YAG followed by QS Nd:YAG laser: multicolored tattoo. Result after four sessions. (Er:YAG: erbium:yttrium aluminum garnet; RTR: rapid tattoo removal; QS Nd:YAG: Q-switched neodymium-doped yttrium aluminum garnet)

This method has two drawbacks, one it is time consuming and secondly, it has not been adequately studied with other wavelengths, like 1,064 nm, which are frequently employed in pigmented skin. There is another issue with this method, as there is a change in the size of the tattoo pigment, which after the first impact will have an altered optical property and size which will change the optical absorption of the pigment. Thus, probably the Q-switched mode may not be ideal for the remnant tattoo particles. Moreover, the 1,064 nm, used in pigmented skin has a higher photothermal impact and depth than the 755 nm laser used originally and repeated passes may cause more thermal injury while using the 1,064 nm device.

R0 Method

A modification of the earlier method has been proposed where application of topical perfluorodecalin (PFD), a highly gas soluble liquid fluorocarbon, that resolves the whitening reaction within seconds, (R0 method) thus obviating the waiting time of 20 minutes.

Imiquimod

Solis et al. used imiquimod to treat freshly applied tattoos on guinea pigs. After 7 days, barely a trace of pigment could be histopathologically detected; however, after 28 days, they observed fibrosis and a loss of dermal appendages. When administered under optimized conditions, imiquimod may be a nonsurgical means of removing fresh tattoos.

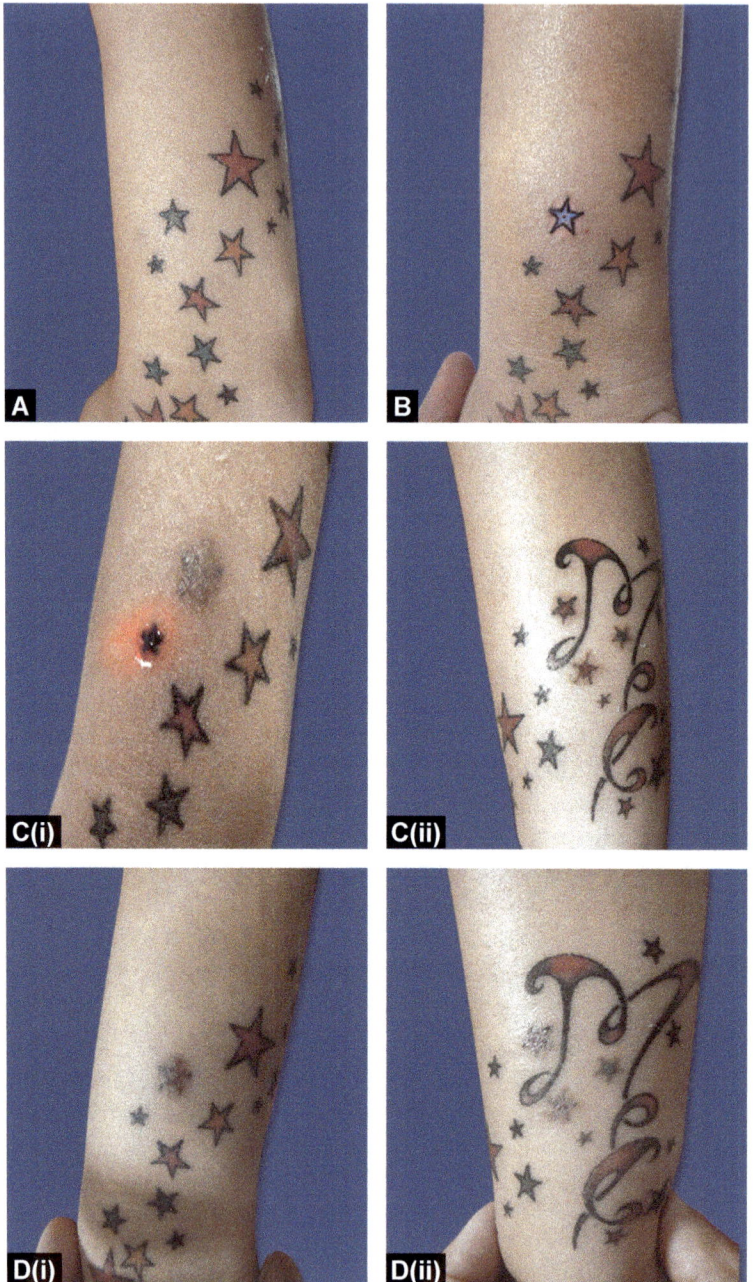

Figs. 3.42A to D

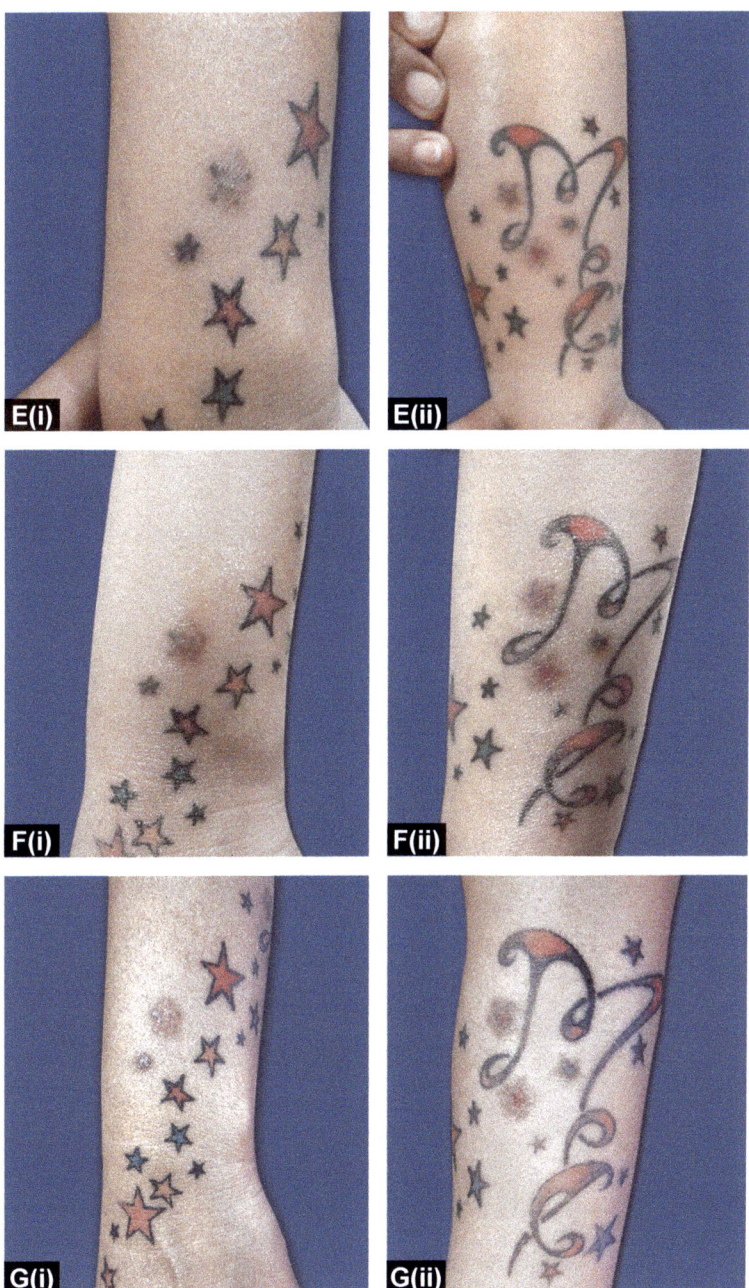

Figs. 3.42A to G: RTR technique for a multicolored tattoo. Here we ablated the epidermis with a Er:YAG followed by Nd:YAG. We choose a spot of the tattoo to predict the response. The series of photographs taken at 2 monthly intervals. This was a difficult cases and after six sessions there is good response on the chosen tattoos. (Er:YAG: erbium:yttrium aluminum garnet; RTR: rapid tattoo removal; QS Nd:YAG: Q-switched neodymium-doped yttrium aluminum garnet)

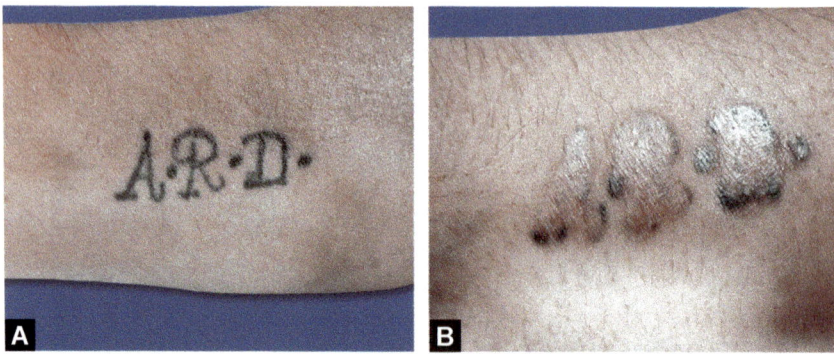

Figs. 3.43A and B: A black amateur tattoo treated by "modified tattoo removal technique" (Up CO_2 followed by QS Nd:YAG). After three sessions there is almost complete removal of tattoo. (CO_2: carbon dioxide; QS Nd:YAG: Q-switched neodymium-doped yttrium aluminum garnet)

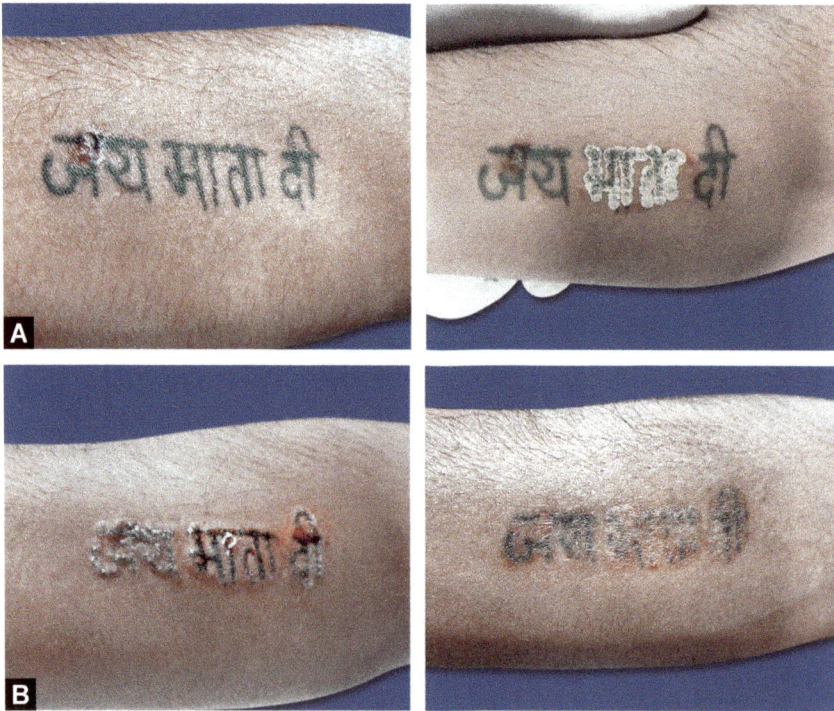

Figs. 3.44A and B: (A) A black amateur tattoo treated with Er:YAG followed by QS Nd:YAG. The center of the tattoo is ablated using Er:YAG set at 2 J/cm^2 and 2 Hz to ablate the epidermis. *Note:* The whitening of the epidermis which is a characteristic transient feature of Er:YAG. (Er:YAG: erbium:yttrium aluminum garnet; QS Nd:YAG: Q-switched neodymium-doped yttrium aluminum garnet); (B) The ablation of the epidermis reveals the visible tattoo pigment and is then treated with QS Nd:YAG at 1,064 nm. The rest of the tattoo is treated with QS Nd:YAG lasers. The "split lesion" view reveals a marked improvement in the combined laser treatment area.
Source: Sardana K, Garg VK, Bansal S, et al. J Cosmet Dermatol. 2013;12:296-305.

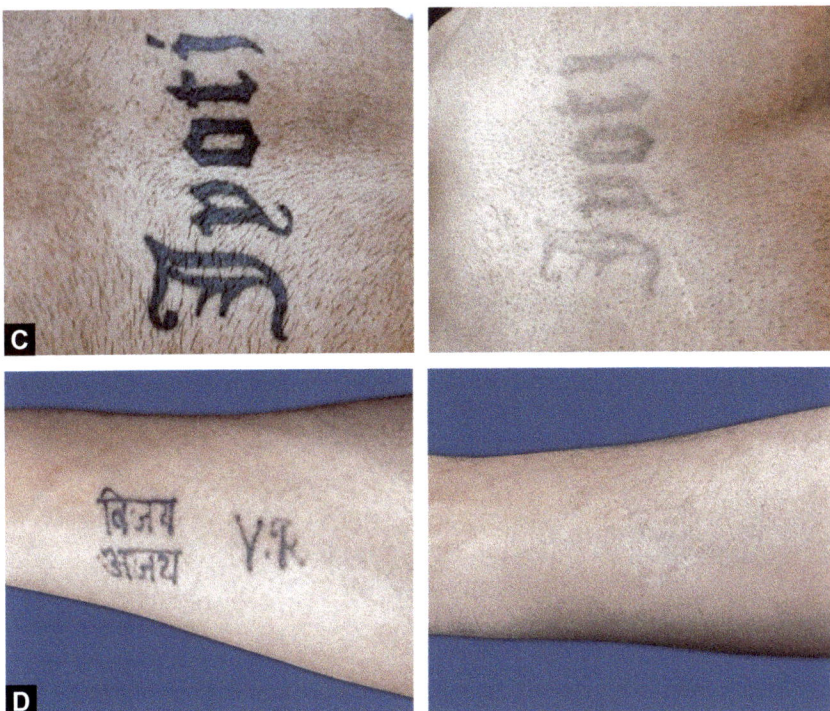

Figs. 3.44C and D: (C) Baseline photograph of a patient with professional tattoo. Response after six sittings of ultrapulse CO_2 laser followed by Nd:YAG laser (1,064 nm); (D) Baseline photograph of a patient with amateur tattoo. Near complete disappearance to tattoo after six sittings of ultrapulse CO_2 laser followed by Nd:YAG (1,064 nm).

Acoustic Shock Wave Therapy

A recent article (Vangipuram R) used a combination of a pico laser followed by ASWT, with an enhanced clearance. The ASWT helped to enhance tattoo clearance by increasing lymphatic drainage and increasing metabolic activity in the treated area, thereby accelerating the clearance of dermal pigment vacuoles produced by the picosecond laser and minimizing epidermal side effects such as erythema, edema, and crusting.

BIBLIOGRAPHY

1. Vangipuram R, Hamill SS, Friedman PM. Accelerated tattoo removal with acoustic shock wave therapy in conjunction with a picosecond laser. Lasers Surg Med. 2018;50(9):890-2.

PREREQUISITES

The prerequisites of laser tattoo removal are described in Table 3.11.

Table 3.11: Preoperative preparation in a patient undergoing laser tattoo removal.

History	Allergy to topical anesthetics; previous isotretinoin use; systemic gold therapy; herpes labialis; sun exposure habits; and keloidal tendencies
Patient counseling	Treatment options; expected outcome; postoperative care; potential risks (blistering, crusting, scarring, hypo and hyperpigmentation, and textural changes); residual outline, and textural changes after treatment
Assessment	Fitzpatrick skin phototype; assessment of tattoo—site, color, amount of ink used, amateur/professional, presence of scarring, and ink layering
Test spots	For patients with dark skin and cosmetic tattoos (risk of paradoxical darkening)
Standardized baseline photographs	–
Informed consent	–

LASER TREATMENT

- Area should be cleansed (avoid using flammable cleansing agents).
- Topical anesthetic should be applied under occlusion for 45–60 minutes. The cream should be removed completely prior to treatment.
- *Methods to reduce discomfort:* Use of cool air, regional nerve blocks, and local infiltration of lidocaine.
- Appropriate eye protection, eye shields (wavelength specific) both for the doctor and the patient.
- *Desired endpoint:* Immediate tissue whitening (lasts for 20 minutes).
- *Fluence:* Lowest possible fluence that causes whitening should be used. Low fluence should be used initially and can be increased as tattoo becomes lighter.
- *Wavelength:* Depends on color of tattoo, previous response, and skin prototype.
- *Spot size:* 3–4 mm spot size used with 10–20% overlap. Alternatively polka-dot technique can be used.
- *Frequency:* 8 weeks.

POSTOPERATIVE CARE

- Cold compresses can be used to decrease discomfort.
- Topical antibiotics to reduce secondary infection.
- Sun protection in the form of broad-spectrum sunscreens.
- Patient should be counseled regarding development of erythema and swelling postprocedure and about the risk of potential complications.

CONCLUSION

Most laser surgeons will graduate to using lasers for tattoos and will face numerous scenarios that make it difficult to produce rapid results. A summary of these scenarios and a suggested approach is given in Table 3.12, though being a dynamic field, some practitioners may adopt other alternative approaches.

Table 3.12: An overview of lasers and modifications used for recalcitrant tattoos (Sardana K, 2013, 2015).

Scenario	Clinical problem	Comments	Laser used
Slow response	Average sittings required vary from 6–10 sittings. Tattoo removal varies from 47.2% after 10 sessions to 74.8% after 15 sessions	Various modifications and combinations have been tried including the picosecond lasers	The various techniques are depicted in Flowchart 3.2
Multicolored tattoos	Colors, like yellow and orange, are known to be highly resistant to treatment, and red and green have a variable response	Absorption spectrum shows variable wavelength requirement; blue (625 nm), green (755 nm), red (575 nm), yellow (<520 nm), orange (<560 nm), tan (<560 nm), and flesh colored (<530 nm). In pigmented skin, the shorter wavelengths used may be absorbed by melanin and thus cause side effects and also prevent degradation of pigment in the dermis	Combination lasers and ablative lasers can be used. A trial and error approach is needed in most cases
Darkening of tattoos	Mild graying to complete blackening of the treated tattoo. Seen in white, flesh-colored, red, brown, yellow, and crimson pigmented tattoo	This is primarily due to the use of ferric oxide (brown, red, and pink) and titanium dioxide (white and flesh-colored green, blue, and yellow pigments)	In most cases, ablative lasers are the only option though in one report a combination of PDL and Q-switched laser has been used
Hypersensitivity to pigments	Pigments used for automobile paint and printer's ink can cause inflammatory, allergic hypersensitivity, granulomatous, lichenoid, and pseudolymphomatous reactions	The Q-switched lasers are of no use in these situations	• Excision of the tissue and ablative lasers are the only option • Recently a combination of AFR with Q-switched laser has been tried in two patients

Contd...

Contd...

Scenario	Clinical problem	Comments	Laser used
Double tattoos	Usually used for masking a previous tattoo	Multiple sittings are required with a high risk of scarring	A combination approach may be a useful modality
Traumatic/Iatrogenic tattoos	These particles are usually gravel, asphalt, dirt, pencil, surgical pen, rework debris, amalgam, or glass	• If pigment is carbon and graphite respond to Q-switched lasers • In case of combustible material scarring may ensue due to combustion in case lasers are used	Usually ablative lasers can be used effectively. Another option could be surgical excision of the particle
Tattoos in pigmented skin	In dark-pigmented skin (Type V/VI), results are slow and incomplete	The epidermal pigment may interfere with the laser wavelength specially for multicolored or colored tattoos due to the shorter wavelength used	Our combination approach may be a simple cost-effective option
Emergent removal of tattoos	In certain situations like interview, marriages, and army recruitment patients are desirous of removal of tattoos in one sitting	Q-switched lasers require multiple sittings and picoseconds laser are pigment specific and expensive	Our combination approach is quick, safe, and removes pigment in 1–2 sittings

(AFR: ablative fractional resurfacing; PDL: pulsed dye laser)

The various aspects that predict successful removal of tattoos are depicted in Figure 3.31 and the wide array of variations means that effective and satisfactory response in tattoos is still an exacting science. Also there are certain side effects that can be seen (Figs. 3.45 to 3.48). Tragically, laser tattoo removal has inevitably led to more tattooing which is unfortunate as a tattoo is never more beautiful than the skin onto which it is placed. Though a permanent solution would entail making tattoos safer and more removable than ever but as the laser industry and the tattoo practitioner are on different poles, the aim of a faster tattoo removal will remain a difficult goal to achieve for laser physicists and practitioners.

CHAPTER 3: Pigmented Lesions and Tattoos **237**

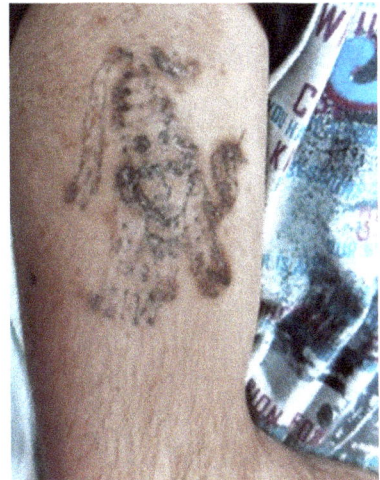

Fig. 3.45: Postinflammatory hyperpigmentation and scarring in a patient treated with neodymium-doped yttrium aluminum garnet (Nd:YAG) laser. Pigmentary changes are common in darker skin due to higher percentage of competing melanocytes.

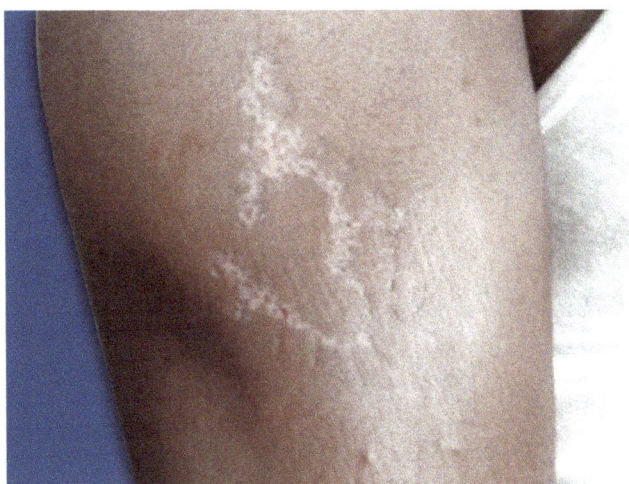

Fig. 3.46: Postinflammatory depigmentation seen in a patient seen after neodymium-doped yttrium aluminum garnet (Nd:YAG) laser treatment.

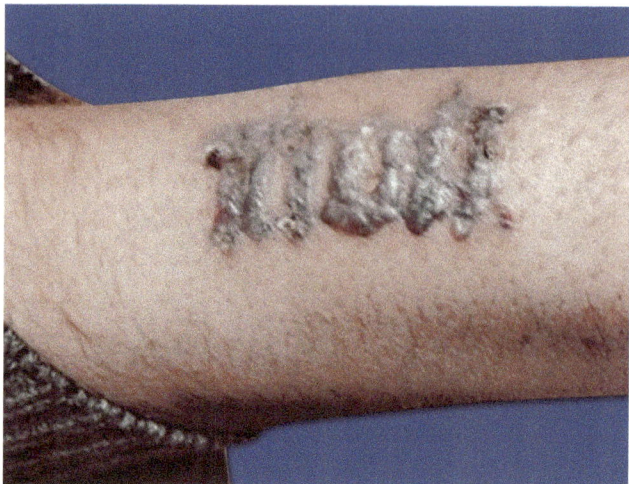

Fig. 3.47: Hemorrhagic blistering in a patient with neodymium-doped yttrium aluminum garnet (Nd:YAG) laser treatment. This occurs due to extensive cytolysis of epidermal cells secondary to thermal injury.

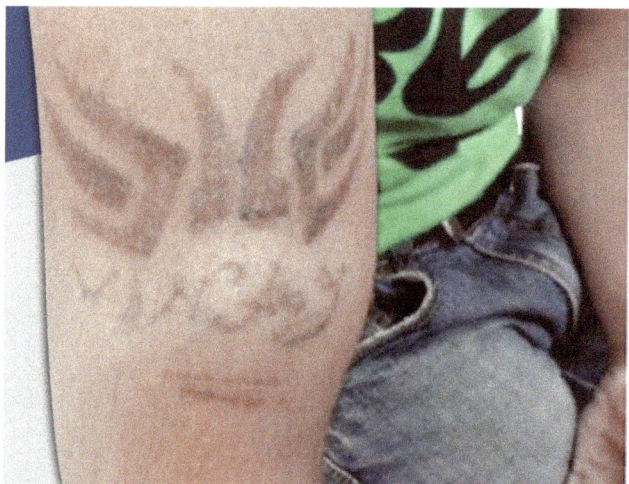

Fig. 3.48: Hypertrophic scarring observed in a patient treated with combination of ultrapulse CO_2 laser followed by Nd:YAG laser treatment. (CO_2: carbon dioxide; Nd:YAG: neodymium-doped yttrium aluminum garnet)

BOOKS

1. Goldman MP, Ehrkich M, Kilmer SL. Treatment of tattoos. In: Goldman MP (Ed). Cutaneous and Cosmetic Laser Surgery, 1st edition. USA: Mosby; 2006. pp. 109-34.
2. Fitzpatrick RE, Goldman MP. Carbon dioxide laser surgery. In: Goldman MP, Fitzpatrick RE (Eds). Cutaneous Laser Surgery, 2nd edition. USA: Elsevier; 1999. p. 302.

BIBLIOGRAPHY

1. Alster TS. Q-switched alexandrite laser treatment (755 nm) of professional and amateur tattoos. J Am Acad Dermatol. 1995;33:69-73.
2. Anderson RR, Geronemus R, Kilmer SL, et al. Cosmetic tattoo ink darkening: a complication of Q-switched and pulsed-laser treatment. Arch Dermatol. 1993;129:1010-4.
3. Bencini PL, Cazzaniga S, Tourlaki A, et al. Removal of tattoos by Q-switched laser: variables influencing outcome and sequelae in a large cohort of treated patients. Arch Dermatol. 2012;148:1364-9.
4. Bernstein EF, Civiok JM. A continuously variable beam-diameter, high-fluence, Q-switched Nd:YAG laser for tattoo removal: comparison of the maximum beam diameter to a standard 4-mm diameter treatment beam. Lasers Surg Med. 2013;45:621-7.
5. Beute TC, Miller CH, Timko AL, et al. In vitro spectral analysis of tattoo pigments. Dermatol Surg. 2008;34:508-15.
6. Fitzpatrick RE, Goldman MP. Carbon dioxide laser surgery. In: Goldman MP, Fitzpatrick RE (Eds). Cutaneous Laser Surgery, 2nd edition. USA: Elsevier; 1999. p. 302.
7. Ho DD, London R, Zimmerman GB, et al. Laser-tattoo removal—a study of the mechanism and the optical treatment strategy via computer simulations. Lasers Surg Med. 2002;30:389-97.
8. Humphries A, Lister TS, Wright PA, et al. Finite element analysis of thermal and acoustic processes during laser tattoo removal. Lasers Surg Med. 2013;45:108-15.
9. Karsai S, Pfirrmann G, Hammes S, et al. Treatment of resistant tattoos using a new generation Q-switched Nd:YAG laser: influence of beam profile and spot size on clearance success. Lasers Surg Med. 2008;40:139-45.
10. Khan MH, Chess S, Choi B, et al. Can topically applied optical clearing agents increase the epidermal damage threshold and enhance therapeutic efficacy? Lasers Surg Med. 2004;35:93-5.
11. Kirby W, Chen CL, Desai A, et al. Causes and recommendations for unanticipated ink retention following tattoo removal treatment. J Clin Aesthet Dermatol. 2013;6:27-31.
12. Klitzman B. Development of permanent but removable tattoos. In: Federal Institute for Risk Assessment, Press and Public Relation. First International Conference on Tattoo Safety. Berlin: BFR Symposium; 2013. p. 23.
13. Kossida T, Rigopoulos D, Katsambas A, et al. Optimal tattoo removal in a single laser session based on the method of repeated exposures. J Am Acad Dermatol. 2012;66:271-7.

14. Leuenberger ML, Mulas MW, Hata TR, et al. Comparison of the Q-switched alexandrite, Nd:YAG, and ruby lasers in treating blue-black tattoos. Dermatol Surg. 1999;25:10-4.
15. McNichols RJ, Fox MA, Gowda A, et al. Temporary dermal scatter reduction: quantitative assessment and implications for improved laser tattoo removal. Lasers Surg Med. 2005;36:289-96.
16. Pinto F, Große-Büning S, Karsai S, et al. Neodymium-doped yttrium aluminium garnet (Nd:YAG) 1064-nm picosecond laser vs. Nd:YAG 1064-nm nanosecond laser in tattoo removal: a randomized controlled single-blind clinical trial. Br J Dermatol. 2017;176:457-64.
17. Prinz BM, Vavricka SR, Graf P, et al. Efficacy of laser treatment of tattoos using lasers emitting wavelengths of 532 nm, 755 nm and 1064 nm. Br J Dermatol. 2004;150:245-51.
18. Reddy KK, Brauer JA, Anolik R, et al. Topical perfluorodecalin resolves immediate whitening reactions and allows rapid effective multiple pass treatment of tattoos. Lasers Surg Med. 2013;45:76-80.
19. Ross EV, Yashar S, Michaud N, et al. Tattoo darkening and nonresponse after laser treatment: a possible role for titanium dioxide. Arch Dermatol. 2001;137:33-7.
20. Ross EV. The picosecond revolution and laser tattoo treatments: are shorter pulses really better? Br J Dermatol. 2017;176:299-300.
21. Ross V, Naseef G, Lin G, et al. Comparison of responses of tattoos to picosecond and nanosecond Q-switched neodymium: YAG lasers. Arch Dermatol. 1998;134:167-71.
22. Saedi N, Metelitsa A, Petrell K, et al. Treatment of tattoos with a picosecond alexandrite laser: a prospective trial. Arch Dermatol. 2012;148:1360-3.
23. Sardana K, Garg VK, Bansal S, et al. A promising split-lesion technique for rapid tattoo removal using a novel sequential approach of a single sitting of pulsed CO_2 followed by Q-switched Nd:YAG laser (1064 nm). J Cosmet Dermatol. 2013;12:296-305.
24. Sardana K, Ranjan R, Ghunawat S. Optimising laser tattoo removal. J Cutan Aesthet Surg. 2015;8:16-24.
25. Sardana K, Ranjan R, Kochhar AM, et al. A rapid tattoo removal technique using a combination of pulsed Er:YAG and Q-Switched Nd:YAG in a split lesion protocol. J Cosmet Laser Ther. 2015;17:177-83.
26. Solis RR, Diven DG, Colome-Grimmer MI, et al. Experimental nonsurgical tattoo removal in a guinea pig model with topical imiquimod and tretinoin. Dermatol Surg. 2002;28:83-6.
27. Tuchin VV, Maksimova IL, Zimnyakov DA, et al. Light propagation in tissues with controlled optical properties. J Biomed Opt. 1997;2:401-17.
28. Ueda S, Imayama S. Normal-mode ruby laser for treating congenital nevi. Arch Dermatol. 1997;133:355-9.
29. Vanarase M, Gautam RK, Arora P, et al. Comparison of Q-switched Nd:YAG laser alone versus its combination with ultrapulse CO_2 laser for the treatment of black tattoo. J Cosmet Laser Ther. 2017;19:259-65.
30. Wang CC, Huang CL, Lee SC, et al. Treatment of cosmetic tattoos with nonablative fractional laser in an animal model: a novel method with histopathologic evidence. Lasers Surg Med. 2013;45:116-22.
31. Weiss ET, Geronemus RG. Combining fractional resurfacing and Q-switched ruby laser for tattoo removal. Dermatol Surg. 2011;37:97-9.
32. Zelickson BD, Mehregan DA, Zarrin AA, et al. Clinical, histologic, and ultrastructural evaluation of tattoos treated with 3 laser systems. Lasers Surg Med. 1994;15:364-72.

CHAPTER 4

Fractional Photothermolysis

Kabir Sardana, Sumit Gupta

OVERVIEW

This technology has its genesis in the attempt to overcome the disadvantages of conventional ablative and nonablative laser therapies. The basic concepts for these studies were introduced in 2003 and reported in full during 2005 (Huzaira M et al.). Manstein and colleagues introduced fractional photothermolysis (FP) in 2004 with their original prototype FP device. The initial studies were restricted to the forearm skin and periorbital rhytides, but the same principles apply to facial skin where the most common indication is acne scarring (Tannous Z et al.).

The *chromophore* for fractional photothermolysis is *tissue water* with targets being epidermal keratinocytes, dermal collagen, and dermal vascular structures. Unlike bulk heating of ablative devices, fractional photothermolysis capitalizes on untreated tissue to accelerate wound healing. This action of the laser, where only a *fraction of the epidermis is damaged*, is the genesis of the term fractional laser.

SCIENTIFIC LOGIC

The scientific concept underlying FP involves the application of microscopic beams of pixelated light, which induce small and focal zones of tissue injury. Because the pixelated zones of treatment spare surrounding normal tissue, reepithelialization occurs at a significantly faster pace. The tissue injury created with FP stimulates the process of collagen remodeling and deposition and promotes elastic tissue formation. These molecular changes are postulated to be responsible for the clinical improvements seen with FP. A comparison of various fractional laser technological systems is given in Table 4.1 and is depicted in Figure 4.1. Nonablative lasers are discussed in a separate chapter.

Arrays of microscopic columns of thermal injury (MTZ) (Fig. 4.1) surrounded by intact tissue are the hallmark of fractional photothermolysis. The *depth* of the MTZ may vary and depends on various *factors* including

Table 4.1: Comparison of the nonablative and ablative fractional lasers with traditional ablative lasers (Narukar et al).

	Nonablative fractional (NAFR) lasers	Ablative fractional (AFR) lasers	Ablative lasers
Wavelength	1,540 nm, 1,550 nm	2,940 nm, 10,600 nm	2,940 nm, 10,600 nm
Type	Fractional, nonablative	Fractional, ablative	100% coverage ablative/pseudofractional, ablative
S. corneum damage	No	Yes	Yes
Downtime	None	48 hours	4–7 days
Avoid Sun	1–3 days	5 days	2.5–4 weeks
Depth	1.4 mm	1.6 mm	1 mm/pass (laser dependent)
Dermal damage	No	Yes	Yes
Number of sitting	3–5	1	1
PIH	No	No	Yes

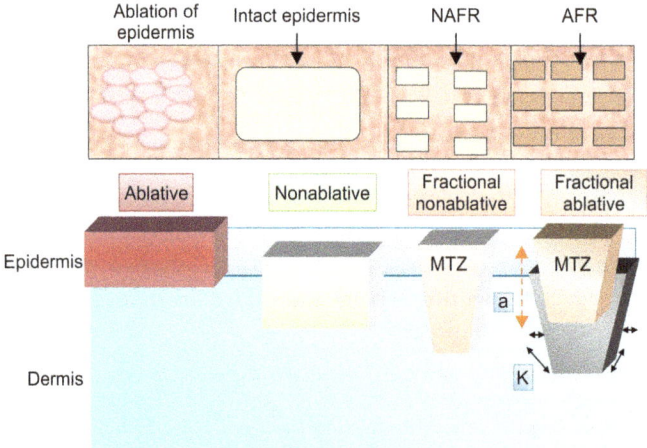

Fig. 4.1: A comparison of various ablative and nonablative lasers. a = zone of ablation, k = zone of coagulation. Ablative lasers (total ablation of epidermis), nonablative lasers (subsurface effect, epidermis is intact), NAFR (columns are formed with intact stratum corneum). AFR (columns with loss of stratum corneum and zone of coagulation) (MTZ: microthermal zone; NAFR: nonablative fractional laser; AFR: ablative fractional laser)

wavelength, dose, pulse duration, density, and temperature of the target tissue. The shape of such MTZs is either an inverted cone or a tapered column extending into the dermis. The histological effect is that of microscopic epidermal necrotic debris (MEND) which shuttles out within 24 hours followed by collagen regeneration, which may take months (Figs. 4.2A and B). The rapid tissue healing is because a fraction of the skin is damaged and thus ensures rapid healing, which forms the basis of fractional lasers (Fig. 4.3). The MTZ zones repair and heal rapidly usually within 24 hours.

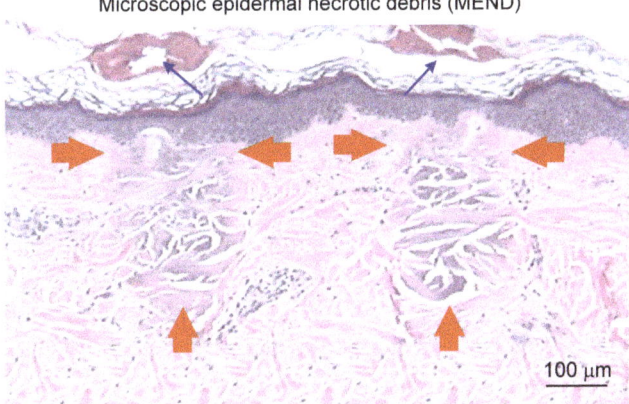

Fig. 4.2A: Controlled zones of denatured collagen in the dermis.

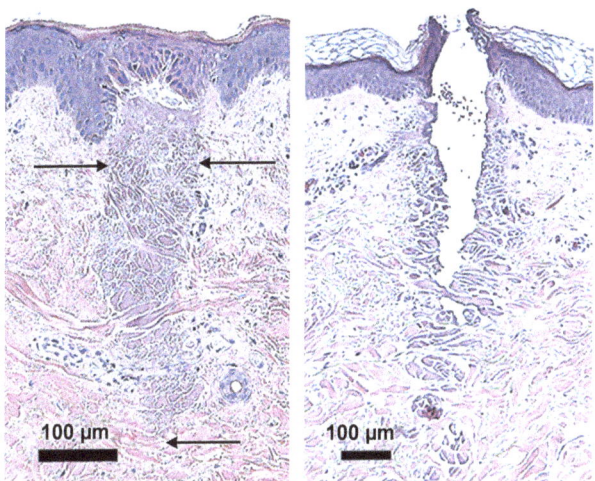

Fig. 4.2B: Histology of treated areas by nonablative fractional resurfacing and ablative fractional resurfacing.

ETHNIC SKIN AND FRACTIONAL LASERS

Ethnic skin is unique in that increased epidermal melanin and melanocyte reactivity results in a pronounced tendency to hyperpigment in response to trauma or light stimuli that can be persistent. Features of aging and cosmetic desires for the Asian population are also distinct from Caucasians. Photodamage is typically manifested as *pigmentary aberration* rather than rhytides. Lentigines, Hori's macules, and melasma are common cosmetic concerns. Wrinkling is encountered about 10–20 years later compared to age-matched Caucasians. With the limited efficacy of nonablative technologies and unacceptably high-risk profile of FA, fractional photothermolysis has found favor.

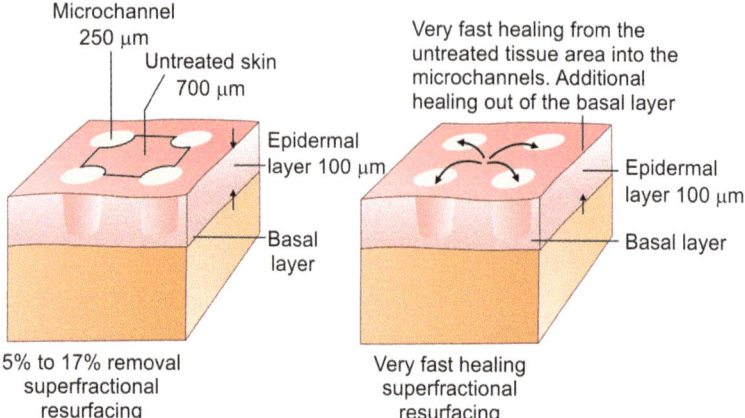

Fig. 4.3: Diagram depicting the regeneration of damaged tissues consequent to fractional laser therapy.
Source: Asclepion Laser Technologies, GmbH.

The formation of microscopic columns of ablative and/or coagulative damage, termed microthermal zones (MTZ), is the fundamental basis of fractional technology. In case of nonablative fractional lasers, columns of coagulative damage are seen traversing the epidermis and dermis but sparing the stratum corneum. By 24 hours, there is formation of microscopic epidermal necrotic debris (MEND) within the epidermis, which serves as shuttles for the transepidermal elimination of coagulated epidermal/dermal material and melanin (Fig. 4.2A).

Genetic analysis of ex vivo skin from Asian patients *24 hours* post-AFL is also demonstrated upregulation of key players in wound healing including metalloproteinases-1 and 3 (MMP-1, MMP-3) and procollagens I and III. Simultaneously, keratinocytes adjacent to each microscopic column migrates and rapidly repopulates the epidermal defect within 24 hours. Preservation of the epidermal barrier allows for greater treatment depths to be achieved safely while also reducing adverse effects and down time. Complete extrusion of MENDs is seen in *7 days*.

The effects of a fractional treatment can be divided under the following steps:
- Repair of the dermal portion of MTZs requires *4–6 weeks*, which corresponds to when clinical benefits first become evident.
- Thermal ablation results in sequentially additive neocollagenesis and collagen contraction that can be seen up to *6 months* following traditional ablative therapies. Procollagens I and III mRNA may reach 8–9 times the baseline levels from 3 weeks up to 6 months post-treatment explaining the prolonged treatment effects.

- Histological studies on Asian patients found significantly increased levels of heat shock protein (HSP)-70 expression, neocollagenesis, and formation of nascent elastic fibers at *1 month* following AFL, which persisted at 6 months following treatment.

FRACTIONAL VERSUS SELECTIVE PHOTOTHERMOLYSIS

Fractional photothermolysis (FP) is distinct and yet similar to the well-known process of selective photothermolysis (SP) originally described over 20 years ago (Manstein D, et al.) (Table 4.2). Both SP and FP cause small, spatially limited zones of photothermal effects within tissue due to local energy deposition. Widespread clinical use of SP for decades has shown that this type of injury is very well tolerated; the same is true for FP. In any photothermal process, including SP and FP, distribution of thermal excitation is proportional to the product of the local optical energy density times and the local optical absorption coefficient. While SP relies on selective absorption of a largely uniform optical field by pigmented target structures, FP relies on optical foci within a largely uniform medium. It should be noted that SP and FP are conceptual descriptions of idealized situations (Table 4.2). In practice, neither the medium nor the optical field is ever completely homogeneous.

Table 4.2: Difference between selective photothermolysis and fractional photothermolysis.

Characteristic	Selective photothermolysis (SP)	Fractional photothermolysis (FP)
Optical field in medium	Homogeneous	Focused beam
Optical properties of medium	Local absorbers	Homogeneous
Confined thermal damage	Target chromophore	Optical focus regions

CLASSIFICATION OF FRACTIONAL TECHNOLOGY

There are broadly two types of fractional lasers:
- Nonablative fractional laser, and
- Ablative fractional lasers.

A list of some of the leading fractional laser manufacturers is given in Table 4.3 for quick reference.

Nonablative Fractional Resurfacing

True NAFR requires three criteria:
1. Nonablative mode of tissue coagulation with the stratum corneum remaining intact and the tissue not being vaporized (Fig. 4.2B)
2. Creation of multiple microthermal zones surrounded by islands of viable tissue, and

Table 4.3: A summary of fractional lasers with their specifications.

Laser company	Wavelength and pulse duration	Mode	Diameter/depth	Energy (mJ/MTZ)	Density/(cm²)	Fractional coverage of skin surface at end of one session (%)
Nonablative Fractional Lasers						
Affirm (Cynosure)	1,320/1,440 nm Nd:YAG	Stamping	100 µm/ 200–300 µm	8–12	1,000 mb/cm²	10–30
Fraxel re:store (Solta)	1,550 nm Nonablative True fractional	Scan	100 µm/ 500–1200 µm	8–40	250 mb/cm²	12–20
Fraxel re: fine (Solta)	1,410 nm Er: Glass	Rolling		5–20		
Fraxel restore DUAL	1,550/1,927 nm Er: Glass/thulium	Rolling	135–600 µm	4–70 5–20		
Lux (Palomar)	1,540 nm Nonablative true fractional Er: Glass	Stamp	125–200 µm/ 125–850 µm	70–100	100–320 mb/cm²	10–25
Lutronic (Mosaic)	1,540 nm Nonablative true fractional Er: Glass	Scanned stamping	220 µm/ Up to 1,000 µm	5–40	100–500 mb/cm²	NA

Contd...

Contd...

Laser company	Wavelength and pulse duration	Mode	Diameter/depth	Energy (mJ/MTZ)	Density/(cm²)	Fractional coverage of skin surface at end of one session (%)
Matisse (Quanta)	1,540 nm Nonablative true fractional Er: Glass	Stamp	100 μm/ 30–150 μm	5–20	1,000 mb/cm²	NA
Protocadmus	1,545 nm Er: Glass	Stamp	NA	NA	NA	NA
Sellas	1,550 nm Er: Glass	Scanned stamping	Size: 312–1,000 μm	1–300		
Ablative Fractional Lasers Er: YAG						
MCL 30 MCL 31 Ascepelion (variable pulse duration)	2,940 nm (100–1,000 μs)	Stamp	100 μm/ 200–300 μm	8–12	1,000 mb/cm²	10–30
Lux 2940 (Palomar)	2,940 nm (0.2–5.0 ms)	Scanned	100 μm/ 500–1200 μm	8–40	250 mb/cm²	12–20
Profractional (Sciton)	2,940 nm	Stamp	125 μm–200 μm/ 125–850 μm	70–100	100–320 mb/cm²	10–25
Pixel (Alma)	2,940 nm (1–2 ms)	Scanned	220 μm/ Up to 1,500 μm	5–40	100–500 mb/cm²	NA

Contd...

Contd...

Laser company	Wavelength and pulse duration	Mode	Diameter/depth	Energy (mJ/MTZ)	Density/(cm²)	Fractional coverage of skin surface at end of one session (%)
Ablative Fractional Lasers CO_2						
Active Fx Lumenis (1.3 mm spot size) Deep Fx (Spot Size = 0.12 mm) SCAAR Fx	10,600 nm (<1 ms)	Scanned paint brush	• 1300 μm/10–300 μm • 120 μm/150–1,600 μm • 120 μm/4,000 μm	60 W		30–60
AcuPulse (SuperPulse)	0.3–0.5 m		0.12 mm and 1.3 mm/1mm	40 W	225 mJ	
Fraxel repair (Solta)	10,600 nm (0.15–3 m) (0.8–1.8 m)	IOTS (paintbrush) continuous motion	140 μm/1,600 μm	40 W		5–50
Smartxide Dot (Deka)	10,600 nm (200 μs-2.0 ms)	Scanned conventional	350 μm/ 500–800 μm	30 W		
Youlaser CO_2 (Quanta)	10,600 nm	paint brush		30 W		
Quadralase (Candela)	10,600 nm	paint brush motion	Ablation depth 30–750 μm	60 W	30–90 mJ	5–30

Contd...

Contd...

Laser company	Wavelength and pulse duration	Mode	Diameter/depth	Energy (mJ/MTZ)	Density/(cm²)	Fractional coverage of skin surface at end of one session (%)
Mixto SX (Lasering)	(2.5–16 ms)	Scanned (four quadrants)	180 µm/200 µm	0.5–30 W		
Multipulse (Ascepelion)	0.2–2.0 ms		350 µm 500–800 µm	30		
ProFrax C₂ Protocadmus	1–50 ms		5–10 µm Up to 5,000 µm/			
eCO₂ (Lutronic)	Variable	Stamping dynamic	120–1,000 µm/ 2,500 µm	30 W		
Ablative Fractional Lasers Fractional YSGG laser						
Pearl (Cutera)	Variable	Scanned	300/1,500		60–320 mJ/ microspots	

*As laser treatment depends on various parameters and novel devices are added, it is advisable to refer to company manuals for device-specific settings to optimize depth and results.

3. Resurfacing with extrusion and replacement of damaged tissue, with reepithelialization within 24 hours (*see* Figs. 4.1 and 4.3).

The major conundrum is to balance the minimal clinical effects, which are usually seen with traditional nonablative modalities resulting in disappointing clinical results, and blistering, which produces an ablative-like response.

In the Asian population, NAFL may be considered a *first line* treatment for atrophic scarring and wrinkle reduction. The favorable side effect profile and low risk of dyspigmentation make it the preferred option for the majority of Asian patients seeking photorejuvenation as well. NAFL may be reserved as a *second-line* modality for the treatment of recalcitrant melasma.

Systems and Devices

The basic concept is to use a wavelength with optimal mid-dermal penetration. These include the 1,320-, 1,410-, and 1,440-nm Nd: YAG laser, the 1,450-nm diode laser, and the 1,535-, 1,540-, and 1,550-nm ytterbium: erbium-phosphate glass (also known as erbium: glass or Er: Glass) laser.

1. ***1,320-nm Nd:YAG Laser:*** It typically leads to an epidermal heating of 40–50°C accompanied by a temperature elevation within the dermis up to 70°C with a fluence of 12–18 J/cm^2 (17–19 J/cm^2 CoolTouch3, CoolTouch⁰ Corp, Roseville, California, USA). It has a fixed spot size of 10 mm and gives six stacked pulses at duration of 50 ms.
2. ***1,410-nm System (Fraxel re:fine):*** This has the facility of a variable spot size and a continuous motion scanner, which enables MTZs of 500 µm in depth.
3. ***1,440-nm Nd:YAG Laser (Affirm, Cynosure, Westford, Massachusetts, USA):*** This uses a microarray of lenses and delivers a 10-mm fractional beam. It also has a spot size of 15 mm (470 microbeams), with a microbeam density of 320 spots per cm^2.
4. ***1,450-nm Diode Laser:*** It provides four stacked pulses (210 ms), interspersed with five cryogen applications to ensure cooling. The 4- or 6-mm spot size provides fluences ranging from 9 J/cm^2 to 14 J/cm^2. The usage of energies above 12 mJ/cm^2 has been reported to lead to an increased production of collagen type III but not collagen type I or elastic fibers (Smoothbeam, Candela, Wayland, Massachusetts, USA). The lower penetration wavelength is especially suitable for patients with thinner skin (400 µm with 1,320 nm vs 200 µm with 1,450 nm).
5. ***1,540-nm Er: Glass Laser (Lux1540, Palomar Medical Technologies, Inc.):*** This is a laser that has been widely used by us and can be used in a normal or single pulse mode. The pulses are delivered with a frequency of up to 3 Hz. The system is equipped with a 4-mm spot size to apply typical fluences of 8–10 J/cm^2 up to 70 mJ throughout a chilled sapphire window. It has two tip size 15 mm for superficial indications like melasma and a 10 mm tip used for deeper pathologies like acne scars (Fig. 4.4).

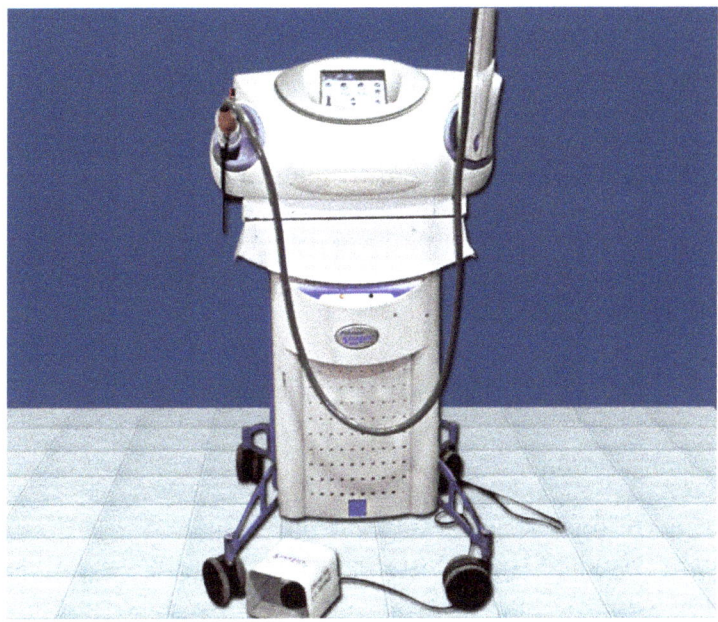

Fig. 4.4: The Star Lux -500 laser system with a Lux 1,540 nm fractional 10 mm handpiece. *Source:* Palomar Medical Technologies, Burlington, MA.

6. ***1,550-nm Erbium Laser (Fraxel, Reliant Technology):*** This was the first device to adopt the concept of fractional photothermolysis. This has been improved upon by the 1,550 nm Er: Glass laser (Mosaic, Lutronic Corporation, Gyeonggi, Korea), which has a large energy range up to 120 mJ. In addition, the system allows for the application of the laser energy in different modes. The so-called static mode, also known as stamp mode, delivers, with the appropriate tips, light to treatment areas of varying sizes (6 × 6, 8 × 8, 5 × 10, and 10 × 10 mm). The system has the advantage of using nonlinear, nonsequential microbeam delivery technology (Controlled Chaos Technology). In combination with variable microbeam delivery and a skin sensing feature within the tips, a decrease of the likelihood of postinflammatory hyperpigmentation in darker skin types is reported (Laubach et al.)

More recently, a CO_2 laser equipped with a scanner has been used for nonablative fractional treatments. In this, a spot density of 8 × 8 spots/cm^2 (64 MTZ/cm^2) was used. The spot size was set to 500 μm, laser power adjusted to 12 W, and pulse duration set to 3–5 ms (36–60 mJ). On histology slides, the microthermal treatment zone was characterized mainly by absence of ablation and display of very superficial epidermal coagulation immediately after exposure, leading to average increases in skin density of 40.2% without any signs of postinflammatory hyperpigmentation.

Ablative Fractional Resurfacing

There are two types of ablative fractional resurfacing (AFR), the Fractional Er: YAG (2,940 nm), which utilizes traditional ablative wavelengths, such as 2,940-nm (Dermablate, Profractional 2940 laser, Lux 2940, Pixel 2940 Laser and Protocadmus) (Figs. 4.5 and 4.6) and the fractional CO_2 (10,600 nm), which utilizes the standard CO_2 wavelength (Active FX, Fraxel Repair, mixTo, Protocadmus) (Figs. 4.7 and 4.8). The Er: yttrium-scandium-gallium-garnet (YSSG) (2,790 nm) laser is also used for AFR, though the experience with that system is limited (Table 4.3).

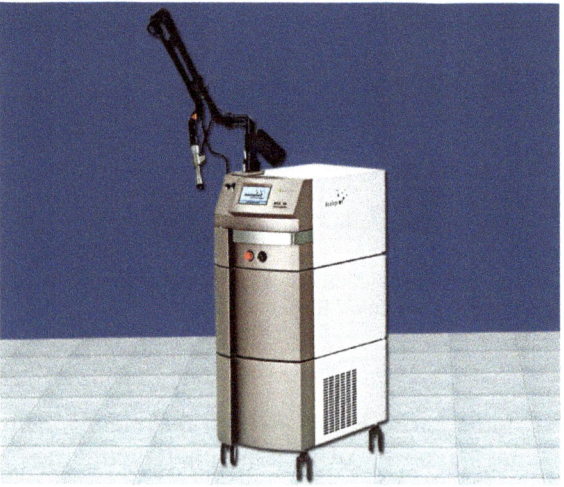

Fig. 4.5: Dermablate (Fractional Er: YAG).
Source: Asclepion Laser Technologies, GmbH.

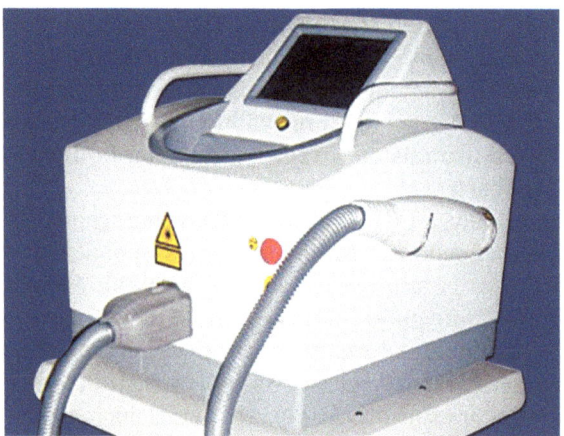

Fig. 4.6: Protocadamus laser system.

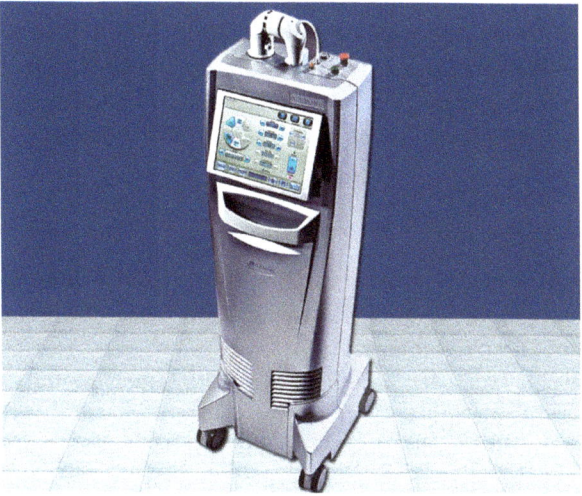

Fig. 4.7: SuperPulse CO_2.
Source: Lumenis.

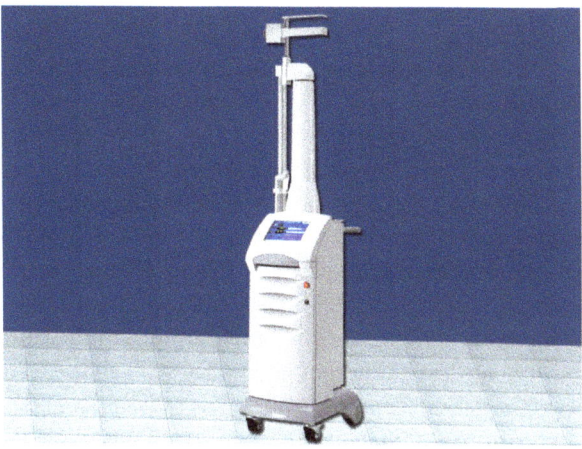

Fig. 4.8: UltraPulse CO_2.
Source: Lumenis.

The rationale for ablative fractional devices is to reduce the number of treatments as compared with nonablative fractional devices and still maintains greater safety than traditional ablative modalities. The depth of the MTZ is primarily dependent on pulse energy and may extend into the deep reticular dermis. The resulting tapered cavity is lined by a thin layer of eschar and surrounded by a cuff of thermal denaturation, which is sufficient to destroy cells and coagulate collagen. Ablative FP results in immediate tissue loss due to the physical removal of portions of the skin by vaporization, and the physical integrity and barrier function of the skin is locally compromised (Fig. 4.2B).

Ablative fractional therapy should be used judiciously in the Asian patient. Areas where AFL may be considered include severe *acne scarring, thick hypertrophic scars,* and *advanced photodamage*. However, the increased risk of both prolonged erythema and PIH tends to favor the selection of a longer series of NAFL treatments over AFL to achieve similar efficacy with less downtime.

Systems and Devices

Fractional carbon dioxide lasers: The first two *microfractional* systems were the rePair (Solta Medical, Inc., Hayward, California, USA) and the Lumenis DeepFx (Santa Clara, California, USA)

- **Solta device:** This uses a continuous paint-brush motion to apply the laser microbeams to the tissue, whereas the Lumenis device employs a *stamped* scanning technology. The Solta re:Pair uses a microprocessor-controlled handpiece to deliver a laser beam with a penetration depth of 300–1,600 mm, which is determined by the pulse energy, up to a maximum of 70 mJ. Treatment densities (or coverage) may be adjusted from 5% to 50% by performing multiple passes and choosing higher treatment densities, which are chosen based on the severity of photodamage or presence of scarring.
- **Lumenis:** The company introduced a macrofractional handpiece (ActiveFX, Lumenis) as an attachment to their CO_2 resurfacing laser in 2006. The macrofractional handpiece scans patterns with a 1.3-mm spot size, at treatment densities providing 50–90% of surface area coverage. Ablation is limited to the epidermis with some coagulation of the papillary dermis, producing a superficial laser peel that heals in 3–4 days. In 2007, a microfractional attachment (Deep FX) was introduced. This microfractional handpiece fractionates the laser beam to a diameter of 0.12 mm and uses a stamping-style microscanning method. The handpiece produces multiple different geometric scan shapes, and treatment densities can be varied from 5% to 50%. The pulse energy determines the depth of tissue injury, with a maximum of 70 mJ providing tissue penetration up to 1 mm.
- The **DEKA system** (SmartXide DOT, Calenzano, Italy) is a low-power (30 W) CO_2 laser used with a scanning handpiece. The scanned microbeam measures up to 350 μm and the pulse duration varies from 200–2,000 ms. The longer pulse durations, used with this system, produce larger zones of coagulation around the ablated channels of tissue.

Fractional Erbium:YAG lasers
- **Palomar fractional Er:YAG:** This has the multiple interchangeable optical tips that provide various densities (170–1,000 microbeams/cm^2) of focused miocrobeam arrays (each ~75–150 mm in diameter) with up to 12 mJ/microbeam of energy. The density of microbeams is fixed for

each optical tip, but the total density of microbeams delivered will vary depending on the number of laser passes. This laser ablates tissue to depths of 1,000 μm without coagulation when used with a pulse width of 0.25 ms, and produces zones of coagulation up to ~70 μm with 5 ms pulse durations.

Another attachment produces a 6-mm spot size with a directional or *groove* pattern of injury, with each groove measuring 100–200 μm in width and 350 μm in depth spaced at 350-μm intervals. The treatment density is increased by performing additional laser passes with varied orientations of the linear pattern.

- ***Sciton, Inc. (ProFractional Palo Alto, California, USA):*** They have developed two microfractional handpieces for their Er:YAG laser base unit. One handpiece uses a 250 μm spot to vaporize tissue from 25 μm to 1,500 μm per pass with treatment densities (coverage) from 1.5% to 60%. The other uses a 430-mm spot with predetermined densities of either 5.5% to 11%. The latter offers the ability to add depth-selectable tissue coagulation for enhanced collagen remodeling by delivering a train of subablative laser pulses that heat the tissue to three selectable depths: level 1, up to 50 μm; level 2, up to 100 μm; and level 3, up to 150 μm.
- ***Alma's fractional Er:YAG laser:*** This is essentially a superficial epidermal ablative laser. It uses a microlens arranged in a matrix of either 9 × 9 microbeams with energies up to 17 mJ or 7 × 7 microbeams with energies up to 28 mJ.

  The channels produced by this laser measure 120–140 μm in depth and 150 μm in diameter, limiting treatment to the epidermis and superficial papillary dermis. The treatment density is increased by performing multiple passes.
- ***Fractional Erbium:YSGG laser:*** Cutera (Brisbane, California, USA) was the first company to develop an Er:YSGG laser for superficial skin resurfacing. With a water absorption coefficient roughly one-third that of the Er: YAG laser and five times that of the CO_2 laser, it vaporizes tissue with a zone of coagulation approximately midway between that of the CO_2 and short-pulsed, or *cold*, Er:YAG laser. In 2008, they developed a fractional Er:YSGG laser (Pearl) with pulse duration of 600 μs and a spot size of 300 μm. It produces scans of variable densities and patterns up to 12 × 14 mm, ablating up to 100 μm in depth with a coagulation zone of ~40 μm.

New Fractional Devices and Technology

When the concept of FP was first introduced, the laser was used as the energy source to generate fractional damage to the skin. The laser is still the most common energy source used in FP procedures. Its ability to quickly deliver energy in the form of focused optical radiation with high precision into small confined zones makes the laser a modality well suited for FP. Recently, other energy sources have emerged for generating fractional damage patterns.

For example, radiofrequency (RF) and ultrasound devices are now commercially available that generate a pattern of small and confined thermal damage zones in skin tissue. The shape and anatomical location of MTZs generated using such modalities typically differ from those induced by focused optical radiation because of a different energy distribution within the tissue. Further investigations are needed to investigate how the size and location of thermal lesions generated using RF and ultrasound sources affect the clinical outcome as compared to laser-generated MTZs. Also more importantly, it is important to compare these technologies with the existing devices for similar indications. These are discussed in detail in **Section 2** of the book.

Fractional ablative radiofrequency: As RF energy quickly diverges with increasing distance from the delivering electrode, it is possible to generate a spatially confined RF-generated thermal injury only within the tissue directly adjacent to the tip of a needle electrode. Depending on the location of the tip of such RF electrode, damage can be generated either at the skin surface, or virtually at any depth by inserting needle electrodes into the skin. The use of stamping techniques with arrays or linear arrangements of multiple needle electrodes allows for coverage of a treatment area within a reasonable time.

Aside from laser modalities, fractionated radiofrequency devices also serve an important role in the treatment of Asian types. Radiofrequency devices deliver *subablative* wavelengths that induce coagulative damage to the dermis with *relative sparing of melanin*. Therefore, the risk of dyspigmentation may be minimized. Studies utilizing fractionated radiofrequency on Asian skin types have demonstrated promising results in the treatment of atrophic acne scarring, periorbital wrinkles, photoaging, and striae.

Results: A study by Trelles MA (2014) used a newly developed high-power device for patient of acne scars (iPixel™ RF, Alma Lasers, Caesarea, Israel). The improvement in scarring was about 57% on the face and 49% on the back and shoulders. More importantly, a comparison study with a fractional erbium-doped glass 1,550-nm device found no significant difference (Rongsaard N, 2014).

This device is discussed in a separate chapter dedicated to this technology.

Intense-focused ultrasound (Ulthera Inc.): Focused ultrasound noninvasive generation of confined lesions, in skin layers, such as, the deep reticular dermis or even the superficial musculoaponeurotic system (SMAS) without causing any surface damage. The MTZ cross-section of RF or ultrasound-generated MTZs are typically larger than that of laser-generated MTZs because laser radiation can be more focused. However, the ability to focus optical radiation decreases with increasing skin depth due to scattering and absorption of optical radiation (Laubach HJ, 2008). The actual utility in acne scars is not established as yet, but it must be noted being a new device, complications may arise as noted recently (Jeong KH et al. 2014). This is discussed in a separate chapter.

Fractional Thulium Laser: The superficial depth of this device makes it useful for removal of superficial pigment, including for nonfacial areas. This system can produce a larger MTZ diameter up to approximately 600 μm. Its wavelength is more superficially absorbed (OPD 100 μm) as compared to the 1,540 nm or 1,550 nm lasers (OPD » 1,000 μm) but less absorbed than the CO_2 lasers (OPD » 10 mm). Thus, it is designed to generate thermal injury in relatively superficially tissue without significant disruption of the epidermal barrier.

Though, a few studies have been published (Ho SG, Lee HM), it is the author's view that unless an objective scoring by a mexameter combined with clinical improvement is seen, mere subjective improvement is not enough to justify its use in melasma, especially in pigmented skin.

Fractionated picosecond laser: Picosecond-pulsed lasers were originally introduced for the treatment of tattoos and have proved to be a significant advancement on the previous generation of nanosecond QS lasers. Additionally, these lasers are also safe and effective for the clearance of benign pigmentary lesions in both Asian and non-Asian skin types.

Recently, fractionated picosecond handpieces have been developed for the purposes of resurfacing and rejuvenation: a diffractive lens array for the 755-nm picosecond alexandrite laser (Picosure, Cynosure) and a holographic lens for the 532/1064-nm picosecond Nd:YAG laser (Picoway, Syneron Medical and Enlighten, Cutera, Brisbane, CA).

HOW TO INTERPRET DEVICE DATA?

During the past 2 years, multiple different fractional CO_2 lasers have been developed, some of them having no FDA/CE approval and little or none histological data. Though the same basic principles apply to all these systems, the power and delivery systems of the individual units vary considerably. Lower power lasers have pulse width longer than the thermal relaxation time of skin and produce larger zones of coagulation beyond the ablated wound, which affects the safe, allowable treatment depth and surface area coverage. Thus, the practitioners should, therefore, be familiar with the histological and clinical correlation of varying parameters with the fractional ablative device, they are using.

- Ask always about *histological data* and the *pulse width*, any pulse width that is markedly high should be used with caution as it will cause more damage than required.
- There is no study to prove that smaller the *pulse* better the results. Thus, it is the author's opinion based on the present data that a superpulse or ultrapulse system may not have a markedly different clinical result from other modes of CO_2 lasers, as far as fractional lasers are concerned.
- There is also little data to prove that NAFR is superior or inferior to AFR.

- It remains unclear what constitutes the ideal combination of ablation and coagulation or treatment depth and density. It is also unclear whether varying the pattern of ablative or coagulative injury or delivering them sequentially or simultaneously will be most beneficial.

In effect, if the laser device has a histological dose depth analysis study and a FDA/CE approval, changing the dose parameters can lead to an adequate clinical result. Thus, instead of running after the latest fractional laser, optimal use of the existing device makes more sense. The data provided in Table 4.3 can help to compare the various devices.

VARIABLES THAT AFFECT FRACTIONAL LASER TREATMENT

Size of Wound

Microwound

In the most common approach, 75–150-μm wide microwounds are created in the skin with densities ranging from 100–1,500 microwounds/cm. In a typical scenario, approximately 3–10% of the surface area of the skin is involved per pass, with typical pass numbers ranging from three to eight, so that total involved surface areas tend to range from 15% to 30% per session. This category has both ablative and nonablative fractional devices.

Ablative devices with microwound approaches are the Profractional laser (Sciton, Palo Alto, CA), equipped with a scanned microbeam, as well as the newly introduced Palomar 2,940-nm handpiece and finally the Pixel Erbium YAG laser from Alma (Alma lasers, Buffalo Grove, IL). Reliant technologies (Mountain View, CA) have a newer fractional CO_2 laser system (Re: Pair) that creates 125 μm diameter *ablative* wounds as deep as 1 mm.

Macrowound

Fractional technologies create wounds greater than 300 μm in diameter. These include the KTP laser with a scanner (with approximately 700 μm wounds) as well as the active FX CO_2 system (Lumenis, Santa Clara, CA), which creates an array of approximately 1-mm wide wounds and covers approximately 60% of the surface area per session. Wound depths range from 80 μm to 150 μm depending on pulse energy. Fluences with these approaches range from 5 to 15 J/cm^2.

Wavelength

Based on the water absorption coefficients of their respective wavelengths, the Er:YAG produces the least amount of coagulation or residual thermal damage (~10 μm), the CO_2 laser produces the greatest amount of coagulation (~100 μm), and the Er:YSSG laser lies somewhere in-between (~40 μm) (Fig. 4.9).

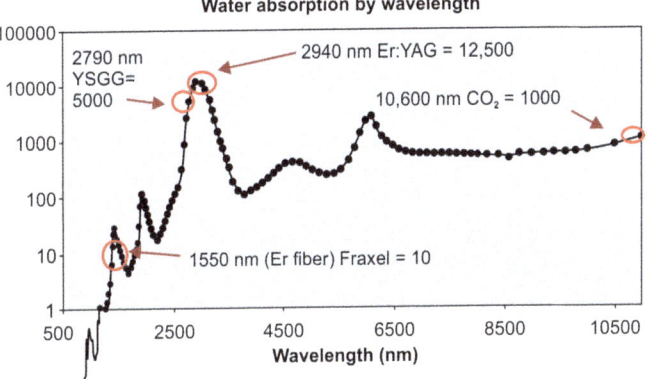

Fig. 4.9: Absorption spectrum of the primary chromophore water. Note that the highest absorption of Er:YAG, which makes it the safest of the 3 lasers.
(CO_2: carbon dioxide; Er:YAG: erbium-doped yttrium aluminum garnet)

As the ablative fractional resurfacing (AFR) are ablative, the depth of the laser created cavity is primarily related to the total energy delivered for a given spot size, and relatively independent of the applied wavelength. It should be noted, that the Er: YAG typically produces less thermal damage in the residual tissue as compared to the CO_2 laser due to the stronger absorption by water.

On the contrary, nonablative fractional resurfacing (NAFR) does not physically remove tissue, the maximum depth of MTZs is thus dependent on the **optical penetration depth** of any particular laser wavelength. Thus, the approximate optical penetration depth (OPD) of Nd: YAG (1,440 nm, 300 μm) is less than Er: Glass (1,540 and 1,550 nm, 1,000 μm), but more than Thulium fiber laser (1,927 nm, 100 μm). These differences in optical penetration lengths indicate why the Thulium laser, with a relatively shallow penetration depth, is often used to treat superficial lesions within the epidermis and papillary dermis, and why the Er: Glass laser with a relatively larger optical penetration depth can generate MTZs extending down into the mid-deep reticular dermis.

Pulse Number/Frequency

Several studies have shown that the depth can be manipulated depending on the number of pulses wherein multiple pulses are superior to single pulse. The delay between the pulses is crucial. To maintain a steady state temperature, the delay should be 3–5 times the TRT (thermal relaxation time) of the target tissue. Thus, the optimal delay ranges from 300 (3 Hz)–500 millisecond (2 Hz) intervals that corresponds to 3–5 times the TRT. As can be seen in the Table 4.3, the pulse duration of most fractional devices does not exceed 3-4 ms.

Practical use of knowing the number of pulses is that there is a nonlinear increase in depth depending on the pulses used (Fig. 4.10) and thus again a gross histological data of the laser should be sought from the manufacturer.

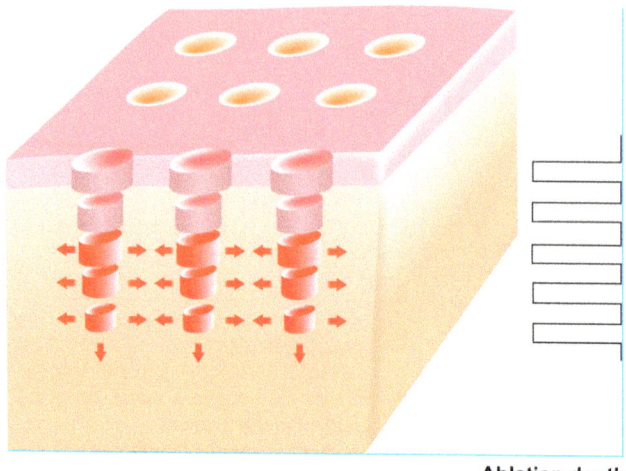

Fig. 4.10: The effect of number of pulses on the depth of the microscopic treatment zone (MTZ). Note the proportionate nonlinear increase in depth of MTZ.
Source: Asclepion Laser Technologies, GmbH.

Pulse Duration

This is another tool employed to cause either ablation or coagulation especially in Er: YAG systems. The purely ablative wounds created by the short-pulsed fractional Er: YAG lasers produce increased bleeding intraoperatively, but may have an advantage in reducing the risk of postinflammatory hyperpigmentation in patients with darker skin types. By lengthening the pulse duration, the wounds produced by the Er: YAG laser can be made to approximate those of the CO_2 laser.

The longer pulse duration results in a larger zone of coagulation (Dierickx et al.). In addition to providing hemostasis, it seems that the large volume of collateral tissue coagulation is beneficial for inducing increased skin tightening. The DEKA system exemplifies this principle as the pulse duration varies from 200–2,000 μs. The longer pulse durations used with this system produce larger zones of coagulation around the ablated channels of tissue. Palomar fractional Er: YAG when used with a pulse width of 0.25 ms leads to an ablation up to 1,000 μm while coagulation up to ~70 mm is produced when the 5-ms pulse durations is used. Sciton Profractional laser offers the ability to add depth-selectable tissue coagulation for enhanced collagen remodeling by delivering a train of subablative laser pulses that heat the tissue to three selectable depths. A similar effect of pulse duration and thermal effects has been seen with CO_2 lasers (Walsh et al.).

A prototype of the fractional Er: YAG (Dermablate MCL 31) has a variable pulse duration from 100–1,000 μs, which creates various patterns of tissue damage, with varying coverage rates (Fig. 4.11A).

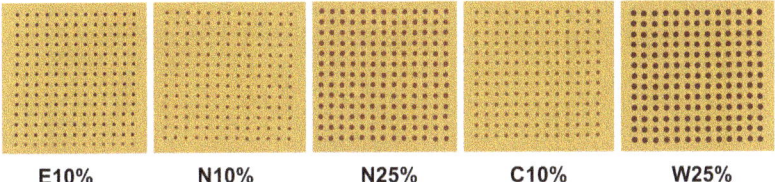

| E10% | N10% | N25% | C10% | W25% |

Parameters for the different settings
E10% (E = Expert, pulse length 300 μs, 10% coverage)
N10% (N = Normal, pulse length 300 μs, 10% coverage)
N25% (N = Normal, pulse length 300 μs, 25% coverage)
C10% (C = Cold, pulse length 100 μs, 10% coverage)
W25% (W = Warm, pulse length 1.000 μs, 25% coverage)

Fig. 4.11A: The effect of pulse duration on the coverage rate and tissue effect. Note that higher the pulse duration, more the heat coagulation and larger the coverage rate. (Dermablate MCL 31:Fr Er:YAG)
Source: Asclepion Laser Technologies, GmbH.

A basic **principle** that must be remembered is that as long as the pulse durations are within the thermal relaxation time of individual MTZs, minor variation of pulse duration should have limited effects on lesion shape. However, variation of pulse duration over an extended range of pulse profiles will affect the MTZ shape, e.g. ablation depth and/or extent of residual thermal damage.

Energy (Fournier et al. and Kono et al.)

The energy is conventionally described in mJ/beam but this is usually an incorrect way of representing the energy that impinges on the skin. As the total energy per beam depends on the density, the total energy is:

Energy (J) = Energy/microbeam (mJ) × total density (100–1,000/cm^2).

To achieve a high dose, we can either increase the energy/microbeam or the density. A simple way to achieve these high doses is to give multiple passes, which has been shown to have more side effects and is histologically nonuniform. Another way is to increase the dose per microbeam.

Hantash et al. had demonstrated that increasing the pulse energy increased the depth of ablation. Similarly, Bedi et al. (2007) examined the effect of NAFR and found that an increase in pulse energy leads to increase in the depth and width of MTZs without compromising the viability of interlesional tissue in vivo and in explant models, provided that the density of the MTZ is low enough (Fig. 4.11B).

Correlation of Energy and Depth (Farkas 2009, Sardana K)

It is a logical conclusion that increased energy would lead to increased depth of penetration. This correlation is essential to quantify the dose required for dermatological indications like acne scars where depth is an important issue.

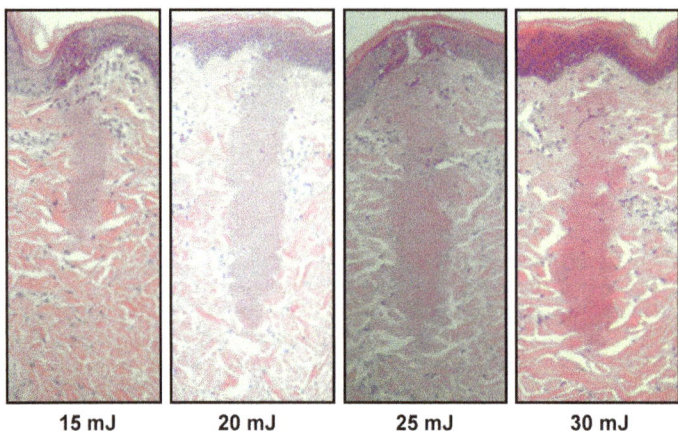

Fig. 4.11B: Relationship of fluence and depth.

Table 4.4: A rough assessment of dose depth ratio of common lasers systems.

Laser	Company	Depth/mJ
Nonablative fractional resurfacing (NAFR)	Lux Palomar Fraxel	12.9 28.5
Ablative fractional resurfacing (AFR) (Er:YAG)	Lux 2,940 nm Profractional 2,940 nm	54.38 3
Ablative fractional resurfacing; AFR (CO_2)	ActiveFX DeepFX Fraxel repair MedArt	6.28 53.66 20 12

(NAFR: nonablative fractional resurfacing; AFR: ablative fractional resurfacing)

Higher energies create deeper columns and disruption of the epidermis and DEJ. Dermal appendages and microvasculature remain anatomically intact, but evidence of thermal damage and streaming of nuclei without total destruction have been demonstrated.

Though not all laser manufacturers have data on the depth a few have well conducted studies and an approximate depth/mJ dose is given in Table 4.4 for quick reference (Sardana K). Thus, if a depth of 1,000 µm is needed using the Lux Palomar, a dose of 70 mJ should suffice. Conversely, a low dose may have little effect.

As discussed in Table 4.4, many factors can affect thermal damage patterns generated in the skin and subsequent wound healing responses. Such factors include laser exposure parameters (e.g. energy per MTZ and focal spot size), the number of passes and time interval between them, mechanical tissue manipulation, use of skin cooling procedures, and others. The treatment interval between individual passes within a single treatment session and the number of sessions can also be varied. This virtually unlimited number of possible treatment combinations provides the possibility of tailoring patient treatment protocols to specific needs, which is still not completely researched.

Density (Fournier et al. and Kono et al.)

The density of the lasers range from 100–1,000 spots/probe. By manipulating the density of the microcolumns, a more aggressive treatment may be achieved in a single treatment. However, when retreating or passing over a treated area multiple times, a nonuniform damage is achieved.

There are two general techniques currently available for generating the desired density of MTZs (number per unit area) within the treatment area: the *stamping technique* and the *rolling technique* (Figs. 4.12A and B).

The *stamping technique* is performed by forming a preset pattern of multiple MTZs on a skin region within a well-defined exposure area of the fixed handpiece and then moving the handpiece to another skin region and repeating until the entire treatment area is covered. The operator has to change the direction of the passes manually (Figs. 4.12A and B). The density of MTZs at the end of a treatment session depends on the preset density within the exposure area of the handpiece and the number of passes performed over each skin region.

The problem with this mode is that gaps or Moire artifacts are often seen when the stamping mode is applied, thus most machines now have a scanning device that produces a randomized treatment pattern with a blended appearance after treatment.

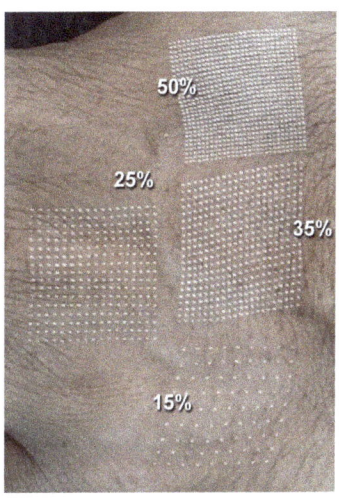

Fig. 4.12A: A depiction of the increased coverage area depending on the density pattern of the fractional handpiece.

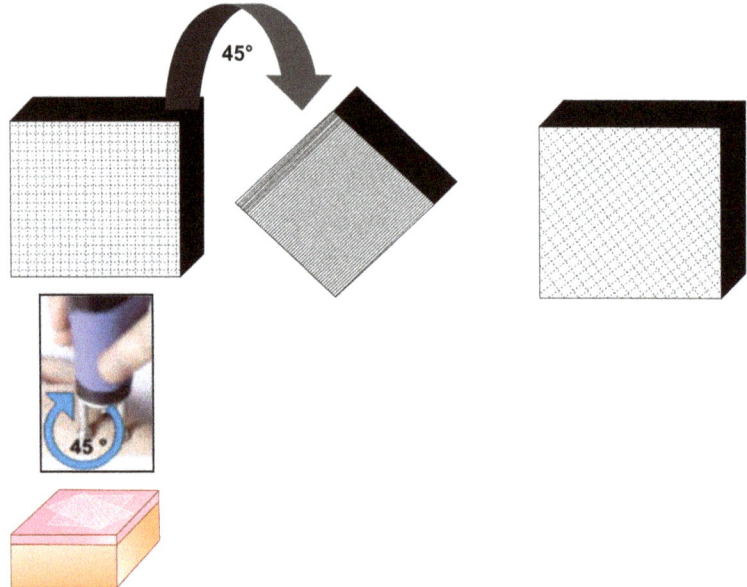

Fig. 4.12B: Stamping technique. The second pass and third pass are given at 45° to the first pass.

The *rolling technique* is performed by continuously rolling the handpiece across the entire treatment area. It is also referred as *brushing* technique, because the movements of the operator are similar to using a paint brush. As the velocity of the handpiece relative to the skin varies during treatment, the delivery rate is adjusted automatically in order to maintain a defined and preset MTZ density per pass. The total density of MTZs at the end of a treatment session can be estimated as the density of MTZs per pass multiplied by the number of passes performed.

There appears to be no single best technique for delivering the desired density of MTZs. The rolling technique can facilitate treatment of larger areas, while the stamping technique can facilitate the precise treatment of smaller areas, in particular areas having an irregular surface profile.

Single/Multiple Pass (Manstein et al. 2009)

During each nonablative fractional treatment session, a variable percentage of the skin surface is thermally damaged as a result of the placement of many individual MTZs.

The so-called *fill factor*, defined as the ratio of thermally damaged surface area to that of the total area, can theoretically vary from 0% to 100%.

It is primarily determined by energy per MTZ, density of MTZs per pass, and the number of passes. The application of multiple passes results in clustering of the lesions [microscopic treatment cluster (MTC)]. The size of MTCs increases

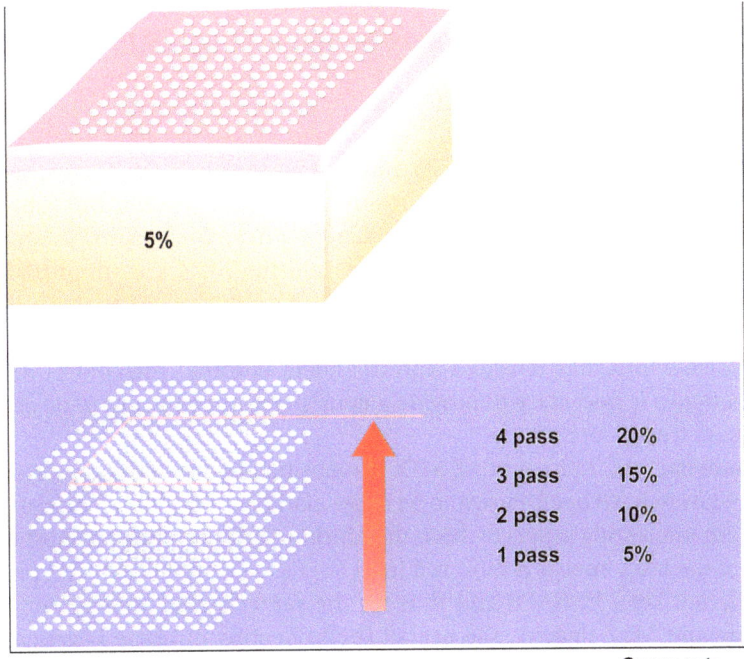

Fig. 4.13A: A figurative depiction of the effect of number of passes and cover rate on the fractional laser effect on the skin (fill factor).
Source: Asclepion Laser Technologies, GmbH.

linearly as a function of the number of passes. Confluent thermal damage may result in prolonged recovery time and a higher frequency of side effects.

The fill factor varies from 10% to 20% for each treatment session. With fractional thermal injury confined to multiple small thermal lesions, migration from surrounding epidermal keratinocytes allows for rapid healing and, therefore, lowers the risk of complications. Therefore, it is important for the clinician to understand how the above-mentioned exposure parameters affect the resulting thermal damage a knowledge of the pattern generated.

This can help as multiple passes can lead to a higher degree of PIH (Fig. 4.13A).

Surface Cooling and Temperature (Laubach H et al. and Fournier et al. 2005)

It has been suggested that microcolumn separation may also be dependent on fluence and skin temperature. It is important to note that the role of contact cooling with fractional nonablative laser treatments and the relationship to microthermal damage, depth, and width of the columns. Cooling of the epidermis can be achieved by two techniques—dynamic and parallel cooling. Parallel cooling is contact cooling provided during a long laser pulse or a sequence of pulses. It can protect the epidermis by a factor of 10. Dynamic cooling is a concomitant cooling process and is seen in the newer fractional lasers. Advanced lasers have a precooling and postcooling concomitant with the contact cooling.

In a study on the importance of cooling, a 1,550-nm fiber laser (Fraxel SR Laser) was used in a dose of 10 mJ on cadaver skin. It was found that the average MTZ diameter exhibits a positive and linear relationship with skin temperature. As the skin temperature increases from 0–45 the MTZ diameter increases from 93 to 147 micron (58%), and the MTZ area from 6,870 to 17,050 micron (148%). Thus, skin cooling is a double-edged tool; while the use of simultaneous skin cooling increases patient comfort, it also decreases MTZ size and it may interfere with treatment efficacy. The control of skin temperature is necessary to provide a consistent outcome and to be able to compare treatments.

Interestingly, reduction of MTZ dimension due to decrease of tissue temperature have been shown to be more marked for NAFR as compared to AFR. An interesting aspect of this is that during AFR procedures, a substantial part of the laser energy is removed from the tissue with the hot laser plume. This is not seen in NAFR and thus for the same applied energy per MTZ energy and MTZ density, the overall (bulk) heating of tissue is greater for NAFR. Thus, NAFR may be better for remodeling collagen.

Depth Width Ratio

The aspect ratio of lasers is basically the area of skin impacted by the laser beam and has a depth and a width (Figs. 4.13B and C). The ratio of depth/width constitutes the aspect ratio. This ratio is more for fractional lasers as they can achieve higher effective depths than conventional ablative lasers (for example CO_2) where the thermal necrosis and coagulation limit their depth (Fig. 4.13C).

This can be varied and depends on the spot size, dose and dosage (Fig. 4.13C). Of courses, there is a variation with different technologies and the aspect ratio of AFL-like CO_2, Er: YAG is not comparable (Figs. 4.13D to F).

The point being that most such technologies are ideally studied in vitro or ex vivo before translating to patients. Clinicians should either ask for such data or buy from reputed manufacturers instead of using preset dose guidelines, which may not translate to effective results.

Practical use of this concept is given in Figures 4.14A to D.

TREATMENT PRINCIPLES

Principles

- For higher energies, the spatial density of MTZs formed in the treatment region should be decreased.

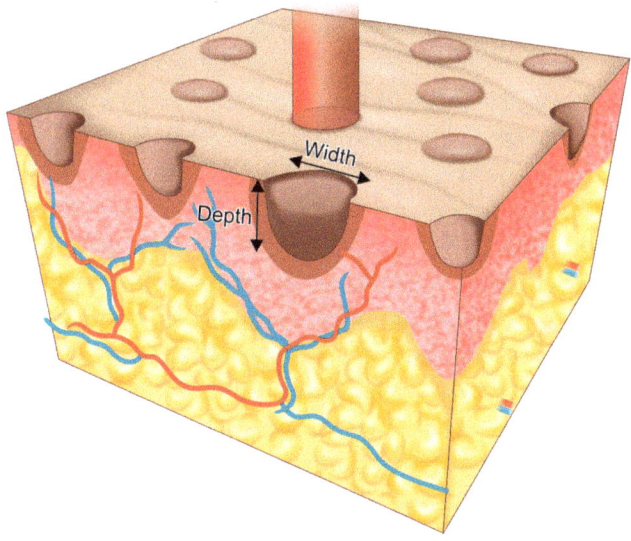

Fig. 4.13B: Depth-width ratio (DWR)/aspect ratio.

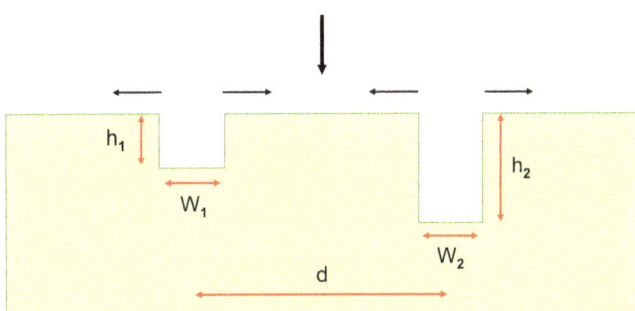

Fig. 4.13C: A comparison of the aspect ratio of an ablative laser (left) and a fractional laser (right) (h: height; w: width).

- When multiple passes are performed on a treatment region, the time interval between passes should be long enough to allow the tissue to cool down between consecutive passes.
- External cooling, e.g. forced air cooling, can be used to remove some heat from the tissue region being treated.
- Individual MTZs should induce wound healing but not fibrosis.
- Confluent damage and bulk heating should be avoided.
- The cumulative MTZ density should be sufficiently high to result in clinical improvement after the completion of a treatment course.

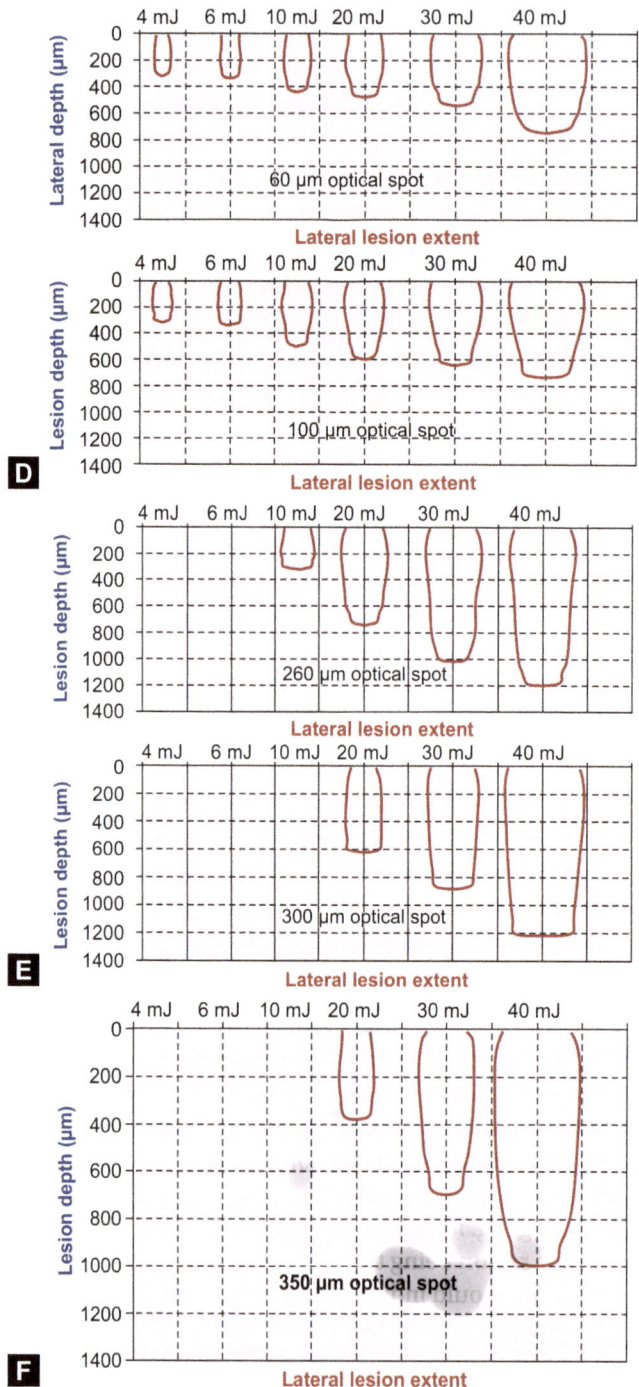

Figs. 4.13D to F: The effect of spot size and energy on the aspect ratio (Depth and width) of fractional lasers.

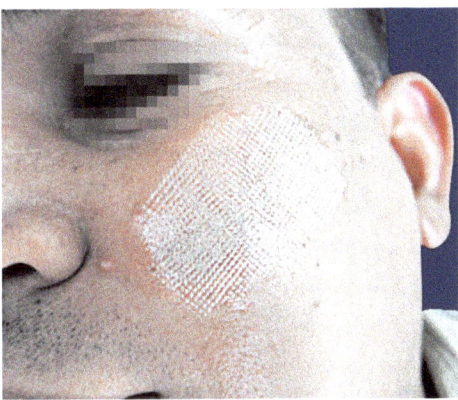

Fig. 4.14A: Overlapping of fractional laser to increase the "aspect ratio" and density (Er:YAG ascepelion 90 J/cm²). This technique can be used to target deep ice pick scars.

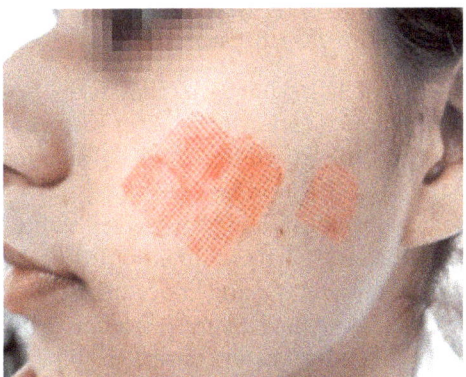

Fig. 4.14B: Postlaser crusting that tends to fall off in 5–7 days. The laser used was the fractional Er:YAG (Dermablate, Ascepelion).

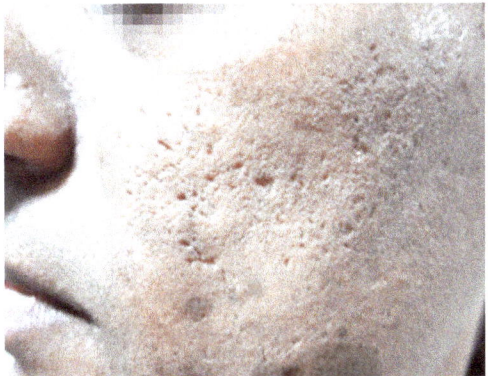

Fig. 4.14C: A male patient with predominantly ice pick and boxcar scars. Plan: Fractional Er:YAG (162 J/cm²; six sessions). The *aspect ratio* of the laser was altered to increase the energy in the areas with deep scars.

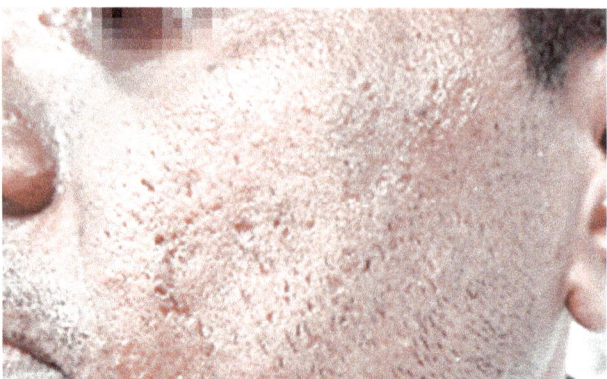

Fig. 4.14D: At 6 months follow-up, there is an improvement of most of the scars except the deep boxcar scars, which remodel with time, thus unnecessary surgical/TCA is unwarranted within the 6 months following a fractional laser.

Preoperative Evaluation/Management

The ideal candidate is a fair-skinned patient (skin type I–III). But the remarkable safety profile makes fractional laser resurfacing ideal even for darker skin types. It can also be used for extrafacial sites like the neck, trunk, and extremities.

A complete medical history should be taken for herpes labialis, keloid or hypertrophic scar formation, postinflammatory hyperpigmentation (PIH), isotretinoin use, topical retinoid use and lidocaine allergy.

Contraindications to NAFR include oral isotretinoin within 6 months to 1 year of surgery, active skin infection and unrealistic patient expectations.

Nonablative fractional resurfacing may occasionally trigger reactivation of herpes simplex infection. Prophylactic antiviral medications is initiated only in patients with a history of recurrent herpes infection and are given the day before the procedure and continued for 3–5 days. Patients with a history of dry skin are advised to discontinue tretinoin cream 1 week before NAFR to prevent skin irritation.

A prophylactic antibiotic course (levofloxacin 500 mg twice a day to be started 2 days before to 3 days after surgery) can be given. An oral analgesic (ibuprofen/ketorolac) half hour before the procedure is better than giving topical anesthesia.

In patients with darker skin types, in particular, use of bleaching creams (hydroquinone 4%), coupled with a sunscreen, can decrease the risk of PIH, though there is little evidence-based literature for this practice.

External eye shields are advisable. A smoke evacuator should be used during laser irradiation because all ablative lasers produce a plume. Patients should have realistic expectations from the procedure. They should be aware that the treatment will improve fine to moderate wrinkles, pigmentation, and superficial scars, but will not completely eliminate deep wrinkles or ice pick scars. As botulinum toxin (BTX) is not deactivated by the laser energy, it may be injected prior to laser therapy (Semchyshyn et al.). Ideally, BTX is administered 10–14 days before laser intervention to enable its full effectiveness. A flattened skin surface may help to treat the dermal compartment more uniformly and to provide access to deeper photodamage. Finally, the muscle relaxation properties of the toxin may contribute to uniform dermal remodeling.

Intraoperative Procedure

Topical anesthesia is not always essential but the use can decrease the discomfort and also helps to track the pattern of passes. It is believed that EMLA can increase the moisture of the skin and as water is the primary chromophore of AFR, this can influence the results. Nevertheless, most clinicians will use topical anesthesia where tetracaine-based topical creams are preferred as they have a faster onset of action. Conventionally, though most clinicians use topical anesthesia but contact cooling, ice packs and even pain killers can suffice in most cases. In case topical anesthesia is used, it is better to *not take* an immediate photograph as the blanching and erythema can alter the surface morphology. Immediately prior to the laser intervention, all makeup, creams, and other substances need to be removed from the skin surface because they may absorb, scatter, or reflect the photons, causing overheating at the epidermis.

Method of Use

There are numerous methods to use the probe. All have a singular aim of providing 3–4 passes.

Scanning Mode

In the new systems, the concept of pitch is used (Figs. 4.15A and B). This can range from 200 µm to 2,000 µm. As a thumb rule, the smaller the pitch, the higher the cover rate (Fig. 4.15B).

Conventionally, three types of pitch can be set in the scanner mode (Fig. 4.15C).

Normal mode: When this scan mode is selected, the area is treated by scanning the lines from left to right and from right to left, starting at the first line from the top to the last line at the bottom.

Interlaced: When this scan mode is selected, the area is treated by first scanning the odd lines and then the even lines from the top to the bottom. Then the even lines are scanned from the bottom to the top. This mode is advisable for reducing the thermal effects during treatment.

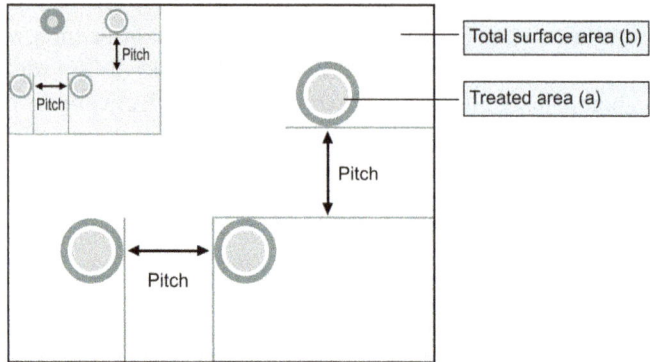

Fig. 4.15A: Correlation of pitch on *cover rate* Pitch = 200 μm to 2,000 μm; the smaller the pitch, the higher the cover rate; density = a/b.

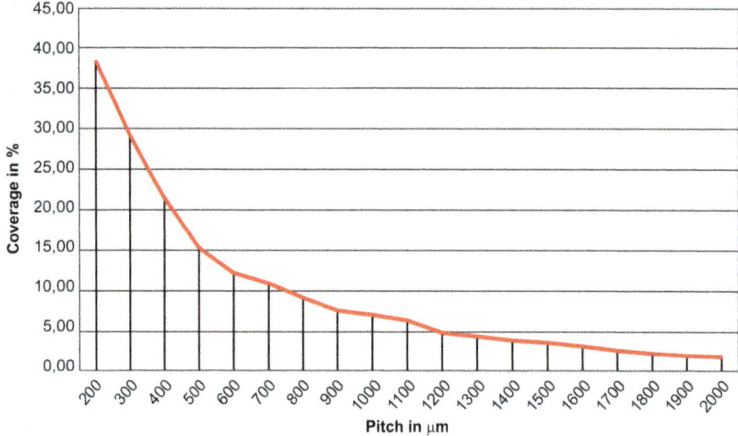

Fig. 4.15B: *Cover rate* is defined as the percentage of treated skin and is dependent on the pitch.

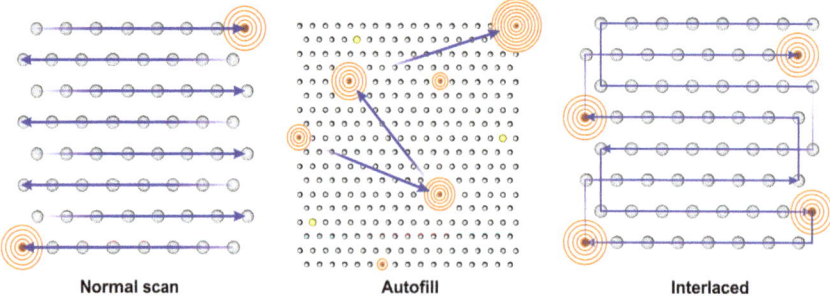

Fig. 4.15C: The patterns of scanning mode in fractional lasers.

Autofill scan mode: When this scan mode is selected, the area is treated and scanning the dots with random order: this minimizes the tissue overheating and then the thermal damage.

Stamping Mode

In this, one pass is given, then the probe is turned by 45° to the right and a second pass is given then the probe is brought back to the initial position. Then a similar pass is given to the left. Unless indicated, multiple passes over the same area should be avoided (Fig. 4.16).

A second method described is as follows:
The handpiece is placed in full contact with the skin, and the foot pedal is depressed. A double pass, 50% overlap technique is used, (a) Deliver 1 pass, (b) come to a complete stop, (c) then pull back to deliver the second pass with 100% overlap and (d) move the handpiece laterally by 50% and repeat steps (a) to (c).

Dose

The dose of each laser varies according to the indication. Almost all US FDA/CE approved lasers have a histological dose depth analysis to predict the dose (Fig. 4.17A). This is especially useful in dermal pathologies like acne scars. A general rule is difficult to detail for the different laser systems available but a few principles are given below:
- As a general rule, *higher densities* and *lower doses* are used for epidermal pathology while a *lower density* and *higher dose* are used for dermal disorders.

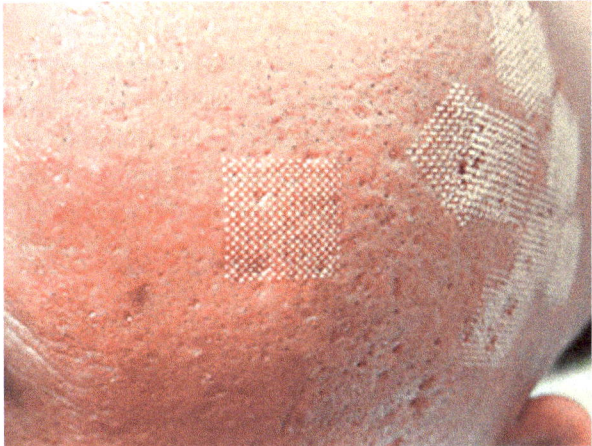

Fig. 4.16: A single pass on the center of the cheek and overlapping passes on the preauricular area using the stamping mode.
(Fractional Er: YAG)

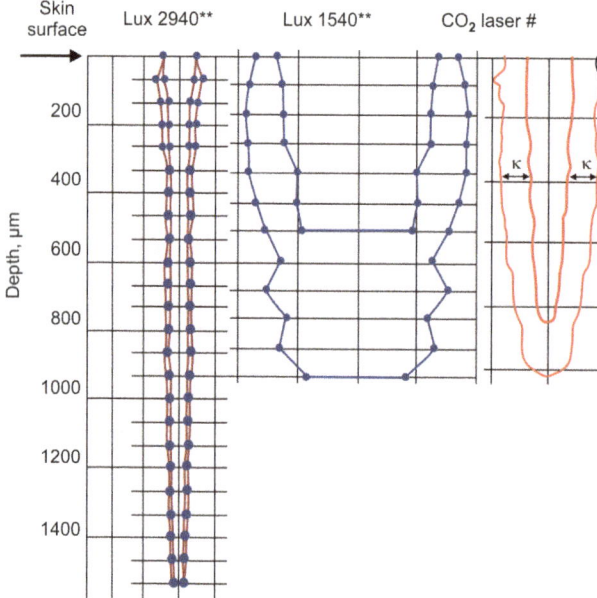

Fig. 4.17A: A comparison of histological depth of 3 fractional systems. Various settings can change the aspect ratio.

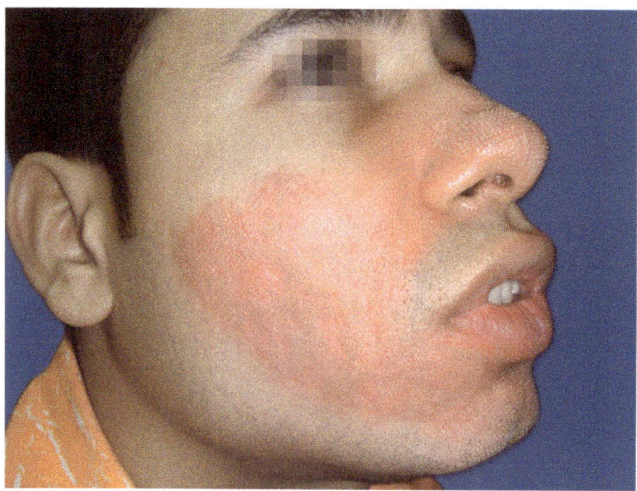

Fig. 4.17B: Immediate post-treatment image after Fr: CO_2

- When treating moderate-severe photodamage or scars, higher pulse energies and treatment densities are required, which may cause intense erythema (Fig. 4.17B).
- Less aggressive treatment parameters are required for eyelid, preauricular, jawline, and neck skin.

- If a combination of treatments is planned, a nonablative laser treatment should precede the fractional ablative treatment, and superficial macro-ablation should follow the deep fractional treatment.

Sittings

About 3-5 sittings are done at an interval of 6-8 weeks. There is a little improvement after the 4th session.

Postoperative Instructions

- In case of AFR, it is useful to apply cold compress for minimum 30 minutes or cold air. Do not apply ice. For NAFR, cooling is not always required.
- We ask the patients to apply aloe vera 40% gel and ask the patient to use a sunblock. Also, till the bronzing peels off, the patient is asked to avoid going out in sunlight without protection. The MTZs, which account for the bronzing (Fig. 4.18) peel off by day 3-7.
- In case of aggressive AFR therapy, anti-inflammatory medication and antibiotic medication can be considered.
- Inflammatory acne flares have been reported, especially with more aggressive settings. For acne prone patients, it is best to initiate an oral antibiotic prior to treatment and continue for 10-14 days post-laser, we prefer levofloxacin 750 mg OD.
- Postoperatively, sun avoidance, compliance with medication, and proper recognition and management of complications are the key.

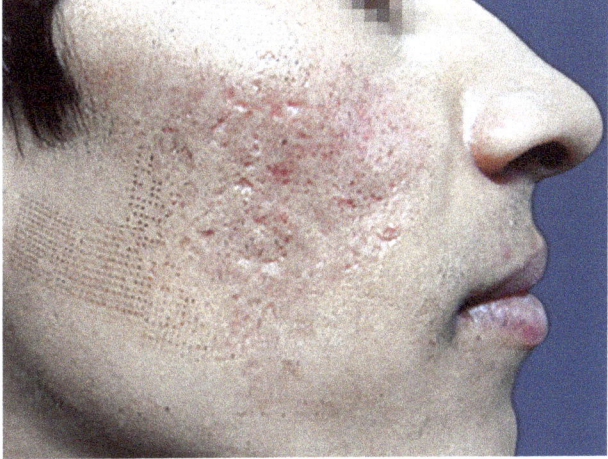

Fig. 4.18: Simultaneous presence of bronzing in the preauricular area with erythema on the other areas of the face. Note the *pattern* of the fractional laser of the facial skin, which is transient and inevitable.

Side Effects

Predictable Side Effects

- Postoperative discomfort, which is generally mild and transient
- Sunburn sensation for approximately 1 hour postoperatively
- Sunburn like erythema that may persist for 3-7 days
- Edema, which is generally minimal and usually resolves in 2-3 days
- The density pattern of the laser manifests after 1 day and lasts for a week
- Bronzing, which is usually noted on the third postoperative day and often lasts for 3-4 days
- Flaking that is often mild and is noted to start on the third postoperative day and persists for 3-4 days
- Occasionally, petechiae may be seen.

Other Adverse Side Effects

- Laser nicks, which are superficial scratches that can occur secondary to incomplete contact of the handpiece with the skin or secondary to tilting or lifting the handpiece while the foot switch is still depressed
- Blistering and crusting, although this is not common
- Reactivation of herpes infection. Antiviral therapy is recommended for patients with a history of herpes labialis
- Postinflammatory hyperpigmentation, especially in darker skin types. It usually resolves over the course of several months and can be prevented or decreased by pretreating the patient with bleaching creams. This can also be avoided by decreasing the density and dose per sitting
- Hypertrophic scarring, although very rare, occurs secondary to bulk heating. Extra caution should be exerted when treating smaller areas such as the upper lip with high fluencies to avoid bulk heating.

Conclusion

There are numerous issues that can be discussed regarding the technology some of which are beyond the scope of this book. We will focus on the needless comparison of AFR and NAFR and detail some of the hitherto unresolved issues that involve the use of fractional lasers.

COMBINATION OF ENERGY MODALITIES

In clinical practice, there is a tendency for combining a variety of long-pulsed, QS, or picosecond lasers for the treatment of benign pigmentary lesions, vascular lasers for redness and telangiectasia, and low-energy, low-density NAFL for full face resurfacing and rejuvenation. Additionally, acne scars with erythema are best targeted by a combination of vascular laser and NAFL.

Fractional resurfacing also produces excellent results in combination with noninvasive skin tightening modalities such as monopolar radiofrequency (Thermage, Solta Medical) and microfocused ultrasound with visualization (Ultherapy, Ulthera, Mesa, AZ).

Combination energy modalities have the potential to synergistically improve cutaneous structure and function. There is a rationale for combining modalities in skin aging where there are pigment and skin textural aberrations. In Indian skin though aging is a less complex problem and the skin pigment helps to prevent age spots and wrinkles. If needed, a pigment laser can be used first for lentigines and freckles, followed by a fractional laser for scars, textural issues, or tightening. Aggressive combination of more than 2 devices has little logic especially in the *same session* as the tissue effects of one can obviate the effects of the other. *Sequential* use though makes sense but the clinicians should know that combining more than 2 devices is a tacit admission on the futility one of the devices and can be misconstrued as an intervention for monetary gain. For examples, skin tightening may be best achieved by an RF device than a fractional laser and hence combining the two is meaningless. Hence, combination of therapies should be based only when the primary skin problem has a chromophore and pathology that is markedly different than the device at hand and not just to add **costs** and *novelty* in conference presentations.

ABLATIVE FRACTIONAL RESURFACING VERSUS NONABLATIVE FRACTIONAL RESURFACING

The question of comparing the two differing technologies frequently leads to a lively discussion without any relevant conclusions. The numerous parameters that can influence the depth and width of the MTZ coupled with the variation in collagen remodeling dynamics further complicates the issues. However, histological analysis indicates that NAFR procedures may even exhibit a greater total volume of denatured collagen, as compared to an AFR process performed with similar energy per MTZ (comparison of data from Hantash et al. and Thongsima et al.) (Fig. 4.17A). The depth of the various laser technologies and their tissue effects is rarely the focus of research and whatever little exists (Thongsima et al. Baily et al. Zelickson et al. Sardana K et al.) have highlighted the fact that given the optimal dose settings of the available technology there may be little to choose between NAFR and AFR (Fig. 4.17A). The two clinical studies addressing this issue (Cho et al. 2009, Manuskiatti W et al.) have found no difference between the two technologies. Considering that most of the major laser manufacturers dabble in both the technologies, clinical comparison studies will be hard to come by considering the cost of possessing both the technologies. This is more so as like companies are not willing to share these data.

We believe that all the present fractional lasers if used in the optimal settings can achieve similar results and the laser practitioner should learn to optimize settings instead of changing technologies (Fig. 4.17).

GRAY AREAS IN FRACTIONAL LASERS

Even though literature is replete with data on fractional lasers, there are numerous issues that have yet to be discussed. A few are pointed below, and instead of buying the *best* available machine, it may better to understand the technology to maximize results with whatever device that is available:

- Tissue effects related to pulse duration and/or temporal pulse profile have not yet been characterized in detail, but these parameters are likely to be the focus of future studies for optimizing fertility preservation (FP) procedures.
- It is a widely held belief that analogous to traditional ablative procedures, the amount of residual thermal injury in AFP procedures may also be affected by the temporal profile of the laser pulse. Typical temporal profiles for energy delivery include continuous wave (CW), superpulsed, and ultrapulsed mode. Although, such dependency of thermal injury on pulse profile appears reasonable, there is currently no investigational data available that specifically relates the extent of thermal damage for AFP procedures to the temporal pulse profiles. Thus, there is no objective clinical advantage of an AFR over an NAFR.
- There appears to be no single best technique for delivering the desired density of MTZs. The rolling technique can facilitate treatment of larger areas, while the stamping technique can facilitate the precise treatment of smaller areas, in particular areas having an irregular surface profile.
- The balance between wound healing, neocollagenesis, coagulation, and remodeling for optimal skin tightening and rejuvenation with fractional technology warrants further investigations. In Asian skin, though it has been confirmed that it is better to increase the dose/microbeam than increase the density to achieve an equivalent energy.
- The optimal settings for coagulation versus ablation and more importantly, the effect of that on the conditions to be treated has not been studied.
- The variations in skin type have been not addressed, as most Asian studies are in skin types (I, II, III) that are not representative of darkly pigmented skin.

The innumerable variables and the choice and control of all possible parameters and factors are rarely the focus of studies. The multivariate complexity of FP procedures explains in part the current lack of clinical studies comparing the effect of many specific FP parameters on patient outcomes. In spite of this complexity, it turns out that most FP treatment regime result in some kind of clinical improvement for appropriate indications.

BOOKS

1. Fractional Photothermolysis. Dieter Manstein and Hans-Joachim Laubach. In: Nouri K (Ed). Lasers in Dermatology and Medicine. Springer-Verlag London Limited; 2011.
2. Kauvar ANB, Warycha MA. Wrinkles and Acne Scars: Fractional Ablative Lasers. In: Raulin C, Karsai S. (Eds). Laser and IPL Technology in Dermatology and Aesthetic Medicine. Springer-Verlag London Limited; 2011.
3. Manstein D, Laubach HJ. Fractional Photothermolysis. In: Nouri K (Ed). Lasers in Dermatology and Medicine. © Springer-Verlag London Limited; 2011.
4. Wrinkles UP. Acne Scars: Fractional Nonablative Lasers. In: Lasers C, Raulin S, Karsai (Eds). Laser and IPL Technology in Dermatology and Aesthetic Medicine. © Springer-Verlag Berlin Heidelberg; 2011.

BIBLIOGRAPHY

1. Bailey SH, Brown SA, Kim Y, et al. An intraindividual quantitative assessment of acute laser injury patterns in facial versus abdominal skin. Lasers Surg Med. 2011;43(2):99-107.
2. Cho SB, Lee SJ, Kang JM, et al. Combined fractional laser treatment with 1550-nm erbium glass and 10 600-nm carbon dioxide lasers. J Dermatolog Treat. 2010;21(4):221-8.
3. Cho SB, Lee SJ, Cho S, et al. Nonablative 1550 nm erbium-glass and ablative 10, 600 nm carbon dioxide fractional lasers for acne scars: a randomized split-face study with blinded response evaluation. J Eur Acad Dermatol Venereol. 2009;24(8):921-5.
4. Farkas JP, Richardson JA, Hoopman J, et al. Micro-island damage with a nonablative 1540-nm Er:Glass fractional laser device in human skin. J Cosmet Dermatol. 2009;8(2):119-26.
5. Fournier N, Mordon S. Nonablative remodeling with a 1,540 nm erbium: glass laser. Dermatol Surg. 2005;31(9 Pt 2):1227-35.
6. Fournier N, Dahan S, Barneon G, et al. Nonablative remodeling: clinical, histologic, ultrasound imaging, and profilometric evaluation of a 1540 nm Er:glass laser. Dermatol Surg. 2001;27(9):799-806.
7. Goodman GJ, Baron JA. The management of postacne scarring. Dermatol Surg. 2007;33(10):1175-88.
8. Ho SG, Yeung CK, Chan NP, et al. A retrospective study of the management of Chinese melasma patients using a 1927 nm fractional thulium fiber laser. J Cosmet Laser Ther. 2013;15(4):200-6.
9. Huzaira M, Anderson RR, Sink K, et al. Intradermal focusing of near-infrared optical pulses: A new approach for non-ablative laser therapy. Lasers Surg Med. 2003;3217-38.
10. Jeong KH, Suh DH, Shin MK, et al. Neurologic complication associated within tense focused ultrasound. J Cosmet Laser Ther. 2014;16(1):43-4.

11. Kono T, Chan HH, Groff WF, et al. Prospective direct comparison study of fractional resurfacing using different fluences and densities for skin rejuvenation in Asians. Lasers Surg Med. 2007;39(4):311-4.
12. Laubach H, Chan HH, Rius F, et al. Effects of skin temperature on lesion size in fractional photothermolysis. Lasers Surg Med. 2007;39(1):14-8.
13. Laubach HJ, Makin IR, Barthe PG, et al. Intense focused ultrasound: evaluation of a new treatment modality for precise microcoagulation within the skin. Dermatol Surg. 2008;34(5):727-34.
14. Lee HM, Haw S, Kim JK, et al. Split-face study using a 1,927-nm thulium fiber fractional laser to treat photoaging and melasma in Asian skin. Dermatol Surg. 2013;39(6):879-88.
15. Manstein D, Herron GS, Sink RK, et al. Fractional photothermolysis: a new concept for cutaneous remodeling using microscopic patterns of thermal injury. Lasers Surg Med. 2004;34(5):426-38.
16. Manstein D, Zurakowski D, Thongsima S, et al. The effects of multiple passes on the epidermal thermal damage pattern in nonablative fractional resurfacing. Lasers Surg Med. 2009;41(2):149-53.
17. Manuskiatti W, Iamphonrat T, Wanitphakdeedecha R, et al. Comparison of fractional erbium-doped yttrium aluminum garnet and carbon dioxide lasers in resurfacing of atrophic acne scars in Asians. Dermatol Surg. 2013;39(1 Pt 1):111-20.
18. Narurkar VA. Nonablative fractional resurfacing in the male patient. Dermatol Ther. 2007;20(6):430-5.
19. Rongsaard N, Rummaneethorn P. Comparison of a fractional bipolar radiofrequency device and a fractional Erbium-Doped Glass 1,550-nm device for the treatment of atrophic acne scars: A Randomized split-face clinical study. Dermatol Surg. 2014;40(1):14-21.
20. Ross EV. Nonablative laser rejuvenation in men. Dermatol Ther. 2007;20(6):414-29.
21. Sardana K, Garg VK, Arora P, et al. Histological validity and clinical evidence for use of fractional lasers for acne scars. J Cutan Aesthet Surg. 2012;5(2):75-90.
22. Tannous Z. Fractional resurfacing. Clin Dermatol. 2007;25(5):480-6.
23. Thongsima S, Zurakowski D, Manstein D. Histological comparison of two different fractional photothermolysis devices operating at 1,550 nm. Lasers Surg Med. 2010;42(1):32-7.
24. Tierney EP, Kouba DJ, Hanke CW. Review of fractional photothermolysis: Treatment indications and efficacy. Dermatol Surg. 2009;35(10):1445-61.
25. Trelles MA, Martínez-Carpio PA. Attenuation of acne scars using high power fractional ablative unipolar radiofrequency and ultrasound for transepidermal delivery of bioactive compounds through microchannels. Lasers Surg Med. 2014;46(2):152-9.
26. Zelickson BD, Walgrave SE, Al-Arashi MY, et al. Semi-automated method of analysis of horizontal histological sections of skin for objective evaluation of fractional devices. Lasers Surg Med. 2009;41(9):634-42.

LASER TREATMENT OF COMMON CONDITIONS

INDICATIONS

Though an elaborate list of conditions has been reported to respond to the technology (Table 4.5) including poikilodermatous disorders, not all patients or dermatoses achieve optimal results (Tierney et al.). Indications that have shown some promise for treatment using NAFR in small case studies are minocycline-induced hyperpigmentation, granuloma annulare, striae, nevus of Ota and alopecia areata. A detailed discussion of the common indications will follow in the next chapter.

Most *importantly*, it must be remembered that there is a risk of *PIH* in our skin type and an NAFR like Er:YAG or Er:Glass is preferred, if a cosmetic effect like tightening or pigmentation is the target. The use of AFR like CO_2 in dark skin type for cosmetic indications (excluding scars) can have the reverse effect and cause PIH.

Acne Scars

There are numerous ways to classify acne scars and the heterogeneity in their classification makes clinical trial comparisons difficult. For practical

Table 4.5: Indications for therapy with fractional lasers.

Fractional lasers	Indications
Ablative fractional lasers	Acne scars (Rolling/boxcar) Other scars (Traumatic, surgical, atrophy scars, burn scars) Striae distensae Moderate and deep wrinkles Skin laxity Solar elastosis Dyschromia* Melasma (Epidermal) Poikiloderma* Photo-induced wrinkles
Nonablative fractional lasers	Acne scars (Rolling/boxcar) Rejuvenation Mild to moderate photodamaged skin Fine wrinkles Pigmentary alterations* (Poikiloderma, dyschromia, hyperpigmentation, melasma, lentigines, tattoos) Vascular abnormalities* Skin texture

*Not effective in Indian skin. In melasma there are side effects and a rapid relapse.

Table 4.6: A practical intervention based on morphological type of scars (Goodman GJ, 2007).

Scar	Treatment modality
Ice pick scars	Punch excision, CROSS Lasers Ablative and nonablative fractional lasers are largely *ineffective* against ice pick scars
Boxcar scars	
(i) Shallow boxcar scars	• Dermabrasion, subcision, dermaroller lasers • Fractional lasers are useful

(ii) Deep boxcar scars	• *With regular base:*
	  – Punch floatation if diameter < 3.5 mm, elliptical excision and suturing, if diameter > 3.5 mm
	• *With irregular base:*
	  – Punch excision with primary closure or graft replacement if diameter < 3.5 mm
	  – Elliptical excision and suturing, if diameter > 3.5 mm
	• *Fractional lasers:*
	  – The volumizing effect is not sufficient for most deep scars

Rolling scars	• Subcision, dermal fillers • Fractional lasers – They consistently respond and are an ideal indication for this technology
Hypertrophic scars	Intralesional steroid, cryosurgery

purposes, a simple classification is based on the morphology, i.e. rolling, boxcar, ice pick, and hypertrophic scars, is ideal as this enables a simple interventional protocol as given in Table 4.6.

How do Fractional Lasers Help in Postacne Scarring?

As we have seen, fractionated photothermolysis produces small vertical zones of full-thickness thermal damage by a mid-infrared laser. This is akin to sinking posts or drilling holes of thermal damage with areas surrounding these posts left free of damage. This is a method of ablative resurfacing without the patient having to experience a pronounced healing phase. Conceptually, it may be the *laser equivalent* of *skin needling* and would be expected to have a significant role in the treatment of scars.

But the effect of the fractional lasers varies depending on the type of atrophic scar treated. This is as in the deep boxcar and ice pick scars, a volumizing effect is needed to fill-up the defect, which requires heat-induced collagen remodeling (Fig. 4.19). This is not easy to achieve as the very purpose of fractional lasers was to minimize damage.

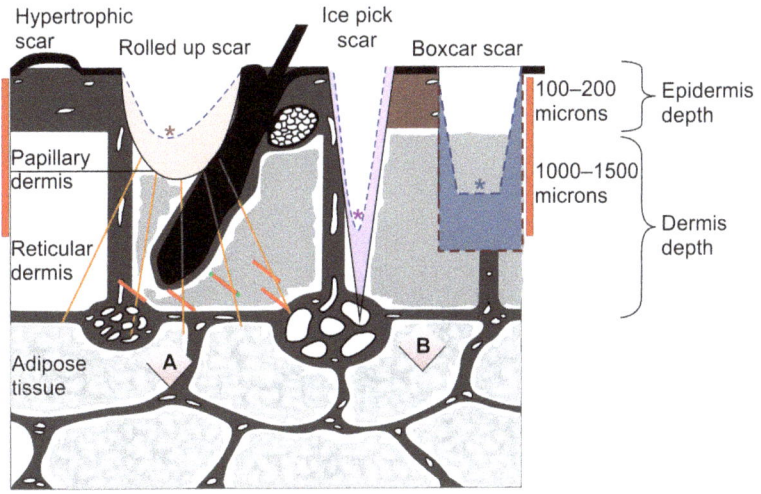

Fig. 4.19: The effect of fractional lasers on acne scars. (A) Rolling scars respond due to snapping of dermal bands; (B) Deep ice pick scars and boxcar scars need collagen remodeling to *fill* the tissue defect which may not completely eliminate the scars.

A very important and often missed aspect is to assess the depth of the laser in relation to the scar. Thus as seen in Figure 4.19, a depth beyond **1,000 μm** is *not required* for most acne scars. Importantly, the clinician should know the dose required for such depths, which should be enquired from the manufacturers.

As the depth of scars varies, a combination of conventional laser (Cho et al.) AFR (Kim et al. 2009), CROSS (Kang et al.), and subcision should be used in conjunction with NAFR for best results. A recent review (Sardana K et al.) has defined the depth of penetration of various systems with NAFR laser (Er: Glass, 679 μm) achieving a depth that was less than that of the AFR lasers (Er:YAG, 825 μm, and CO_2 895 μm; $P < 0.05$). But this difference may not be relevant on the facial skin as the total depth is 2,196 μm.

Rolling Scars

Rolling scars occur deep in the follicle and are the end products of inflammation that causes destruction of the subcuticular fat. Abnormal fibrous anchoring of the dermis to the subcutis leads to superficial shadowing and a rolling or undulating appearance to the overlying skin (Figs. 4.19 to 4.21).

They are amenable to fractional lasers (Figs. 4.20 and 4.21) as the MTZ *snap* the tethered fibrotic bands.

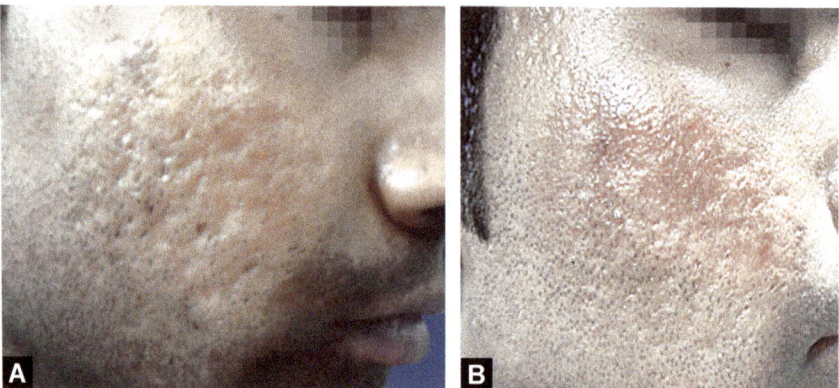

Figs. 4.20A and B: (A) A case with predominantly rolling scars treated with the Er: Glass (Lux Palomar); (B) Post-therapy improvement using the Lux Palomar after 6 sittings (70 mJ/4 passes/10 mm).
Source: Sardana K, et al. Which type of atrophic acne scar (ice pick, boxcar, or rolling) responds to nonablative fractional laser therapy? Dermatol Surg. 2014;40(3):288-300.

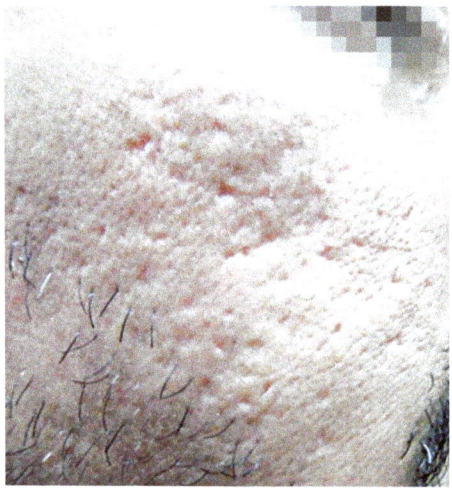

Fig. 4.21A: A case with predominantly rolling scars. Plan: Fractional Er:YAG (126 J/cm^2; six sessions).

Ice Pick Scars

Ice pick scars are narrow (<2 mm), deep, sharply marginated epithelial tracts that extend vertically to the deep dermis or subcutaneous tissue. The surface opening is usually, but not always, wider than the deeper infundibulum, as the scar tapers from the surface to its deepest apex (Fig. 4.19). They do not respond effectively to most fractional lasers even though the laser may help to *fill* some of the defect.

Boxcar Scars

Boxcar scars may be shallow (0.1–0.5 mm) or deep (>0.5 mm) and are most often 1.5–4.0 mm in diameter (Fig. 4.19). Shallow boxcar scars are within the dermal reach of skin resurfacing treatments (such as laser skin resurfacing), but deeper boxcar scars are resistant to improvement in the absence of full-thickness treatment of the scar. For boxcar scars, fractional technologies should be considered, depending on the patient's expectations and tolerance for downtime. This can be appreciated in Figures 4.22 and 4.23.

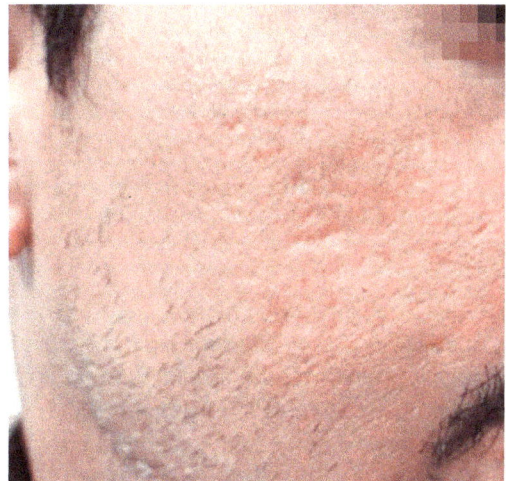

Fig. 4.21B: Marked improvement in rolling scars which respond to most fractional lasers.

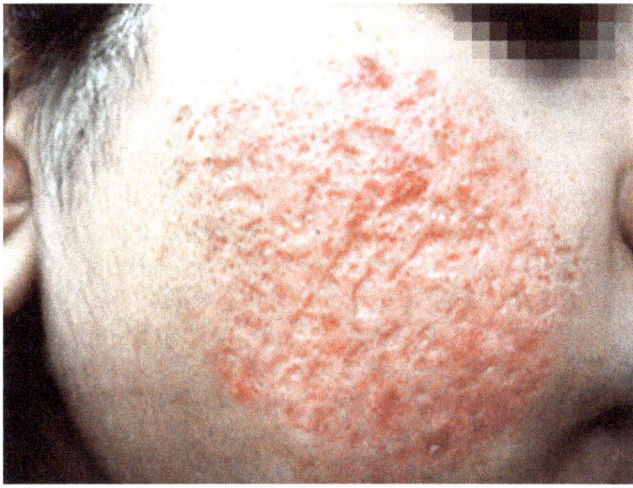

Fig. 4.22: A case with large *Boxcar* atrophic acne scars treated with the Lux Er: Glass (70 mJ).

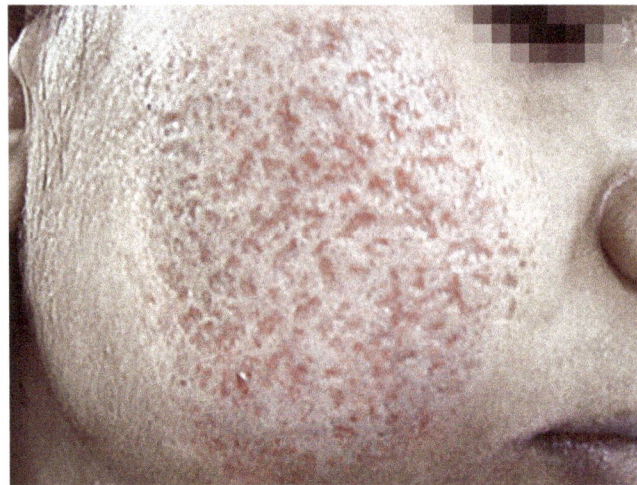

Fig. 4.23: After 6 sessions, an appreciable improvement is seen, but the volume defect in the scars may require non-laser modalities.

Literature Overview and Critique

The numerous studies published on acne scars, entice the practitioner into believing in the superlative efficacy of lasers. No doubt that there are certain advantages like the fast procedure and less downtime, but the results have to be interpreted cautiously, as most studies neither do not subclassify the types of scar nor do they use an objective tool to quantify results (Tables 4.7 and 4.8).

Thus, the plethora of data has to be understood in respect to the following points:
- Very few studies have used an *objective scoring pattern*. Thus, a quartile improvement is highly subjective and can mean little as assessment of depth improvement is difficult as it is requires a 3D aspect.
- Objective analysis has shown a realistic improvement of 43–79.9% with a mean level of improvement of 66.8% (Anne M Chapas). In fact, subjective improvement is always more than objective improvement.
- These results are even less impressive, if we look at individual scars. *Deep ice pick scars* rarely respond to the fractional laser (Sardana K, 2014).
- Some authors have combined modalities, thus it is difficult to determine which modality has helped in scar improvement (Table 4.7).
- Most importantly, a comparison of NAFR and AFR has shown that the results are not markedly different (Table 4.7).

Devices vary in their penetration capacities, and optimal parameters still need to be defined (Taub et al.) and thus there is still a need for optimal device usage to achieve satisfactory results.

Table 4.7: Summary of studies of ablative fractional resurfacing (AFR) fractional laser in acne scars.

Authors/Number of patients studied	Scars treated	Laser	Dose/sessions	Assessment subjective	Assessment objective*	Results/improvement
Anne M Chapas, (2008) 13 patients	Moderate-to-severe acne scars	Fraxel repair	Energies of 20–100 mJ/pulse, spot size = 120 mm, 10–400 MTZ/cm² total densities of 200–1,200 MTZ/cm² 2–3 sittings	Quartile scale	Primos imaging	The result ranged from 43% to 79.9% with a mean level of improvement of 66.8%
Susan E Walgrave (2009) 30 patients	Moderate-to-severe acne scars	Fraxel repair	20–100 mJ/pulse, 600–1,600 MTZ/cm², 4 sittings	Quartile scale	Photography (but subjective observer evaluation)	1–25% at 3 months 23/25 –improved
Elliot T Weiss (2010) 15 patients	Nonacne scars	Fraxel repair	20–100 mJ/pulse, 100–300 MTZ/cm² per pass, density of 100 to 900 MTZ/cm² 1–3 passes, 3 sittings	No	Yes, Primos	Volume improvement = 26.8–57.5% Mean improvement in scar volume = 38.0%. Maximum depths of reduction 26.3% to 40.9%, with a mean reduction of 35.6% (at 6 months)
Sung Bin Cho (2009) 20 patients	Acne scars	Deep Fx Active Fx	10–20 mJ, density 2, and 300 Hz using the Deep FX mode 2 sittings	Yes	No	1 = 76–100% 9 = 51–75% 7 = 26–50% 3 = minimal to no improvements

Contd...

Contd...

Authors/Number of patients studied	Scars treated	Laser	Dose/sessions	Assessment subjective	Assessment objective*	Results/improvement
Manuskiatti W (2010) 13 patients	Atrophic acne scars	Fraxel repair	3 sessions	Subjective (clinical evaluation by two blinded dermatologists)	Objective (ultraviolet A-light video camera)	85% of the subjects had 25–50% improvement of scars. While 62% of subjects had a 50% improvement in their scars (6 months)
Chan NP (2010) 9 patients	Acne scars	Fraxel repair	30–70 mJ Fraxel repair 30–45% coverage 1 treatment	No	Photographic evaluation	Only mild-to-moderate improvement after a single treatment 86% had a subjective improvement
Wang YS (2010) 5 patients	Moderate-to-severe acne scars		Energy 28 J/cm^2; pulse width 2.5 ms; spot size, 300 μm; penetration depth up to 500 μm; degree of skin coverage, 20%; single pass 2 treatment	Quartile scoring	Photographic evaluation	At 2 months post-treatment, all five subjects showed some clinical improvement (four: mild improvement; one: moderate improvement)

*Though photography is touted an objective measure its evaluation by visual comparison is never accurate as depth analysis requires a 3D perspective. Only Primos is a truly objective tool.

Table 4.8: Summary of studies of fractional Er: Glass laser in acne scars.

Authors	No.	Scars treated	Types of laser	Sittings	Results‡ (Improvement/ Assessment)
Geronemus 2006*	17	Ice pick† Boxcar Rolling	Fraxel	3–5	Results 22–66% Ice pick—25–50% boxcar, 22–62% Rolling scars 29–67% Assessment Digital photography, high-resolution typographic imaging, and patient-completed questionnaires
Hasegawa 2006 III/IV	10	Not stated	Fraxel SR 1,500 nm	3	Results 4 patients—excellent 3 patients—good 3 patients—fair Assessment Subjective
Alster 2007	53	Mild-to-moderate atrophic scar	Fraxel SR 1,500 nm (1st generation)	2–3	Results 51–75% Assessment (Subjective/ Photography with quartile scoring)
Glaich 2007	2	Atrophic scars	Fraxel SR 1,500 nm	5	Results Physician clinical assessments: Moderate-to-marked improvement in atrophic acne scarring in all patients Assessment Subjective
Lee HS 2008 IV/V	27	Rolling† Boxcar Ice pick scars	1550 nm Fraxel	3–5	Results All types of scars improved Patients assessment= Excellent improvement in 8 (30%), significant improvement in 16 patients (59%), and moderate improvement in three patients (11%) Mean = 51–75% Assessment (Subjective/ Photography-Quartile)

Contd...

Contd...

Authors	No.	Scars treated	Types of laser	Sittings	Results[‡] (Improvement/ Assessment)
Weiss 2008	500	Mild-to-moderate scars	1,540 nm Lux Palomar	NA	Results Physician evaluation: 50–75% median improvement Patient evaluation: 85% of patients rated their skin as improved Assessment Subjective
Chrastil 2008	29	Mild-to-severe	Second-generation 1,550 nm laser	2–6	Results 50–75% improvement in facial and back acne scarring 5 > 75% 5 = 25–50% 1 <25% response Assessment Photographic evaluation
Cho SB 2009 * IV	12	Mild/moderate atrophic scars and pores	Mosaic LC 1,550 nm	3	Results: 3 patients-76–100% 5 patients-51–75% 2 patients-26–50% 2 patients-0% Mean improvement =26–50% Assessment (Subjective/Photography with quartile staging)
Yoo KH 2009*	16	Acne scars	Lux 1,540 m	3	Mild-to-moderate improvement in acne scars Increase in collagen and elastin Assessment Subjective
Hu S 2009[§] Type III/IV	45	Mild-to-moderate atrophic scars	Fraxel 750 Fraxel 1,500	1	Results 60% patients-good to excellent 40% patients-none to fair No significant difference between two lasers Assessment Subjective

Contd...

Contd...

Authors	No.	Scars treated	Types of laser	Sittings	Results[‡] (Improvement/ Assessment)
Cho SB 2009 ‖ II/IV	1	Atrophic scars	Fraxel SR1,500 Combined with AR (ultraPulse CO_2)	1	Scars Improved
Kim HJ 2009[§] IV/V	20	Rolling and Ice pick[†]	Mosaic LC, 1,550 nm VS CROSS	3	Results Rolling scars and ice pick both improved By 25–75% For Rolling scars Er:Glass is better Ice pick CROSS Assessment (Subjective/ Photography Quartile)
Kang HW 2009 ‖ IV/V	10	Atrophic scars	Mosaic LC 1,550 nm + TCA + Subcison	4	Results All subjects improved by 55% Assessment (Objective scar evaluation but subjective improvement scores)
SB Cho 2010[§]	8	Mild-to-severe scars	Fraxel SR1500 versus Fractional CO_2	1	Results Both lasers were equally good All patient improved 26–50% Assessment Subjective
Hedelund 2010 (RCT split face study)	10	Atrophic scars	StarLux 1,540 nm	3	Results Moderate—marked improvement in 50% patients. No PIH The observer score came down from moderately even to mildly even scar texture. Assessment Subjective

Contd...

Contd...

Authors	No.	Scars treated	Types of laser	Sittings	Results[‡] (Improvement/ Assessment)
Mahmoud 2010[§] Type 4–6	15	Acne scars	1,550 nm laser (Fraxel) With Trilumina-cream	5	Results Equal response in both groups, significant improvement seen by patients but with PIH Observer = 1–25% No difference in doses *Assessment* Photography Quartile
Sardana K 2014[†]	30	Ice pick Boxcar Rolling scars	StarLux 1,540 nm	4-6	Ice pick scar improved by 25.88% Boxcar scars improved by 52.9% Rolling scars improved by 43.14% *Assessment* Subjective improvement 46.7% of patients = 25–49% improvement 30% >50% improvement

*Studies where histology was done, [†]Studies where acne scars were subclassified as, ice pick, boxcar, and rolling, [‡]Though photography is touted as a objective measure its evaluation by visual comparison is never accurate as depth analysis requires a 3D perspective. Only Primos is a truly objective tool, [§]Comparative studies, [||]Studies where NAFR was combined with other modalities.

Based on the available evidence, an approach to treating acne scars is given here (Fig. 4.24).

Here, it must be emphasized that initially a single device should be used (Figs. 4.25A and B) to first complete the required sessions (6-9) and then target the remnant scars by other means, instead of unnecessary combining modalities as is the practice (Figs. 4.25C and D). Needling, subcision, fillers should be done after the sessions of laser are over. The use of the non-laser interventions can wait as the full effect of the fractional lasers is seen after 6 months. The often discussed combination makes little rationale sense as they may actually do little over the existing effect of lasers.

Summary of Literature

Nonablative fractional resurfacing is an effective treatment for atrophic acne scarring. *Higher fluences* with *lower densities* are considered the optimal

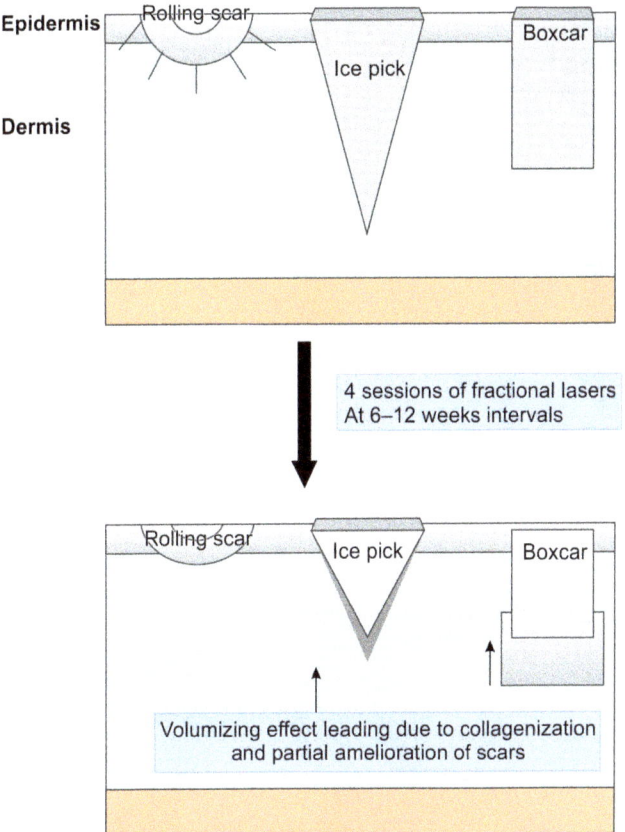

Fig. 4.24: A diagrammatic depiction of the volumizing effect on deep atrophic scars. The tethered rolling scars respond well to fractional lasers.

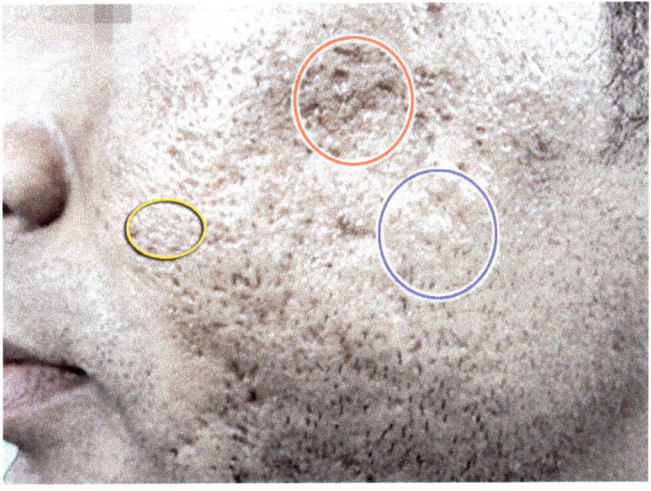

Fig. 4.25A: A topography of a patient with acne scar, ice pick scar (yellow circle), boxcar scar (red circle), and rolling scar (blue circle).

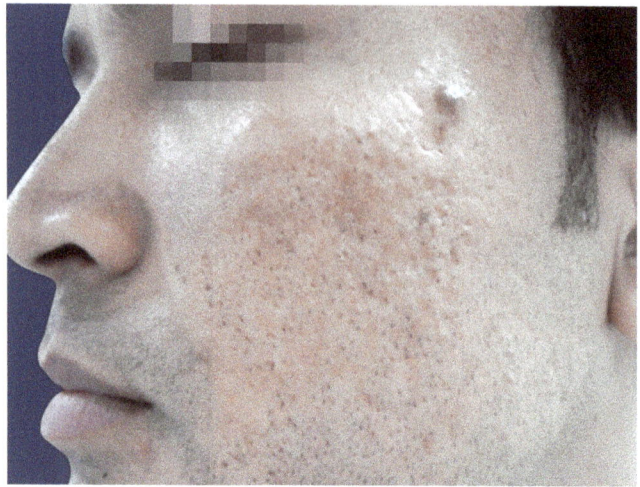

Fig. 4.25B: Follow-up photograph of the patient after five sessions of fractional Er:YAG with substantial amelioration of all types of scars.

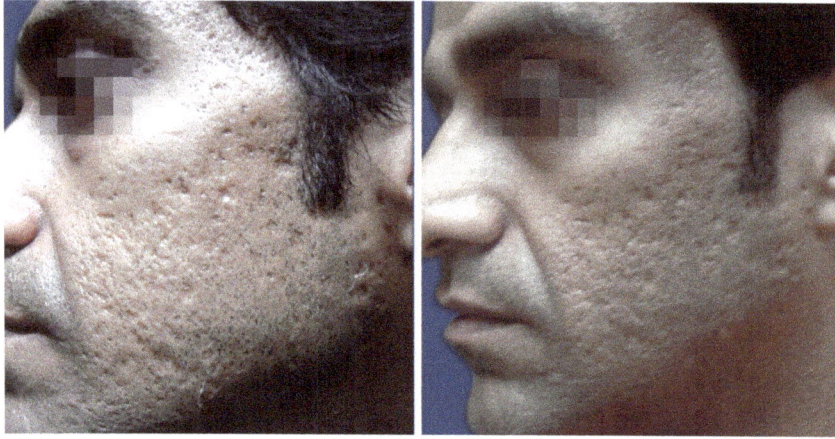

Fig. 4.25C: Modest improvement after 4 sessions of Er:Glass (1,540 nm).
Courtesy: Dr Anil Ganjoo, Skinnovation Clinics

parameters to maximize efficacy and minimize complications. A longer series of low-density treatments can dramatically reduce rates of PIH and erythema without compromising clinical efficacy and is the preferred approach for NAFL resurfacing in Asian patients.

Ablative fractional lasers (AFL) can be an excellent treatment for atrophic acne scarring. However, patients undergoing these treatments must accept the need for dedicated healing time and an increased risk of unwanted complications—particularly PIH. Thus, its excessive use in Indian patients may not be always advisable and especially in female patients.

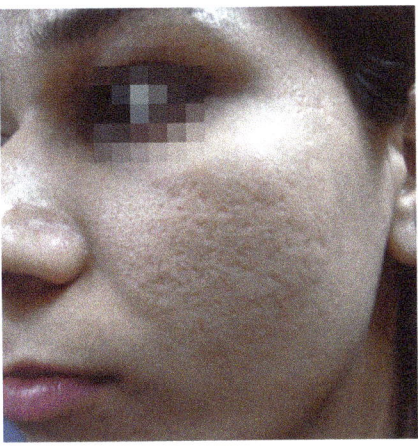
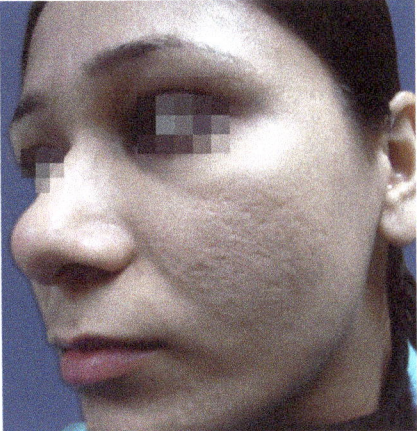

Fig. 4.25D: Modest improvement after 5 sessions of Er:Glass (1540 nm)
Courtesy: Dr Anil Ganjoo, Skinnovation Clinics

BIBLIOGRAPHY

1. Alster TS, Tanzi EL, Lazarus M. The use of fractional laser photothermolysis for the treatment of atrophic scars. Dermatol Surg. 2007;33(3):295-9.
2. Chan NP, Ho SG, Yeung CK, et al. Fractional ablative carbon dioxide laser resurfacing for skin rejuvenation and acne scars in Asians. Lasers Surg Med. 2010;42(9):615-23.
3. Cho SB, Lee JH, Choi MJ, et al. Efficacy of the fractional photothermolysis system with dynamic operating mode on acne scars and enlarged facial pores. Dermatol Surg. 2009;35(1):108-14.
4. Cho SB, Lee SJ, Cho S, et al. Nonablative 1550-nm erbium-glass and ablative 10, 600-nm carbon dioxide fractional lasers for acne scars: a randomized split-face study with blinded response evaluation. J Eur Acad Dermatol Venereol. 2009;24(8):921-5.
5. Cho SB, Lee SJ, Kang JM, et al. The efficacy and safety of 10,600-nm carbon dioxide fractional laser for acne scars in Asian patients. Dermatol Surg. 2009;35(12):1955-61.
6. Cho SB, Lee SJ, Kang JM, et al. Combined fractional laser treatment with 1550-nm erbium glass and 10, 600-nm carbon dioxide lasers. J Dermatol Treat. 2009;1:1-3.
7. Chrastil B, Glaich AS, Goldberg LH, et al. Second-generation 1,550-nm fractional photothermolysis for the treatment of acne scars. Dermatol Surg. 2008;34(10):1327-32.
8. Friedman PM, Skover GR, Payonk G, et al. 3D *in vivo* optical skin imaging for topographical quantitative assessment of non-ablative laser technology. Dermatol Surg. 2002;28(3):199-204.
9. Geronemus RG. Fractional photothermolysis: current and future applications. Lasers Surg Med. 2006;38(3):169-76.
10. Glaich AS, Goldberg LH, Friedman RH, et al. Fractional photothermolysis for the treatment of postinflammatory erythema resulting from acne vulgaris. Dermatol Surg. 2007;33(7):842-6.

11. Goodman GJ, Baron JA. The management of postacne scarring. Dermatol Surg. 2007;33(10):1175-88.
12. Hasegawa T, Matsukura T, Mizuno Y, et al. Clinical trial of a laser device called fractional photothermolysis system for acne scars. J Dermatol. 2006;33(9):623-7.
13. Hedelund L, Moreau KE, Beyer DM, et al. Fractional nonablative 1,540-nm laser resurfacing of atrophic acne scars. A randomized controlled trial with blinded response evaluation. Lasers Med Sci. 2010;25(5):749-54.
14. Kang WH, Kim YJ, Pyo WS, Park SJ, Kim JH. Atrophic acne scar treatment using triple combination therapy: Dot peeling, subcision and fractional laser. J Cosmet Laser Ther. 2009;11(4):212-5.
15. Kim HJ, Kim TG, Kwon YS, et al. Comparison of a 1,550 nm Erbium:Glass fractional laser and a chemical reconstruction of skin scars (CROSS) method in the treatment of acne scars: A simultaneous split-face trial. Lasers Surg Med. 2009;41(8):545-9.
16. Kim S, Cho KH. Clinical trial of dual treatment with an ablative fractional laser and a nonablative laser for the treatment of acne scars in Asian patients. Dermatol Surg. 2009;35(7):1089-98.
17. Lee HS, Lee JH, Ahn GY, et al. Fractional photothermolysis for the treatment of acne scars: a report of 27 Korean patients. J Dermatolog Treat. 2008;19(1):45-9.
18. Mahmoud BH, Srivastava D, Janiga JJ, et al. Safety and efficacy of erbium-doped yttrium aluminum garnet fractionated laser for treatment of acne scars in type IV to VI skin. Dermatol Surg. 2010;36(5):602-9.
19. Manuskiatti W, Triwongwaranat D, Varothai S, et al. Efficacy and safety of a carbon-dioxide ablative fractional resurfacing device for treatment of atrophic acne scars in Asians. J Am Acad Dermatol. 2010;63(2):274-83.
20. Park GH, Rhee DY, Bak H, et al. Treatment of atrophic scars with fractional photothermolysis: short-term follow-up. J Dermatolog Treat. 2011;22(1):43-8.
21. Sardana K, Garg VK, Arora P, et al. Histological validity and clinical evidence for use of fractional lasers for acne scars. J Cutan Aesthet Surg. 2012;5(2):75-90.
22. Sardana K, Manjhi M, Garg VK, et al. Which type of atrophic acne scar (Ice-pick, Boxcar, or Rolling). Responds to nonablative fractional laser therapy? Dermatol Surg. 2014;40(3):288-300.
23. Taub AF. Fractionated delivery systems for difficult to treat clinical applications: acne scarring, melasma, atrophic scarring, striae distensae, and deep rhytides. J Drugs Dermatol. 2007;6:1120-8.
24. Walgrave SE, Ortiz AE, MacFalls HT, et al. Evaluation of a novel fractional resurfacing device for treatment of acne scarring. Lasers Surg Med. 2009;41(2):122-7.
25. Wang YS, Tay YK, Kwok C. Fractional ablative carbon dioxide laser in the treatment of atrophic acne scarring in Asian patients: a pilot study. J Cosmet Laser Ther. 2010;12(2):61-4.
26. Weiss ET, Chapas A, Brightman L, et al. Successful treatment of atrophic postoperative and traumatic scarring with carbon dioxide ablative fractional resurfacing: quantitative volumetric scar improvement. Arch Dermatol. 2010;146(2):133-40.
27. Weiss R, Weiss M, Beasley K. Long-term experience with fixed array 1540 Fractional erbium laser for acne scars. Abstract presented at American Society for Laser Medicine and Surgery Conference. Kissimmee: Florida; 2008.

28. Yoo KH, Ahn JY, Kim JY, et al. The use of 1540 nm fractional photothermolysis for the treatment of acne scars in Asian skin: a pilot study. Photodermatol Photoimmunol Photomed. 2009;25(3):138-42.

PHOTODAMAGE SKIN

The desire to reverse aging is a universal desire and fractional lasers are one of the many tools employed for this purpose. The basic premise of the technology is based on the principles of targeting the dermis (and/or deeper epidermis) and can be achieved either by:
- Targeting chromophores in the dermis
- Using devices that are not avidly absorbed by water, like the mid-infrared lasers in the range of 1.3–1.55 µm.

Thus, numerous devices can be used from visible (400–760 nm), near-infrared (760–1400 nm), or mid-infrared (1.4–3 µm) ranges, radiofrequency (RF) devices (Gold MH, 2014), intense pulsed light (IPL) devices, as well as light-emitting diode (LED) devices.

Clinical Morphology

Given the increased risk of PIH, a greater number of treatments with lower density are the preferred approach in treating skin of color. Both density and fluence contribute to risk of PIH, but *density* has been shown to be the predominant factor: type and degree of photodamage. Photoaging in Asian patients typically manifest as pigmentary alteration, lentigines, and seborrheic keratoses rather than fine lines and deep rhytides as seen in Caucasian counterparts (Wat H et al.)

Asian patients between the ages of *30 and 60* exhibit *far less* fine lines and rhytides compared to age-matched Caucasians, but reach equivalent rates of wrinkling beyond age 60.

Common esthetic concerns in the young to middle-aged Asian population typically include *enlarged pore size, skin textural irregularities, and dyspigmentation.*

Mode of Action

The photothermal heating of the dermis leads to increases collagen production by fibroblasts and induces dermal matrix remodeling by altering glycosaminoglycans as well as other components of the dermal matrix.

Richard Glogau, MD, developed a classification scale to chart the progression of clinical photoaging (Table 4.9), which is a prerequisite for the use of lasers. It should be remembered that the fractional lasers are primarily useful in Glogau grade I/II patient and may not affect the pigmented and vascular changes.

Fractional Lasers Used

Almost all the fractional lasers have been used from nonablative lasers (1,440 nm, 1,550 nm) to fractional ablative lasers (Er: YAG, CO_2, thulium). Recently, fractional Nd: YAG has also been used successfully (Gold MH). The spate of data has to be understood objectively (Table 4.10) even though the results may seem impressive. As the main mode of action is collagen remodeling, this depends on multiple factors, such as the grade (Table 4.9), dose, density, type of lasers, and the aspect ratio of the laser. The last is the depth and width of the MTZ that has been discussed in the previous chapter.

The nonablative fractional resurfacing (NAFR) is ideal in this condition and various lasers have been used (Wat H et al.)

- More pronounced issues with acne scarring, skin texture, dyschromia as well as pore size can be simultaneously improved with low-density *mini* treatments utilizing 1,550 nm erbium glass (Fraxel Re:store, Solta Medical) over six sessions as discussed previously (*Chan NP*).
- When patients present predominantly with discrete or diffuse, mottled superficial dyspigmentation characterized mainly by macular seborrheic keratoses and solar lentigines, the fractionated 1,927-nm thulium fiber laser (Fraxel Dual, Solta Medical) has proven to be a treatment of choice (Poler KD). The 1,927 nm wavelength can be combined with 1,550 nm to achieve both superficial and deep treatment depths, respectively, in a single session.
- A series of NAFL treatments is also effective for reducing periorbital and forehead wrinkles and may even approach the clinical efficacy of AFL with the appropriate settings (Moon HR, Wattanakrai P).

Literature Overview

- Sadly, there is little standardization of trial data (Table 4.10) and except for a few studies (Ross et al.) histological data is lacking.
- As the major chromophore for most fractional lasers is water, it is logical to presume that lesser the absorption coefficient better the results, thus the 1,540 nm, 1,550 nm would be better than the ablative fractional lasers. This is as the primary component of the dermis is water, and thus lesser the absorption more would be the potential for thermal remodeling.
- As little objective scoring is done in studies, in mild-to-moderate cases (Table 4.9), the results of all the fractional lasers would largely be similar.
- Also with little data in pigmented skin, aggressive settings (Pardo et al.) should be avoided.
- Most important is the persistence of the effect, which has been studied by Lapidoth et al. and found to persist for 6–9 months. In the rest of the studies (Table 4.10), long-term follow-up has not been done.

Table 4.9: Glogau photoaging classification.

Grade	Classification	Typical age	Description	Skin characteristics
I	Mild	20s or 30s	No wrinkles	*Early photoaging:* Mild pigmentary change, no keratoses, minimal wrinkles, minimal or no make up
II	Moderate	30s or 40s	Wrinkles in motion	*Early to moderate photoaging:* Early solar lentigines, keratoses palpable but not visible, parallel smile lines begin to appear, wears some foundation
III	Advanced	50s	Wrinkles at rest	*Advanced photoaging:* Obvious discolorations, visible telangiectasias, visible keratoses, wears heavier foundation always
IV	Severe	60s and older	Only wrinkles	*Severe photoaging:* Yellow-gray skin color, prior skin malignancies, wrinkles throughout—no normal skin, make up *cakes and cracks*

Table 4.10: Literature overview of fractional lasers in photodamage skin.

Author	Laser used	Results
Rahman et al., 2009	Fractional CO_2 laser	(50–100%) improvement was observed in 83% of subjects
Pardo et al., 2009	Fractional CO_2 laser	Higher-density coverage (10.1% ablated tissue) produces a greater inflammatory response and improved results compared to a lower density of ablation (3.5%)
Weiss et al., 2008	1,550 nm versus fractional CO_2	75% improvement compared to a 25% improvement in periocular rhytides
Lomeo et al.	Fractional CO_2 versus Er:YAG laser	CO_2>Er: YAG
Lapidoth et al, 2008	Fractional Er: YAG laser	Excellent improvement in 75% (n = 21) and good improvement in 25% (n = 7)
Ross et al. 2009	Fractional 2,790-nm Er:YAG laser	Wrinkle and fine lines improved
Doherty, 2009	Fractional Er:YAG laser	50% or greater reduction in perioral and periorbital wrinkles in 76% of patients (n = 17) and a more than 25% reduction in dyschromia in all patients
Kohl E, 2013	Fractional CO_2 laser	Site periorbital, perioral, forehead, cheeks. Wrinkles were significantly reduced in all facial areas, and the best results regarding wrinkle size and depth were found for the cheeks

Conclusion

Fractional lasers can be considered as one of the tools to treat photodamaged skin and as an extension rhytides, actinic keratosis (Lapidoth M) and blepharochalasia (Balzani A 2014). Patient selection is important to obtain the best expectation–outcome match. Thus, a combination of intense pulsed light (IPL) and potassium titanyl phosphate (KTP) lasers, photodynamic therapy (PDT), mid-infrared lasers, and fractional lasers may be required in exemplifying the complexities inherent in treating photodamaged skin. Thus, studies on lasers should be interpreted both by the amount of improvement and the type of improvement! A detailed discussion is given in **Chapter 12**.

In Asian skin, AFR have been used ranging from fractioal CO_2, Er:YAG but adverse sequelae (particularly PIH) are frequent and patients generally require dedicated healing time postprocedure. Because of these risks and associated downtime, AFR are ideal for elderly patients with advanced photodamage. If there is *photoaging* with greater *dyspigmentation* as *opposed* to *wrinkles* and therefore less aggressive NAFR tends to be more suitable.

In a retrospective review of 362 patients undergoing a total of 856 NAFL treatments with either 1,550-nm Erbium or 1,927-nm thulium fiber laser, significant adverse events occurred in only 5%. This included prolonged erythema (> 7 days) in 1.8%, PIH in 1.1%, and worsening of melasma in 0.9%. Nonablative fractional resurfacing can be considered among first line therapy for the reduction of fine lines and wrinkling, textural abnormalities, and pore size in Asian patients.

Summary

- A series of treatments with lower densities and adequate recovery intervals provides optimal results.
- In our opinion, ideal patients are those presenting with mild-to-moderate photodamage, in the *absence* of other significant clinical features such as melasma, severe acne scarring, and/or thick hypertrophic scars.
- In particular, very low-density and low-energy fractionated diodes produce minimal adverse effects and short recovery times making it a popular choice for patients.

BIBLIOGRAPHY

1. Balzani A, Chilgar RM, Nicoli M, et al. Novel approach with fractional ultrapulse CO_2 laser for the treatment of upper eyelid dermatochalasis and periorbital rejuvenation. Lasers Med Sci. 2013;28(6):1483-7.
2. Chan NP, Ho SG, Yeung CK, et al. The use of nonablative fractional resurfacing in Asian acne scar patients. Lasers Surg Med. 2010;42(10):710-5.
3. Doherty S, Seckel B, Ross EV. Advantages of a groove pattern of microfractional ablation for facial skin resurfacing. Lasers Surg Med. 2009;41:S21 (abstract 84).

4. Gold MH, Adelglass J. Evaluation of safety and efficacy of the TriFractional RF technology for treatment of facial wrinkles. J Cosmet Laser Ther. 2014;16(1):2-7.
5. Gold MH, Biron JA. Combined superficial and deep fractional skin treatment for photodamaged skin: a prospective clinical trial. J Cosmet Laser Ther. 2012;14(3):124-32.
6. Kohl E, Meierhöfer J, Koller M, et al. Fractional carbon dioxide laser resurfacing of rhytides and photoaging: a prospective study using profilometric analysis. Br J Dermatol. 2013;6(1):30-2.
7. Lapidoth M, YAGima Odo ME, Odo LM. Novel use of erbium:YAG (2,940–nm) laser for fractional ablative photo-thermolysis in the treatment of photodamaged facial skin: a pilot study. Dermatol Surg. 2008;34(8):1048-53.
8. Lapidoth M, Adatto M, Halachmi S. Treatment of actinic keratoses and photodamage with non-contact fractional 1540-nm laser quasiablation: an *ex vivo* and clinical evaluation. Lasers Med Sci. 2013;28(2):537-42.
9. Pardo A, Ciscar E, Alvarez-Suriaca GB. Microablative fractional CO_2 resurfacing: non-invasive objective *in vivo* assessment using reflectance confocal microscopy. Lasers Surg Med. 2009;41:S21 (abstract 70).
10. Rahman Z, MacFalls H, Jiang K, et al. Fractional deep dermal ablation induces tissue tightening. Lasers Surg Med. 2009;41(2):78-86.
11. Ross EV, Biesman B, Green R. Clinical and histological results with a novel 2.79 UM fractionated YSGG laser. Lasers Surg Med. 2009;41:S21 (abstract 100).
12. Weiss R, Weiss M, Beasley K. Prospective split-face trial of a fixed spacing array computed scanned fractional CO_2 laser versus hand scanned 1550 nm fractional for rhytides. Abstract presented at American Society for Laser Medicine and Surgery Conference. Kissimmee: Florida;2008.

RHYTIDES

To achieve satisfactory results with deep or dynamic rhytides, ablative lasers are usually necessary and ideally a combination of fillers and neurotoxins are used. A few basic principles are given below which are applicable to the use of fractional lasers in rhytides:
- Sessions should be given at 4-week intervals.
- About 4–6 treatments are required for results.
- Mean improvement seems to be higher in facial than in nonfacial skin.
- Perioral wrinkles are the most difficult to treat.

NONACNE SCARS

Post-traumatic and surgical scars can be treated by multiple methods and lasers should be used as an adjunct to standard therapies (*see* Chapter 12).

At a fundamental level, there is little justification of using fractional lasers in all cases, as the mode of action of these lasers does not lead to collagen reduction but increase in collagen. In case of hypertrophic scars, a combination with topical steroids may be a useful adjunct (Waibel JS). We feel that the use of *fractional lasers* should be largely restricted to *post-traumatic*

Table 4.11: Literature overview of fractional lasers in nonacne scars.

Author	Fractional lasers used	Indications	Results
Kim SG, 2012	2,940-nm erbium: yttrium-aluminum-garnet (Er: YAG)	Traumatic scars	Treat early within 4 weeks of scar
Choi JE, 2014	Er: YAg versus CO_2	Hypertrophic scars	Average percentage changes of VSS was 28.2% for Er:YAG and 49.8% for CO_2
Lee SH, 2013	CO_2	Surgical scars	Treat within the first 3 weeks
Weiss ET, 2010	CO_2	Atrophic postoperative and traumatic scarring	Image analysis revealed a 38.0% mean reduction of volume and 35.6% mean reduction of maximum scar depth

and surgical scars and *not keloids*. The studies published on this topic throw up some basic principles that are enshrined in Table 4.11.

- Treat scars early ideally within the first *3–4 weeks*. A combination therapy with topical agents may help to augment the results of the laser therapy.
- A *combination* of pulsed-dye laser (Hultman CS) and fractional CO_2 may prove to be a better option as the pulsed-dye laser can target pruritus and erythema, whereas the fractional CO_2 laser works on the *stiffness* and abnormal texture.
- *Ablative fractional lasers* are superior due to the greater penetration depths and the delivery of a more powerful remodeling stimulus.
- Among ablative fractional lasers, there is an advantage in using fractional CO_2 over Er:YAG.
- Objective improvement is modest (36%) (Weiss et al.).

Remember, energy devices for hypertrophic scarring impact primarily on scar pliability and thickness. *Low-density* and *high-energy* per treatment session is necessary to achieve the desirable outcome. Pulsed-dye laser (PDL) is superior to AFL for addressing the erythema component of scars, while quality switched (QS) or picosecond lasers can be used to improve the pigmentary component.

An overview of scar improvement in a case of post-traumatic scar is depicted in Figures 4.26A to D.

Conclusion

It has been proposed that the scar treatment paradigms should include extensive integration of fractional resurfacing and other combination therapies but the research and studies as yet cannot give any firm guidelines (Anderson RR).

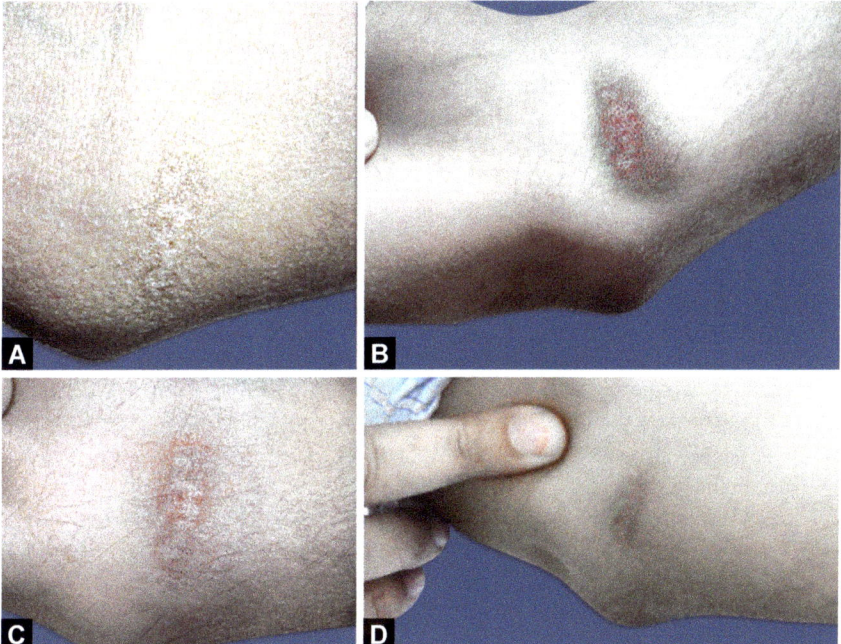

Figs. 4.26A to D: (A) Preoperative view of traumatic scar; (B) Immediately after Er: Glass, note the MENDs seen on the surface; (C) Appearance after 1 month, note the edema in the scar; (D) After 6 months marked improvement in the scar.

Some important aspects should guide the reader before using the fractional technology for scars. How many studies use an objective assessment of improvement? How many studies have compared lasers with established conventional methods of therapy like topical steroids, silicone dressing, and occlusion? And lastly with very few split lesion studies (Lee SH), it is likely that a certain degree of scar remodeling may ensue on its own and is credited to lasers!

Most importantly, no single laser can help in scars and in most hypertrophic scars a combination is required, a vascular-specific pulsed-dye laser (PDL) to reduce hyperemia, ablative fractional CO_2 laser to improve texture and pliability of the scar, and intense pulsed light (IPL) to correct scar dyschromia and alleviate chronic folliculitis (Hultman CS, 2012). Do not forget the topical or injectable cytostatic agents such as 5-fluorouracil and triamcinolone acetonide (Anderson RR).

If a single choice is needed, due to obvious cost, the motto is *hit early with ablative fractional laser* with IL steroids for hypertrophic scars *(see* **Chapter 12B***).*

BIBLIOGRAPHY

1. Anderson RR, Donelan MB, Hivnor C, et al. Laser treatment of traumatic scars with an emphasis on ablative fractional laser resurfacing: consensus report. JAMA Dermatol. 2014;150(2):187-93.
2. Choi JE, Oh GN, Kim JY, et al. Ablative fractional laser treatment for hypertrophic scars: comparison between Er:YAG and CO_2 fractional lasers. J Dermatol Treat. 2014;25(4):299-303.
3. Hultman CS, Edkins RE, Wu C, et al. Prospective, before-after cohort study to assess the efficacy of laser therapy on hypertrophic burn scars. Ann Plast Surg. 2013;70(5):521-6.
4. Hultman CS, Edkins RE, Lee CN, et al. Shine on: Review of laser- and light-based therapies for the treatment of burn scars. Dermatol Res Pract. 2012;2012:243651.
5. Kim SG, Kim EY, Kim YJ, et al. The efficacy and safety of ablative fractional resurfacing using a 2,940-nm Er:YAG laser for traumatic scars in the early post-traumatic period. Arch Plast Surg. 2012;39(3):232-7.
6. Lee SH, Zheng Z, Roh MR. Early postoperative treatment of surgical scars using a fractional carbon dioxide laser: a split-scar, evaluator-blinded study. Dermatol Surg. 2013;39(8):1190-6.
7. NS, Waibel JS. Laser treatment of traumatic scars with an emphasis on ablative fractional laser resurfacing: Consensus report. JAMA Dermatol. 2013;39(8):1190-6.
8. Waibel JS, Wulkan AJ, Shumaker PR. Treatment of hypertrophic scars using laser and laser-assisted corticosteroid delivery. Lasers Surg Med. 2013;45(3):135-40.
9. Weiss ET, Chapas A, Brightman L, et al. Successful treatment of atrophic postoperative and traumatic scarring with carbon dioxide ablative fractional resurfacing: quantitative volumetric scar improvement. Arch Dermatol. 2010;146(2):133-40.

ACTINIC KERATOSES

Apart from the 1,550 nm, the thulium laser has also been used for this condition. The concept of fractional 1,927-nm thulium laser is based largely on the superficial depth of penetration. Importantly though studies have shown a clinical improvement, histological persistence has also been noted, and as a result, it has been recommended that NAFR should not be used as a single treatment modality for actinic keratoses.

BIBLIOGRAPHY

1. Lapidoth M, Adatto M, Halachmi S. Treatment of actinic keratoses and photodamage with non-contact fractional 1540 nm laser quasi-ablation: an ex vivo and clinical evaluation. Lasers Med Sci. 2013;28(2):537-42.
2. Pearce DJ, Williford PM. Another approach to actinic keratosis management using nonablative fractional laser. J Dermatol Treat. 2014;25(4):298.
3. Weiss ET, Brauer JA, Anolik R, et al. 1927-nm fractional resurfacing of facial actinic keratoses: a promising new therapeutic option. J Am Acad Dermatol. 2013;68(1):98-102.

STRIAE

It must be understood that the treatment of striae depends on the stage of the disease and in the initial stage almost nothing would work. In the later stage also called striae alba when most therapies fail, lasers have been tried. This is the stage where a meaningful intervention will have therapeutic consequences.

In our experience even after multiple sessions of fractional CO_2 lasers, majority have a mild response.

The progressive evolution of striae and its natural course of resolution mean that studies on lasers in the condition should account for this natural course. Without comparing lasers with other topical agents, a firm conclusion of its efficacy cannot be concluded. But the collagen remodeling action of fractional laser is an elegant way of buttressing claims of its use. More importantly, we feel that a combination of PDL, excimer, and fractional lasers may help more than a single device alone.

Generally, striae rubra are more responsive to therapy and can be treated successfully with a variety of lasers without major adverse effects. Fractional lasers exhibit the strongest results for striae alba repigmentation and collagen induction, and several other lasers produce temporary repigmentation. Lasers in combination with other modalities such as topical agents and additional energy devices have also demonstrated promising preliminary results; however, large comparative studies are necessary to validate these outcomes. Most importantly, a control group is essential to understand what effect natural healing has on the results credited to the fractional lasers (*see* Chapter 12C).

BIBLIOGRAPHY

1. Alexiades-Armenaka M, Sarnoff D, Gotkin R, et al. Multicenter clinical study and review of fractional ablative CO_2 laser resurfacing for the treatment of rhytides, photoaging, scars and striae. J Drugs Dermatol. 2011;10(4):352-62.
2. Aldahan AS, Shah VV, Mlacker S, et al. Laser and light treatments for striae distensae: A comprehensive review of the literature. Am J Clin Dermatol. 2016;17(3):239-56.
3. De Angelis F, Kolesnikova L, Renato F, et al. Fractional nonablative 1540-nm laser treatment of striae distensae in Fitzpatrick skin types II to IV: clinical and histological results. Aesthet Surg J. 2011;31(4):411-9.
4. Gauglitz GG, Reinholz M, Kaudewitz P, et al. Treatment of striae distensae using an ablative Erbium: YAG fractional laser versus a 585 nm pulsed-dye laser. J Cosmet Laser Ther; 2013.
5. Yang YJ, Lee GY. Treatment of striae distensae with nonablative fractional laser versus ablative CO_2 fractional laser: A randomized controlled trial. Ann Dermatol. 2011;23(4):481-9.

MELASMA

Though this topic has been discussed extensively in the previous chapters, we will give a brief overview of the same here with a specific focus on fractional lasers.

Mechanism of Action

An elegant concept has been propounded for the action of fractional lasers, whereas the melanin present within the MEND helps to remove the pigment. In fact as the MEND sheds off, it *shuttles* out the pigment. Also, the optical clearance is believed to take place via melanophage rupture with consecutive dispersion of melanin within the dermal tissue. In addition, a relative decrease in melanocytes and a reduction in melanin within keratinocytes have also been reported.

But there are three important facts that explain the *lack of marked clinical results*:
1. The diameter of the MEND is in μm and even if a high density is employed the melanin that is removed is miniscule.
2. If melasma was a static condition, which it is not, there may have been sustained results, but being a dynamic disorder, the pigment production compensates for the loss in the MEND. This is more so in pigmented skin in tropical countries.
3. As discussed previously, only when combined with triple combination (TC) creams and peels do lasers have some results (Sardana K). In fact, a moot point is that where is the need to combine with other agents if lasers are so effective?

Lasers Used

Apart from fractional ablative and nonablative lasers, thulium and fractional Qsw ruby have also been used for melasma and have been discussed previously.

Results

Despite individual reports documenting successful treatment of melasma with NAFR, long-term efficacies of such treatments is still uncertain. The first pilot study by Rokhsar and Fitzpatrick demonstrated an astounding 75–100% clearance of melasma in 60% of the patients at 3 months. There are numerous cases of worsening of melasma and Wind et al., have shown that probably a TC cream would be a better option. Our own results have been largely disappointing (Figs. 4.27A and B).

A few facts are given here, which highlight the futility of lasers in melasma:
- Most results are temporary in nature and there is a risk for potential rebound worsening. Lee et al. treated 25 melasma patients with four

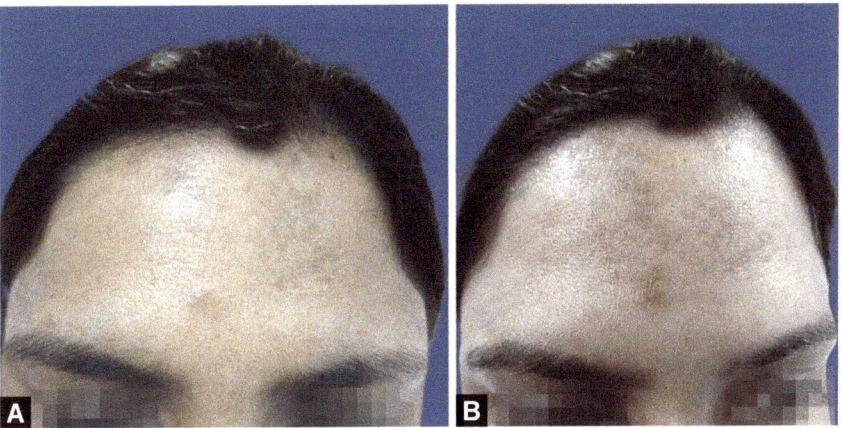

Figs. 4.27A and B: (A) A case of melasma treated with fractional Er:YAG (Dermabalte); (B) Minimal response, note the PIH that leads to an *aggravation* of the condition.

sessions of 1,550 nm NAFL (Fraxel SR, Solta Medical) at 15 mJ, 1,000 MTZ/cm^2, and eight passes at 4-week intervals and found that 24% had definite improvement at 1 month. However, by the 6-month follow-up, only 17% had definite improvement and 13% had worsened *(Lee HS)*.
- One study showing no difference between 1,550-nm NAFL (Fraxel Re:store, Solta Medical) and sunscreen for the treatment of melasma *(Karasi S)*.
- With the superficial depth of 1,927-nm thulium fiber NAFL (Fraxel Dual, Solta Medical), new hope arose but once again recurrence and rebound were observed.
- The risk of pregnancy-induced hypertension (PIH) with acute fatty liver (AFL) is generally too high to justify its use in pigmentary problems like melasma. A small split face trial in Thai patients explored whether pretreatment with AFL may allow a secondary pigment laser to penetrate deeper and reach dermal melanocytes. PIH developed in 50% (3/6) of cases on both sides, which persisted for 3 months (Angsuwarangsee S).

Conclusion

While initial nonablative fractional resurfacing (NAFR) reports showed promise in the treatment of melasma, it remains unclear how truly effective these lasers are in treating this chronic, stubborn condition, and whether lasers alter the natural history of the condition.

The most complimentary endorsement for fractional lasers comes from a study by Kroon et al. where they found that nonablative fractional laser therapy is safe and comparable in efficacy and recurrence rate with triple topical therapy. It may be a useful alternative treatment option for melasma when topical bleaching is ineffective or not tolerated. Different laser settings and long-term maintenance treatment should be tested in future studies.

Our own experience with fractional lasers (Er: Glass, CO_2 and Er: YAG) has not been as favorable and we do not find any justification in using this device for melasma. *If* this technology has to be used, always use a *low energy* and *high density*.

Pigmentary clearance is typically temporary with 1,550-nm erbium and 1,927-nm thulium devices with the potential even for rebound hyperpigmentation at 3–6 months following treatment. In light of these findings, fractional resurfacing with 1,927-nm thulium fiber may be considered *a last resort therapy* or an adjunct to a combination regimen involving topical skin lightening agents, light chemical peel, and strict sun protection. The use of that ablative fractional resurfacing is an absolute blunder in Indian skin as the PIH can be an issue.

BIBLIOGRAPHY

1. Kroon MW, Wind BS, Beek JF, et al. Nonablative 1550 nm fractional laser therapy versus triple topical therapy for the treatment of melasma: a randomized controlled pilot study. J Am Acad Dermatol. 2011;64(3):516-23.
2. Rokhsar CK, Fitzpatrick RE. The treatment of melasma with fractional photothermolysis: a pilot study. Dermatol Surg. 2005;31(12):1645-50.
3. Sardana K, Chugh S, Garg VK. Which therapy works for melasma in pigmented skin: lasers, peels, or triple combination creams? Indian J Dermatol Venereol Leprol. 2013;79(3):420-2.
4. Taub AF. Fractionated delivery systems for difficult to treat clinical applications: acne scarring, melasma, atrophic scarring, striae distensae, and deep rhytides. J Drugs Dermatol. 2007;6:1120-8.
5. Wind BS, Kroon MW, Meesters AA, et al. Nonablative 1,550 nm fractional laser therapy versus triple topical therapy for the treatment of melasma: a randomized controlled split-face study. Lasers Surg Med. 2010;42(7):607-12.

OTHER PIGMENTARY DISORDERS

There are reports of the use of fractional lasers in postinflammatory hyperpigmentation (Lee SJ, 2013), Beckers nevus (Ablative CO_2; Glaich AS and Meesters AA), nevus of Ota (Kouba DJ; 1440 nm), lichen amyloidosis (Anitha B, 2,940 nm), and even blue minocycline pigmentation, but till more reports or studies are published they cannot be recommended for use in these disorders.

The removal of *Becker's nevi (BN)* poses a significant challenge due to limited available therapeutic options and increased risk of adverse effects, including scarring and dyspigmentation. BN may be further classified as hypertrichotic or atrichotic, and this may help guide treatment selection. The latter is easier to treat. Though various pigment-specific lasers have been used, there are frequent recurrences. One major issue with Indian skin is that QS lasers, LPAL, normal-mode ruby laser (NMRL), and ablative lasers may further induce undesired scarring, and hypo- or hyperpigmentation.

Principle

Microscopic epidermal necrotic debrises (MENDs) comprised of melanin and degenerated epidermal and dermal components are an outcome of fractional laser therapy. MENDs ultimately facilitate the transepidermal elimination of epidermal and dermal melanin, the so-called *melanin shuttle*. A novel approach utilizes a combination nonablative FP and laser hair removal for the treatment of hypertrichotic Becker's nevus exploits the *melanin shuttle* phenomenon and further reduces the risk of follicular repigmentation. Furthermore, nonablative FP has a relatively excellent safety profile and is well tolerated in all skin types.

Protocol

First two sessions of laser hair removal with the 1,064-nm LP Nd: YAG (18 mm, 10 J/cm^2, 3-5 ms, 30/20 dynamic cooling) delivered at 8-week interval followed by nonablative fractional photothermolysis utilizing the 1,550-nm erbium-doped laser (15 mm, 9–40 mJ, 14–20%, cold-air cooling 5, 8 passes) for a total of eight sessions delivered at 4–8 week intervals.

Conclusion

The result in the recent study by Balaraman B was favorable but in the three cases none had a complete amelioration.

BIBLIOGRAPHY

1. Anitha B, Mysore V. Lichen amyloidosis: Novel treatment with fractional ablative 2,940 nm Erbium: YAG Laser Treatment. J Cutan Aesthet Surg. 2012;5(2):141-3.
2. Balaraman B, Friedman PM. Hypertrichotic Becker's nevi treated with combination 1,550 nm non-ablative fractional photothermolysis and laser hair removal. Lasers Surg Med. 2016;48(4):350-3.
3. Glaich AS, Goldberg LH, Dai T, et al. Fractional resurfacing: a new therapeutic modality for Becker's nevus. Arch Dermatol. 2007;143(12):1488-90.
4. Kouba DJ, Fincher EF, Moy RL. Nevus of Ota successfully treated by fractional photothermolysis using a fractionated 1440-nm Nd: YAG laser. Arch Dermatol. 2008;144(2):156-8.
5. Lee SJ, Chung WS, Lee JD, et al. A patient with cupping-related post-inflammatory hyperpigmentation successfully treated with a 1,927 nm thulium fiber fractional laser. J Cosmet Laser Ther; 2013.
6. Meesters AA, Wind BS, Kroon MW, et al. Ablative fractional laser therapy as treatment for Becker nevus: a randomized controlled pilot study. J Am Acad Dermatol. 2011;65(6):1173-9.
7. Trelles MA, Allones I, Moreno-Arias GA, et al. Becker's nevus: A comparative study between erbium: YAG and Q-switched neodymium: YAG; clinical and histopathological findings. Br J Dermatol. 2005;152(2):308-13.

POIKILODERMA OF CIVATTE

Poikiloderma of Civatte is characterized by hyper- and hypopigmentation, atrophy, and telangiectasia. As the clinical spectrum suggests, a single laser will rarely help and ideally a pulsed-dye lasers, intense pulse light, and KTP will have to be combined with a fractional nonablative devices in improving the overall color and texture in this condition.

BIBLIOGRAPHY

1. Behroozan DS, Goldberg LH, Glaich AS, et al. Fractional photothermolysis for treatment of Poikiloderma of Civatte. Dermatol Surg. 2006;32(2):298-301.
2. Tierney EP, Hanke CW. Treatment of Poikiloderma of Civatte with ablative fractional laser resurfacing: prospective study and review of the literature. J Drugs Dermatol. 2009;8(6):527-34.

VITILIGO

In difficult to treat vitiligo, various modalities have been tried including Er:YAG laser ablation followed by 5 fluorouracil application and NB-UVB phototherapy, combined dermabrasion with 5-fluorouracil, combined Er:YAG laser ablation plus topical steroids and NB-UVB phototherapy, combined microdermabrasion and pimecrolimus cream, and combined fractional ablative CO_2 laser and narrow-band ultraviolet B (NB-UVB).

A recent study compared the efficacy and safety of combined ablative fractional CO_2 laser, narrow-band ultraviolet B (NB-UVB) phototherapy, and topical 0.05% clobetasol propionate cream with combined NB-UVB phototherapy and topical 0.05% clobetasol propionate cream in difficult-to-treat areas in vitiligo. Here, it is obvious that it is not claimed to be a stand-alone modality for vitiligo!

Fractional Lasers and the Rationale there in?

Despite the promising effects of the preceding ablative treatments, the depth produced by laser resurfacing and dermabrasion can sometimes be difficult to control. Delayed healing and scarring is possible following these modalities, especially in areas with atrophic skin, for example, lesions previously treated with topical corticosteroids.

The randomized prospective study by Vachiramon et al. demonstrated that combined ablative fractional CO_2 laser, NB-UVB, and 0.05% clobetasol propionate give significantly higher mean improvement score than the combination of NB-UVB and 0.05% clobetasol propionate for the treatment of vitiligo in difficult-to-treat areas.

Here, it is important to use the correct settings. The laser-treated side was treated with fractional CO_2 laser 10,600 nm at a 1-week interval for

> **Box 4.1:** Protocol of using fractional laser for vitiligo.

Fractional CO_2 laser
(Once a week × 10 sessions)
NB-UVB phototherapy
(Twice a week × 20 sessions)
0.05% clobetasol propionate cream
(Twice a day × 22 weeks)

10 consecutive weeks. The treatment settings were as follows: a pulse energy of 100 mJ and a spot density of 150 spots cm^2 in the static mode; two passes were delivered using a 300-density tip. The laser was irradiated to the entire vitiliginous lesions, plus a 2-mm margin beyond the lesional border.

Immediately after the laser treatment, both hands were treated with NB-UVB using a phototherapy system (Box 4.1).

The maximal ablation depth was approximately 1,500 μm, while the epidermal thickness on the dorsum of extremities is approximately 70–140 μm. Also the ablation was deep enough to induce wound healing, secretion of cytokines and growth factors, and migration of melanocytes from adjacent normal skin and hair follicles. The effect of ultraviolet and topical medications was enhanced through the removal of superficial layer of the skin, allowing for their more potent stimulatory effects on the regeneration of new melanocytes. In addition, the extension of ablative laser treatment from the lesional border into the adjacent normal skin could probably trigger melanocyte migration from the normal skin to the lesion. This migration is important in creating repigmentation in areas with low hair density, for example, acral skin.

Conclusion and Literature Review

This is not the first study in this regard but a well-performed study nevertheless. Previous studies by Shin et al. have also shown that the combination of fractional CO_2 laser therapy at a 2-month interval combined with twice weekly whole-body NB-UVB phototherapy results in significantly higher improvement rate compared to the contralateral side, which did not receive fractional CO_2 laser treatment. A more practical study in Indian settings was done by Helou et al. who found that 3-monthly session of fractional CO_2 laser treatment followed by 2 hours sunlight exposure on daily basis results in improvement in vitiligo. Another study reported by Li et al. also confirms the superior result of triple combination of fractional CO_2 laser, NB-UVB, and topical steroids. These findings prove the benefit of adding fractional CO_2 laser in the treatment of vitiligo, particularly in cases not responsive to other treatments.

Issues with Fractional Lasers

- The problem is that the difficult sites like the palms, soles, acral areas, and lips still defy treatment and that remains the problem with most work on vitiligo, which either looks are cytokines or well-treaded path of treating hairy areas, which respond very well to conventional photochemotherapy (PUVA)-Sol!
- Autologous noncultured cell suspension transplantation is an effective treatment for repigmentation in segmental vitiligo and piebaldism. Full surface laser ablation is frequently used to prepare the recipient site before cell suspension transplantation, even though the optimal laser settings and ablation depth are unknown. A study by Lommerts JE, found that superficial full surface ablation with a depth of 144 μm is an effective recipient-site preparation before cell suspension transplantation, while fractional CO_2 laser is not.
- El-Zawahry MB in a study in nonsegmental vitiligo, combining fractional CO_2 laser with NB-UVB for the treatment of nonsegmental vitiligo did not show any significant advantage over treatment with NB-UVB alone.

Hence, fractional lasers might be a decent **add-on** therapy but may not be a trend setter in vitiligo therapy. A thesis done using fractional Er:YAG by us did not mirror the salutary effects of previous studies, but we did not used phototherapy but melanocyte suspensions in combination with Er: YAG ablation, which like the Lommert's study, were not found to be useful.

BIBLIOGRAPHY

1. El-Zawahry MB, Zaki NS, Wissa MY, et al. Effect of combination of fractional CO_2 laser and narrow-band ultraviolet B versus narrow-band ultraviolet B in the treatment of non-segmental vitiligo. Lasers Med Sci. 2017;32(9):1953-8.
2. Helou J, Maatouk I, Obeid G, et al. Fractional laser for vitiligo treated by 10,600 nm ablative fractional carbon dioxide laser followed by sun exposure. Lasers Surg Med. 2014;46(6):443-8.
3. Li L, Wu Y, Li L, et al. Triple combination treatment with fractional CO_2 laser plus topical betamethasone solution and narrowband ultraviolet B for refractory vitiligo: A prospective, randomized half-body, comparative study. Dermatol Ther. 2015;28(3):131-4.
4. Lommerts JE, Meesters AA, Komen L, et al. Autologous cell suspension grafting in segmental vitiligo and piebaldism: a randomized controlled trial comparing full surface and fractional CO_2 laser recipient-site preparations. Br J Dermatol. 2017;177(5):1293-8.
5. Shin J, Lee JS, Hann SK, et al. Combination treatment by 10,600 nm ablative fractional carbon dioxide laser and narrowband ultraviolet B in refractory nonsegmental vitiligo: A prospective, randomized half-body comparative study. Br J Dermatol. 2012;166(3):658-61.
6. Vachiramon V, Chaiyabutr C, Rattanaumpawan P, et al. Effects of a preceding fractional carbon dioxide laser on the outcome of combined local narrowband

ultraviolet B and topical steroids in patients with vitiligo in difficult-to-treat areas. Lasers Surg Med. 2016;48(2):197-202.
7. Yan R, Yuan J, Chen H, et al. Fractional Er: YAG laser assisting topical betamethasone solution in combination with NB-UVB for resistant nonsegmental vitiligo. Lasers Med Sci. 2017;32(7):1571-7.

SKIN TIGHTENING

It is obvious that ablative fractional laser treatment does not compare with face lift, as AFR does not reduce skin laxity as much as a face lift. Histological studies of human skin after ablative fractional CO_2 laser treatment show that the deep, laser-induced ablation channels remain open, then subsequently fill in with new epidermal and dermal tissue in approximately the same size and shape of the channels. The filling-in of ablative fractional laser channels appears to account for the relatively *less* skin tightening observed clinically after ablative fractional laser treatment. The residual thermal damage layer surrounding each hole after ablative fractional laser treatment consists of thermally denatured, desiccated dermal tissue. Dermal collagen shrinks upon thermal denaturation, which is thought to somewhat tighten the dermis. However, clinically, it is apparent that skin tightening is *minimal* after treatment with fractional ablative laser devices.

This is as the cuff of desiccated tissue that surrounds the opening of each laser-induced hole prevents spontaneous hole closure. In addition, there are rapidly forming fibrin plugs, which fill up the laser holes.

A recent study showed that immediately following laser exposure, the resulting holes can be closed using a stretched elastic adhesive dressing, which, when applied, recoiled and compressed the diameter of the ablation hole. This lead to significant skin tightening by immediate temporary noninvasive wound closure.

What are the implications?

The first and most obvious is a fact not admitted or not realized by most dermatologists is that the skin tightening effect of fractional lasers does not match surgical procedures and thus it is no use promising the patients. Secondly, a commentary by Christopher Zachary has summarized the often hidden fact that *it was one of the great disappointments of the fractionated ablative laser that 50% vaporization did not result in 50% tightening.* The body is just too good at repairing itself. Thus, it is obvious that the natural healing process cannot be subverted by external means.

The cylinders of vaporized tissue have a *sponge cuff* of coagulated tissue, which tends to hold them open until they are filled with coagulum and other healing elements. This will inherently lead to less tightening. Hence, AFL should not be used as a primary tightening procedure.

BIBLIOGRAPHY

1. De Bruler DM, Blackstone BN, Baumann ME, et al. Inflammatory responses, matrix remodeling, and reepithelialization after fractional CO_2 laser treatment of scars. Lasers Surg Med. 2017;49(7):675-85.
2. Russe E, Purschke M, Limpiangkanan W, et al. Significant skin-tightening by closure of fractional ablative laser holes. Lasers Surg Med; 2017.
3. Zachary C. Commentary on significant skin tightening by closure of fractional ablative laser holes. Lasers Surg Med; 2017.

MISCELLANEOUS CONDITIONS

Nonablative fractional resurfacing (NAFR) has also been used to treat a host of other conditions including matted telangiectasias, residual fibrofatty tissue after hemangioma involution, recalcitrant disseminated superficial actinic porokeratosis, disseminated granuloma annulare, colloid milium, pearly penile papules, postinflammatory hypopigmentation, alopecia areata, and pattern alopecia. This list will certainly grow but we feel that the most useful indications at present are acne scars and photodamaged skin.

BIBLIOGRAPHY

1. Cho S, Choi MJ, Zheng Z, et al. Clinical effects of non-ablative and ablative fractional lasers on various hair disorders: a case series of 17 patients. J Cosmet Laser Ther. 2013;15(2):74-9.
2. Glaich AS, Goldberg LH, Dai T, et al. Fractional photothermolysis for the treatment of telangiectatic matting: a case report. J Cosmet Laser Ther. 2007;9(2):101-3.
3. Glaich AS, Goldberg LH, Friedman RH, et al. Fractional photothermolysis for the treatment of postinflammatory erythema resulting from acne vulgaris. Dermatol Surg. 2007;33:842-6.
4. Lee GY, Lee SJ, Kim WS. The effect of a 1550 nm fractional erbium-glass laser in female pattern hair loss. J Eur Acad Dermatol Venereol. 2011;25(12):1450-4
5. Yoo KH, Kim MN, Kim BJ, et al. Treatment of alopecia areata with fractional photothermolysis laser. Int J Dermatol. 2010;49(7):845-7.

FUTURE OF FRACTIONAL LASERS

Using lasers can be an effective drug permeation enhancement approach for facilitating drug delivery into or across the skin. This is known as **Fractional Drug Delivery**. The controlled disruption and ablation of the stratum corneum, the predominant barrier for drug delivery are achieved by the use of lasers. The possible mechanisms of laser-assisted drug permeation are the direct ablation of the skin barrier, optical breakdown by a photomechanical wave, and a photothermal effect.

It has been demonstrated that ablative approaches for enhancing drug transport provide some advantages including increased bioavailability, fast treatment time, quick recovery of stratum corneum (SC) integrity, and the fact that skin surface contact is not needed.

The laser can be used in enhancing the permeation of a wide variety of permeants, such as small-molecule drugs, macromolecules and nanoparticles. This method has been tried in Non-Melanoma Skin Cancer (NMSC) IB; photodamage scars, for topical anesthetics and onychomycosis. Ablative frcational lasers are ideal and the highest uptake potential was within the first 30 minutes after AFL and then dissipates gradually over the next 6 hours and just after 24–48 hours it stops. Deeper the channel better the response.

This potential use of the laser affords a new treatment for topical/transdermal application with significant efficacy.

STEP-BY-STEP APPROACH

PRINCIPLES

The fundamental principles of FP that guide the selection of treatment parameters are relatively simple and can be summarized by three basic rules:
- The dimensions of individual MTZs should not exceed certain dimensions, such that the induced wound-healing results in tissue repair rather than inducing fibrosis.
- The overall density of MTZs should not be excessively high to maintain sufficient undamaged tissue between the MTZs and facilitate tissue repair.
- The cumulative density of MTZs should be sufficiently high to induce sufficient clinical improvement after a completed course of FP treatments.

PATIENT SELECTION

The preoperative consultation is crucial to maximize outcomes while minimizing complications. The clinician should assess the patient expectations and goals for treatment during this encounter, individuals with unrealistic expectations should not be treated. Showing patients before and after photos of a typical result can help to set the patient expectations regarding the efficacy of treatment. Even so, the patient must also understand that individual responses can vary.
- To achieve satisfactory results about four to six treatments is required that are spaced at 4–6-week interval and thus require 6 months or more to complete.
- Importantly in acne scars, deep ice pick and boxcar scars do not respond as well as rolling and superficial boxcar scars.

- Rule out history of keloids, herpes simplex infection, postinflammatory hyperpigmentation (PIH), current medications, lidocaine allergy, pain tolerance, and anxiety level.

Women who are pregnant or lactating, those with active infection, particularly herpes simplex, and patients with a history of isotretinoin use in the past 6 months. The last recommendation is debatable as there is evidence of dermabrasion being undertaken, while on isotretinoin and even within 3 months of stopping the therapy (Picosse et al., Bagatin et al.).

PREOPERATIVE STEPS

- *Sunscreens:* It is advisable to use a broad-spectrum sunscreen (SPF > 30) and to avoid sun exposure before, during and immediately after their treatments. There is *no evidence* that treating with topical hydroquinone for 1–2 months prior to nonablative fractional resurfacing decreases the risk of postinflammatory pigmentation in individuals with darker skin types (type IV–VI). There is no scientific evidence that topical retinoids need to be discontinued prior to treatment in those with sensitive skin.

  We though prefer using topical retinoids in cases of acne scarring and a non-HQ/Steroid based, depigmenting cream in our patients (Melaglow™/Clearz Plus™).
- Antiviral prophylaxis should be given only if there is history of herpes labialis.
- *Anesthesia:* There are two options—either using prilocaine-based creams or tetracaine based creams. Anesthetic agents with tetracaine induce significant erythema leading to patient dissatisfaction. Thus, another option is to use 30% lidocaine.
- *Baseline photograph:* In case topical anesthesia is used, it must be noted that some patients have a *blanched appearance* thus making photographic evaluation difficult. Thus, a photograph should be taken before applying the anesthesia.

INTRAOPERATIVE STEPS

Safety

- For any laser skin resurfacing procedure, the treatment room should have the appropriate eye protection for all persons present.
- A smoke evacuator should be used to remove aerosolized debris and surgical masks are also essential for operating personnel.
- External eye shields are sufficient for patient protection during most nonablative procedures and the skin can be retracted and treated over the bony orbital rim.
- Any laser or light procedure that involves treatment within the orbital rim requires placement of ocular metal shields.

Procedure

Always test spot an area or two with two different dose settings and evaluate after 3–4 weeks. This helps the patient to gain confidence, tells about PIH, and also gives realistic expectations.

- Ensure that the laser handpiece is applied perpendicular to the skin.
- *Scanning handpiece:* While using the Fraxel systems (Solta Medical, Hayward, CA) the protocol is eight passes when treating acne scars, rhytides, and photoaging of the face. A double-pass, 50% overlap technique is used.

  One linear pass is delivered, the handpiece is brought to a complete stop, lifted, repositioned, and then returned along the same path for a second pass. The handpiece is then moved laterally by 50% and the technique is repeated until the treatment area is completed. As a result, each area is treated with four passes. For the next four passes, the passes are given perpendicular to the first treatment to ensure complete and even laser coverage.
- *Stamping handpiece:* For stamping handpieces, the fractionated energy is delivered according to the tip size. The Lux system (Palomar Medical Technologies Inc. Burlington, MA) and the Acepelion Er: YAG is example. Here, three to four passes are generally delivered with a 50% overlap in both directions. The handpiece should be lifted off the skin between each pulse, and pulse-stacking is not recommended. The number of passes and treatment parameters vary with the different machines and is discussed in the chapter of fractional lasers.
- For rhytides, stretch the skin so that the cutaneous base is treated evenly.
- Periorbital skin is treated with decreased fluences while using a moistened gauze piece to protect the lashes and brows.
- The perioral area should be treated while covering the teeth with moist gauze to protect from laser-induced etching of dental enamel.
- The transition of the mandible to the neck should be feathered with lower fluence and/or fewer passes to prevent a sharp demarcation line between treated and untreated skin.

POSTOPERATIVE CARE

- Erythema develops immediately afterward in all treated patients and typically resolves in 3 days.
- Use of noncomedogenic moisturizers is recommended (Sebamed clear gel, Cetaphil cream).
- Icing regularly and maintaining head elevation helps to minimize edema, but in the case of severe edema, particularly when periorbital swelling is significant enough to impair vision, a 3–5 days course of systemic corticosteroids should be prescribed.
- After the first few days when re-epithelialization is complete, the transition from ointment to a cream-based moisturizer is possible.

- Patients are advised to wear sun protection for several weeks after their treatment to reduce the risk of hyperpigmentation. A useful option is to use a depigmenting cream with a sunscreen.
- In Indian skin, it is advisable to start a lightening cream after 7 days, though others wait till 21 days by which time PIH appears. A nonsteroidal nonhydroquinone (HQ)-based cream is preferred (Melaglow™, Clearz Plus™).

PITFALLS/PEARLS

- The response to most fractional lasers is *curvilinear and delayed*. This is for the simple reason that scars remodeling takes *6–9 months*. Thus, giving eight sittings give better results.

    The first two treatments yield very little visible improvement, the next two a bit more, and the final two show the greatest degree of change. Sometimes in patients with bad scarring an additional two treatments help but it is advisable better to wait for 6 months to see the maximum improvement from the first six before deciding.

    This has another important implication and that is unnecessary procedures like chemical reconstruction of skin scars (CROSS), subcision, dermaroller, and ascribing improvement to them can wait for at least 6 months after laser therapy! This is as they are credited with the improvement, which the laser would have induced, if enough time had elapsed postsurgery.

    A simple *protocol* is—fractional laser (6–8 sessions) followed by 6 months of follow-up, which should be followed by surgical procedures. Thus, an average of 1 *year* may be required for an acne scar patient.
- Patients with significant photodamage, sagging, and deep rhytides are *not* a primary candidate for fractional lasers, as this requires other techniques like fillers and botox, the combination of which with lasers is strictly *off label*.
- To minimize the risk of systemic toxicity from the topical anesthetics, areas no greater than 300–400 cm^2 should be treated during each session. In case, the patient complains of agitation, anxiety, nausea, and perioral paresthesias, it indicates toxicity. An infusion of normal saline is helpful. To avoid this problem, topical anesthesia application should be limited to no more than 1 hour.
- In general, in Indian skin postinflammatory pigmentation is less common using *lower density settings, fewer passes, and longer treatment intervals*.

    A set of commonly used settings for a prototype fractional laser is depicted in Figures 4.28A and B.
- Decrease the MTZ areal density, if higher energies are applied per MTZ to keep the areal fraction of damaged skin surface constant.

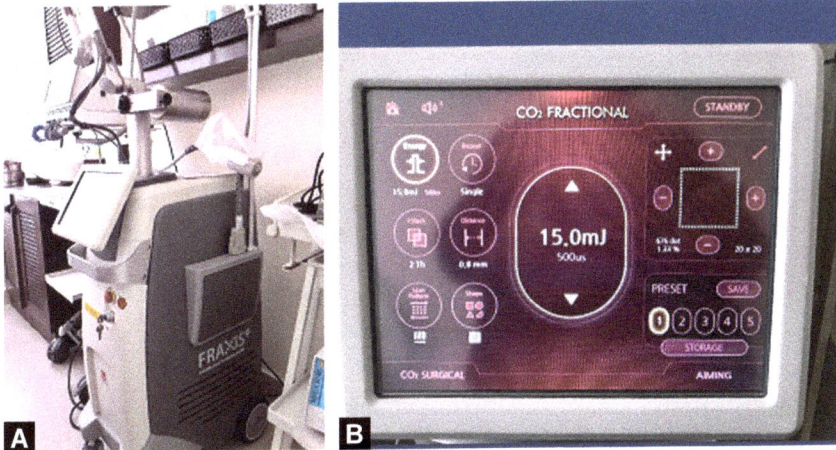

Figs. 4.28A and B: (A) Fraxis Duo fractional CO_2; (B) Acne scarring 'Th' = pulse stacking 18–21 mJ for fair skin, density can be reduced to 0.6 mm for traumatic scars.
Courtesy: Dr Vivek Nair, New Delhi.

There is little difference between the various fractional lasers as long as you have the histological depth data of the lasers and know the art of manipulating the dosimetry. Remember that conference talks represent what a speaker has used and when a technology is new everyone gloats over it. I still remember the times when fractional Er: Glass was the flavor of the year and showed *great results* in conference talks within 6 months of their launch dates! Even after the whole axis of fractional lasers has come and we have progressed to fractional RF, some scars just do not respond. Ice pick scars among them. So at the end of the day, choose your lasers with care and do not promise the sky or hope for miracles!

BIBLIOGRAPHY

1. Bagatin E, dos Santos Guadanhim LR, Yarak S, et al. Dermabrasion for acne scars during treatment with oral isotretinoin. Dermatol Surg. 2010;36(4):483-9.
2. Picosse FR, Yarak S, Cabral NC, et al. Early chemabrasion for acne scars after treatment with oral isotretinoin. Dermatol Surg. 2012;38(9):1521-6.

CHAPTER 5

Vascular Lasers

Tanvi Pal, Sujay Khandpur, Kabir Sardana

BACKGROUND

Cutaneous vascular lesions, especially those occurring on the face, produce devastating cosmetic impact and psychological distress, besides being associated with pain, bleeding, ulceration, infection, and obstruction of vital functions. This necessitates prompt treatment with good cosmetic results. Earlier, vascular lesions were treated with radiation, cryotherapy, excision and grafting, and camouflage, with unsatisfactory results and poor aesthetic outcomes. The introduction of lasers, with the immense convenience of being used in an outpatient setting, has allowed for easier patient access with more reliable and cosmetically pleasing results.

Laser treatment for cutaneous vascular lesions was initiated by Dr Leon Goldman in 1963 at the Children's Hospital Research Foundation in Cincinnati, Ohio, with the treatment of port-wine stains (PWS) and cavernous hemangiomas using ruby, neodymium: yttrium-aluminum-garnet (Nd:YAG), and argon lasers.

The treatment of vascular lesions is one of the most commonly requested cutaneous laser procedures. Since the introduction of the argon laser, a variety of laser and light sources are being used for the treatment of vascular lesions. These include visible and infrared lasers, as well as broadband light sources.

THEORY OF SELECTIVE PHOTOTHERMOLYSIS

The theory of selective photothermolysis was developed by Anderson and Parish (Anderson RR et al.). They proposed that, to limit thermal damage to the intended target, the *pulse duration* of laser must be shorter than the thermal relaxation time of the target tissue. The thermal relaxation time of tissue is defined as the time taken by target tissue to transfer its 50% heat to the surrounding tissue through thermal diffusion. The thermal relaxation time of vessels with diameter of 10–50 μm is 0.048–1.2 ms (Anderson RR et al.). Typical natural chromophores in skin include water, melanin, hemoglobin, protein, lipid, etc. Artificial chromophores that can be used include dyes, ink, carbon particles, etc. In vascular lesions, the targeted structure is oxyhemoglobin within blood vessels. When hemoglobin is heated, it also heats up and destroys the endothelial cells of blood vessel walls.

The success of selective photothermolysis depends on **three major factors:** (1) wavelength of the light source; (2) duration of light pulse; and (3) amount of energy (fluence) delivered. The importance of knowing the above three factors is that it explains, the complexity of vascular treatment and also explains why it is so difficult to achieve consistent and good results. Remember that the laser physics is based on the skin being an optical window and in Indian skin that is never the case.

Wavelength

Wavelength is selected to target oxyhemoglobin. Oxyhemoglobin strongly absorbs light between 400 nm and 600 nm, and has absorption peaks at 418 nm, 542 nm, and 577 nm. Therefore, lasers with wavelengths between 488 nm and 600 nm are useful for the treatment of vascular lesions.

To achieve desirable photothermolysis, the wavelength of the light source must be able to *penetrate* adequately into the skin (to reach the target structure) and be *absorbed* preferentially by the target chromophore. Optic penetration varies with wavelengths: light with shorter wavelengths (300–400 nm) is largely scattered by dermal collagens and is only able to penetrate less than 0.1 mm into the skin. In contrast, longer wavelengths (600–1200 nm) penetrate deeper, with less scattering.

The major target chromophores in skin are hemoglobin, melanin, and water. The absorption spectra of important skin chromophores are shown in Figure 5.1. Hemoglobin has a few absorption peaks, whereas melanin has a broad spectrum of absorption, which gradually diminishes with longer wavelengths. Water absorption dominates in the far-infrared range while protein absorption dominates in the far-ultraviolet range. Such properties render wavelengths in the visible light spectrum the choice for vascular lasers.

Principle: To target a vascular lesion, the ideal wavelength chosen must be well-absorbed by oxyhemoglobin and poorly absorbed by epidermal melanin.

Oxyhemoglobin has major absorption peaks at *418 nm, 542 nm, and 577 nm,* corresponding to *blue, green, and yellow* wavelengths, respectively (Fig. 5.1). Melanin normally presents in the epidermis and hair follicles, and absorbs broadly across the visible light spectrum. Despite strong absorption by blood in the blue band (418 nm), wavelengths in this region are less desirable because of limited penetration and interference by high melanin absorption. The yellow band (*577 nm*) of oxyhemoglobin

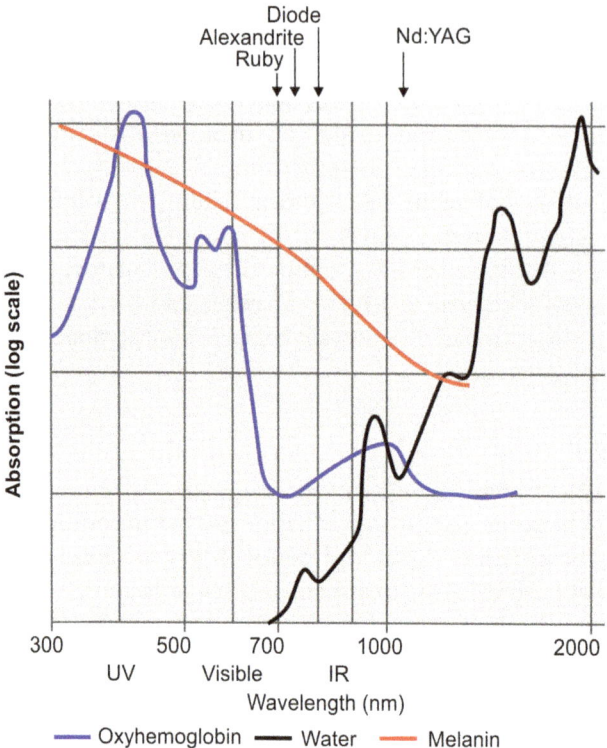

Fig. 5.1: Absorption spectra for the three major chromophores: hemoglobin, melanin, and water.

absorption was chosen initially for targeting superficial vessels using the flashlamp-pumped pulsed-dye laser. The wavelength of this laser was subsequently increased to *585 nm* and later *595 nm*, to provide deeper penetration. Pulsed potassium titanyl phosphate (KTP) lasers emit at 532 nm (green light spectrum). Green light is absorbed by hemoglobin nearly as well as yellow light, and has roughly the equivalent optic penetration through fair skin.

There is also a broad oxyhemoglobin band at around 900 nm, which features advantages of preferential hemoglobin absorption, minimal interference from melanin absorption, and good optic penetration. Lasers in this near-infrared region have been applied to treat cutaneous vascular lesions. They include the alexandrite (755 nm), diode (800 nm), and Nd:YAG (1,064 nm) lasers.

Intense-pulsed light (IPL) sources use high-intensity pulsed flashlamps. The broad emission spectrum provides selective absorption by hemoglobin and deep penetration for large, deep-seated vessels.

Why do We Use 585/595 nm?

While 585-nm absorbs light about one-half as efficiently as it absorbs 577-nm light, 585-nm light will coagulate *larger* vessels better than 577-nm light at a given depth because of *deeper penetration* of laser energy. In addition, deeper vessels absorb laser energy at longer wavelengths. The 595 nm would be better than 585 nm by the same logic.

The tissue depth to which a given fluence will coagulate the target vessel depends largely on the blood volume of vessels above the target vessels. Superficial vessels containing blood will absorb laser light before it reaches deeper target vessels. This explains why *multiple* treatments are necessary for complete PWS resolution.

Why not 532 nm ?

Because blood also has an absorption peak at 532 nm, the frequency doubled Nd:YAG laser is also effective in treating superficial vascular lesions. However, to obtain a degree of selectivity over the high melanin absorption at 532 nm and to penetrate to clinically useful depths, cooling the overlying epidermis is important.

Optical Penetration

Fluence

Energy of electromagnetic radiation is measured in units of joules (J). The amount of energy delivered per unit area is the fluence, which is measured in J/cm^2. Power is the rate at which light energy is delivered and is measured in watts (W). By definition, 1 Watt is 1 Joule per second (W = J/s).

- High fluences are used when less target chromophore is present either due to sparse blood vessels or faintly colored vessels.
- Lower fluences are used when more target chromophore is present either due to dense blood vessels or intensely colored vessels.

In practice, sufficient fluence must be supplied such that the light beam is able to reach (adequate optic penetration) and produce irreversible damage to the target.

Spot Size

In addition to wavelength, optical penetration is also determined by spot size. With smaller spots, a greater fraction of photons scatter outside the beam and may render the treatment ineffective. Larger spots allow more photons to remain within the diameter of incident beam and hence offer greater optic penetration. Lower treatment fluence is required with larger spots when compared to smaller ones. For instance, 7- and 10-mm spots require only one-half to two-thirds of the fluences required for a 5-mm spot with the 585-nm pulsed-dye laser.

Pulse Width

To limit thermal damage to the intended target, the pulse duration must be shorter than the thermal relaxation time of the target tissue. The thermal relaxation time of tissue is defined as the time necessary for target tissue to cool down by 50% through transfer of its heat to surrounding tissue through thermal diffusion (Tables 5.1 and 5.2). If a targeted tissue can be heated sufficiently to affect it irreversibly before its surrounding tissue is damaged by thermal diffusion, selective photocoagulation occurs.

- Pulse width selection is based on vessel size and depth, and erythema intensity.
- *Short pulse widths* are used to treat small, superficial red vessels that are faintly colored.
- *Longer pulse widths* are used to treat large, deep vessels that are intensely colored.
- In addition, the deeper cutaneous penetration of long pulse widths makes them safer on the epidermis and preferable on darker skin types (IV–VI).

For vascular lesions, the exposure time should be long enough to conduct heat from the red blood cell (RBC)-filled lumen to the entire blood vessel wall. The thermal relaxation time of vessels 10–50 µm in diameter is 0.1–10 ms, averaging 1.2 ms. However, pulse durations less than 20 ms result in vessel rupture and hemorrhage secondary to RBC explosion. This will lead to hemosiderin pigmentation. Therefore, with single laser pulses, the therapeutic window is small. This argues for the development of a *wider single pulse* or a *multipulsed laser* that is able to transfer absorbed heat to the endothelium without causing its rupture.

Hence, the logic for the settings employed, wherein the pulse duration of the PDL has increased from *0.45 ms to over 1.5 ms* which limits purpura

Table 5.1: Approximate thermal relaxation time (Tr) for vessels of different diameters.

Diameter (µm)	Tr (ms)
10	0.048
20	0.19
50	1.2
100	4.8
200	19.0
300	42.6

Table 5.2: Thermal relaxation time (Tr) of laser targets.

Target	Diameter (µm, approx)	Tr
Epidermis	60	2 ms
Basal layer	20	400 µs
Melanosome	1	0.2 µs
Erythrocyte	5	5 µs

without decreasing efficacy. The immediate purpuric threshold increases from 6.2 to 8, 10.4, and 13.8 J/cm^2 with an increase in the pulse duration from 0.5 to 2.0, 20 and 40 ms.

In 1995, Dierickx and colleagues performed a landmark in-vivo study, which demonstrated that the thermal relaxation time for PWS vessels (approximately 60 μm in diameter) was between 1 ms and 10 ms for a 585-nm PDL. Since the 1990s, newer generation PDL systems with longer pulse durations greater than *1 ms* have been developed. They offer the additional advantage of reduced incidence of prolonged, unsightly purpuras.

Longer pulse durations minimize photomechanical injury and hence reduce post-treatment purpura. Pulse durations greater than 1 ms produce gentle vaporization of blood rather than explosive vessel rupture. Controlled evacuation of blood produces an empty, thermally coagulated blood vessel. Lengthening the pulse duration of PDL to 1.5 ms further reduces the intensity and duration of purpura significantly. Kauvar and associates demonstrated that in treating adult PWS, a *595-nm, 1.5-ms PDL* resulted in reduced purpura when compared with the 585-nm, 450-μs system.

Moreover, lengthening the pulse duration also minimizes epidermal damage, as melanosomes are less effectively heated with longer pulses. They cool significantly during laser pulse delivery due to small size.

Spot Size

Larger spot sizes have deeper penetration of laser energy compared to smaller spot sizes. Larger spot sizes are used to treat larger blood vessels and smaller spot sizes to treat smaller vessels heated with longer pulses. They cool significantly during laser pulse delivery due to small size.

Skin Cooling

Although higher fluence produces more thermal injury, it can also lead to more adverse events. Absorption by epidermal melanin and heat transfer from dermal targets can result in serious epidermal injury. Ideally, the epidermis should remain unaffected during light treatments. Effective skin cooling methods were developed over the past decade to minimize tissue injury by extracting heat from the epidermis.

Skin cooling can be achieved before, during, and after successful laser pulse impacts. Skin cooling, before and after laser exposure, with ice can reduce pain and swelling, which in turn enhances patient tolerability. Cooling the skin during laser treatment (dynamic skin cooling) effectively decreases epidermal heating by the laser pulses (Fig. 5.2). The various measures include, by application of a cold gel, a liquid medium, or a liquid cryogen spray during treatments.

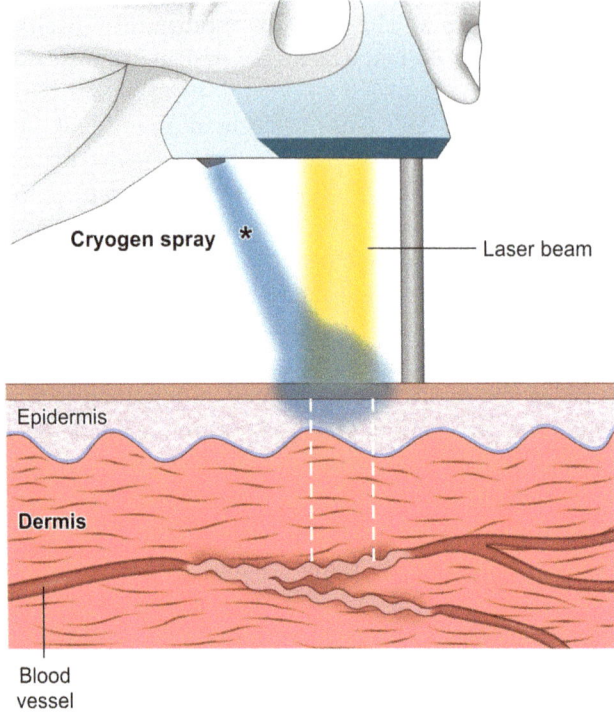

Fig. 5.2: The Dynamic Cooling Device (DCD; Candela Laser Corp) provides a brief spurt of cryogen that selectively cools the epidermis during Vbeam laser application.

LASERS COMMONLY USED TO TREAT VASCULAR LESIONS

Flashlamp-pumped Pulsed Dye Lasers

Flashlamp-pumped pulsed dye lasers (PDL) were first successfully used by Tan et al. in 1989 for PWSs. PDL was the first laser developed based on the principle of selective photothermolysis. Three manufacturers produce this type of laser. Candela Corporation (Wayland, MA) manufactures the SPTL line of machines, which originally emitted a wavelength of 585 nm and now can emit wavelengths of 590 nm, 595 nm, and 600 nm. The flashlamp-pumped PDL has as its active medium an organic dye energized by a short pulse of light from a flashlamp. PDL emits a pulsed beam of yellow light at 585–600 nm powered by flash lamp. *The dye's chemical structure, solvent and additives used, dictate the operating lifetime, which is limited (around 6 months); due to decomposition of the above, when exposed to heat and intense light.* This is a very important factor that makes the operation of the machine a drain coupled with the fact that multiple sessions are required with inconsistent results.

The PDL *beam profiles* may be different between laser companies. With the Candela PDL a 10-20% overlapping spot provides for an even distribution of energy fluence. This is because of the Gaussian distribution of beam output. An 18% overlap has been found to cover the largest surface area with the least overlap. In contrast, the Cynosure PDL has a "top hat" distribution of energy fluence (Figs. 5.3 and 5.4). In addition, when the 5-mm diameter spot size of

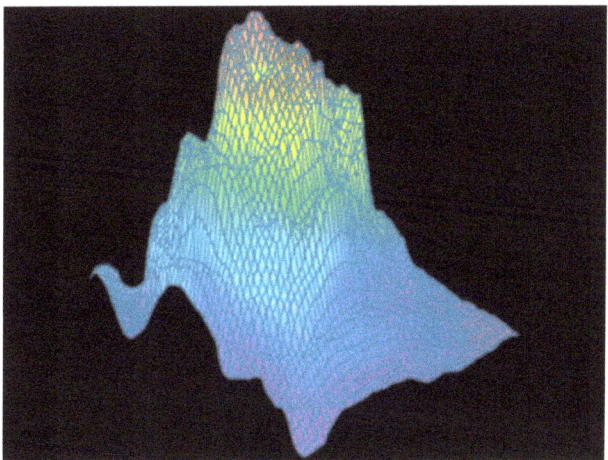

Fig. 5.3: Beam profile of Candela SPTL-1 from laser head. It exhibits Gaussian-like distribution of energy with some irregularities.
Source: Jackson BA, Arndt KA, Dover JS. Journal of the American Academy of Dermatology. 1996;34(6):1000-4, with permission from the American Academy of Dermatology.

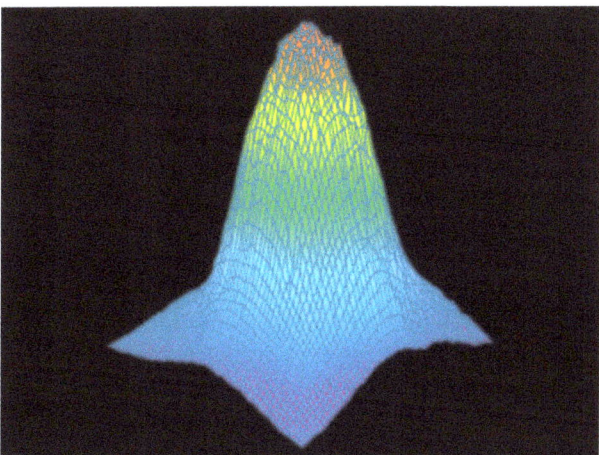

Fig. 5.4: Cynosure PhotoGeniaca V laser from laser head. Like the Candela SPTL-1 (see Fig. 5.3), it exhibits Gaussian energy distribution with irregularities.
Source: Jackson BA, Arndt KA, Dover JS. Journal of the American Academy of Dermatology. 1996;34:1000-4, with permission from the American Academy of Dermatology.

the two lasers were tested, the Candela laser spot size was up to 35% larger than 5 mm while the Cynosure laser was up to 8% smaller.

Therefore, it is prudent to check the diameter of the spot with burn paper before switching from one PDL machine to another.

Majority of the PDLs have an integrated cooling system, and with maximal achievable energy fluence of 20 J/cm^2 which targets oxidized hemoglobin in superficial blood vessels. The brief pulse duration of 300–500 μs can cause vascular rupture. After treatment, there are histologic findings of agglutinated red blood cells, fibrin, and platelet thrombi within the vessels of the papillary and superficial reticular dermis (average depth of 1.2 mm) with little or no damage to the surrounding tissue.

Near Infrared Lasers

More recently, the near-infrared wavelengths have been used to treat vascular lesions. Alexandrite (755 nm), diode (800 nm, 940 nm), and Nd:YAG (1,064 nm) lasers use the broad oxyhemoglobin absorption band in the 800–1,000-nm spectrum, and features the advantage of greater optic penetration. These longer wavelength lasers are being used to treat larger vessel vascular anomalies, as well as larger *leg veins* (1–5 mm).

Neodymium:yttrium-aluminum-garnet (Nd:YAG) laser: The 1,064 nm wavelength has been used for various pigmentary diseases and vascular dermatoses. With the advent of lasers capable of achieving longer pulse durations and longer wavelengths, deeper (depth of 5–6 mm) and larger caliber vessels can be treated more effectively with fewer treatment sessions and less purpura. The absorption coefficient of blood at 1,064 nm is 0.4/mm, which is much higher than that of the surrounding dermis (0.05/mm) at the same wavelength. This difference in absorption coefficients provides treatment selectivity of deeper blood vessels. Increasing the fluence may compensate lower absolute values of blood absorption at 1,064 nm. The increase in fluence does not necessarily damage the epidermis, because the absolute absorption of melanin is lower at 1,064 nm.

Potassium Titanyl Phosphate Laser

Potassium titanyl phosphate with a wavelength of 532 nm is an alternative laser for superficial cutaneous vascular lesions. This laser emits green light and produces pulse durations ranging from 1 ms to 100 ms. These longer pulse durations gradually heat the blood vessel, without vessel wall rupture and subsequent purpura. Side effects frequently seen with the KTP are edema, crusting, and atrophic scarring (particularly using smaller spot sizes to treat nasal telangiectasias).

Because of the shorter wavelength, there is greater absorption by epidermal melanin in darker skin types and this limits the laser's use in Fitzpatrick skin types III–VI.

Hybrid Lasers

Newer techniques involve *hybrid laser systems*, which emit a dual band of wavelengths (e.g. Nd:YAG/KTP, 1064/532 nm; Nd:YAG/PDL, 1064/595 nm) in a sequential manner.

The combined technology of PDL with Nd:YAG laser treats more effectively than conventional wavelength platforms. Sequential emission means that subpurpuric, pulsed-dye laser fires millisecond before the Nd:YAG laser. This first pulse converts oxyhemoglobin to methemoglobin, which increases the absorption coefficient for Nd:YAG wavelength by 300–500%. Next, the Nd:YAG laser fires and is more effectively absorbed by the converted target, enabling reduced Nd:YAG fluence for enhanced patient safety. Since greater penetration depth is achieved, outcome results are also optimized.

Hybrid lasers can be used to treat resistant PWS with lower laser fluences.

Argon Lasers

The development of the argon laser with wavelengths between 488 nm and 577 nm allowed successful treatment of vascular lesions. However, it carries the disadvantage of damaging the surrounding tissue including epidermis, which produces depigmentation, epidermal atrophy, and scarring.

Intense-pulsed Noncoherent Light

Intense-pulsed noncoherent light systems are high-intensity flashlamps that emit a broad spectrum of polychromatic lights from 500 nm to 1,200 nm. Cut-off filters are used to match the spectrum of lights that are capable of penetrating to the desirable depth in skin and to maximize absorption by target chromophores. By filtering the shorter wavelengths, deeper or larger-diameter blood vessels can be targeted effectively. Energy is delivered by single or multiple synchronized pulses with exposure times of 0.5–80 ms. The pulse duration is also matched to the thermal relaxation time of the vessels being treated. The inter-pulse delays allow cooling of the epidermis and smaller vessels, whereas heat is retained in larger vessels (Fig. 5.5).

The ability of the epidermis to cool more quickly than the target vessel is a function of the vessel size. When one combines the **longer** wavelength, **longer** pulse duration, **larger** spot size, and ability to deliver **multiple** pulses within the thermal relaxation time of the target vessel, treatment efficacy is enhanced.

Photodynamic Therapy

This is another effective modality in treating vascular lesions. PDL uses intravenous photosensitizer and, upon activation by the appropriate light source, generates reactive oxygen species and causes desirable vessel damage. Photodynamic therapy (PDT) alone or in combination with PDL has been proven effective in blanching PWS.

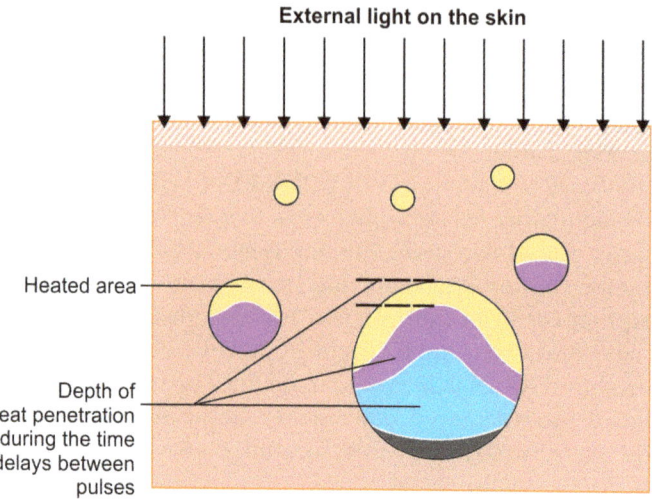

Fig. 5.5: Diagram of effect of repetitive pulses of intense pulsed light on 2-mm vessel, 1 mm below epidermis.
Courtesy: ESC Medical, Inc.

Fractional Lasers

Fractional photothermolysis (FP) is a new technology developed over the past decade. By using focused, high-energy laser microbeams, distinct columns of thermal injury are created. Skin tightening effects are achieved via tissue healing and collagen remodeling. In contrast to the traditional ablative laser, FP allows a rapid healing time and has much better patient tolerance. Ablative and non-ablative FP were reported to be successful in treating the unsightly fibrofatty residuum of involuted hemangiomas.

INDICATIONS FOR VASCULAR LASERS (BOX 5.1)

Port-wine Stains

Introduction

Port-wine stains are the most common cutaneous vascular malformations, involving the postcapillary venules, and affect 3 children per 1,000 live births with no gender predilection. It is believed that PWSs develop within the first 2–8 weeks of gestation (Schneider BV et al.), appear as flat and pink-red to violaceous patches and later turn dark purple in color. They are present for life and have no tendency toward involution. The subsequent hypertrophy of underlying bone and soft tissue further disfigures the facial features of many patients. PWSs may be localized, segmental, diffuse or extensive and occur anywhere on the body, but commonly involve the head and neck region, classically following the trigeminal nerve distribution on the face.

Box 5.1: Practical applications for vascular lasers and light sources.

Capillary malformations
- Infantile PWS
- Macular PWS in adults
- Hypertrophic PWS in adults

Hemangiomas
- Superficial hemangiomas
- Mixed-type hemangiomas
- Involuting hemangiomas

Venous malformations

Telangiectasias
- Spider angiomata
- Actinic telangiectasia
- CREST syndrome
- Essential telangiectasia
- Hereditary hemorrhagic telangiectasia
- Radiation dermatitis
- Rosacea

Facial erythema
- Associated with rosacea
- Flushing and blushing

Cherry angiomas

Venous lakes

Poikiloderma of Civatte

Other lesions treated with vascular lasers
- Angiokeratomas
- Glomus tumors
- Pyogenic granulomas
- Adenoma sebaceum
- Blue rubber bleb nevi
- Hypertrophic and erythematous scars
- Striae distensae
- Warts

Also *see* Chapter 12

Vascular endothelial growth factor (VEGF) and VEGF-R2 expression are significantly increased in capillary malformation skin tissue, suggesting that VEGF and VEGF-R could contribute to the pathogenesis of capillary malformations by inducing vessel proliferation (Vural E et al.). PWSs are associated with syndromes such as Sturge-Weber syndrome, Klippel-Trenaunay syndrome, Cobb syndrome, and Proteus syndrome.

Pulsed Dye Laser for PWS

Though many lasers have been tried in PWS, we will largely focus on PDL.

Pulsed dye laser was specifically designed to treat small vessels found in childhood PWSs. Controversy exists about treating PWS in early versus late stage. However, there are certain advantages of *early treatment*:

- In early stage, the lesion is small in size so fewer spots and sessions are required
- Resolution is quick as compared to older lesions, so fewer treatments are required (Alster TS et al.)
- Early clearance produces less psychological effect on child (Lanigan SW).

Morelli and Weston (Morelli JG et al.) demonstrated that early treatment of PWS gives better results. They proposed that therapy can be started as early as 7–14 days of age and three treatments may be undertaken before the infant reaches 6 months of age. They noted a 50% resolution with this protocol by the third treatment. In another study, Goldman et al. treated 43 children with 49 lesions of capillary malformation between ages of 2 weeks and 14 years. A total of 28 lesions treated in children under age of 4 years had greater overall improvement with less treatment sessions as compared to those over age of 4.5 years (Goldman MP et al.). Alster and Wilson reported 87% clearance rate in patients less than 2 years of age, 78% clearance in those aged 3 years to 8 years, and 73% clearance in patients 16 years and older. All these studies demonstrate a better treatment outcome in younger patients (Alster TS et al.). Nguyen CM et al. evaluated the predictors of improvement of PWS and proposed that younger patients with small PWS (less than 20 cm^2) that are located over bony areas of the face, show greater response when compared to others (Nguyen CM et al.).

Settings: The common starting parameters are fluence of 5.0–5.5 J/cm^2, with increase by 0.5 J/cm^2 with each subsequent treatment, using a 7-mm diameter spot size. About 8–10 sessions are required to achieve significant improvement/clearance. Superficial lesions clear more quickly, with around four sessions, reaching a level of 95% clearance (Goldman MP et al.). When compared with adult PWS, in children, a lower fluence and larger spot size is recommended. Larger spot size prevents cobble stone appearance.

With regard to the number of sittings required for complete or near complete clearance, Koster PHL et al. proposed a mathematical factor of *10% clearance* with each session for the *first five or six treatments*. Additional treatments result in lesser therapeutic response so that **20 treatments** are required to produce **90% clearance**. Lesions present on the lateral side of forehead and cheeks, proximal part of arms and chest respond better as compared to central area of face and limbs (Alster TS et al.).

Response Summary (Adamič M et al.): Only 25% of lesions have complete clearing after multiple treatments. According to our experience, average clearing of 50% could be reached after multiple sessions. Some individuals appear to be able to tolerate long treatments without distress.

Adverse events are usually temporary and include purpura and epidermal crusting. Purpura is more common with PDL compared to other lasers and IP lights. The most common long-term sequelae are pigmentary changes since melanin is a competitive chromophore with hemoglobin in patients with higher Fitzpatrick skin types. Other less common complications are "checkerboard" pigmentation, hypopigmentation, atrophic and hypertrophic scarring, and keloid formation. According to a study, discoloration and purpura were seen in almost all patients, crusting in 52%, and scaling or peeling in 19.6% cases (Ruiz-Esparza J et al.).

Factors Affecting Treatment Response

1. *Age*: Studies have shown an overall better lightening outcome and fewer treatment sessions required in patients of a younger age. The greater lesional clearance observed in young children can be attributed to the smaller lesional surface area, smaller vessel diameter, and thinner skin (i.e. better laser penetration).
2. *Site of lesion*: Regarding PWS over the head and neck region, lesions that are present on the central face or in V2 dermatome respond more slowly than those located elsewhere on the head and neck (Figs. 5.6A and B, Renfro L, et al.). PWS located on the extremities respond more slowly to laser therapy than lesions on the trunk, and lesions on the distal extremities respond the slowest. A conference paper at the ELDS focused on extra facial PWS (Cretu S et al.). They used LP Nd:YAG laser for vascular

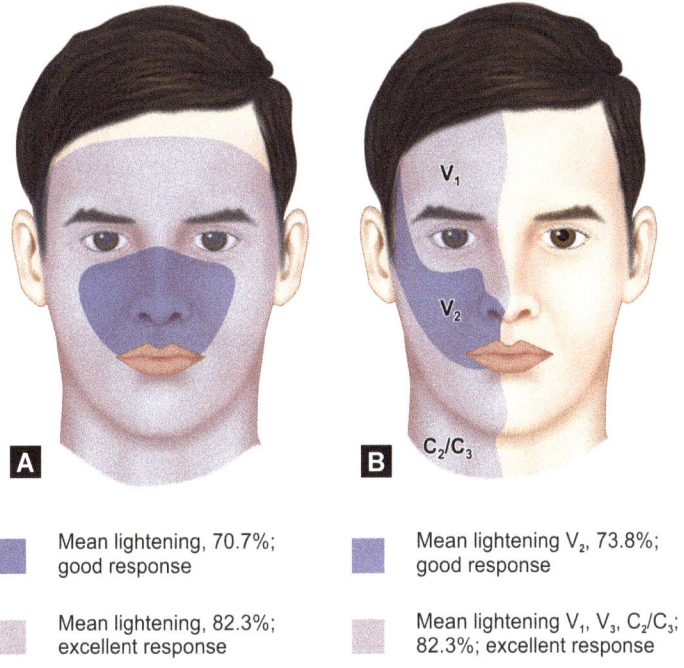

Mean lightening, 70.7%; good response

Mean lightening, 82.3%; excellent response

Mean lightening V_2, 73.8%; good response

Mean lightening V_1, V_3, C_2/C_3; 82.3%; excellent response

Figs. 5.6A and B: (A) Anatomic subdivision of therapeutic response of port-wine stain (PWS) to pulsed dye laser (PDL) treatment; (B) Dermatomal distribution of therapeutic response of PWS to LPDL treatment.
Source: Arch Dermatol. 1993;129:182.

nodules, PDL for the rest of lesions surface, and additional tacrolimus 0.1% ointment in 2 cases. The settings used were, for the LP Nd :YAG : 10-40 ms, 3 to 7 mm spot diameter, 120–140 J/cm^2; for the PDL 595 nm : 0.45–3 ms, 7 mm (7.25–10 J/cm^2), 10 mm (5–12 J/cm^2) or 3 × 10 mm (10–14 J/cm^2) spot size.

Clearance of vascular nodules was obtained after an average of 4 sessions. More than 50% clearance was achieved after an average of 8 sessions for the rest of the lesions. No scarring was observed. The rationale of using the LP Nd:YAG was as the vessels are deeply placed on the extremities.

3. *Size/Morphology of lesion*: Lesions larger than 20 cm^2 respond poorer as compared to smaller lesions (Nguyen CM et al.). Also increased nodularity responds less favorably to PDL treatments.
4. *Color of lesion*: In a histological study, Fikerstrand and co-workers showed that lesions with a poor response to a 585-nm, 450-µs PDL had small vessels. Moderate responses were observed for PWS with deeper and larger vessels. The best response was seen in lesions with superficially located, larger-diameter vessels.

   Videomicroscopy has demonstrated two patterns of vascular abnormality: type 1 consists of tortuous superficial, dilated capillary loops (blobs); type 2 consists of dilated ectatic vessels in the superficial horizontal vascular plexus (rings) (Figs. 5.7A and B). Patients with type 1 vascularity have a better response to PDL treatment because type 2 PWS lesions are more deeply situated and consist of freely anastomosing dilated vessels of the superficial horizontal vascular plexus.

   Vessel size and morphology correlates with the color of the PWS lesions. Pink lesions had the smallest diameter vessels, while purple lesions had the largest. Red lesions were composed of more superficially located vessels than pink or purple ones. *Red color* predicted a *good response*, while pink and purple color predicted a poor response to laser therapy.
5. *Skin types:* Fairer skin types respond better than dark skin (Sharma VK et al.; Ernest Tan et al.).
6. *Depth of lesion:* Lesions with deeper vessels respond poorly.

   Pulsed dye lasers at 585 nm and 6–8 J/cm^2 have been found to coagulate the vessels up to 0.65 mm (mean 0.37 mm). 585 nm dye is more effective in pink or red PWS whereas blue or dark red PWS respond well with 595 nm dyes. In our practice, for treating PWS with the 595 nm PDL, the laser parameters that we use are a spot size of 7 mm, starting fluence of 7–8 J/cm^2 with increase up to 12 J/cm^2 (for hypertrophic PWS) and pulse durations ranging from 0.45 ms to 6 ms.

   Some malformations may have a deep vascular component that cannot be reached with an LPDL, but only by Nd:YAG laser or IPLS.

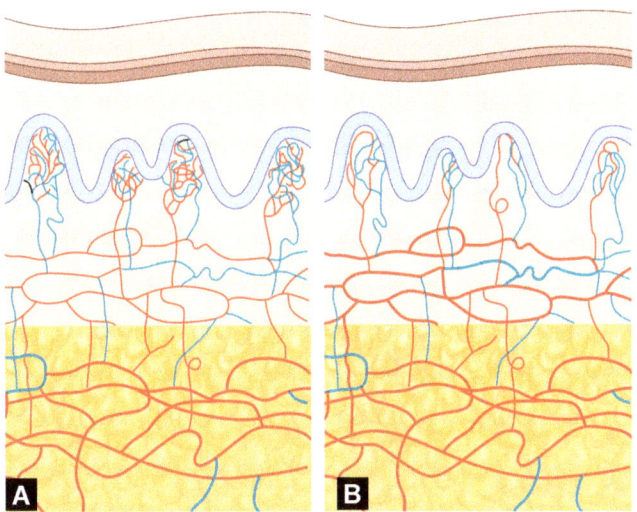

Figs. 5.7A and B: Diagrammatic representations of vascular abnormality found with videomicroscopy. (A) Tortuous, dilated papillary tip vessels; (B) Dilated vessels of superficial horizontal vascular plexor. Note that type 1 abnormality (A) presents a superficial target with limited blood supply. Type 2 abnormality (B) is more deeply situated, and vessels anastomose freely.
Source: Reprinted from Arch Dermatol. 1997;133:921. Copyright © 1997 American Medical Association. All rights reserved).

Technique Tips to Maximize Response to PDL

1. Use higher fluences, increase the spot size of the PDL
2. Change from a 585 nm to a 595 nm wavelength (Chang CJ et al.; Greve B et al.)
3. Increase the pulse duration from 0.45 ms to 1.5–20 ms (Greve B et al.)
4. Perform multiple passes at the same session with variable pulse durations
5. *Combination of lasers*: 595 nm and 1,064 nm laser, PDL and diode laser (Alster TS et al.).

   In our experience we use PDL 595 nm, with spot size at 7 mm, 7 J/cm^2; pulse duration ranging from 0.5–10 ms, and in Nd:YAG 25–40 J/cm^2, pulse width 10–15 ms. A set of images from two different centers is shown here. The results are highly variable as they are dependent on multiple factors (see above) (Figs. 5.8 to 5.16). A study from India (Khandpur S) summarizes the results, with a mean lightening of 54% in flat and 40% in hypertrophic PWS after 10 treatments.

Recurrence

Recurrence of PWS after laser treatment is not uncommon. In general, the size of the recurring lesion is usually a fraction of the initial lesional area and

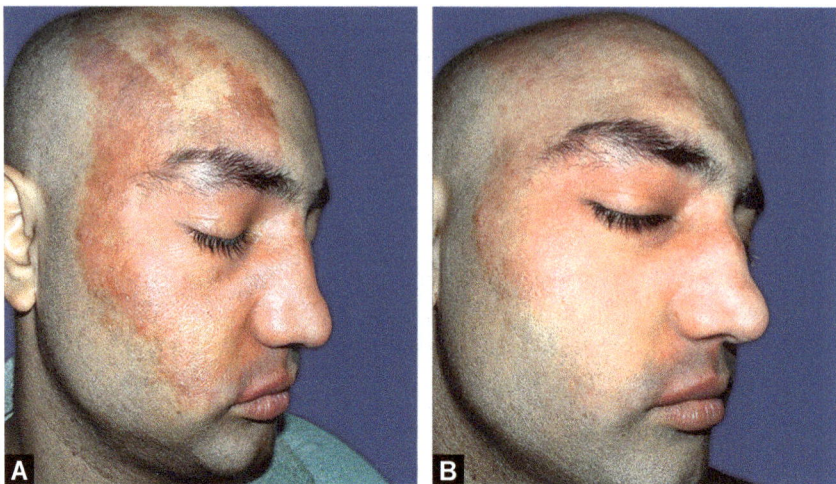

Figs. 5.8A and B: (A) Pretreatment image of PWS over right face; (B) 80% clearance after 7 sessions of 595 nm PDL.

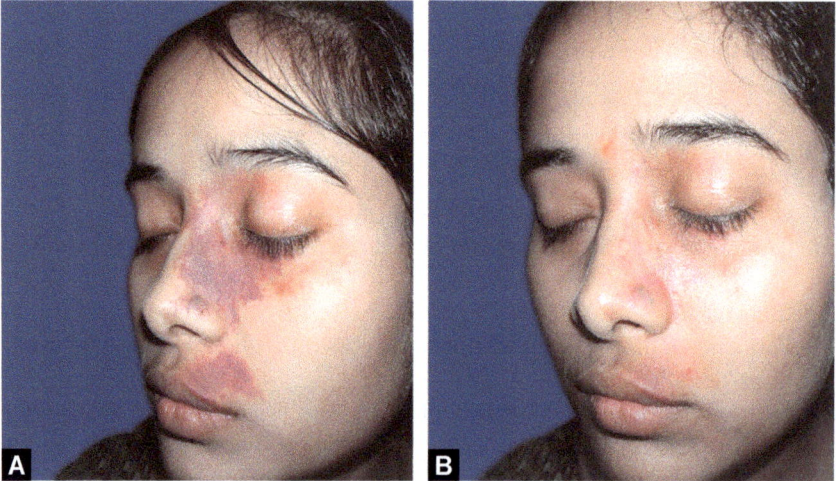

Figs. 5.9A and B: (A) Pretreatment image of PWS over left paranasal region; (B) 90% clearance after 10 sessions of 595 nm PDL.

the color is significantly lighter. In practice, these recurring lesions require only a few additional treatments to achieve satisfactory clearing. Good cosmetic outcome can be maintained with periodic laser treatments.

Anti-angiogenesis

Revascularization of lesional vessels after photocoagulation leads to lesional recurrence and remains the major hurdle of sustained, long-term therapeutic

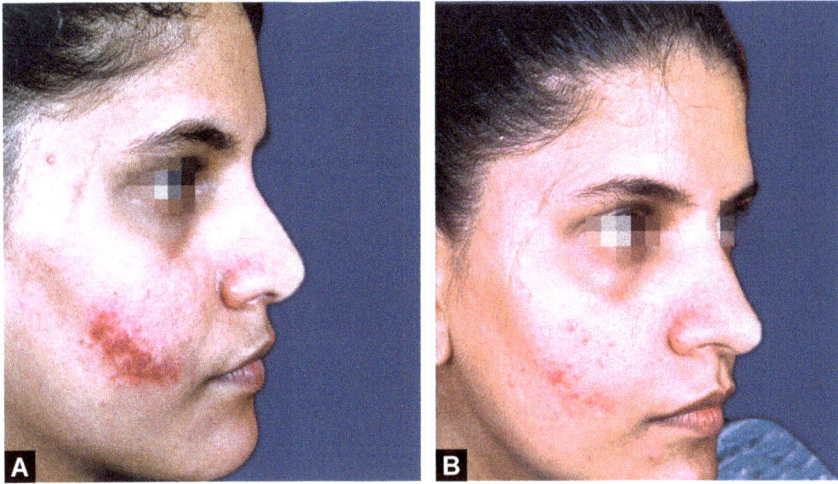

Figs. 5.10A and B: Pretreatment image of PWS over right face; (B) More than 90% clearance after 10 sessions of 585 nm PDL.
Courtesy: Sharma VK, Khandpur S. Efficacy of pulsed dye laser in facial portwine stains in Indian patients. Dermatol Surg. 2007;33(5):560-6.

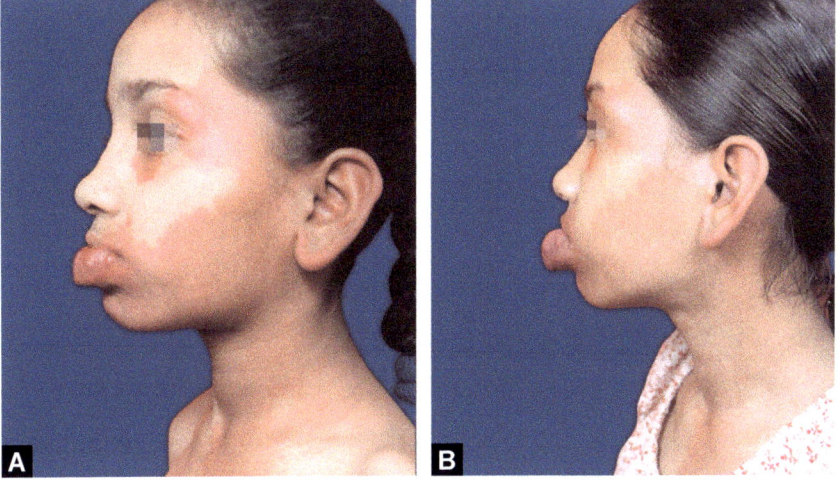

Figs. 5.11A and B: (A) Pretreatment image of PWS over left face and neck; (B) ≥ 90% clearance after 10 sessions of 585 nm PDL.
Courtesy: Sharma VK, Khandpur S. Efficacy of pulsed dye laser in facial portwine stains in Indian patients. Dermatol Surg. 2007;33(5):560-6.

outcome in PWS. Jia and colleagues demonstrated that intense laser injury to the blood vessels would in turn activate angiogenesis pathways. During acute vascular injury, tissue hypoxia would trigger the upregulation of hypoxia-inducible factor-1 alpha (HIF-1α). As a result, transcription of

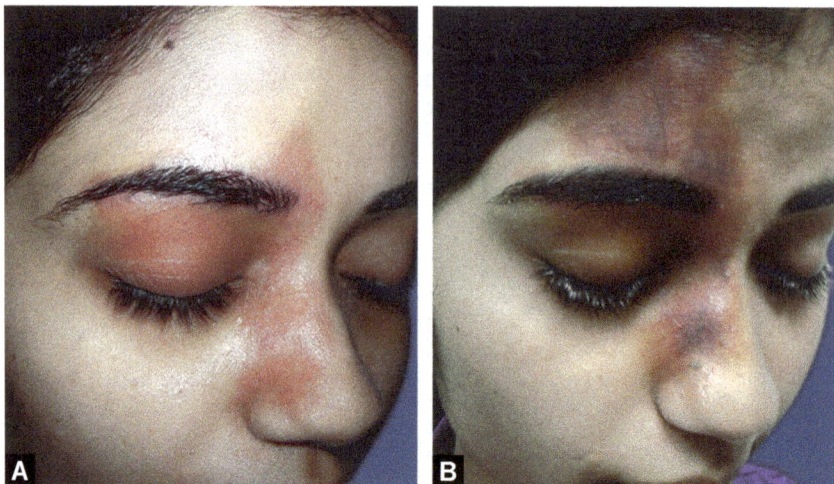

Figs. 5.12A and B: (A) Dusky-red flat PWS over right side of forehead and dorsum of nose before treatment; (B) More than 75% lightening after 10 sessions of PDL.
Source: Khandpur S, Sharma VK. Assessment of efficacy of the 595-nm pulsed dye laser in the treatment of facial port-wine stains in Indian patients. Dermatol Surg. 2016;42(6):717-26.

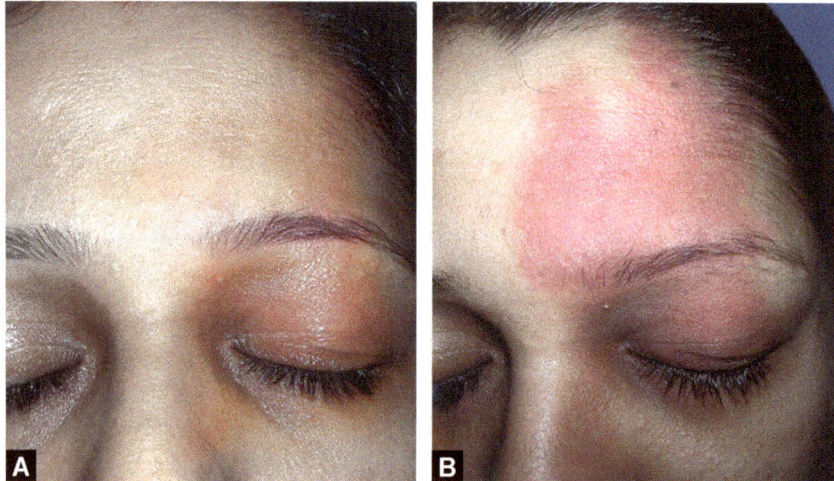

Figs. 5.13A and B: (A) Red flat PWS over right side of forehead and upper eyelid before treatment; (B) More than 75% lightening after 8 sessions of PDL.
Source: Khandpur S, Sharma VK. Assessment of efficacy of the 595-nm pulsed dye laser in the treatment of facial port-wine stains in Indian patients. Dermatol Surg. 2016;42(6):717-26.

numerous angiogenic genes including the VEGF are enhanced, which in turn lead to activation of several downstream signaling pathways, including the mammalian target of rapamycin (mTOR). mTOR is the key mediator involved in regeneration and revascularization of blood vessels in PWS. Based on

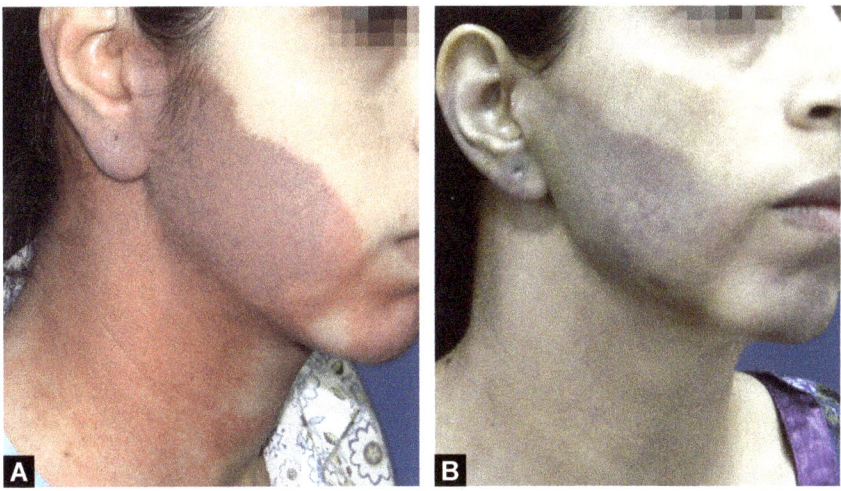

Figs. 5.14A and B: PWS—After 14 sessions. (A) Pretreatment image of PWS over right face and neck; (B) >90% clearance after 14 sessions of Cynergy™.
Courtesy: Dr Latika Arya.

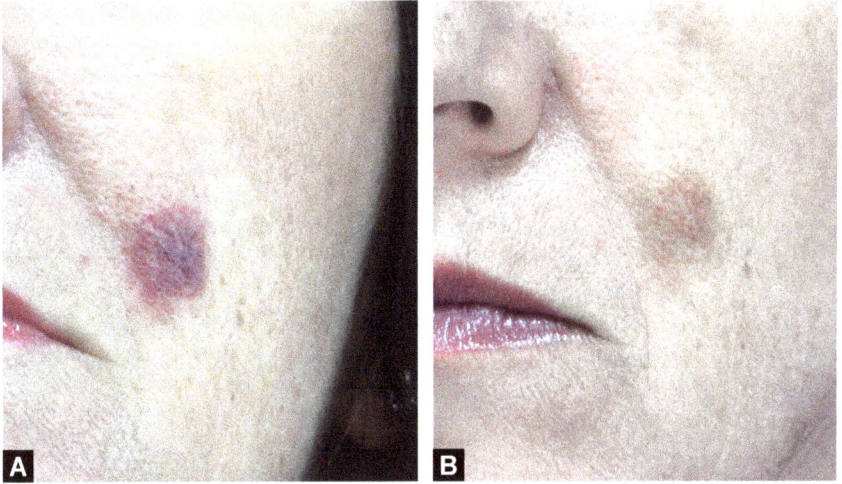

Figs. 5.15A and B: PWS—After 6 sessions. (A) Pretreatment image of PWS over the left cheek; (B) >80% clearance after 6 sessions of Cynergy™.
Courtesy: Dr Latika Arya.

this knowledge, there is a potential role for topical rapamycin to prevent revascularization of PWS after treatment by blocking the mTOR activities. In animal models, Jia and colleagues were able to show reduced frequency of vessel reperfusion in combination treatments with laser and post-treatment application of topical rapamycin. Clinical trials are ongoing to evaluate the efficacy and safety of this combination approach.

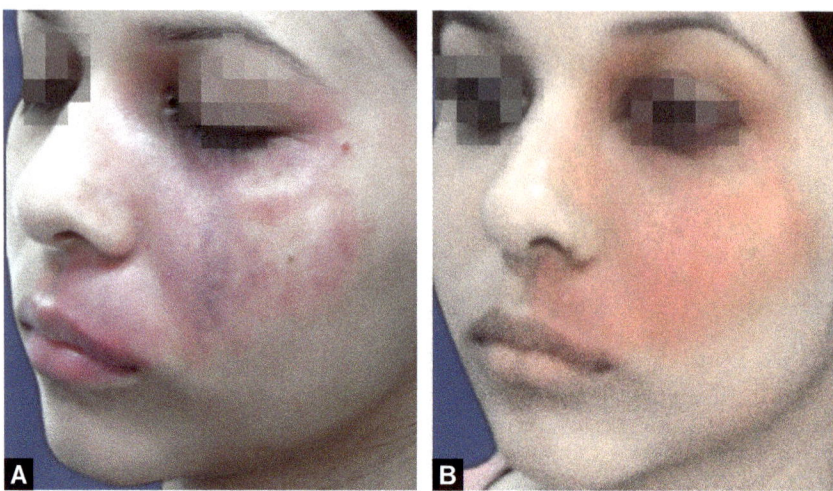

Figs. 5.16A and B: PWS—After 8 sessions. (A) Pretreatment image of PWS over the right cheek; (B) >80% clearance after 8 sessions of Cynergy™.
Courtesy: Dr Latika Arya.

Box 5.2: Lasers for port-wine stain (PWS).

- Treatment of PWS should be done early in life
- Treatments intervals may be shortened to 2–3 weeks in order to enhance efficacy at least when PDL (595 nm) is used
- Multiple treatments are needed and can be done until no treatment results are achieved
- *First choice:* FPDL (585 nm) or LPDL (595 nm) (GRADE 1B), for flat lesions also large spot KTP (532 nm) and IPLS may be tried
- *Treatment-resistant and/or hypertrophic PWS:* millisecond Nd:YAG (1,064 nm), dual wavelength systems (595 nm and 1,064 nm), alexandrite (755 nm) and diode lasers as well as IPLS.

A summary of guidelines is given above as a ready reckoner (Adamič M) (Box 5.2).

Lasers in Hemangiomas

Introduction

Hemangiomas affect up to 4–10% of infants, with 60% occurring on the head and neck, 25% on the trunk, and 15% on the extremities (Finn MC et al.). 80% of hemangiomas are single, well-circumscribed lesions, 0.5–5.0 cm in diameter, while the rest are multiple, cutaneous, and visceral lesions (Mulliken JB).

Infantile hemangiomas present at birth or in neonatal period, as small macule or patch of erythema, which later rapidly proliferate, then stabilize, and slowly involute. The course of individual hemangiomas is heterogeneous, making it difficult to predict outcomes reliably. Approximately 20% of hemangiomas may develop complications in form of ulceration, bleeding, infection, functional impairment with visual, feeding, and respiratory difficulties, which may require active intervention. 50% of infantile hemangiomas completely involute by age of 5 years and 90% by 9 years of age. The remainder may take additional 2-4 years to complete the process (Bowers RE et al.).

They can be classified as superficial, deep, and mixed hemangiomas. Superficial lesions are raised and bright red, and upon regression, leave a flaccid, pedunculated, waxy, yellow-colored skin. Deeper dermal lesions appear as bluish subcutaneous nodules with overlying skin having a fine network of telangiectasia and resolve leaving smooth skin surface with overlying telangiectasia.

According to a study, the lesions that involuted by age 6 years had 38% residual evidence and hemangiomas that completely involuted after age 6 years exhibited cutaneous residua in 80% instances including scar formation, telangiectasia, or redundant skin (Finn MC et al.). Hence, it has been shown that infantile hemangiomas that take longer to involute have a higher incidence of residual changes.

Lasers Used for Hemangioma

Laser treatment of infantile hemangiomas (IH) is still controversial and should only be done by experienced laser surgeons who have a vast knowledge in vascular anomalies as well. The management of patients with potentially problematic hemangiomas should involve a multidisciplinary approach.

The *argon laser* has been effectively used to treat hemangiomas. The potential drawbacks of argon laser are its depth of penetration into the dermis (<1 mm) and its tendency to cause hypertrophic scarring by nonspecific thermal injury. In one study, children under age 12 years were treated with argon laser and the results were poor in more than 50% cases, therefore, authors do not recommend argon laser treatment in children under the age of 12 years, except for infants with complications of capillary hemangiomas (Smith JD).

The *Nd:YAG laser*, with 1,064 nm wavelength, can penetrate into deeper dermis (up to 8 mm) but produces widespread tissue injury and scar formation by its nonspecific absorption (Apfelberg DB et al.). The tissue injury can be minimized by using 3-4 mm diameter spot size with 6-8 mm untreated area between spots. Preeyanont et al. on treating 160 patients with the Nd:YAG laser at fluences of 400-1,600 J/cm^2 and pulse durations of 0.5 second, found excellent results in 13% cases, 55% had a reduction in hemangioma size by more than 50%, 35% had less than 50%, reduction in lesion size and 2% had poor response. Ten percent of patients developed scarring (Preeyanont P et al.).

Potassium titanyl phosphate is an intralesional laser in which the laser fiber is passed through a needle that is positioned in the center of the hemangioma and then laser energy is delivered. The end point of therapy is shrinkage of overlying skin that later becomes warm to touch. KTP laser is indicated for voluminous or large hemangiomas where deeper penetration with conventional lasers is not possible, although it has higher chance of scar formation.

The long-pulse *PDL*, with a wavelength of 595 nm has proven effective in the treatment of superficial (macular) and ulcerated hemangiomas. A retrospective analysis of 60 pediatric patients conducted by Kim et al. showed that in 37% of ulcerated hemangiomas treated with PDL, 50% showed definite improvement, 18% showed no response, and 5% showed worsening of lesions (Kim HJ et al.). Morelli and Weston concluded that ulcerated painful hemangiomas are the best indication for PDL (Morelli JG et al.). Various studies confirm the efficacy of PDL in early hemangiomas. Most authors report cessation of the proliferative phase as a consequence of treatment with the PDL (Glassberd E et al.; Sherwood KA et al.; Garden JM et al.). Maier et al. treated 100 hemangiomas within 12 weeks of their development and found that 73 lesions required a single treatment and 27 up to five treatments; 23% of lesions showed complete remission, 55% showed partial remission, and 14% stopped growing. Only 8% of lesions continued to grow despite treatment (Maier H et al.). Diode laser is also useful in treating residual telangiectasia following spontaneous resolution of hemangiomas, for improving cosmetic results.

A combined therapy of medical management, debulking surgery and PDL has been used in treatment of large or extensive hemangiomatosis and shown faster resolution of infantile hemangiomas. Studies have shown better response of infantile hemangiomas when medical management was combined with PDL as compared to medical therapy alone. Poetke et al. in their prospective, observational study of large facial hemangiomas on 23 patients with age ranging from 2 months to 3.5 years, of which 14 patients received propranolol in combination with laser therapy, reported that only one case receiving the combination therapy experienced rebound hemangioma growth. Nine patients were treated with propranolol (2 mg/kg/day) alone and six had rebound growth when treatment was stopped. This study suggests that propranolol plus PDL may be more effective than propranolol alone.

Carbon dioxide laser is also useful as a debulking tool for large hemangiomas, oral hemangiomas and laryngeal lesions producing airway obstruction. Scarring is significant so it is usually not recommended for facial hemangiomas.

Intense-pulsed light with a cut-off filter at 550 nm, 570 nm or 590 nm has shown excellent results for multiple hemangiomas. Foster and Gold treated an ulcerated cavernous hemangioma in an 11-week-old black infant with setting of 550 nm cut-off filter at a fluence of 38 J/cm^2 resulting in 90% involution (Foster TD et al.).

Treatment of hemangiomas should be decided on the basis of individual circumstances such as the size and location of the tumor, complications, the phase at the time of evaluation, involvement of other organs and psychological factors.

A summary of guidelines as a ready reckoner (Adamič M) is given in Box 5.3.

Facial Telangiectasia and Diffuse Facial Erythema

Telangiectasia is a clinical entity of superficial dilated venules, capillaries or arterioles with average diameter of 0.1–1.0 mm. Telangiectasias that are arteriolar in origin have a smaller diameter, are bright red in color and do not protrude above the skin surface. Those that arise from venules are wider, blue in color and often protrude above skin surface.

Telangiectasias can be treated with PDL using 3 mm, 5 mm, 7 mm or 10 mm spot size, fluences ranging from $5 J/cm^2$ to $8 J/cm^2$ with a 0.45 ms pulse duration or higher. Purpura can be minimized by giving two to three pulses over the telangiectasia at lower fluences (pulse stacking), using spot size 10 mm diameter at $4-5 J/cm^2$ and undertaking therapy with the 595 nm PDL as compared to 585 nm. Telangiectasias on the ala are resistant and often require repetitive pulsing with high settings.

Summary: In general, LPDL and KTP lasers are more effective in the treatment of smaller diameter telangiectasia and diffuse erythema, whereas longer wavelength devices might be more useful for wider, blue, deep-seated telangiectasia. These devices, in general, have a higher potential for side effects. An overview of guidelines as a ready reckoner (Adamič M) is given in Box 5.4 **(Also *see* Chapter 12E)**.

Box 5.3: Lasers for hemangioma.

- Treatment of IH should be considered in tumors which cause functional or structural abnormalities (e.g. airway obstruction, ophthalmologic disturbances), which ulcerate and bleed, are secondarily infected, or may result in disfigurement or scarring
- Laser treatment of large cervicofacial segmental hemangiomas is not advised
- *Ulceration:* They may require as a first choice 595-nm PDL followed by Nd:YAG laser (1,064 nm) or hybrid lasers. The use of Nd:YAG should be with caution as it may cause burns
- As propranolol is a safer option only in cases where it cannot be administered we recommend the use of vascular lasers, especially when hemangioma is ulcerated or residual erythema and telangiectasias persist after involution
- Treat IH early if hemangioma is potentially in a site to cause problems.
    a. First choices are LPDL (595 nm) or millisecond Nd:YAG (1,064 nm) lasers with cooling
    b. Second choice, alexandrite (755 nm) or KTP (532 nm; for superficial lesions) lasers may be used

Box 5.4: Lasers for telangiectasia and facial erythema.

- *First choice*: LPDL (595 nm) and KTP (532 nm) lasers, and IPLs
- *Second choice*: Millisecond or microsecond Nd:YAG (1,064 nm) or diode (940-nm or 980-nm) lasers may be used
- Adequate cooling should be used to protect epidermis from thermal damage.

Rosacea

Patients with rosacea often complain of facial flushing and erythema. Removal of superficial telangiectasia, which does not contain a smooth muscle layer, can be performed only with lasers and light sources (Figs. 5.17A and B).

The telangiectasias are frequently present and are unresponsive to classic topical or systemic therapy. The treatment of these vessels probably contributes to attenuation of inflammation and disease progression in rosacea **(Also *see* Chapter 12E)**.

Summary

1. Diffuse erythema and telangiectasia of rosacea can be effectively and safely reduced by the use of LPDL (595 nm) and KTP (532 nm) lasers, and IPLS.
2. Pretreatment with topical niacin safely enhanced the effect of 585-nm PDL treatment of rosacea-associated erythema overcoming the relatively lower effect of subpurpuragenic PDL in dark-skinned Asians.
3. The 595-nm LPDL and IPL (a filter set at 560 nm) showed a similar efficacy and safety in patients with erythematotelangiectatic rosacea; they are first choice for the treatment of diffuse erythema.

Poikiloderma of Civatte

Poikilodermatous skin is characterized by atrophy, hyper- and hypopigmentation, and telangiectasia. Poikiloderma of Civatte occurs on the sides of neck, more commonly in middle-aged women with a fair complexion. Several lasers have been tried including argon, KTP, pulsed dye laser and intense pulsed light devices with variable results (Goldman et al.; Oldbricht et al.;

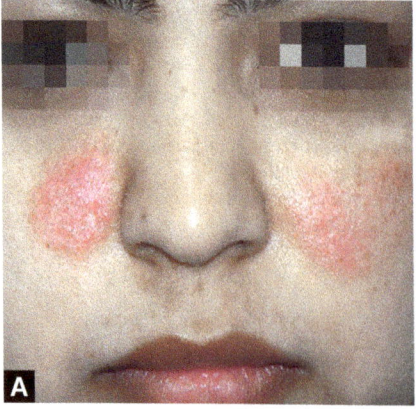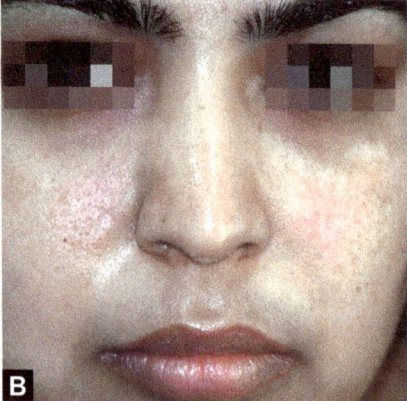

Figs. 5.17A and B: Rosacea—after three sessions. (A) Pretreatment image of rosacea; (B) Clearance > 80% in three sittings of Cynergy™.
Courtesy: Dr Latika Arya.

Batta K et al.; Wheel and RG et al.; Clark RE et al.). Multiple sessions are usually necessary to obtain optimal clearance.

A consensus guideline (Adamič M et al.) recommended the use of IPLS, KTP (532 nm), and LPDL (595 nm) lasers). Generally, two to three treatment sessions are required for satisfactory response. It is important to reduce the radiant exposure by 20–30% when treating scar-prone areas such as the neck and upper chest, to avoid overlapping pulses and to use larger spot sizes, such as 10 mm.

Good results have been obtained with an ablative fractional laser for all aspects of skin lesions (dyschromia, pigmentation and textural changes). In Indian skin though the non-ablative laser is preferred.

Venous Lakes

Venous lake is usually a solitary, soft, compressible, dark blue to violaceous, 0.2–1 cm sized papule caused by dilatation of venules. These are commonly found on sun-exposed surfaces of the vermilion border of lip, face and ears. Lesions generally occur in the elderly. Venous lakes have clinical importance because of their mimicry to malignant lesions, such as melanoma and pigmented basal cell carcinoma. Various surgical and laser modalities have been tried for venous lakes.

Numerous modalities have been tried like: surgical excision, cryosurgery, infrared coagulation, argon lasers, intense pulsed light, pulsed dye lasers, Nd:YAG laser, dual PDL-Nd:YAG laser, diode lasers, carbon dioxide lasers, and sclerosing agents. The long-pulsed Nd:YAG laser is superior to most and achieves fast and safe results.

Hence, the *ideal lasers* include millisecond Nd:YAG (1,064 nm), dual PDL-Nd:YAG laser, alexandrite (755 nm) and diode (800 nm, 808 nm and 980 nm) lasers (**Also** *see* **Chapter 12E**).

Granuloma Telangiectaticum (Pyogenic Granuloma)

Pyogenic granulomas (PGs) are benign vascular tumors that often ulcerate and bleed with trauma and are most commonly seen in children.

Pyogenic granulomas may be treated with surgical excision (necessary in case of any diagnostic doubt to avoid confusion with cutaneous tumors including melanoma), cryotherapy, electrocautery, intralesional sclerotherapy or corticosteroids, topical agents (silver nitrate, phenol and imiquimod) and/or lasers.

Amongst lasers LPDL (595 nm), carbon dioxide (10,600 nm), and millisecond Nd:YAG lasers (1,064 nm) are ideal. Another option is the use of bipolar electrocautery in the coagulation mode. In children, multiple (2–6) sequential PDL or Nd:YAG laser treatments are typically required for clearance, compared to a single CO_2 laser vaporization procedure, but the former are easier for children to undergo because they are practically painless (**Also** *see* **Chapter 12E**).

Cherry Angiomas

It is characterized by a central feed arteriolar vessel with radiant fine red telangiectasia. The spider angiomas should be removed by millisecond Nd:YAG (1,064 nm), KTP (532 nm) and LPDL lasers and IPLS. Sometimes, several treatment sessions are needed because of its high flow nature. Rarely, as a second choice, argon or copper vapor lasers may be used for treatment of spider angioma.

Another option is to destroy the central vessels with a pulsed CO_2 laser, prolonging the pulse duration to 50 ms, in a defocused mode, to coagulate the central vessel. This is a cheaper and much faster method in the authors' opinion.

Leg Veins

A complex venous network is found in the lower limbs, which consists of the superficial and deep systems. They are interconnected by perforating veins. Venulectases are larger vessels (compared with the bright-red telangiectases) with diameters of 0.4–2 mm that are purple or blue in color. Although sclerotherapy is the standard treatment for dilated leg veins, not all vessels can be cannulated practically. Laser therapy provides an alternative option to the treatment of leg veins, which can also be used as an adjunctive therapy.

An *Nd:YAG laser* is often chosen to treat dilated leg veins. The long wavelength offers good optic penetration, which allows targeting of deep-seated vessels in the reticular dermis. In a single-treatment study, a 1,064-nm Nd:YAG laser operating with a 50-ms pulse duration and fluence of 100 J/cm^2 was evaluated. Two-thirds of the target vessels (1–3 mm) were cleared more than 75% after single treatment. The treatment end point was either immediate vessel disappearance (stenosis) or bluing of the vessel (thrombosis).

Although *Alexandrite laser* (755 nm) was reported to be highly effective in treating dilated leg vessels (87% had more than 50% improvement), persistent hyperpigmentation (more than 12 weeks) has been reported in 26% of treatment sites.

Pulsed dye laser can be used to treat superficial, smaller leg vessels. A 3 mm × 10 mm spot was especially designed to target visible, dilated vessels. It has the advantage of minimizing collateral tissue damage. In a study of 15 patients, a long-pulsed 595-nm PDL (V-Beam Perfecta prototype laser, Candela Corporation) has been proven effective in clearing dilated leg veins. The treatment fluences ranged from 17.5–25.0 J/cm^2 and a pulse duration of 40 ms was used. In the study, 44% of the patients had at least 50% improvement.

STEP-BY-STEP APPROACH

Patient Selection

Appropriate treatment of vascular lesions begins with a correct diagnosis. A misdiagnosis can lead to ineffective and potentially harmful treatment. Proper patient selection is mandatory for good success rates. Patients presenting for treatment with vascular lasers are treated with the following goals:
1. Improving overall appearance, with an ideal target to clear the lesions without any complications
2. Improvement in functionality
3. Prevention of disfigurement
4. Avoiding aggressive procedures
5. Preventing or treating ulcerated lesions
6. Minimizing psychological distress.

Preoperative

- A written informed consent of the patient is taken.
- Avoidance of direct sun exposure and daily use of broad-spectrum sunscreen with SPF 30 prior to and throughout the course of the treatment is advised.
- Lightening background skin is a controversial concept, but some authors consider it useful in dark skin types (IV–VI) to reduce risk of postinflammatory hyperpigmentation.
- Patients with unrealistic expectations should be avoided. Doctor or staff should always explain about the procedure to the patient. Multiple laser treatments are usually necessary to remove a vascular lesion necessitating multiple sessions at regular intervals. Although laser treatment has fewer side effects as compared to surgical procedure, there is a small risk of the following which needs to be explained to the patient: Hypopigmentation, hyperpigmentation, mottled discoloration, infection, pain, swelling, activation of herpes simplex infection, allergic reaction to local medications, atrophy or mild scarring, and lesion persistence despite treatment. Baseline and subsequent pre-session photographs are taken:
- Test spots may be considered for patients with darker skin types prior to the initial treatment.
- Topical anesthetics (such as 2.5% lignocaine + 2.5% prilocaine) should be applied under occlusion for at least 45 minutes before the procedure to reduce local discomfort.
- The area to be treated should be shaved in the morning of treatment and rinsed well. No hair removing creams or lotions should be used. No creams, lotions or sprays should be applied to the area.
- The area being treated should be cleansed with mild soap and alcohol.

Intraoperative

- The correct laser parameters are chosen and recorded.
- Wearing especially designed protective goggles during the procedure ensures laser safety of the doctor and patient.
- A test shot is given before procedure to check for any significant pain.
- The patient is advised not to move his head or flinch with each pulse of light delivered as the machine makes a popping sound.
- Place the laser tip firmly on the skin, making certain that the handpiece is perpendicular to the skin surface and the entire tip is in contact with the skin. **Avoid** excessive downward pressure as this can cause vessels to blanch, diminishing target for the laser and reducing treatment efficacy.
- The laser is delivered concomitantly with cryogen cooling to prevent nonspecific thermal damage to surrounding tissue.
- Perform a single pulse at the lateral margin of the treatment area and assess for patient tolerance and clinical endpoints.

Desirable Clinical End Points and Therapy Pearls

- *Telangiectasias*: Increased erythema
    - Vessel clearance
    - Darkening with a grayish discoloration
    - Purpura
- *Background erythema*:
    - Decreased erythema
- *Spider and cherry angiomas*:
    - Darkening with a purplish discoloration
- If there is no apparent change to a vessel, compress the vessel using a fingertip and observe for vessel blanching and refilling once the pressure is removed. Adequately treated vessels will not blanch. Partially treated vessels refill sluggishly
- If areas with rosacea or background erythema do not have adequate endpoints, consider performing a second pass with the same settings, or use a shorter pulse width and slightly lower fluence, to enhance the clinical end points.

Postoperative

- Immediately after procedure, the patient is advised to apply cold compresses to the treated site.
- A topical steroid-antibiotic cream is applied.
- The patient is explained about immediate post-treatment appearance. After treatment, the area may be discolored (purpura) and swollen. Following this, a blister and/or crust may form which can last up to 7–14 days. To reduce swelling and discomfort, cool water compresses may be applied to the area. Do not apply ice directly to the treated area.

- The rate of response to treatment is explained.
- In case of pain and discomfort, acetaminophen is preferred over aspirin or ibuprofen during the healing phase (1 to 2 weeks) as this can increase bruising.
- Showers are permitted but prolonged hot baths are not advised for 1-2 weeks. Patients are advised not to rub but dab the treated area with a towel because the area is extremely delicate while healing.
- Make-up and moisturizers may be applied as usual if there is no blister/ulceration. Otherwise, wait until the crusting has come off. If make-up is applied to cover up the bruising, do not use make-up remover or cleanse harshly while the skin is still healing as this may injure or abrade the treated area.
- Avoid sunlight exposure to the treated areas. Use a sunscreen with SPF 30 or higher for several months following treatment to avoid prolonged redness or pigmentary changes.
- Avoid swimming and contact sports while the skin is healing.
- *Posttreatment precautions*: Patients should avoid:
  - Exercise for 3 days after treatment
  - Consumption of alcohol or any blood thinners for 5 days
  - Taking hot showers or baths, use of hot tubs or saunas for 5 days.
- The subsequent sessions should be undertaken at 6–8 weeks interval. Prior to the next session, thoroughly examine the treated site and compare with baseline photograph to look for improvement and side effects following previous therapy in order to decide the next laser parameter.

CONCLUSION

There are multiple vascular disorders that can be treated by laser, with varying degree of efficacy. Some may respond to ablative lasers (pyogenic granuloma) and others may not require lasers in all cases (hemangioma). One of the biggest drawback is the financial cost of the laser and the dye. The dye is an expensive consumable (around 2.25 lakhs INR) and has a shelf-life of 6 months. Also the Indian skin pigment can make a mess of established skin optics of most vascular lasers. More acquired vascular disorders and their interventions are discussed in Chapter 12E.

BIBLIOGRAPHY

1. Adamič M, Pavlović MD, Troilius Rubin A, et al. Guidelines of care for vascular lasers and intense pulse light sources from the European Society for Laser Dermatology. J Eur Acad Dermatol Venereol. 2015;29(9):1661-78.
2. Alster TS, Tanzi EL. Combined 595-nm and 1,064-nm laser irradiation of recalcitrant and hypertrophic port-wine stains in children and adults. Dermatol Surg. 2009;35:914-8.

3. Alster TS, Wilson F. Treatment of port-wine stains with the flashlamp-pumped dye laser: Extended clinical experience in children and adults. Ann Plast Surg. 1994;32:474.
4. Anderson RR, Parish JA. Microvasculature can be selectively damaged using dye lasers: a basic theory and experimental evidence in human skin. Lasers Surg Med. 1981;1:263-76.
5. Anderson RR, Parrish JA. Selective photothermolysis: Precise microsurgery by selective absorption of pulsed radiation. Science. 1983;220:524.
6. Apfelberg DB, Greene RA, Maser MR. Results of argon laser exposure of capillary emangiomas of infancy: Preliminary report. Plast Reconstr Surg. 1981;67:188.
7. Batta K, Hinson C, Cotterill JA, et al. Treatment of poikiloderma of Civatte with potassium titanyl phosphate (KTP) laser. Br J Dermatol. 1999;140:1191-2.
8. Bowers RE, Graham EA, Tomlinson KM. The natural history of the strawberry nevus. Arch Dermatol. 1960;82:667.
9. Chang CJ, Kelly KM, van Gemert MJ, et al. Comparing the effectiveness of 585-nm vs. 595-nm wavelength pulsed dye laser treatment of port wine stains in conjunction with cryogen spray cooling. Lasers Surg Med. 2002;31:352-8.
10. Clark RE, Jiminez-Acosta F. Poikiloderma of Civatte: Resolution after treatment with pulsed dye laser. N Carolina Med J. 1994;55:234-5.
11. Dierickx CC, Casparian JM, Venugoplan V, et al. Thermal relaxation of port-wine stain vessels probed in vivo: the need for 1-10 millisecond laser pulse treatment. J Invest Dermatol. 1995;105:709-14.
12. Dixon JA, Gilbertson JJ. Argon and noedynium YAG laser therapy of dark nodular port-wine stains in older patients. Laser Surg Med. 1986;6:5-11.
13. Dixon JA, Huether S, Rotering R. Hypertrophic scarring in argon treatment of portwine stain. Plast Reconstr Surg. 1984;73:771-7.
14. Fikerstrand EJ, Svaasand LO, Kopstad G, et al. Photothermally induced vessel-wall necrosis after pulsed dye laser treatment; lack of responses in port wine stains with small sized or deeply located vessels. J Invest Dermatol. 1996;107:671-5.
15. Finn MC, Glowacki J, Mulliken JB. Congenital vascular lesions: Clinical application of a new classification. J Pediatr Surg. 1983;18:894-900.
16. Foster TD, Gold MH. The successful use of the PhotoDerm VL in the treatment of a cavernous hemangioma in a darkskinned infant. Minim Invas Nurs. 1996;10:102.
17. Garden JM, Babus AD, Paller AS. Treatment of cutaneous hemangiomas by the flashlamp-pumped pulsed dye laser: Prospective analysis. J Pediatr. 1992;120:555.
18. Glassberg E, Lask G, Rabinowitz LG, et al. Capillary hemangiomas: Case study of a novel laser treatment and a review of therapeutic options. J Dermatol Surg Oncol. 1989;15:1214-23.
19. Goldman L, Bauman WE. Laser test treatment for postsolar poikiloderma. Arch Dermatol. 1984;120:578-9.
20. Goldman MP, Fitzpatrick RE, Ruiz-Esparza J. Treatment of port-wine stains (capillary malformation) with the flashlamp-pumped pulsed dye laser. J Pediatr. 1993;122:71-7.
21. Greve B, Raulin C. Prospective study of port wine stain treatment with dye laser: Comparison of two wavelengths (58 nm vs. 595 nm) and two pulse durations (0.5 milliseconds vs. 20 milliseconds). Lasers Surg Med. 2004;34:168-73.

22. Jia W, Sun V, Tran N, et al. Long-term blood vessel removal with combined laser and topical rapamycin antiangiogenic therapy: Implications for effective port wine stain treatment. Laser Surg Med. 2010;42(2):105-12.
23. Kauvar AN. Long-pulse, high energy pulsed dye laser treatment of PWS and hemangiomas. Lasers Surg Med. 1997;9:36.
24. Khandpur S, Sharma VK. Efficacy of pulsed dye laser in facial port-wine stains in Indian patients. Dermatol Surg. 2007;33:560-66.
25. Kim HJ, Colombo M, Frieden IJ. Ulcerated hemangiomas: Clinical characteristics and response to therapy. J Am Acad Dermatol. 2001;44:962-72.
26. Koster PH, van der Horst CM, Bossuyt PM, et al. Prediction of portwine stain clearance and required number of flashlamp pumped pulsed dye laser treatments. Lasers Surg Med. 2001;29:151-5.
27. Lanigan SW. Port-wine stains on the lower limb: Response to pulsed dye laser therapy. Clin Exp Dermatol. 1996;21:88.
28. Maier H, Neumann R. Treatment of strawberry marks with flashlamp-pumped pulsed dye laser in infancy. Lancet. 1996;347:131.
29. Morelli JG, Weston WL, Huff JV, et al. Initial lesion size as a predictive factor in determining the response of port-wine stains in children treated with the pulsed dye laser. Arch Pediatr Adolesc Med. 1995;149:1142.
30. Morelli JG, Weston WL. Pulsed dye laser treatment of hemangiomas. In: Tan OT (Ed). Management and Treatment of Benign Cutaneous Vascular Lesions. Philadelphia: Lea and Febiger; 1992.
31. Mulliken JB. Diagnosis and natural history of hemangiomas. In: Mulliken JB, Young AE (Eds). Vascular Birthmarks, Hemangiomas and Malformations. Philadelphia: WB Saunders; 1988.
32. Nelzen O. Prevalence of venous leg ulcer: The importance of the data collection method. Phlebolymphology. 2008;15(4):143-50.
33. Nguyen CM, Yohn JJ, Huff C, et al. Facial port wine stains in childhood: Prediction of the rate of improvement as a function of the age of the patient, size, and location of port wine stain and the number of treatments with pulsed dye laser. Br J Dermatol. 1998;138:821-5.
34. Oldbricht SM, Stern RS, Tang SV, et al. Complications of cutaneous laser surgery: A survey. Arch Dermatol. 1987;123:345-9.
35. Preeyanont P, Nimsakul N. The Nd:YAG laser treatment of hemangioma. J Clin Laser Med Surg. 1994;12:225.
36. Rabe E. Epidemiology of varicose veins. Phlebolymphology. 2010;17(1):21.
37. Redisch W, Pelzer RH. Localized vascular dilatations of the human skin: Capillary microscopy and related studies. Am Heart J. 1949;37:106.
38. Renfro L, Geronemus RG. Anatomical differences of port-wine stains in response to treatment with the pulsed dye laser. Arch Dermatol. 1993;129:182-8.
39. Ruiz-Esparza J, Goldman MP, Fitzpatrick RE, et al. Flashlamp-pumped dye laser for port-wine stains. Lasers Surg Med. 1993;19(11):1000-3.
40. Schneider BV, Mitsuhashi Y, Schnyder UW. Ultrastructural observations in port wine stains. Arch Dermatol Res. 1988;280:338-45.
41. Sherwood KA, Tan OT. Treatment of a capillary hemangioma with the flashlamp-pumped dye laser. J Am Acad Dermatol. 1990;22:136.
42. Smith JD. Argon laser treatment of hemangiomas in children. Int J Pediatr Otorhinolaryngol. 1984;2:153-8.

43. Smoller BR, Rosen S. Port-wine stains. A disease of altered neural modulation of blood vessels? Arch Dermatol. 1986;122(2):177-9.
44. Tan E Vinciullo. Pulsed dye laser treatment of port-wine stains: A review of patients treated in Western Australia. Med J Aust. 1996;164(6):333-6.
45. Vural E, Ramakrishnan J, Cetin N, et al. The expression of vascular endothelial growth factor and its receptors in port-wine stains. Otolaryngol Head Neck Surg. 2008;139(4):560-4.
46. Wheeland RG, Applebaum J. Flashlamp pumped pulsed dye laser therapy for poikiloderma of Civatte. J Dermatol Surg Oncol. 1990;16:12-6.

CHAPTER 6

Lasers for Hair Removal

Shivani Bansal, Soni Nanda, Kabir Sardana, Shikha Bansal, Tarang Goyal

INTRODUCTION

Human skin contains hair follicles all over the body except palms, soles, and lips. All of these follicles contain and produce hair, either vellus or terminal. The complaints of excess hair are subjective and strongly influenced by the prevailing society and cultural norms. Laser hair reduction (LHR) has proved to be a safe and effective means of getting rid of unwanted hair. The term permanent hair reduction is more appropriate and informative than the term permanent hair removal.

Different laser systems including the alexandrite, ruby, diode, and neodymium-doped: yttrium aluminum garnet (Nd:YAG) and now intense pulsed light (IPL) have been tried in all skin types. It is one of the most commonly done cosmetic procedures. It is performed by a whole range of people: by the patient at home, beauty salons, technicians, and dermatologists. The results vary according to technique, expertise, patient's medical condition, and the machine employed. If LHR is done for the correct indication, with proper laser machine, with right fluence and pulse width, it can be quite rewarding for the patient.

History of lasers for hair reduction: Variety of lasers is now available to successfully reduce unwanted hair. In 1996, 694-nm ruby lasers were the first to be formally studied for laser hair removal. Then Nd:YAG carbon based topical suspension became the first LHR system to be approved by FDA for the same, carbon particles serving to damage the hair follicles. But it caused hair growth delayed only up to 3 months. This technique is still used as topical carbon suspension based Q-switched treatment for treating open pores and decreasing sebum. However, there is now a wide array of lasers including alexandrite, diode and Nd:YAG as well as a variety of broad spectrum IPL devices giving lasting results.

Under the FDA's definition, "permanent" hair reduction is the long-term, stable reduction in the number of hair regrowing after a treatment regime. Indeed, many patients experience partial regrowth of hair on their treated areas in the years following their last treatment. This means that although laser treatments with these devices will permanently reduce the total number of body hair, they will not result in a permanent removal of all hair.

Improvements in lasers since 1997, in terms of more effective means of epidermal cooling and ergonomically-designed handpieces, have made treatment more tolerable for both patient and operator and reduced the chances of side effects. Ongoing clinical research has led to more optimized treatment parameters, but understanding of lasers and their long-term effects on hair and other skin structures are still in the early stages.

In 2008, two manufacturers launched FDA-approved laser hair removal devices for at-home use that are compact and portable. Ever since, many more such devices have been launched in the market. These are low energy devices. Eye protection remains a major area of concern for these home use devices.

Hair Growth Cycle

Relevant Basics of Hair Anatomy and Physiology

Hair has a well-described growth cycle. Each hair follicle consists of a permanent (upper) and nonpermanent (lower) part, with the follicular bulge forming the lowermost aspect of the permanent part.

Anagen: In periods of active growth, the rapidly developing bulbar matrix cells differentiate into the hair shaft and the hair lengthens. Anagen hairs, if pulled, have a white glistening dot. Plucking of anagen hairs is painful.

Catagen: A transition period follows in which the bulbar part of the hair follicle undergoes degradation through apoptosis. The glistening root of anagen hair is replaced by small, dark bulb "club-hair". Telogen hairs are painless on plucking.

Telogen: A resting period (telogen phase) ensues with hair eventually falling out, and regrowth is started once again in early anagen.

The hairs are fully loaded with melanin only in anagen phase of development and thus are susceptible to injury. During a particular point of time, not all hair are in anagen phase, hence multiple treatments are necessary to treat all the hair follicles. Laser works on the hair in the anagen phase. The spacing between the sessions is done on the basis of the hair cycle particularly telogen duration of that particular area (Table 6.1).

Recently, a marker of follicular stem cells (keratin 15) has been identified and noted to be detectable using immunohistochemical techniques. In addition, several other immunohistochemical markers for various components of the hair follicle are available.

An ideal patient is the one with coarse, dark, terminal hair in absence of underlying hormonal imbalance and has realistic expectations (Figs. 6.1 and 6.2).

Table 6.1: Regional variation in the percentage of hair in the anagen phase.

Body area	% Telogen hair	% Anagen hair	Telogen duration	Follicles density (1/cm^2)	Depth of follicle
Scalp	13	85	3–4 months	350	3–5 mm
Beard	30	70	10 weeks	500	2–4 mm
Upper lip	35	65	6 weeks	500	1–2.5 mm
Axillae	70	30	3 months	65	3.5–4.5 mm
Trunk				70	2–4.5 mm
Pubic area	70	30	12 weeks	70	3.5–4.5 mm
Arms	80	20	18 weeks	80	
Legs and thighs	80	20	24 weeks	60	2.5–4 mm
Breasts	70	30		65	3–4.5 mm

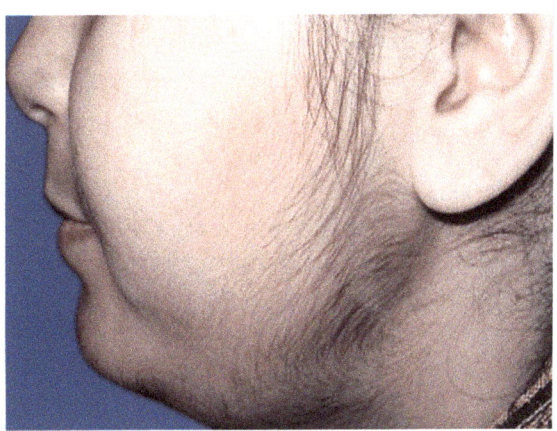

Fig. 6.1: An ideal patient with dark terminal hair.

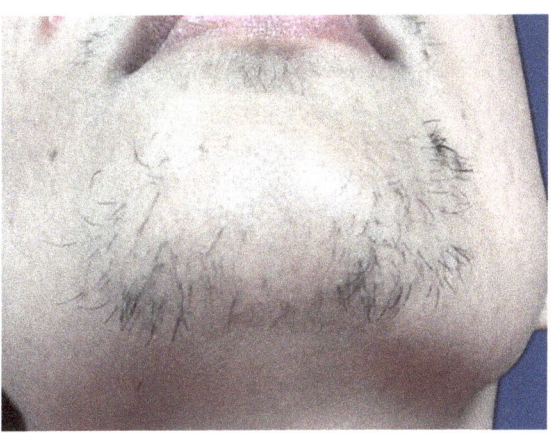

Fig. 6.2: A patient with coarse thick black hair on the chin, an ideal case for laser intervention.

INDICATIONS OF LASER HAIR REDUCTION

- Unwanted body hair in individuals with more than 15 years of age [Indian Association of Dermatologists, Venereologists and Leprologists (IADVL) task force recommendation].
- Hirsutism.
- *Male hair reduction*: This is an emerging subset of patients who want hair removal for various body regions like ears, malar area, glabella, beard shaping, chest, back, fingers, nasal area, etc.
- Hair reduction in transgenders.
- *For special conditions*: Pseudofolliculitis barbae and pilonidal sinus.
- *Reconstructive flaps hair reduction*: Transfer of hair bearing pectoralis flap in aerodigestive tract may lead to dysphagia and halitosis due to hair, pudendal thigh flaps in vagina, scrotal flaps in urethral reconstruction may lead to functional impairment. Similarly, reconstruction of hair by temporal scalp flap, and breast reconstruction using transverse rectus abdominis muscle may also require hair reduction due to cosmetic concerns.

Hirsutism

Hirsutism is defined as the presence of terminal coarse hairs in females in a male pattern (androgen dependent) distribution as face, chest, linea alba, lower back, buttocks, and anterior thighs. Hirsutism results from androgenic effects on the pilosebaceous unit and is commonly associated with acne, hair loss, and oily skin. In addition to being a source of social embarrassment, hirsutism may also be a cutaneous sign of a systemic disease. It affects around 5–10% of women overall. Given the subjectiveness of this perception, Ferriman and Gallwey developed a scoring system. Nine body areas are used to grade hair growth on a scale of 0–4. The scores for the 9 body parts are added, and a total score of 8 or more defines hirsutism.

Basic Definitions Pertaining to Hirsutism and Hair

- Adult hairs are of two types: (1) vellus and (2) terminal.
    1. Vellus hair can be found over the entire body and are nonmedullated, soft, fine, short hair that are nonpigmented or light pigmented.
    2. Terminal hairs are medullated, coarse, long and dark and are present on scalp, under arms, eyebrow, beard, chest, knuckles, and pubic region. The color derives from pigment keratin in the medulla of the hair shaft. Terminal hairs are ones, which respond to laser therapy.
- **Virilization** is extreme degree of hirsutism that may include male pattern balding, voice deepening, increased muscle bulk, and clitoral enlargement and is a sign of high and often rapid androgen production which suggests an androgen-secreting tumor.

- **Clitoromegaly** is defined as clitoral diameter greater than 4 mm.
- **Sexual ambiguity** in female; the most sensitive manifestation is beginning fusion of the labioscrotal folds at the posterior commissure or fourchette.

Hypertrichosis

Definition

Hypertrichosis is nonhirsute excessive hair growth over and above the normal for age, sex, and race of any person. Hypertrichosis can be generalized or localized, congenital and acquired.

Acquired hypertrichosis hair is usually unpigmented vellus hair but may be pigmented terminal hair also.

- *Causes of acquired generalized hypertrichosis*:
  - Malignancy associated (malignant down)—hair may be see on nose and eyelids
  - Porphyria
  - POEMS syndrome
  - Drugs
  - Hypothyroidism
  - Juvenile dermatomyositis
  - Central nervous system-related disorders (head injury, anorexia nervosa, schizophrenia, and after encephalitis)
  - Malabsorption syndromes
- *Causes of acquired localized hypertrichosis*:
  - Becker's nevus
  - Site of immunization
  - Stasis/lymphedema
  - Congenital AV-fistula
  - Repeated trauma
  - Reflex sympathetic dystrophy
  - HIV.

Several congenital disorders are associated with hypertrichosis and are present at birth. Most common among them is congenital hypertrichosis lanuginosa. Both localized as well as generalized congenital hypertrichosis is known and lasers offer a good treatment solution for them.

Approach to a Case of Female Presenting with Excess Hair

Hirsutism can be due to many causes; broadly classified into gonadal hyperandrogenism, adrenal hyperandrogenism, and other causes including drugs, lifestyle factors, and idiopathic (Flowchart 6.1) and thus need a thorough clinical, biochemical, and radiological examination wherever indicated.

Flowchart 6.1: Hirsutism.

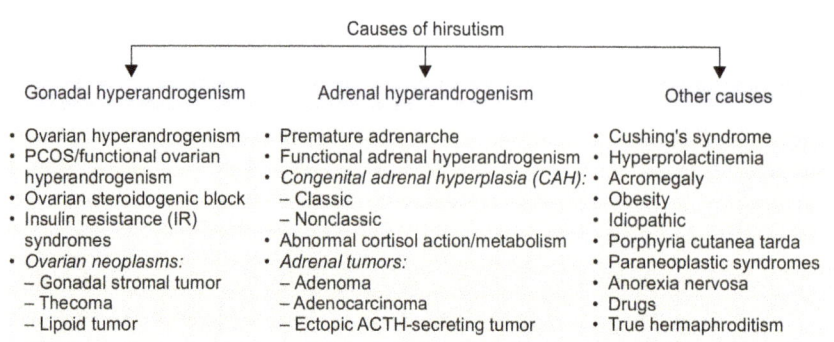

Hirsutism is most often the consequence of androgen excess associated with polycystic ovarian disease (PCOD) which is also the most common cause encountered by clinical practitioner, with idiopathic hirsutism being the second most common cause. Latter is likely caused by subtle forms of ovarian or adrenal hypersecretion, alterations in serum androgen-binding proteins or androgen metabolism, or excessive genetic sensitivity of hair follicles to normal androgen levels.

Many females who complain of hirsutism are endocrinologically normal. Thus in order for long-term treatment, establishing the cause and formulation of treatment plans is of utmost importance (Flowchart 6.2, Boxes 6.1 and 6.2).

Box 6.1: Drugs causing hirsutism.

A. *Vellus hair:*
- Cyclosporine
- Minoxidil
- Diazoxide
- Penicillamine
- Interferon
- Phenytoin
- Cetuximab
- Dexamethasone

B. *Terminal hair:*
- Cyclosporine
- Minoxidil
- Diazoxide
- Androgen creams, patches, tablets or injections
- Progestins
- Estrogen antagonists (tamoxifen and clomiphene)
- Oral contraceptives (OCs) that contain levonorgestrel, norethindrone, and norgestrel induce more powerful androgen activity, while those that include ethynodiol diacetate, norgestimate, and desogestrel have lesser androgenic activity
- Reserpine
- Metoclopramide

Flowchart 6.2: Approach to a case of female with excess hair.

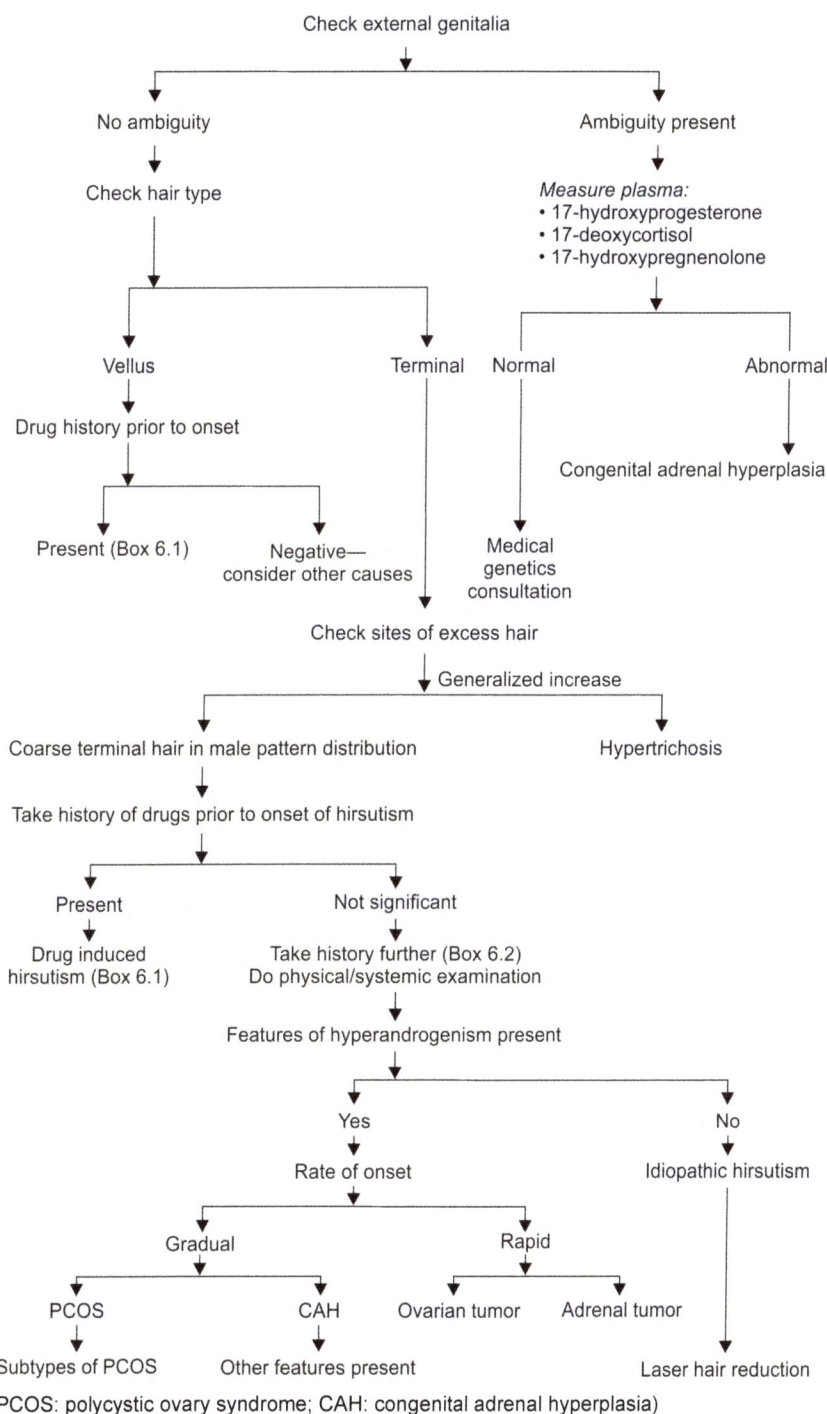

(PCOS: polycystic ovary syndrome; CAH: congenital adrenal hyperplasia)

Box 6.2: Clinical approach to hirsutism.

History points
- Onset of menarche ⎤
- Age of thelarche
- Onset of hirsutism
- Menstrual irregularities ⎬ PCOS
- Weight loss/gain
- Increase in libido
- Hoarseness of voice
- Hair fall ⎦

- Family h/o infertility/PCOS/hirsutism → PCOS/CAH (nonclassic)
- Easy bruising tendency → Cushing's syndrome
  Weakness

Drugs ——————————————→ Drug-induced hirsutism
Galactorrhea ————————————→ Hyperprolactinemia/hypothyroidism

Clinical examination
- Ambiguity of external genitalia ———— Virilizing forms of CAH

- Oily skin ⎤
- Acne
- Male pattern baldness
- Deepening of voice ⎬ Features of hyperandrogenism
- Increased muscle mass
- Clitoral enlargement > 4 mm diameter
- Evidence of fusion of posterior labioscrotal folds ⎦

- Hypertension ⎤
- Striae ⎬ Cushing's syndrome
- Centripetal weight gain ⎦

- Centripetal weight gain with scant
  s/c adipose tissue in upper ⎬ Lipodystrophy
  and lower extremities

- BMI >25 kg/m^2
       >30 kg/m^2 is taken as marks of hyperandrogenemia

- ↑BP Acanthosis nigricans ⎤
       Skin tags   ⎬ IR or androgen excess
- Ferriman-Gallwey score ————→ 8 ± Pustular/resistant comedones
                                Acne on jawline – ↑ androgens

(PCOS: polycystic ovary syndrome; CAH: congenital adrenal hyperplasia).

First of all, determining the type of hair, vellus or terminal is important. Drugs can be a cause of both vellus and terminal hirsutism. Anabolic steroids, testosterone, and glucocorticosteroids are said to be the most common drugs causing hirsutism, thus careful history and withdrawal of offending drug with reduction of hair leads to satisfactory treatment in most cases.

BASIC PRINCIPLES OF LASER HAIR REDUCTION

Laser-assisted hair removal was introduced to reduce hair from large body areas with minimum possible side effects. Laser hair removal can be done in three possible ways; nonselective laser injury, photodynamic therapy (PDT), and selective photothermolysis. Selective photothermolysis is the preferred treatment modality in present times.

Selective Photothermolysis

The concept of selective photothermolysis introduced by Parish and Anderson in the 1980s redefined the way in which lasers are performed.

Selective photothermolysis states that selective thermal damage to a pigmented target structure will occur when a specific wavelength is delivered at a sufficient fluence level during a time equal to or less than the thermal relaxation time (TRT) of the target.

Photothermal destruction of hair follicles is based on the concept of selective photothermolysis. Thus, the concept of **thermal damage time (TDT)** has, therefore, been introduced for hair removal wherein pulse durations are longer than the TRT, allowing dissipation of thermal damage to the follicular stem cells.

Laser emits light on the skin surface, which is reflected, scattered, transmitted or absorbed. At red to near-red infrarange of electromagnetic radiation (600–1,100 nm), the absorbed light heats the target chromophores in the skin.

The hair follicle is unique in that there is a spatial separation of melanin (chromophore) within the hair shaft and the biological target "stem cells" in the **bulge**. For most people, the bulb is approximately **4 mm** beneath the surface of skin, can be deeper in some individuals. Therefore, a considerable laser penetration depth is required to remove the bulb. However, recent evidence suggests that the goal of laser hair removal is to damage cells in the **outer root sheath**, which requires diffusion of heat from melanin in the hair shaft.

Ideal Wavelength

Melanin absorbs light broadly across the optical spectrum ranging from 250 nm to 1,200 nm. In wavelengths less than 690 nm oxyhemoglobin becomes a strong competing chromophore and above 1,000 nm, affinity of light for water increases significantly. Hence, **690–1,000 nm** becomes the optimum wavelength for lasers targeting melanin in hair follicles.

While melanin affinity for light is higher at 690 nm, safety becomes an issue at such low wavelengths, especially in dark-skinned individuals as the epidermal melanin also has a high probability of absorbing light and causing burns. Longer wavelengths have deeper penetration, hence these reach the bulb and bulge area of the hair and are safe even in dark-skinned individuals. Hence, the wavelengths ranging from **800 nm to 1,000 nm** are considered **optimum** for hair reduction in *dark-skinned* individuals.

Selecting Important Parameters

A unique issue with all lasers, so relevant to pigmented skin, is that all lasers have to traverse the epidermis, which is by no means an optical window, hence, the epidermis faces the brunt of the optical energy. In Indian skin, the pigment attenuates the energy. Thus, the ideal laser patient is the Western or the Southeast Asian skin type, with thick and pigmented hair. One option is to use intensive cooling systems and high energy.

An overview of the ideal parameters is given in Table 6.2 and are discussed further.

Table 6.2: Ideal parameters for laser hair removal.

Thin and light hair	Higher fluence
Thick hair skin type V-VII	Lower fluence
Thin hair	Short pulse duration (7–10 ms)
Thick hair	Increase pulse duration (30–40 ms)
Large areas	Higher "spot size"

Sources:
1. Dawber RP. Guidance for the management of hirsutism. Curr Med Res Opin. 2005;21:1227-34.
2. Dierickx C. Laser-assisted hair removal: state of the art. Dermatol Ther. 2000;13:80-9.
3. Macedo F. Luz intense pulsada versus laser. In: Mateus A, Palermo E (Eds). Cosmiatria e Laser: Prática no consultório médico. São Paulo: GEN; 2012. pp. 508-18.

Wavelength

Shorter wavelengths are absorbed more strongly by melanin than longer wavelengths. Longer wavelengths penetrate deeper and are safer to use in individuals with darker skin types. Accordingly, shorter wavelengths can be used for patients with fair skin types and longer wavelengths for patients with darker skin types at the risk of adverse effects.

Thus, a wavelength ranging from 600 nm to 1,000 nm of the electromagnetic spectrum can penetrate to the appropriate depth of the dermis (up to 2–4 mm) and cause selective photothermolysis of the target chromophore, which is the melanin pigment of hair follicle.

Pulse Duration

Thermal relaxation time of human terminal hair follicles is estimated to vary between 10 ms and 100 ms, depending on the size of the hair. The ideal pulse duration should be longer than the TRT for the epidermis (3-10 ms) and adjusted to the TRT/TDT for hair follicles. Devices for hair removal, therefore, operate with pulse durations in the long millisecond range, and the pulse durations between 10 ms and 50 ms is optimal to target hair follicles. Super long pulse heating (>100 ms) may allow for long-term hair removal.

Fine/thin hair need shorter pulse widths as compared to coarse/dense hair who need longer pulse widths. For example, with the light sheer desire pulse width can vary from auto mode (5-30 ms) to 30 ms to 100 ms.

Fluence

Optimum fluence or energy is such, which would cause effective thermal destruction of the hair follicle melanin without causing any damage to the epidermis. This would be different for different individuals depending on the skin and hair type. This is the most important parameter responsible for long-term reduction achieved with lasers.

Highest tolerable fluence gives better results by causing effective thermal destruction of hair follicle melanin in the dermis but heat damage to the epidermal melanin, which may result in adverse effects of burns, blistering, dyspigmentation and scarring, especially in dark-skinned patients. Maximum tolerated fluence is generally inversely proportional to melanin content in skin for a given pulse width.

Spot Size

A small spot size is useful for doing small areas such as upper lips, side locks, etc. A larger spot size has better penetration and is more comfortable and quick for large body parts. Larger the spot size of the laser beam, deeper and more even is the penetration.

Skin Cooling

This is one aspect of lasers and light devices, which is being constantly improved. Adequate skin cooling significantly increases the patient comfort, decreases the chances of burns and improves the results as higher energy levels can be delivered to the patient safely.

Cooling mechanism: Cooling can be obtained before, during, and after laser treatment (pre-, parallel level, and post-cooling) as contact cooling (cooled sapphire, metal or glass plates integrated into the handpiece, cooled gel layer); cold air ventilation; and dynamic cooling devices when pulsed cryogen spray is used as a cooling agent.

The various methods of *cooling* include:

Cryogen sprays: These are more useful when working with low pulse width lasers.

Chill tip cooling: This is now seen in majority of the lasers. The temperature of chill tip is 4°C before and after shot and 0°C during the shot. This is a very practical and convenient means of pre- and post- and cooling during the session.

Ice packs: These can be used for post-cooling while doing large body parts and also with the laser/light machines which do not come with the option of chill-tip cooling. Using of ice packs can be very cumbersome at times and are at best adjunctive measure.

Forced refrigerated air (Zimmer): This is now gaining popularity as means of cooling with all laser procedures including the LHR. It gives chilled air and can be used throughout the procedure to increase the patient comfort.

The least effective type of cooling is the use of an aqueous cold gel, which passively extracts heat from the skin and then is not capable of further skin cooling. Alternatively, cooling with forced chilled air can provide cooling to the skin before, during, and after a laser pulse. Currently, most of the available LHR devices have a built-in skin cooling system, which consists of either contact cooling or dynamic cooling with a cryogen spray.

Contact cooling, usually with a sapphire tip, provides skin cooling just before and during a laser pulse. It is most useful for treatments with longer pulse durations (>10 ms). Dynamic cooling with cryogen liquid spray pre-cools the skin with a millisecond spray of cryogen just before the laser pulse. A second spray can be delivered just after the laser pulse for post-cooling, but parallel cooling during the laser pulse is not possible as the cryogen spray interferes with the laser beam. Dynamic cooling is best suited for use with pulse durations shorter than 5 ms.

Compression

Compression with handpiece reduces competing chromophore, oxyhemoglobin. It blanches vessels, which eliminates energy lost into target. Moreover, compression helps to ensure that the hair follicle is localized closer to the surface targeted by laser light.

HAIR REMOVAL: AN EVIDENCE-BASED OUTLOOK

Various studies have reported on the efficacy of different laser systems to reduce hair growth, and reduction in the number of hair counts is the end point most often evaluated. To make meaningful comparisons between treatments, it is important to consider under which circumstances the treatment results are reported, because huge diversities are seen in terms of study design (randomized and nonrandomized controlled studies, uncontrolled studies, retrospective studies, and case reports); patient inclusion; treatment settings, including specific devices; number of treatment sessions; and follow-up periods.

To demonstrate the true effectiveness of laser and IPL devices, two definitions can be employed:

Hair reduction estimated up to 6 months after treatment is considered as *"short-term efficacy"* and beyond 6 months postoperatively as *"long-term efficacy."*

Results of Laser Hair Reduction

Evidence for Short-term Efficacy (up to 6 Months after Epilation)

Substantial evidence exists for a short-term efficacy of hair removal up to 6 months after treatment with the ruby laser, alexandrite laser, diode laser, Nd:YAG laser, and IPL.

The efficacy is improved when repetitive treatments are given and there is considerable evidence that the short-term efficacy from photoepilation is superior to conventional treatments with shaving, wax epilation, and electrolysis.

Overall, the short-term efficacy is reported between **30% and 70%** hair reductions up to 6 months **after** the last treatment; the treatment outcomes depend on the treatment settings.

Evidence for Long-term Efficacy (Beyond 6 Months after Epilation)

Evidence was found for a long-term efficacy of hair removal after repetitive treatments with the alexandrite laser, the diode laser, and the long-pulsed Nd:YAG laser. It may be possible that repetitive treatments with the ruby laser (3–4 treatments) and IPL (5 treatments) are capable of inducing long-term hair reduction as well, although the actual evidence is sparse. The overall results from long-term studies with the alexandrite, diode, and Nd:YAG laser vary a lot, but show on average a **50%** hair reduction from repetitive treatments with these devices (*see* Table 6.3).

Hair Removal Devices

The current market for LHR is growing so rapidly that the FDA has not maintained an up-to-date listing of all approved laser devices. Currently used lasers fall into one of four categories: The long-pulsed ruby laser (694 nm), the long-pulsed alexandrite laser (755 nm), the long-pulsed semiconductor diode laser (800–810 nm), and the long-pulsed Nd:YAG laser (1,064 nm). Additionally, the IPL system (515–1,200 nm) is approved as a safe and effective method for hair reduction. ELOS has been used but is not as effective as other systems (Figs. 6.3 and 6.4).

Other devices that have not been included in the Table 6.3, include fluorescent pulse light, optical light energy combined with RF (eMax/eLight of Syneron), and diode combined with RF (eLaser Syneron and MeDiostar Effect Asclepion).

Home Use Devices

They have recently gained popularity due to the low cost involved and convenience of the patient. Home use devices have their own set of safety concerns as they are being used by untrained professionals.

Table 6.3: Overview of some of the Food and Drug Administration (FDA) approved devices for hair removal.

Laser	Devices	Patient type	Hair reduction	Hair removal
Long-pulsed ruby lasers (694 nm)	E2000 Epitouch Ruby Ruby Star Sinon	I–III (SPT) Hair: Dark to light brown Fine and coarse	38–49% hair reduction	Long-term hair removal
Long-pulsed alexandrite lasers (755 nm)	Apogee Arion Epicare Epitouch ALEX Gentelase Ultrawave II/III	I–IV (SPT) Hair: Dark to light brown Fine and coarse	74–78% hair reduction	Long-term hair removal
Pulsed diode laser (800 nm)	Apex-800 F1 Diode Laser LightSheer MedioStar SLP 1000 Soprano Ice (diode plus alexandrite) (see Fig. 6.3)	I–IV (SPT) Hair: Dark to light, brown and coarse	70–84% hair reduction	Long-term hair removal
Long-pulsed Nd:YAG lasers (1,064 nm)	Acclaim 7000 Athos CoolGlide (see Fig 6.4) Dualis Gentle Yag Lyra Mydon Profile Smartepil II Ultrawave I/II/III Varia Vasculight Elite	I–VI (SPT) dark and coarse hair	29–53% hair reduction	Long-term hair removal
Intense pulsed light source (515–1,200 nm)	Ellipse EpiLight Estelux PhotoLight ProLite Quadra Q4 Quantum HR Spatouch SpectraPulse	I–VI (SPT) Dark to light brown and coarse hair	49–90% hair reduction	Long-term hair removal

Home-based devices are based on IPL and laser technologies but operate at lower fluences than comparable in-office devices. The 810-nm diode Tria laser (Tria Beauty, Inc, Dublin, CA) and 475 to 1,200 nm IPL Silk'n device (Home Skinovations, Kfar Saba, Israel) are the current FDA-approved home use hair removal systems.

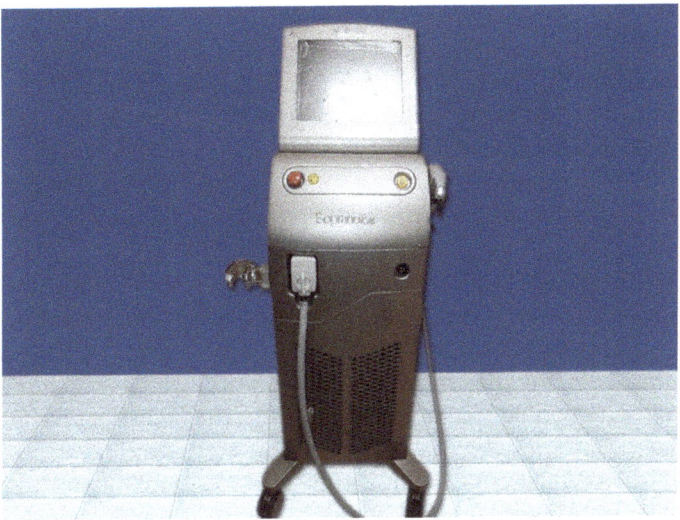

Fig. 6.3: Soprano ICE laser.

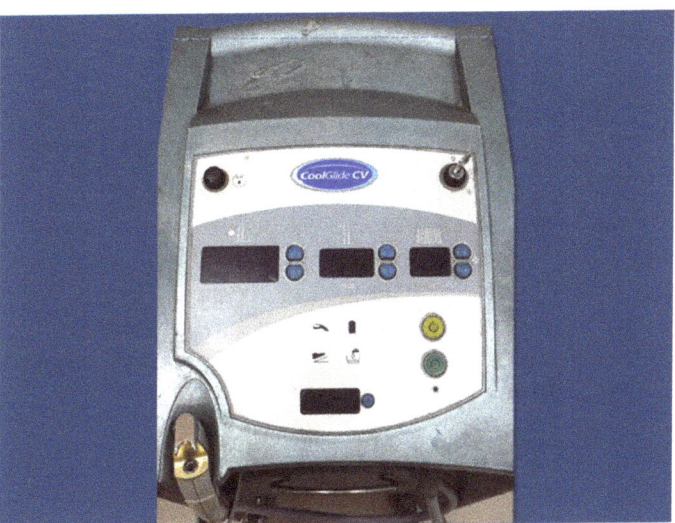

Fig. 6.4: Long-pulsed neodymium-doped: yttrium aluminum garnet (Nd:YAG) 1,064 nm—CoolGlide laser, with parameters to be set fluence and pulse duration.

One safety feature on most home-use devices is a skin contact sensor that prevents the beam from firing when not on the skin. Light is supposedly self-contained within the device, and special protective goggles are not required, but if eye precautions are breached, irreversible corneal burns, lens cataracts, and retinal damage may result. Aside from ocular damage, unintentional misuse by individuals with darker skin type or a tan or inappropriate treatment of moles or tattoos may lead to thermal burns.

Ideal Lasers

The literature on this is varied and most clinicians would prefer one over the other. In the absence of any comparative trials from India, a summary of the present data is summarized here:

- **Diode** and **alexandrite** lasers are considered, in general, the most effective for hair removal, followed by IPL and Nd:YAG devices (Campos and Pitassi 2012).
- For SPT I-V, the diode laser (800 nm) is the ideal laser (Campos et al. 2000). The pulse duration varies between 5 ms and 400 ms and their fluences, in general, between 10 J and 60 J.
- For **thin hair**, the **Alexandrite laser** (755 nm) which has shorter pulse durations than diode laser is better. This is better suited for the fairer skin types.
- The **Nd:YAG** (1,064 nm) with its inherent lower affinity for melanin is ideal for **richly pigmented skin**.
- **Intense pulsed light** for its merits of emitting shorter wavelengths that do not penetrate so deeply into the skin, are believed to be safer to use in fairer skin types but is found to be better for thin light hair (Campos and Pitassi 2012).

PROCEDURE

Preoperative

- *Patient counseling, and informed consent*: The patient should be clearly informed in the beginning and before every subsequent session that the laser would ensure delay of growth, decrease the number of hair and make the hair finer but it will not cause removal of all the hair.

    The patient has to be informed regarding the gap between the sessions (according to the body part being treated).

    In between the sessions, the patient can theoretically use hair removing creams or shave the area. The authors preferably avoid using hair removal creams as irritant reactions are very common.

    The patient should also be informed regarding the number of sessions, session time, requirement of maintenance sessions, side effects encountered, and the total cost of the procedure. In case of any hormonal imbalances, concomitant therapy may be needed.

- *History and examination*: A detailed history including age of onset of hair growth, menstrual history, and any concomitant drug intake should be taken (Box 6.2). Any previous treatments taken for the same should be recorded. If the patient is suspected to be having hirsutism due to underlying polycystic ovarian disease, a complete work up should be done including the ultrasound pelvis to rule out PCOD along with hormonal profile. An endocrinological opinion can be sought for the same, if required. Appropriate medical therapy should be initiated and patient should be informed regarding the more number of sessions that would be required and also for reduction in efficacy results due to PCOD. Patients with a sudden onset of hypertrichosis should be evaluated for paraneoplastic etiologies.

History of any photosensitizing drugs, colloid, and hypertrophic scars, history of recent sun exposure and tanning, parlor activities, occupations involving prolonged exposure to sun, history of herpes simplex in treatment area should be recorded. Patient should be asked regarding photosensitive conditions, such as the autoimmune connective tissue disorders, or disorders prone to the Koebner phenomenon. A history of recurrent cutaneous infections at or in the vicinity of treatment area might warrant the use of prophylactic medications. History of hair dye application in male beard should be also taken to exclude any white/gray hair.

Topical retinoids used in the treatment area should be discontinued at least **4 days** prior to treatment. There are divided opinions regarding use of oral retinoids along with laser treatment. Majority of clinicians recommend a washout period of 6 months to 1 year after stopping the drug. However, authors have not seen any side effects with concomitant use of low dose retinoid.

The patient is assessed for the Fitzpatrick skin type, as darker skin types are more prone to adverse effects related to laser therapy, e.g. burns or postinflammatory hyperpigmentation.

Examination is done for the presence of tan. If present, the treatment should be deferred till subsidence of tan. Tanned type 4 skin is more prone to burns than type 5 skin. All topical depigmenting and exfoliating creams should be discontinued **3 days** prior to treatment.

One of the most important steps in evaluation of patient for LHR is assessment of patient's hair color. It is important as the chromophore for LHR is melanin. Black and brown hairs contain sufficient amounts of melanin to serve as a chromophore for LHR. In contrast, the lack of melanin, paucity of melanin, or presence of eumelanin in the hair follicle, which clinically correlates to white or gray, is predictive of a poor response to LHR. Treatment should be also deferred, if patient's hair are bleached.

- The individual's skin type, hair color, and hair coarseness are important as these factors will determine which device is most suitable (Table 6.4).
- *Investigations*: Ideally all females with hirsutism in the reproductive age group should be investigated between 2 days and 5 days of cycle.

Free testosterone is usually the best marker but, as this requires sensitive assays, is rarely reliable.

17 α-OH-progesterone test done during the luteal phase, is good for investigating females with normal cycles with a suspicion of NCCAH.

Table 6.4: Laser source, skin type, hair color, and hair thickness of individual patient.

Laser source	Skin type	Hair color	Hair thickness
Normal mode ruby	I–III	Dark to light brown	Fine and coarse
Normal mode alexandrite	I–IV	Dark to light brown	Fine and coarse
Pulsed diode	I–IV	Dark to light brown	Coarse
Normal mode Nd: YAG	I–VI	Dark to light brown	Coarse
Q switched Nd: YAG	I–VI	Dark to light brown	Fine
IPL	I–VI	Dark to light brown	Coarse

The LH:FSH ratio of 1.6 or more has been proposed to be a marker for evolving PCOS, especially in young females, but is not useful in obese PCOS patients and NIH criteria has *removed* it from the preferred tests for diagnosing PCOS.

The AMH with a value of more than five is a highly reliable and sensitive marker for PCOS and does not require the bother of USG. This can replace the LH/FSH ratio which is considered unreliable in obese PCOS case. Altered ratio is also a marker for end-organ hypersensitivity. The only issue is that it is better in older females (>25 years) and there may be an interassay difference.

Ultrasonographic string of pearl appearance is considered a useful investigation.

- *General advice to patients*: The patients are advised not to carry out parlor activity like waxing, threading, plucking or bleach **3 weeks** before the first session and in between the sessions. Use of hair removing creams should be discouraged due to the chances of irritant reaction. The patients are allowed to shave in between the sessions.

  The patients can use bleach with 2 months gap before and after the session, when the gap between sessions is more than 3 months and during the maintenance phase. Ideally, bleach can be recommended only during the maintenance phase. Patient should also be counseled regarding laser hair shedding.
- *Informed consent*: A detailed consent form should be developed which should include details regarding the procedure, the expected results and rare side effects that can be expected with the treatment. The consent form should be get signed before every session.
- *Pre- and post-procedure photographs*: Keeping a photographic pre-, post-procedure, and in-between sessions in comparable setting is important. It helps the patient as well as the treating physician to compare the response/nonresponse. TrichoScan images can prove to be extremely useful for monitoring the results.
- Patient's records should be updated including the exact area treated, skin and hair type, the fluence used and wavelengths used during all sessions and treatment response.

- Patients should be aware that the average number of hair removal treatments to achieve a significant reduction of hair is between **five and seven** performed at 1-3 months intervals.

Intraoperative

Topical Anesthesia

Topical anesthetic creams are available. They are used especially for sensitive areas, e.g. pubic region. However, the authors do not prefer the use of topical anesthetic preparations as they have a high potential of causing irritant reactions and subsequently burns with laser. They also increase the cost of a given session and the time required to complete a session. Also cooling is a very effective alternative.

The need for topical anesthesia is variable among patients and anatomic sites. Various topical anesthetics including lidocaine, lidocaine/prilocaine, and other amide/ester anesthetic combinations can be used to diminish the procedural discomfort, and should be applied 30 minutes to 1 hour before treatment under occlusion. Care should be taken when using lidocaine or prilocaine to apply these medications to a limited area to diminish the risk of lidocaine toxicity or methemoglobinemia, respectively. Deaths have resulted from lidocaine toxicity resulting from occlusion of the back as well as lower extremities with topical lidocaine. Likewise, systemic toxicity can occur with the use of any topical anesthetic in large amounts.

Calibration

The laser should be calibrated before treatment. Ideal treatment parameters must be individualized for each patient. The **largest** spot size and the **highest** tolerable fluence based on both pain and epidermal injury should be used.

Test Patch

A small test patch area should ideally be done before the first session to determine any skin reaction to the laser.

Procedure

Procedure is re-explained to the patient in brief. The skin is checked for any sensitive areas, to determine hair type, tanning or any cuts under adequate light with a magnifying glass. Patient should be instructed to wash the face to remove any dust and make-up. Depending on the area to be treated, the patient can be in a supine or sitting position chairs or adjustable operation tables.
- *Marking*: The area to be lased is marked with a white pencil under adequate light. Red pencil can be used with IPL. Small grids should be made for large areas. Marking should be reconfirmed in patients especially in beard shaping hair reduction procedure.

- *Shaving*: Cleansing gel is applied and the area is shaved taking care not to leave any hair behind and at the same time avoid any cuts on the skin due to vigorous shaving. Magnifying glass should be used to ensure proper shaving. Shaving against the direction of hair should be avoided (Figs. 6.5A and B). Site should be re-examined to see any hair left to avoid skin burn.
- *Cooling*: Pre-cooling, post-cooling, and cooling during the session are absolutely mandatory. Chill tip is very effective for this. Ice packs can be used for large body parts.
- *Gel application*: Cool gel in a thin layer needs to be applied in all lasers except the big handpiece of lightsheer duet.
- *Eye protection*: Patient and operator should wear glasses.
- *Parameters and procedure*:
  - The parameters are decided on the basis of hair and skin type (Figs. 6.5D to F).
  - The handpiece of the system should be placed perpendicularly to the skin surface and it should be pressed gently to displace blood from capillaries and to bring the hair follicle nearer to the aiming source (this is particularly important, if you are using Nd:YAG laser).
  - Overlapping of handpieces in treating adjacent areas (10%) in stamping mode is ideal as it avoids skipping of areas.
  - Cooled gauze packings should be used in adjacent areas to avoid paradoxical hair stimulation.
  - During treatment session, laser handpiece tip should be checked for any singed hair.
  - Cleaning of handpiece can be done with gauze piece moistened with distilled water.
  - Any melanocytic nevi in laser treated area should be covered with micropore.
  - Laser should be done around one-fourth inch away from tattoo border if any tattoo is present at treatment site.
  - Marked or confluent erythema, whitening, blistering, or purpura indicates acute epidermal injury from overly aggressive treatment. If there is a sign of epidermal damage, the fluence should be reduced by 20–30%.

Standard parameters of a representative device are detailed in Figures 6.5D to F.

Postoperative

Postprocedure Care

Positive clinical end points are perifollicular edema and erythema. There can be odor of singed hair or they can be visualized also. Patient can be given ice packs to cool the laser treated area. After cooling, sunscreen is applied on the site.

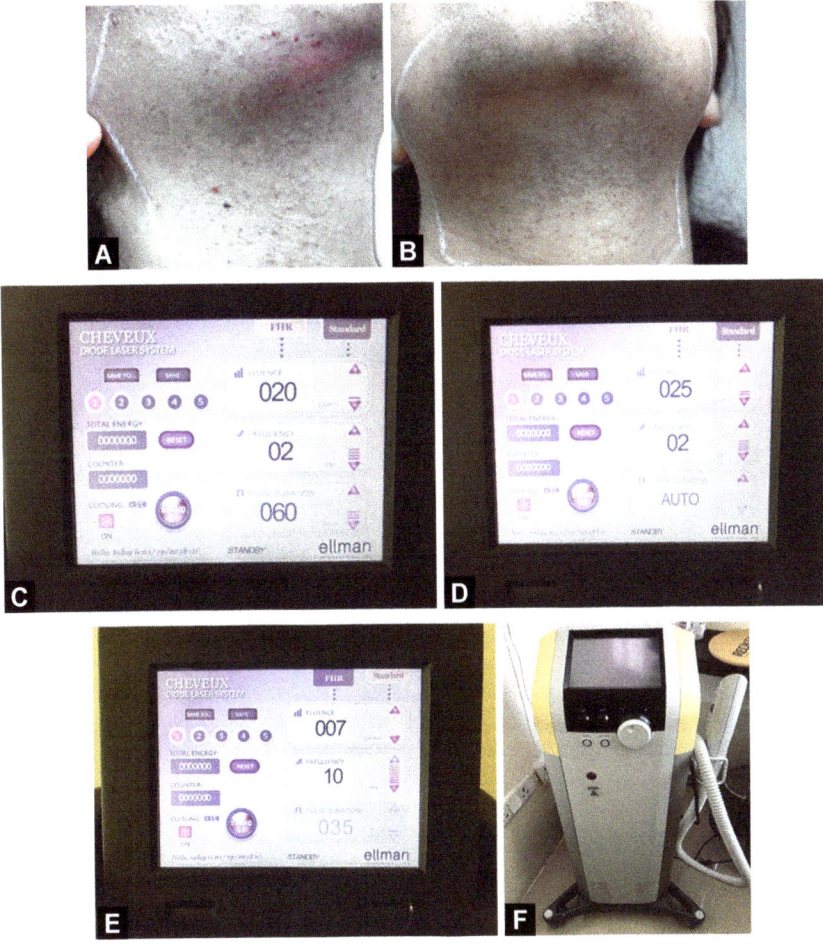

Figs. 6.5A to F: (A) Shaving against the "grain" leading to erythema and bleeding points; (B) Perifollicular redness postexcessive shaving—this is to be avoided before a hair removal sitting; (C) For fine hair use short pulse widths (3–7 ms) with long intervals (15–20 ms) and 2–3 pulses per shot. 1–2 passes; (D) Common settings for a new case, second setting 25 J/15 ms PW is for fine hair—single pass; (E) Settings (7 J/10 Hz/35 ms), this is the fast painless mode for body hair, it needs 2–4 passes per area; (F) BTL Exilite intense pulsed light (IPL) system, 640 nm (fair skin), 690 nm (dark skin). (*Courtesy:* Dr Vivek Nair, MD).

A steroid antibiotic cream can be used. Oral antiallergic or rarely oral steroids might be needed in case of a burn. All the patients are advised regular use of sunscreen and use of a moisturizing cream for 5 days after any laser session.

Patient Follow-up

The best time to evaluate the effect of laser session is 2–3 weeks post the session (Figs. 6.6 and 6.7).

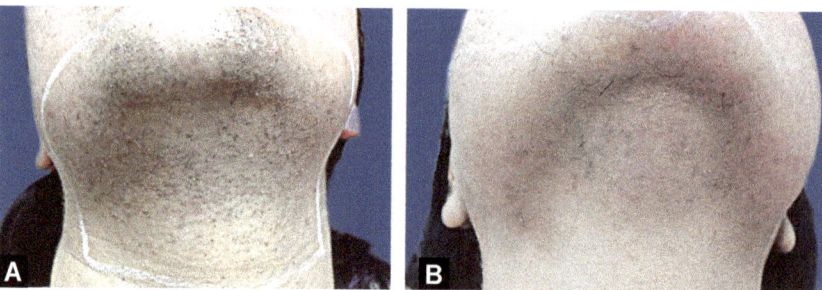

Figs. 6.6A and B: (A) A patient treated with long-pulsed neodymium-doped: yttrium aluminum garnet (Nd:YAG) laser; (B) Treatment response after 6 sessions of long-pulsed Nd:YAG laser.

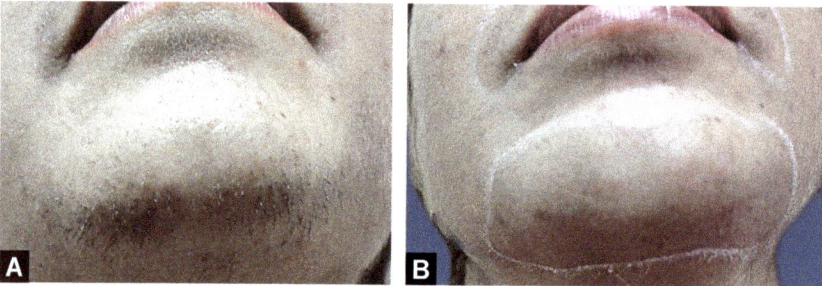

Figs. 6.7A and B: Treatment response after six sessions of long-pulsed neodymium-doped: yttrium aluminum garnet (Nd:YAG) laser. (A) Preoperative; and (B) Postoperative.

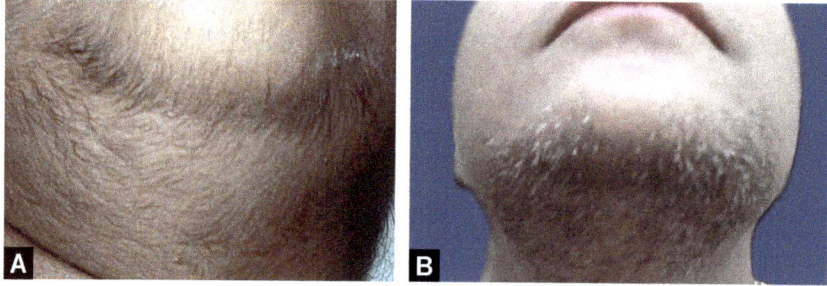

Figs. 6.8A and B: (A) A patient with a few gray hair it must be emphasized that the nonpigmented hairs are unresponsive; and (B) A patient with multiple gray hair, which is not a candidate for laser hair reduction (LHR).

Nonresponsive cases:
- Patients with fine (Fig. 6.8A), gray (Figs. 6.8B and 6.9A)/blonde/light brown hair have inadequate pigment in hair hence do not respond well.
- If very low fluences are used, patients do not get the desired response.
- Low energy machine which is not delivering the right energy is another factor for nonresponse.

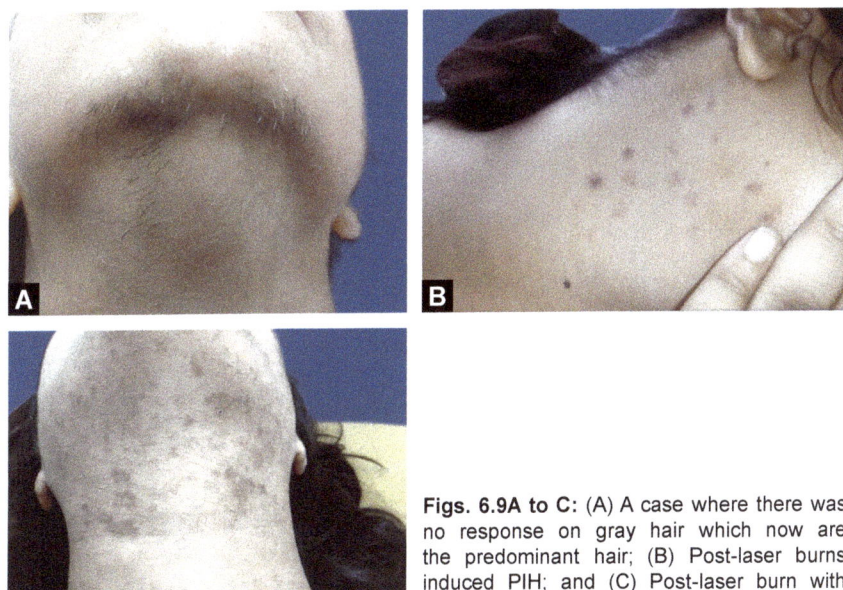

Figs. 6.9A to C: (A) A case where there was no response on gray hair which now are the predominant hair; (B) Post-laser burns induced PIH; and (C) Post-laser burn with hyperpigmentation.

- Underlying hormonal disturbances is also a reason for suboptimal response.
- Session done on patchy hair growth is also one of the common reason for nonresponse.

SIDE EFFECTS

In majority of cases, the side effects are transient and easily remediable. Sun protected regions are less likely to suffer from side effects as compared to photoexposed areas, e.g. face and arms.

- The *most common* skin reactions are pain during session, mild burning, transient erythema post-session, perifollicular erythema, acneiform eruptions, and folliculitis.
- In few cases, persistent erythema, vesiculation, crusting, hyperpigmentation, (Figs. 6.9B and C) hypopigmentation, and permanent scarring can occur. Pruritus may occur in rare cases.
- Thermal burns can occur which can be superficial or deep. This may result either from selecting a nonoptimal wavelength, pulse duration, fluence, nonfunctional epidermal cooling, or by treating a tanned patient. Superficial burns (Fig. 6.10) are more prone to occur in patients with tan, dry skin or rigorous shaving. They need counseling, mild topical steroids and moisturizers. If a patient has extreme burning sensation, there is high probability that a deep burn (Fig. 6.11) has occurred.

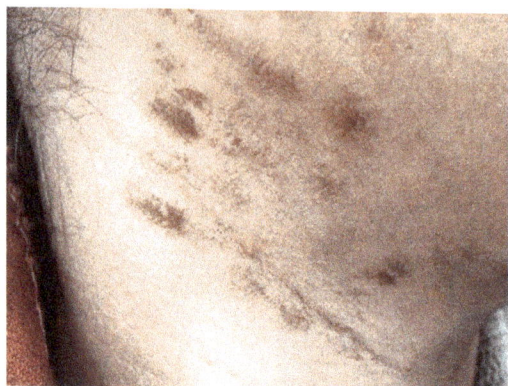

Fig. 6.10: Superficial laser burns, consequent to inadequate cooling.

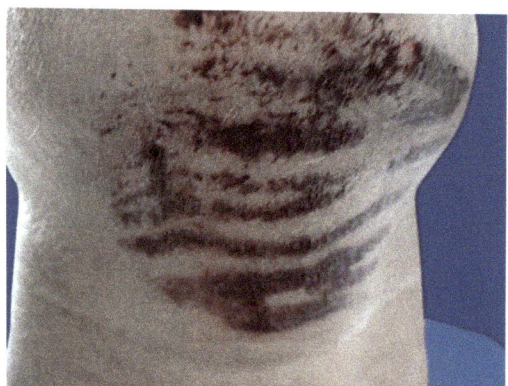

Fig. 6.11: Deep laser burns in a patient of laser hair removal.

For this, the patient should start oral steroids (dose of 1 mg/kg body weight) for 3 days. After 3 days, advice the patient to use a steroid antibiotic combination and bland moisturizers. Hyperpigmentation can be treated with mild agents such as topical vitamin C and strict sun protection. Acneform eruptions can be treated by giving antibiotic course.

- *Paradoxical hair stimulation* (Fig. 6.12) can occur as a side effect. Few patients have increased hair growth at sites surrounding previously treated sites or increase in hair growth over the treated site.
  a. Paradoxical hair stimulation is most commonly seen at chin and upper neck.
  b. It is seen more frequently in patients of skin types III or higher, more commonly with IPL and in an adjacent area of untreated skin.
  c. It is commonly reported in individuals with previously undiagnosed hormonal conditions, such as polycystic ovarian syndrome, emphasizing the importance of history taking and proper patient selection in laser hair removal.

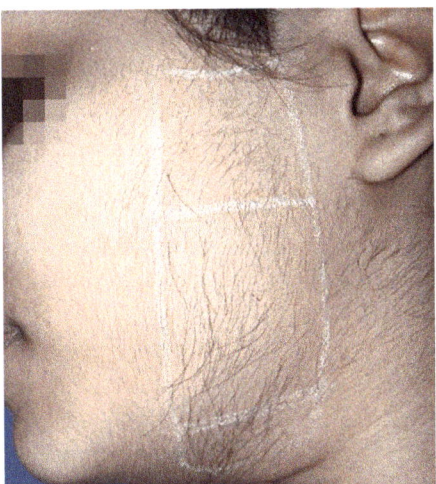

Fig. 6.12: Paradoxical hair stimulation seen in a pigmented skin patient.

    d. A lower-range fluence is also implicated in its causation. Use of higher fluences reduces this side effect.
    e. Increasing the area to be lased in the maintenance sessions is another very common cause of paradoxical hair stimulation.
    f. Inadequate cooling can also lead to paradoxical hair stimulation. Especially when working with IPL, the surrounding area should also be cooled as unlike lasers, IPL is not a coherent beam and heat can lead to increased hair growth.
    g. The treatment for paradoxical hypertrichosis is to continue laser hair removal and to increase the energy just a little bit.
- Ocular injury is another potential complication of laser hair removal.
- Acne aggravation, development of lesions similar to those of rosacea, early follicles depigmentation, diffuse erythema, and inflammatory or pigmentary changes of preexisting nevi are rare side effects.

PEARLS AND PITFALLS

Spacing between Sessions

Face

The authors recommend that the first two sessions can be done at an interval of 4–6 weeks to target the hair in the early anagen phase, after that the gap can be increased. This is as the resting phase of facial hair is around 4–6 weeks. One of the most prominent effects of laser is the prolongation of the resting phase. Hence, we recommend that the sessions should be spaced out from the third session itself to target the hair in the anagen phase. Preforming the sessions frequently might lead to a temporary suppression rather than destruction of hair follicle.

If large body parts are to be treated the authors recommend that the gap between first and sessions should be 6-8 weeks and gradually the gap can be further increased in subsequent sessions.

Maintenance Sessions

These are regular laser sessions done at frequency of 1-3 times per year. The frequency depends on the area treated and the response of laser sessions and associated medical condition.

Long Hair (Fig. 6.13)

This process is known to happen with all kinds of hair reduction technologies. The lased hair is pushed into a prolonged anagen phase. The patient should be informed about this in the beginning and proactively advised to use scissors to cut these long hairs in the maintenance phase.

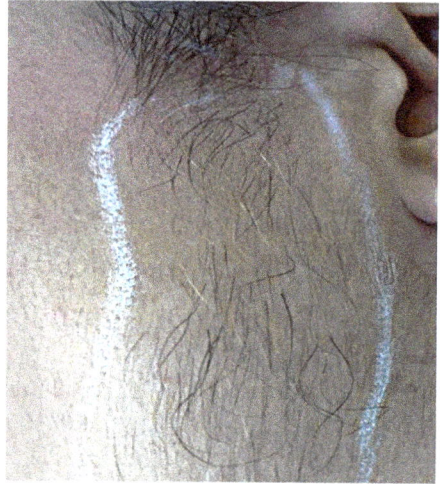

Fig. 6.13: Persisting long hair—a process known to occur with all kinds of hair reduction technologies.

SPECIAL SITUATIONS

Role of Eflornithine along with Laser Hair Reduction

The role of topical eflornithine is still controversial. It is being used by some practitioners in the maintenance phase to delay hair growth. Twice a day application is suggested and the results are usually seen after 4-6 weeks. This can lead to acne in patients with acne prone skin and it also significantly increases the cost of therapy for the patient.

Polycystic Ovarian Disorders and Laser Hair Reduction

In case of clinical signs suggestive of PCOD (like abnormal cycles, acne over lower face, obesity and thinning of frontal hair), a hormonal profile should be carried out between the second and fifth day of the cycle and an ultrasound of the lower abdomen is advised. As stated previously the AMH is a sensitive and specific test better than LH/FSH for diagnosing PCOS.

In cases where PCOD is documented, an endocrinological opinion should be sought. The patients are started on medical therapy followed by laser treatment from the second month onward ideally. Many practitioners start medical and laser therapy simultaneously. These patients should be counseled regarding the requirement of increased number of sessions and long-term efficacy results.

Laser and EBD for Gray Hair

Melanin is the chromophore targeted by laser. Gray hair lack melanin, hence, the treatment is unsuccessful. The patient should be informed in advance that these hairs will not respond to laser and as the number of black hair decreases, the patient would feel that number of gray hair has increased. Few gray hair can be managed by electrolysis. If the percentage of gray hair is **more than 50%,** laser should be avoided.

Removal of nonpigmented hairs with a combined light/bipolar radiofrequency device with or without pretreatment with a topical photosensitizer has shown little success. Integrated radiofrequency and optical energy technology might represent a new photoepilatory technique for the long-term removal of white hair. Although results may not be quite as efficient as with chromophore targeting primarily light-based technologies.

A recent alternative approach to treat white, blond and gray hair with laser hair removal has been the external application of melanin to the hair through the use of liposome technology. Melanin-encapsulated liposomes have demonstrated to selectively deliver melanin to the follicle and hair shaft. The effectiveness of these modalities for gray hair still needs to be proved.

Lasers for Fine Hair

In Indian skin due to the high melanin content and the risk of burns, very high energies cannot be used with any laser systems. For patients, who are left with fine hair after receiving a number of laser sessions, the **pulse width** needs to be decreased and **high fluence** levels are needed. Hence, patients with fine hair should be **dissuaded** for LHR.

Pseudofolliculitis

Laser hair reduction is a very effective treatment for pseudofolliculitis seen post-waxing in females and post-shaving in males. The laser should be done

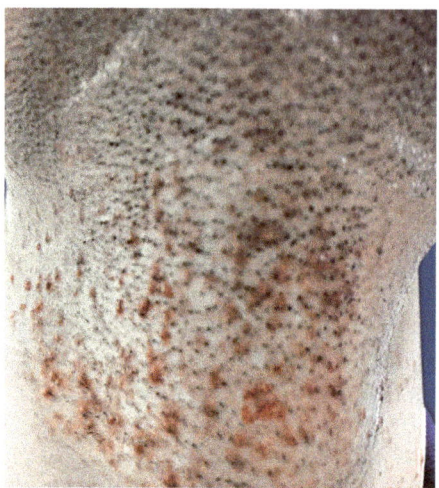

Fig. 6.14: Patient with pseudofolliculitis barbae treated with hair reduction lasers.

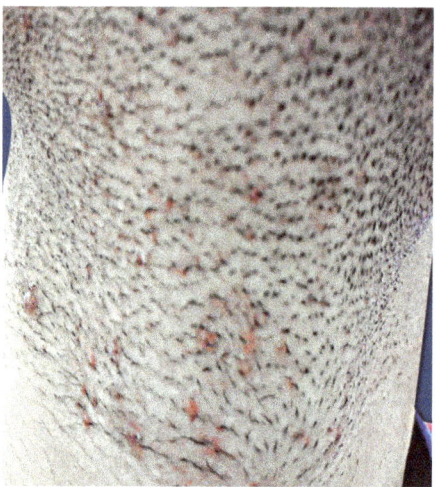

Fig. 6.15: Same patient after 2 months after first session with neodymium-doped: yttrium aluminum garnet (Nd:YAG) laser.

at low energy levels and usually 3–4 sessions are sufficient to make the hair **fine** and hence solve the problem of pseudofolliculitis (Figs. 6.14 and 6.15).

Lasers in Dark Skin Types

There are several characteristics, which make skin of dark color more susceptible to laser-related complications. There are several factors, which can be taken into account to minimize the complications:
- *Wavelength*: Use *longer* wavelengths as they are associated with less epidermal absorption and hence greater safety.

- *Treatment parameters*: Use **lower** (optimum) fluences and **longer** pulse durations for laser hair removal. These can be determined by doing a patch test.
- *Pre- and post-treatment advice*: *Sun protection* is an important aspect to prevent any complications, e.g. postinflammatory hyperpigmentation.
- *Epidermal cooling*: *Adequate* cooling is one of the key factors in determining the safety.
- *Topical corticosteroids*: Consider using in patients with post-treatment erythema or edema to reduce chances of postinflammatory hyperpigmentation.

Laser in Pregnant and Lactating Women

Treatment of a pregnant woman for nonurgent conditions is discouraged, although there is no evidence suggesting a potential risk to pregnant women undergoing LHR. The hormonal changes of pregnancy and breastfeeding may interfere with the results of laser hair removal. There are also concerns about hyperpigmentation that is more likely under the influence of hormones.

SAFETY ISSUES

Standard Precautionary Measures

Eye Protection

The recommended eye protection devices should be used at all times by any person present in the laser room.
- *Clinician's eyewear*: Appropriate protective eyeglasses according to the wavelength of laser being used have to be worn by the clinician.
- *Patient's eyewear*: Opaque or metal goggles, corneal shields, or protective wet eyepads should be used by the patient during the procedure.

The clinician/patient should never look directly into laser aperture, even when wearing laser safety glasses. Avoid directing laser beam anywhere other than within holster or at intended treatment area. Remove mirror-like surfaces from vicinity of laser beam path. Do not treat eyebrows, eyelashes, or other areas within bony area surrounding orbit.

Fire Protection

Flammable or explosives should not be used in the laser room. Acetone or alcohol-based skin preparations should not be used. Fire-retardant drapes and gowns should be used. Fire extinguisher and water should be readily available in the clinic.

Electrical Safety

Many lasers use high voltage and high current electrical power, ensure proper grounding. Proper cables should be used instead of extension cords.

Good wiring and proper stabilizers should be used. Appropriate room cooling should be there for better functioning of laser machines.

ADVANCES IN LHR

- *Pain-free lasers*: A novel technique to reduce LHR-associated pain is **pneumatic skin flattening (PSF)**. PSF works by coupling a vacuum chamber to generate negative pressure and to flatten the skin against the handpiece treatment window. Based on the gate theory of pain transmission, it stimulates pressure receptors in the skin immediately prior to firing of the laser pulse, thereby blocking activation of pain fibers. Less energy is absorbed by the epidermis and lower fluence is required. Light sheer "duet" has pneumatic skin flattening in which vacuum is used for decreasing the pain. But this handpiece can only be used in larger body areas like back, abdomen, legs, and arms.

    Alma Lasers' unique IN-Motion™ SHR technology combines concurrent cooling with a gradual thermal rise to the target's therapeutic temperature applying low fluencies at high repetition rate, without the risk of injury and with much less pain for the patient. In this technology, the temperature achieved in hair follicle reaches 50°C as compared to epidermis with temperature around 25°C (Figs. 6.16A and B). This is in contrast to the high-peak energies used in traditional photoepilation technology that requires high cooling before, during and after each pulse, and requires that the handpiece remains stationary during the energy delivery. The sweeping technique of IN-Motion™ technology enables continuous administration in a larger treatment area for increased comfort and fewer missed spots with less time. This technique was promoted as pain-free technology but due to heat felt during treatment sessions it makes it less painful but not pain free.

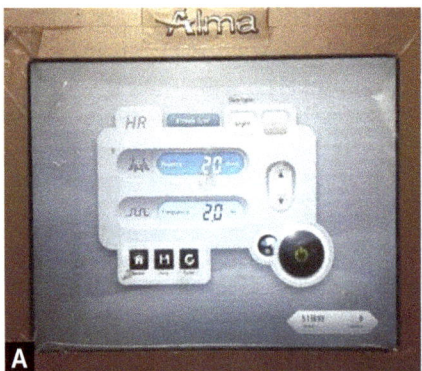 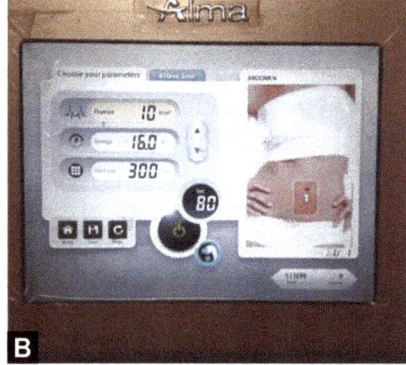

Figs. 6.16A and B: Two modes of functionality of Soprano ICE. (A) HR mode—fluence and frequency parameters to be set depending upon type of hair; (B) SHR mode—fluence and energy parameters to be set depending upon area, type of hair treated. After settings, automatically it will show the total time to be taken.

- **Meladine**, a topical melanin chromophore, has been studied in Europe with interesting results. The liposome solution dye, which is sprayed on, is selectively absorbed by the hair follicle and not the skin. This gives the follicles a temporary boost of melanin to optimize laser hair removal treatments. Clinical studies in Europe have shown permanent hair reduction in patients who used meladine prior to treatment.
- Studies have shown that eflornithine in combination with the alexandrite or Nd:YAG laser (*see* Fig. 6.15), may increase the efficacy of laser hair removal and that topical melanin improves the efficacy of the diode laser.
- Sienna Biopharmaceuticals has developed Topical Photoparticle Therapy which, according to its website, uses "silver particles to absorb laser light and converts the light energy into heat to facilitate local tissue injury". This may be useful for unwanted light or mixed pigment hair, which cannot be removed with lasers alone.
- Laser machines are coming up with unique **facial tips** with spot size around 6 mm allowing treatment of hard to reach areas, including the ears, glabella, and nostrils. Also for pubic regions, disposable tips are also available (Figs. 6.17A to D).
- **Photodynamic therapy** with aminolevulinic acid (ALA) has been shown in a small pilot study to result in up to 40% hair reduction with a single treatment, although wax epilation was performed prior to treatment in this study.

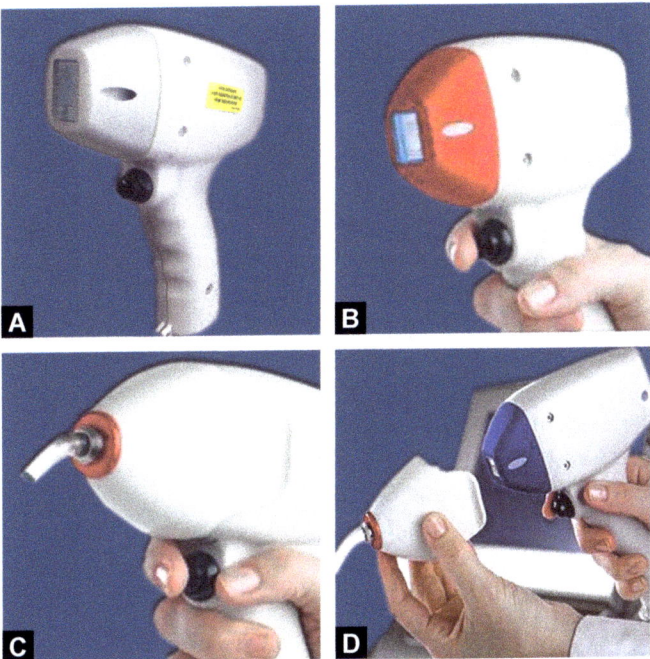

Figs. 6.17A to D: Handpiece of Soprano ICE laser: (A) Diode 810 nm handpiece with spot size 20 × 10 mm; (B) Alex 755 nm handpiece with spot size 15 × 10 mm; (C) Facial tip diode probe with spot size 6 mm; and (D) Detailed view of facial tip.

- **Electro-optical synergy (ELOS)** technology combines electrical (conducted radiofrequency) and optical (laser/light) energies. A handful of devices based on this technology have been produced. The theory behind ELOS is based on the optical component (laser or IPL) heating the hair shaft, which then is thought to concentrate the bipolar radiofrequency (RF) energy to the surrounding hair follicle. Based on this combination, lower fluences are needed for the optical component, thereby suggesting it might be well tolerated in all Fitzpatrick skin phototypes, and potentially effective in the removal of white and poorly pigmented hair.

  In a study 40 patients (Fitzpatrick skin phenotypes II–V) with varied facial and non-facial hair colors were treated with combined IPL/RF ELOS technology. An average clearance of 75% was observed at 18 months following four treatments. No significant adverse sequelae were noted and there were no treatment differences between patients of varying skin types or hair color. Pretreatment with ALA prior to use of a combined IPL and radiofrequency device has been shown to further augment the removal of terminal white hair.
- *Scanners*: Many systems now have automated scanners which direct a series of laser pulses uniformly over the are to be treated, hence improving efficiency especially in treating large areas.
- *Diode 1060 nm (Ross Ev, 2018)*: A recent study has used the novel 1060 nm to target darker skin subjects. This device had the added advantage of a large handpiece, and suction. The specifications were a spot size of 22–35 mm, pulse duration 30 ms, with a variaton from 30–400 ms, and fluence: 4.5–14 J/cm^2. The highlight was the vacuum pressure ranging from low (8 in Hg) to high (18 in Hg). The results were impressive with 93.5% of large spot size vacuum-assisted—treated subjects and 86.4% of the chilled sapphire—treated subjects showing a 50% hair clearance at 6 months following the last treatment session. Treatment with the large spot size vacuum-assisted handpiece, was most effective in axillae and calves, with a 77.9% and 78.5% hair count.

CONCLUSION

Literature reveiws by Zandi et al. (2013) and Haedersdal et al. have opined that the best available evidence was found for the alexandrite and diode lasers, followed by the ruby and Nd:YAG lasers, whereas limited evidence was available for IPL sources. Thus, the data on LHR can be summarized under the following heads:
- Epilation with lasers and light sources induced a partial short-term hair reduction up to 6 months postoperatively.
- Efficacy was improved with repeated treatments.
- Efficacy was superior to conventional treatments like shaving, waxing epilation, and electrolysis.

- Evidence existed for a partial long-term hair removal efficacy beyond 6 months postoperatively after repetitive treatments with alexandrite and diode lasers and probably after treatment with ruby and Nd:YAG lasers, whereas evidence was lacking for long-term hair removal after IPL treatment.
- At present there is no evidence for a complete and persistent hair removal efficacy.
- The occurrence of postoperative side-effects is reported low for all the laser systems.

The majority of adverse effects with LHR are transient and minor. They are more common in darker skin and can be minimized by using longer wavelength devices.

Laser hair removal removes one of the most predictable, cost effective and largely replicable procedures and will remain a target of active research and continual improvement.

BIBLIOGRAPHY

1. Buddhadev RM. IADVL Dermatosurgery Task Force. Standard guidelines of care: laser and IPL hair reduction. Indian J Dermatol Venereol Leprol. 2008;74:S68-74.
2. Campos V, Pitassi L. Epilação no rosto e no corpo. In: Mateus A, Palermo E (Eds). Cosmiatria e Laser: Prática no consultório médico. São Paulo: GEN; 2012. pp. 489-503.
3. Campos VB, Dierickx CC, Farinelli WA, et al. Hair removal with an 800-nm pulsed diode laser. J Am Acad Dermatol. 2000;43:442-7.
4. Dawber RP. Guidance for the management of hirsutism. Curr Med Res Opin. 2005;21:1227-34.
5. Dierickx C. Laser-assisted hair removal: state of the art. Dermatol Ther. 2000;13: 80-9.
6. Faurschou A, Haedersdal M. Photoepilation of unwanted hair growth. In: Raulin C, Karsai S (Eds). Laser and IPL Technology in Dermatology and Aesthetic Medicine. Berlin Heidelberg: Springer-Verlag; 2011. pp. 124-46.
7. Ferriman D, Gallwey JD. Clinical assessment of body hair growth in women. J Clin Endocrinol Metab.1961;21:1440-7.
8. Haedersdal M, Wulf H. Evidence-based review of hair removal using lasers and light sources. J Eur Acad Dermatol Venereol. 2006;20:9-20.
9. Macedo F. Luz intense pulsada versus laser. In: Mateus A, Palermo E (Eds). Cosmiatria e Laser: Prática no consultório médico. São Paulo: GEN; 2012. pp. 508-18.
10. Murphy MJ, Torstensson PA. Thermal relaxation times: an outdated concept in photothermal treatments. Lasers Med Sci. 2014;29:973-8.
11. Nanda S, Bansal S. Long pulsed Nd:YAG laser with inbuilt cool sapphire tip for long term hair reduction on type-IV and V skin: a prospective analysis of 200 patients. Indian J Dermatol Venereol Leprol. 2010;76:677-81.
12. Ross EV, Ibrahimi OA, Kilmer S. Long-term clinical evaluation of hair clearance in darkly pigmented individuals using a novel diode1060 nm wavelength with

multiple treatment handpieces: A prospective analysis with modeling and histological findings. Lasers Surg Med. 2018;50(9):893-901.
13. Sachdeva S. Hirsutism: evaluation and treatment. Indian J Dermatol. 2010;55: 3-7.
14. Sardana K, Khurana A. Hirsutism in Hair Loss. Disorders, Restoration and Management Disorders, Restoration and Management, 2nd edn. CBS Publishers. New Delhi. 2018. pp. 388-405.
15. Tierney EP, Goldberg DJ. Laser hair removal pearls. J Cosmet Laser Ther. 2008;10:17-23.
16. Zandi S, Lui H. Long-term removal of unwanted hair using light. Dermatol Clin. 2013:31:179-91.

CHAPTER 7

Cosmetic Use of Radiofrequency in Dermatology

Vivek Nair, Kabir Sardana, Apratim Goel

INTRODUCTION

The first electrosurgical device was discovered by William T Bovie and was used by Dr Harvey Williams Cushing on October 1, 1926, at Peter Bent Brigham Hospital in Boston, to remove a tissue mass from a patient's head. Since then, radiofrequency (RF) electrosurgical devices have become an indispensable part of the surgical armamentarium. Recently, RF has experienced a resurgence in aesthetic medicine with applications for ablative and nonablative indications.

With an aging population and the desire to retain a youthful appearance the demand for skin tightening procedures has seen a surge over the last two decades. Given the excellent safety profile and minimal downtime of these procedures, most patients prefer the modest improvement they afford to going under the knife. According to the 2015 statistics published by the American Society of Aesthetic Plastic Surgery, nonsurgical aesthetic procedures increased by 44% compared to 2014, and in this group nonsurgical skin tightening showed the maximum increase (58%).

Typically, sine RF voltage is used in medical devices. The RF energy can be delivered in continuous wave (CW) mode, burst mode, and pulsed mode (Fig. 7.1).

Continuous wave: It is used for gradual treatment of large areas, as it allows a slow increase in temperature in bulk tissue. This is used for targeting *cellulite, subcutaneous fat, and skin tightening.*

Burst mode: This is used in applications where peak power is important while average power should be limited. This application is used in *blood vessel coagulation.*

Pulsed mode: This is used when the goal is to heat a small tissue volume while limiting heat conduction to the surrounding tissue, similar to the rationale of applying short pulse duration in laser treatments. It is used for *fractional skin ablation* and is characterized by pulse durations which do not exceed the thermal relaxation time (TRT) of the treated zone.

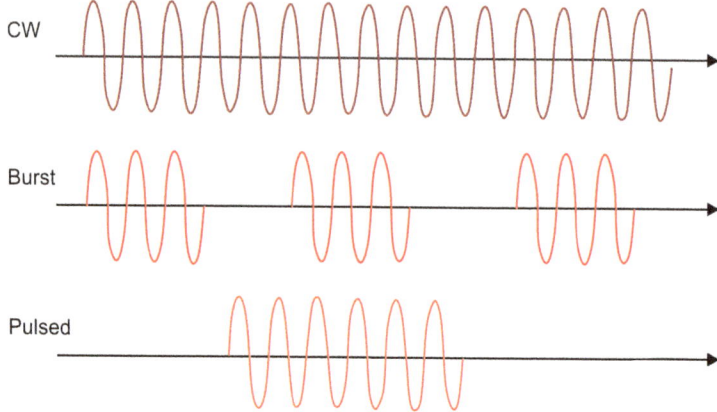

Fig. 7.1: Three patterns of radiofrequency waves.

SCIENTIFIC PRINCIPLE

Characteristics of an aging face include surface pigmentary and vascular changes, deepening wrinkles, facial sagging, ptosis of the muscular aponeurotic system, as well as bony resorption. It is a testament to todays' technology how all of these problems can be helped significantly without surgery. A combination of different techniques gives the best outcomes.

The treatment effect is based mostly on collagen remodeling and local metabolism acceleration. Skin tightening, which is often desired in noninvasive treatments, requires heating of the reticular dermis and subdermal structures. The required heating depth for these indications is 3-6 mm, a range that light energy does not reach well; therefore, RF is currently the main tool or these kinds of treatments (Emilia del Pino M).

With aging there is an alteration of dermal substrate—namely the fibrous part (functional collagen, elastin) as well as the ground substance (viz. hyaluronic acid, glycosaminoglycans, proteoglycans, etc.). This alteration may be an actual loss or a change in the character of the dermal component. Senescent fibroblasts produce less functional collagen and a lack of this main structural protein of the dermis causes wrinkle formation. The epidermis tends to thicken in contrast. There is also a decrease in the subcutaneous fibrous tissue and periosteal resorption—all of these leading to externally visible changes like prominent nasolabial and mentolabial folds, elongation of the lid-cheek junction, hollowing of the mid-face, and jowl formation.

Collagen has a triple helical structure consisting of three polypeptide chains. There are various types of collagen and in the dermis type III is predominant. Collagen fibrils are stabilized by the cross linking of specific lysine and hydroxy-lysine moieties; these bonds are heat sensitive and rupture when dermal temperatures exceed 55°C for 3-4 minutes (57-61°

is the ideal range). This breakage of intramolecular bonds is visible on electron microscopy and results in denaturation of the protein with the result that collagen loses its typical highly organized crystalline structure and assumes a random gel-like state. These fibers are shorter and this shrinking is responsible for the immediate tightening seen after RF skin tightening procedures. The dermis treats this collagen denaturation as an injury and sets into action the body's wound healing mechanism ultimately resulting in neocollagenesis over the course of 3-6 months resulting in the final clinical benefit. The precise heat-induced behavior of connective tissue is very variable though and dependent on several factors such as the maximum temperature reached, exposure time, tissue hydration, and age.

The heating of collagen can be modeled along the Arrhenius equation in the sense that the reaction rate is dependent on both time and temperature (Nelson AA). At a temperature of 85°C an exposure time of 1 ms is sufficient to induce structural changes in collagen while at a temperature of 43°C an exposure time of 90 seconds to 5 min is necessary. The former risks full thickness burns of the skin and is very painful; hence devices have gravitated to the latter approach.

Several studies have tried to define the surface skin temperature that correlates with the aforementioned dermal temperatures to achieve collagen denaturation. DiBernado showed a temperature correlation of 40-42°C on the surface equated to 50-55°C in the subreticular dermis using Nd:YAG laser delivered subcutaneously using a fiber-optic cable. A study (Jason Bentow) with the Pelleve device recommended skin surface treatment temperatures between 40°C and 44°C; temperatures below 40°C were not sufficient for the desired therapeutic effect according to the authors. Manufactures of the Exilis device recommend a temperature range of 40-42°C. The subjective **pain threshold** is *43.2°C*—therefore skin surface temperatures should be kept *below this* to avoid patient discomfort.

The RF energy can be derived in a stamping or in-motion technique—the latter is usually less painful with most patients just describing a heat like sensation during treatment. The stamping techniques (e.g. with Thermage) were associated with significant pain with the earlier high energy low pass protocols, this has improved with the newer low fluence high-pass protocols which also achieve better clinical results.

Because skin damage is an exponential function of the temperature, it is challenging to get to the maximal point of the temperature range without the risk of a burn. It is much easier—and safer—to obtain optimal results by *extending* the treatment time and maintaining a safe temperature longer.

Radiofrequency was the first technology which showed significant improvements in noninvasive skin tightening with Thermage; (Lolis MS) 15 years later RF machines still remain the most widely used for this purpose. The last few years have seen an explosion in the number of RF devices available for wrinkle reduction and skin tightening, all claiming to be better than the other.

RF energy has also been combined with optical energy and infrared energy to deliver synergistic benefit. It remains to the astute physician to choose the best machine for his/her practice.

Current noninvasive skin tightening devices produce a broad thermal injury 1–3-mm below the surface of the skin. Most have a cooling apparatus to protect the epidermis. Monopolar and bipolar RF devices have been used alone or in combination with broadband and laser light sources. Precise subsurface thermal profiles are source specific, but the local mechanisms of action are all based on heat generation. For example, monopolar devices have been shown to selectively heat fibrous septae (where present) and fat deeper in the dermis, somewhat regardless of the depth of the "electrical field" anatomical plane. Outside of RF devices, most skin tightening tools heat poorly defined volumes with water as the chromophore, such that the boundaries of the heated regions reflect the pulse duration, wavelength range, and cooling type.

There are two newer devices, fractionated broadband light and focused ultrasound, which produce a different subsurface energy profile.

Unlike more superficial laser procedures, where rapid assessment of clinical endpoints is possible, in skin tightening, erythema, and edema are often the only immediate outcomes. At times these phenomena obscure any immediate contraction. Despite an immediate "shrinkage" response, final clinical results may not occur until weeks to months later. This delayed tissue tightening is due to wound healing. While studies show that partially denatured contracted collagen can persist for up to 6 months, the inflammatory response contributes largely to the final clinical outcome. In general, deeply heated collagen fibers persist longer than superficially heated ones, which typically are degraded and "cleared" by the skin in less than 2 weeks.

PHYSICS OF RADIOFREQUENCY

Dermal and subcutaneous heating is the mode of action of RF energy when applied to the skin. Unlike lasers there is *no chromophore* for RF waves and heat is generated due to the *resistance* to the flow of the RF waves—this makes RF energy **"color-blind"** and suitable to all skin colors. This is one of the reasons that this technology makes a lot of sense in *Indian patients* as complications like PIH are much less than lasers that were primarily developed using Western skin types.

Energy

Energy is delivered to the tissue according to Ohm's law which states: E (energy in joules) = I (current in amps) × Z (impedance/resistance in ohms) × T (time). I and T can be controlled by the operator, however, the impedance of tissues is their basic nature to resist the flow of energy through them and is characteristic to each particular type of tissue, e.g. dry skin, fat, and bone have high impedance while wet skin has low impedance. Energy tends to flow *around* areas of high impedance instead of through them. Furthermore, impedance drops by 5% for every 1°C increase in temperature.

Impedance

Impedance is a central concept to understanding how RF energy heats up tissue. Impedance refers to the fundamental resistance of a tissue to the passage of energy through it and is measured in *ohms*. RF waves alternate at a given frequency—this causes cellular molecules in the path of the RF wave to vibrate at the same frequency.

For example, an RF wave of 6 MHz will cause molecules to vibrate at 6 million times per second while that of 1 MHz will cause vibration at 1 million times per second. Obviously, the first will generate more heat than the second but this higher frequency wave will also penetrate less into the skin (i.e. a 1 MHz wave will penetrate deeper than a 6 MHz wave). The depth of this penetration as well as of the heat generated will also depend on the impedance of the tissue.

As Table 7.1 shows different tissues have different impedance. However, this is **not** a static value—it changes with change in skin temperature or humidity, shape of the RF electrode, and RF coupling mechanism to the skin (resistive vs capacitive). Impedance also varies between individuals (according to age, gender, race, etc.). Basically, tissue with higher water and blood content has high electrical conductivity. Tumescent anesthesia may significantly increase tissue conductivity by increasing water and salt content.

Harth and Lischinsky studied impedance and RF interaction in a group of 30 patients using the EndyMed Pro RF device. This device is equipped with real time impedance monitoring (measured every 50 ms during an RF pulse). They found a large range for impedance in the studied subjects with 584 ohm being the maximum and 215 ohm being the minimum with a median of 356 ohm and a standard deviation of 39 ohm. They also found a 5-18% reduction in impedance during the course of a single 30 seconds RF pulse.

Table 7.1: Dielectric properties for human tissue at 1 MHz and room temperature.

Types of tissue	Electrical conductivity (Siemens/m)
Bone	0.02
Fat	0.03
Dry skin	0.03
Nerve	0.13
Cartilage	0.23
Wet skin	0.22
Muscle	0.50
Thyroid	0.60

This *variability* in impedance is responsible for the *variation in clinical results* with RF devices with some patients not improving at all. The need of the hour is for devices to continuously adjust their energy delivery based on measured impedance to provide uniform energy delivery to the dermis and subcutis. This will ensure more homogeneous results.

Penetration Depth

Penetration depth is a parameter broadly used in laser dermatology to mean the distance below the skin, which laser waves penetrate. In contrast to optical energy, which is attenuated with distance of travel through tissue as a result of scattering and absorption, RF current *decreases* at a distance from the *electrode* due to the divergence of current lines.

This is dependent on various *factors* including the topology of the skin and the electrode system. In aesthetic medicine, the most common configurations of electrode systems are monopolar, bipolar, and multipolar including fractional, where the effect is achieved by superposition of RF current paths between paired electrodes.

Penetration depth can also be affected by the anatomical structure of treated area. For example, penetration depth over bone can be limited by low conductivity of bone tissue. For this reason, treatment parameters over bone, for example, the forehead and hip are lower than the parameters applied in adjacent areas.

Classically, the *depth of penetration* is estimated to be half the diameter of the active electrode in a monopolar system and half the distance between adjacent electrodes in a bipolar system (Fig. 7.2A). The major disadvantage with bipolar RF energy delivery is that it does not penetrate very deep into the skin and is unable to produce uniform, volumetric heating unlike monopolar RF energy.

As penetration depth of RF for bipolar devices is a function of electrode size and the distance between them, thus by increasing the distance between the electrodes, electrical current can go deeper, but divergence is also increased. For the case when the distance between the electrodes is much larger than the electrode size, the heating profile will be similar to two monopolar electrodes. Thus, there should be an ideal distance between the electrodes to enable uniform heating of the tissue. The most uniform distribution of RF current is obtained in planar geometry when the area of parallel electrodes is larger than the distance between them (Fig. 7.2B). If the skin is folded between electrodes, by applying negative pressure (in the form of vacuum) to elevate and pinch the skin between two parallel electrodes, uniform heating to the tissue can be delivered.

With a tripolar system (e.g. TriPollar RF), the depth of heat penetration is close to the average distance between the three electrodes and capable of heating the dermal and subcutaneous layers. A unipolar device (e.g. Alma Accent) is similar to a monopolar device but with the patient return electrode

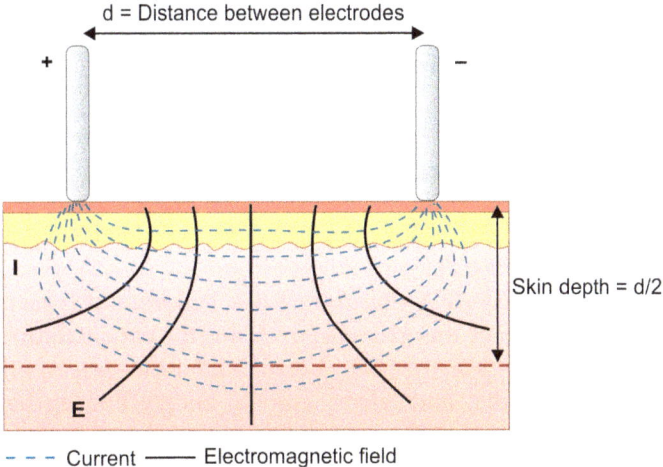
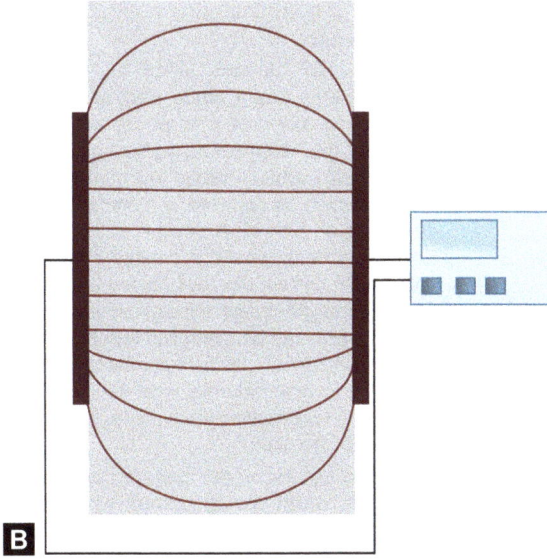

Figs. 7.2A and B: (A) A depiction of the depth of penetration in bipolar radiofrequency (RF); and (B) Uniform distribution of RF current in case of planar geometry. Here the area of parallel electrodes is larger than the distance between them.

built into the RF active electrode tip. These devices have a unique side effect known as **"arcing"**, i.e. RF energy can jump across an air gap to cause skin burns if the active electrode is not properly in contact with the skin when engaged.

Pulse Duration Effect

Like in lasers, pulse duration remains a critical parameter when utilizing RF energy (bipolar RF) in order to achieve a clinical response. It affects treatment results because timing influences the thermochemical process in tissue. The other effect of pulse duration is energy dissipation away from the treatment zone due to heat conductivity from the exposed area to the surrounding tissue.

TYPES OF RADIOFREQUENCY DEVICES

Radiofrequency devices can be categorized into monopolar, bipolar, tripolar, and multipolar (Table 7.2).

A *monopolar* device (e.g. Thermage, Exilis, Pelleve, and TruSculpt) has RF energy flowing between the active electrode and the patient return electrode/plate placed elsewhere on the body. A *bipolar* RF device (e.g. Aluma, Ematrix, ePrime, Infini, Scarlet, and Secret) has RF energy flowing between two adjacent electrodes—these electrodes may or may not penetrate into the skin (Fig. 7.3A).

Table 7.2: Basic radiofrequency system classification.

Radiofrequency system	Characteristics
Monopolar radiofrequency (RF) system	Monopolar RF devices utilize an active electrode in the treatment area and a return electrode, usually in the form of a grounding pad with a large contact area, which is placed outside of the treatment zone; "grounding" here does not refer to the energy system having any connection to ground—it is a closed system as opposed to hyfrecation which utilizes actual grounding as part of its design. In this electrode geometry, a high RF current density is created near the active electrode, and the RF current diverges toward the large return electrode. The ultimate treatment effects depend on the *density* of RF energy, which can be controlled with RF power, and the *size* of active electrode. In *cutting* instruments, a *needle type* electrode is used to concentrate electrical current on a very small area whereas in *bulk heating* instruments the probe has a *large* skin surface contact area
Bipolar RF system	Bipolar configuration is characterized by the use of two electrodes which are in contact with the treated area. RF energy flows from one electrode to the other. No grounding pad is required. This geometry creates uniform heating in a small amount of tissue—the depth of penetration is *superficial* unless transcutaneous needle electrodes area used. Bipolar devices are used to create focused thermal zones in *nonablative* application. The advantage of bipolar systems is the localization of RF energy in the treatment area making it safe for almost all patient subgroups
Tripolar RF system	Tripolar configurations have a *deeper* depth of penetration than bipolar systems due to the use of three active electrodes. The RF waves can reach the *subcutaneous layer*
Multipolar RF system	This category includes systems with more than three active RF probes. The *depth* of penetration is a complex interaction between the electrodes and can *vary* from superficial to deep depending on the electrode array

CHAPTER 7: Cosmetic Use of Radiofrequency in Dermatology

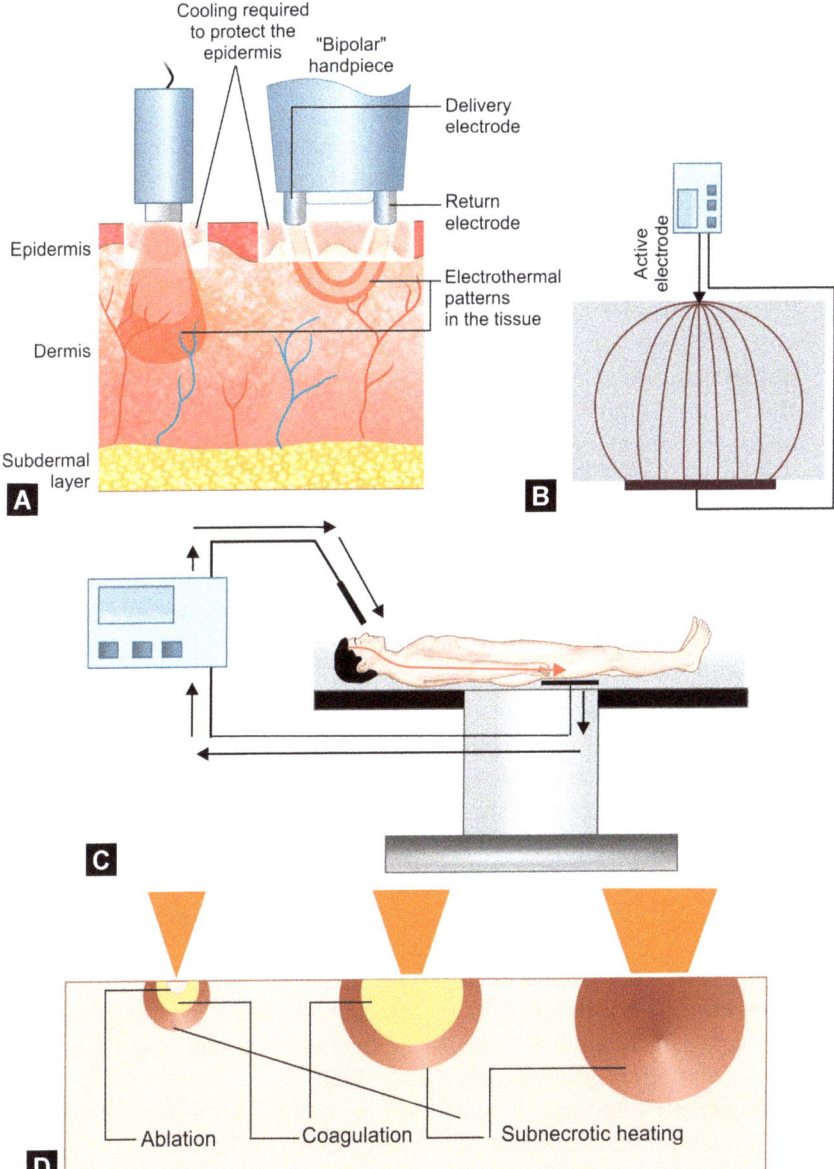

Figs. 7.3A to D: (A) A depiction of monopolar and bipolar radiofrequency (RF); (B) Schematic diagram of monopolar RF; (C) A depiction of the electric current flow in a unipolar RF; and (D) Treatment effects with monopolar devices depend on the density of RF energy, which can be controlled with RF power, and the size of active electrode.

Monopolar devices like Thermage and Exilis require skin surface cooling to prevent burns as well as to drive the RF energy deeper into the skin. *Pelleve* is also a monopolar system but only requires cooled contact gel during treatment. Bipolar and tripolar systems have more focused energy delivery and typically do not require surface cooling.

Monopolar Radiofrequency Systems

Monopolar RF devices utilize an active electrode in the treatment area and a return electrode, usually in the form of a grounding pad with a large contact area, which is placed outside of the treatment zone. In this electrode geometry, a high RF current density is created near the active electrode, and the RF current diverges toward the large return electrode (Fig. 7.3B). In this mode:

- Radiofrequency current is concentrated on the RF electrode and rapidly diverges toward the return electrode.
- Heat generated by RF current near the active electrode does not depend on the size, shape, or position of the return electrode when the return electrode is much *larger in size* than the active electrode and is located at a distance which is much greater than the size of the active electrode.
- Heating decreases dramatically as distance increases from the electrode. At a distance equal to the electrode size, heating becomes insignificant. In other words, most of the RF energy applied in monopolar systems is converted into heat near the active electrode. Therefore, the heat zone can be estimated as a radius equal to half the size of the active electrode.

Traditionally monopolar devices were most commonly used for tissue cutting. Schematically, the RF current flow for monopolar devices is shown in Figure 7.3C. RF current always flows in a closed loop via the human body. Treatment effects with monopolar devices depend on the *density* of RF energy, which can be controlled with RF power, and the *size of the active electrode* (Fig. 7.3D).

- **For tissue ablation**, very high energy density is required. In cutting instruments, a **needle-type** electrode is used to concentrate electrical current on a very small area (Fig. 7.3D).
- **Coagulation handpieces** have a **larger surface** area than ablative devices, usually a few square millimeters, to generate heat on a larger area, creating coagulation rather than ablation.
- **Subnecrotic heating** is usually used for treatments related to collagen remodeling, and in this case, the spot size is about **1 cm^2**.
  This is depicted in Figure 7.3D.

Thus, the main features of **monopolar devices** are:
- Predictability of thermal effect near the active electrode
- Ability to concentrate energy on a very small area
- High nonuniformity of heat distribution, with very high heat at the surface of the active electrode and dramatic reduction at a distance exceeding the size of electrode, thereby limiting penetration depth.

Bipolar Radiofrequency

Bipolar configuration is characterized by the use of two electrodes, which are in contact with the treated area. This geometry is better able to create uniform heating as compared to a monopolar system, albeit in a smaller volume of tissue. The basic principles are:
- For any geometry, RF current density is highest along the line of shortest separation between the electrodes and reduced with distance from the electrodes.
- Heating is greater near the electrode surface and drops with distance because of current divergence.
- RF current is concentrated on the part of the electrode that has high curvature creating hot spots.

In bipolar devices, both electrodes create an equal thermal effect near each of the electrodes, and the divergence of RF current is not strong because of the small distance between the electrodes. For bipolar systems shown in Figure 7.3A, most of the heat is concentrated between electrodes.

Combined Electrical and Optical Energy

Combined electrical and optical energy, or selective electrothermolysis, is another type of RF technology that combines RF energy with optical energy from laser or light sources. Whereas the *Thermage* tightening device delivers RF energy to the skin using *monopolar* electrodes, the RF component of the *combined* electrical and optical energy units currently available uses *bipolar* electrodes. The effect contributed by each of the energy sources, light versus RF, has not, however, been demonstrated.

Uses: This technology has shown efficacy in hair removal, skin tightening, wrinkle reduction, and the treatment of both pigment and vascular disorders.

Devices: There are several devices currently on the market using combined RF and laser or light technology including the Aurora, Polaris, Galaxy, and ReFirme systems (Syneron Medical Ltd, Yokneam, Israel).

Hybrid Monopolar and Bipolar Radiofrequency

A relatively new RF system uses two RF-configured handpieces (one monopolar, one bipolar) in a single device (Accent RF, Alma Lasers Ltd, Caesarea, Israel). The device theoretically takes advantage of two mechanisms of RF-induced tissue heating. The monopolar handpiece achieves heating via the rotational movement of water molecules in the alternating current of the electromagnetic field.

The end result is volumetric heating at deeper levels in the skin (up to 20 mm). The bipolar handpiece, on the other hand, has more superficial

(2-6 mm), localized (nonvolumetric) heating based on tissue resistance to the RF conductive current.

Vacuum-assisted Bipolar Radiofrequency

Another relatively new device (Aluma, Lumenis Inc., Santa Clara, CA, USA) combines bipolar RF and vacuum technology in what has been termed ***FACES*** technology (functional aspiration controlled electrothermal stimulation). The device has incorporated a vacuum into the handpiece to suction a fold of skin in alignment between two electrodes.

Fractional Radiofrequency

Fractional skin treatment was introduced in aesthetic medicine about a decade ago and has been touted as a superior technology than lasers. This procedure is based on heating or ablation of multiple small foci with a spot size of 100-400 μm. This allows the procedure to be very tolerable and with relatively short downtime.

The RF fractional technologies can be administered from the surface, using a grid of electrodes, or intradermally, using a grid of microneedles which deliver the RF energy within the dermis.

The *surface electrodes* provide a more superficial effect improving texture and fine lines while *longer needles* penetrate deeper, providing deeper dermal remodeling (Mulholland RS). Though there are two types of needles used (insulated and noninsulated) they do not markedly effect the treatment results (Fig. 7.4).

The RF is often touted as being safe for all skin types due to its "color-blind" nature. It should be noted that while RF interaction with skin is not affected by the presence of melanin, darker skin types, and tanned skin are still susceptible to **postinflammatory pigmentary** changes. Since RF exerts its tissue effects by heating and in most applications will induce some degree of wound healing response, it is better to exercise appropriate caution when treating pigmented skin.

Noninvasive fractional RF can be delivered in several modalities: **monopolar**, **bipolar**, or a technology, which applies bipolar RF in what has been termed **sublative** treatment (Table 7.3 and Figs. 7.5A and B). Bipolar RF is unique in the sense that there are various ways in which it can be delivered to the target tissue. The electrodes can be on the surface of the skin (noninvasive bipolar RF) or they can be needles inserted to varying depths in the skin (minimally invasive RF). These needles can be insulated or noninsulated. Furthermore, there may be a 1:1 ratio of the active and return electrodes or there may be one return electrode for many active electrodes—all of these factors affect the depth of penetration of the RF waves.

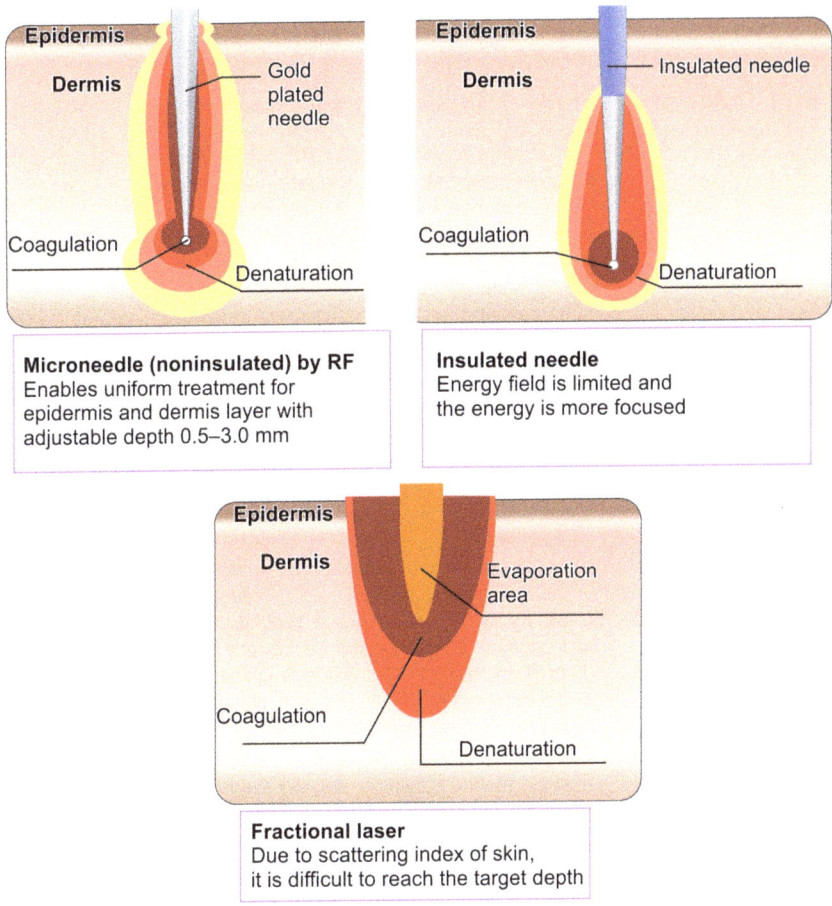

Fig. 7.4: Differences between insulated and noninsulated radiofrequency (RF) needles as compared to a CO_2 laser beam.

Table 7.3: Characteristics of different fractional radiofrequency (RF) systems.

Fractional RF system	Characteristics
Unipolar fractional RF	RF energy is applied with a single active electrode, whose contact with the skin is made with a series of pinpoint extensions from the handpiece electrode An example of unipolar frequency response function (FRF) is the Pixel RF (Alma Lasers, Israel). The device utilizes handpieces which have either a grid of pins or a rolling wheel with pins; these pins allow the transfer of current to the skin when placed in gentle, direct contact with the skin. The tissue effect of unipolar RF is very similar to that of lasers since the majority of the energy is absorbed at the point of contact, and heating decreases with distance from the electrode

Contd...

Contd...

Fractional RF system	Characteristics

Bipolar fractional RF	RF energy is applied with a series of active and return electrodes (Fig. 7.5A)
	   In straight forward bipolar RF, the current is limited to the tissue between the active and return electrodes
	   The distance between the electrodes affects the depth of penetration of the current. As a rough rule of thumb, the depth of penetration with marketed bipolar RF devices is one-half the distance between the electrodes. The frequency of the RF generator also impacts the depth of penetration. Therefore, by varying the RF frequency and the distance between electrodes, the pattern of RF current can be modified to allow superficial or deeper heating when one is preferable to the other for a particular clinical indication

Sublative RF	This is a variant of bipolar RF in which the epidermal effect is small and the dermal effect greater Sublative RF is offered by the Matrix RF and eMatrix handpieces (Syneron-Candela, Israel). In contrast to fractional lasers and fractional unipolar RF, which induce a "V"-shaped lesion in the skin, sublative RF generates a *pyramid-shaped* effect, by limiting the extent of heating in the uppermost layers and promoting the transfer of current in the deeper dermis (Figs. 7.5A and B). This effect is produced by staggering the active electrodes in a matrix with variable distances from the return electrodes. This inverted geometry allows mild treatment of epidermal defects with a more aggressive treatment of the deeper dermis. Because the epidermal effect is localized to small foci, the approach allows a dermal treatment with more rapid epidermal healing and therefore shorter downtime and reduced risks of infection, pigmentary change, and scars

OVERVIEW OF AVAILABLE DEVICES (TABLE 7.4)

Thermage (Solta Medical, CA, USA)

Thermage was the first RF device to be commercially marketed for noninvasive skin tightening in 2002. To date it remains the most widely studied device with the maximum publications in peer reviewed journals (Alster TS, Fisher GH, and Weiss RA). The initial study was a multicenter, blinded trial by Fitzpatrick et al. which led to FDA approval for skin tightening in 2003. It was FDA approved for periorbital wrinkling in 2004 and for body contouring in 2006.

Thermage is a *monopolar device* and has undergone significant modifications over the last 15 years. The original device was called Thermage ThermaCool NXT and initial treatment protocols involved the use of high intensity RF energy with few passes. The results were suboptimal with only

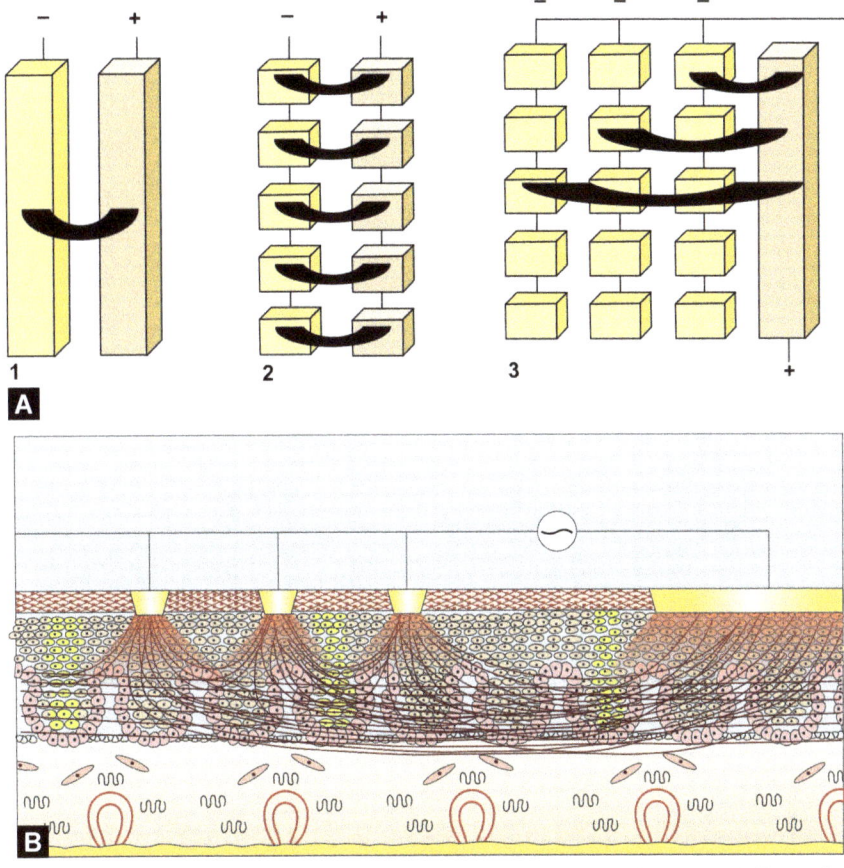

Figs. 7.5A and B: (A) Different forms of bipolar radiofrequency (RF) energy delivery: the current low in traditional bipolar RF (1), fractional bipolar RF (2), and sublative RF (3); and (B) The unique pyramid-shaped RF effector zones in sublative RF application.

50–60% patients showing objective skin tightening after 6 months. The procedure was also very uncomfortable with only about 70% patients finding the treatment results met their expectations. New Thermage *multiple-pass algorithms* with a larger tip and shorter RF pulse configurations showed that almost 90% of patients observed immediate tightening and that more than 90% of patients had visible and measurable moderate skin tightening 6 months after treatment. Only 5% of patients now find the procedure too painful and more than 94% find the treatment meets their expectations.

The *ThermaCool NXT device* employed 400, 600, and 900 REP (radiofrequency energy pulse) disposable tips. Efforts to make the treatments more comfortable led to the development of the Thermage CPT which has a redesigned tip and utilizes TENS (transcutaneous electrical nerve stimulation)

Table 7.4: Comprehensive classification of radiofrequency (RF) devices.

Company and device	Energy specifications	Tips/electrodes	Comments
Monopolar devices			
Thermage (Hayward, CA)	6.78 MHz; 400 W		New handpiece (CPT: Comfortable Pulse Technology) with vibrations to improve patient comfort. Pain nerval interceptors get confused and busy (vibrations, cooling, heating)
Cutera (Brisbane, CA)	1 MHz	4" handpiece	Handpiece reads out once optimal temperature is reached of 43–45°C
Ellman® (Oceanside, NY)	4 MHz	(7.5, 10, 15, and 20 mm)	Several handpieces for smaller areas. Can use unit as an electrocautery unit also RF + cautery
Exilis Elite, BTL Industries (Prague, Czech Republic)	90 W		Two handpieces—larger cooled, smaller uncooled, Inbuilt impedance and temperature monitoring
Intragen, Jeisys Medical, (Seoul, Korea)	6 MHz	2 handpieces (KT-07, KT-15)	Impedance monitoring
Bipolar RF			
Accent family (Caesarea, Israel)	40.68 MHz; Up to 300 W		Unipolar + bipolar + fractionated RF
Aluma (Yokneam, Israel)	up to 300 W	Bipolar and unilarge handpiece	FACES technology using functional aspiration
Aurora SR (Candela, San Jose, CA)	Up to 25 J/cm²	400–980 nm; 580–980 nm; 680–980 nm	RF + IPL (intense pulsed light)
Elos Plus (San Jose, CA)	~3 Hz (Variable)		RF + Infrared light
eMatrix (Candela, San Jose, CA)	Up to 62 mJ/pin	Matrix of electrodes Fractional RF	Disposable tip, which can prove to be a disadvantage over conventional fractional lasers

Contd...

Contd...

Company and device	Energy specifications	Tips/electrodes	Comments
EndyMed PRO 3 Deep 3 Pole (EndyMed Medical, Caesarea, Israel)	1 MHz 65 W	4 handpieces	3 Deep RF, handpieces: skin tightening, body contouring, facial tightening, fractional skin resurfacing
ePrime (Syneron/Candela, San Jose, CA)	460 kHz 84 VRMS	Microneedles	20° delivery angle, injected into dermis, fractional skin resurfacing
eTwo (Candela, San Jose, CA)	62 mJ sublative; 100 J/cm^3 sublime	Matrix of electrodes	RF + IR
Ray Life (Ascepelion)	0.5–1 MHz	3 handpieces	Suction and three modes
Reaction (Jersey City, NJ)	MHz Body 50 W Face 20 W	4 modes—0.8, 1.7, 2.45, and multichannel	SVC (suction, vacuum, cooling) devices
TiteFx (Israel)	1 MHz 60 W		Bipolar w/suction real time epidermal temperature monitor
VelaShape II/Candela, (San Jose, CA)	Infrared—up to 35 W RF Up to 60 W	Handpiece with bipolar infrared laser, suction	

Contd...

Contd...

Company and device	Energy specifications	Tips/electrodes	Comments
Velasmooth (Syneron/Candela)	700–2,000 nm		RF/infrared light with mechanical manipulation
V-Touch Viora, Jersey City, NJ		3 handpiece—0.8, 1.7, and 2.45	SVC (suction, vacuum, cooling) devices
Tripolar RF			
Apollo-TriPollar	1 MHz 50 W	3 handpieces	
Unipolar RF			
Accent RF Caesarea, Israel	Up to 200 W	1 handpiece	Unipolar energy to heat fat, bipolar to deliver energy to dermis
Multipolar devices			
Vanquish Aesthetics, Prague, CR		Noncontact	Operator independent
Venus Concept-8 Circular Poles (Toronto, ON)	RF: 1 MHz Magnetic pulse: 15 Hz RF: up to 150-W Magnetic flux: 15 Gauss	Large handpiece 8 Poles, 5 mm apart, dual mode = bipolar magnetic field	Multipolar RF and magnetic pulse

as well as vibration to minimize pain based on the gate control theory of pain mitigation. The treatment protocol involves making square grids on the area to be treated so that the requisite amount of overlap can be done to ensure complete coverage. The epidermis is protected during treatment using cryogenic cooling. The heat sensation from a single shot lasts 2–7 seconds.

Current protocols favor lower energy and multiple passes. The Thermage tips have built in contact monitoring to ensure proper contact during treatment. These tips are disposable and need to be changed per patient. The high cost of these tips (~ $ 400) makes treatments expensive. Benefit from one session usually takes 3–6 months to manifest; second sessions if required should be done after this time.

Exilis Elite (BTL Industries, Prague, Czech Republic)

The BTL Exilis Elite is a *monopolar RF system*, which has the unique advantage of being able to treat skin laxity as well as reduce underlying fat. This is accomplished with the help of built in cooling in the handpiece of the device, this drives the energy deeper reaching depths of 2.5–3 cm thus heating fat. The powerful 90W handpiece enables the target fat reaching the desired temperature of more than 44°C (which is the temperature at which fat apoptosis occurs when this temperature is maintained for 4–6 minutes). The smaller uncooled handpiece delivers the energy in the superficial and mid-dermis thereby stimulating neocollagenesis in the traditional RF model. The cooling of the handpiece is adjustable from 30–10°C with a proportional increase in the depth of RF energy delivery, e.g. with no cooling the depth is about 0.7 cm, at 20° the depth is 1.6–1.8 cm and at 10° the depth is 2.5–3 cm. A veterinary study (Fritz K) showed increase in collagen content of porcine tissue from an average of 9.0% before the therapy up to 25.9% after the 3-month follow-up period following a single 10 min session targeting a skin surface temperature between 39° and 43°C.

Any part of the body can be treated and there are no costly consumables (only the disposable return electrode pad needs to be changed with every patient). The system comes with a built-in impedance monitor which continuously varies RF delivery to provide uniform energy delivery and avoid hot spots. A sensor automatically shuts of the probe when not in contact with the skin and this prevents arcing and burns. The older 50 W Exilis system needed 4–5 sessions spaced 2–4 weeks apart for optimum results in lower face treatment; compared to this the 90 W Exilis Elite usually only requires 2 sessions for the face and neck area spaced 14 days apart.

Pelleve (Ellman International, NY, USA)

The Pelleve system was initially a modification of the company's workhorse Surgitron 4.0 brand. The Surgitron is an RF system used for cutting and coagulation purposes and has both monopolar and bipolar functionality.

Bulk heating of tissue was made possible by the development of special ball-shaped handpieces made with an advanced alloy matched to the radio-wave circuit—this functions as a thin capacitative membrane distributing RF energy over a volume of tissue beneath the membrane surface. A frequency of 4 MHz was recommended for skin tightening and the first electrode available was 0.5 cm in size. This was the system used by Rusciani et al. in their 2007 study using the Surgitron 4.0 system; they treated 93 patients and after one session found an average improvement between 25% and 30% at the end of 6 months.

Since then the device has been refined and is now available as the Pelleve S5 system using 4 MHz and variously sized tips (7.5 mm, 10 mm, 15 mm, and 20 mm). A 2013 study by Chipps et al. using this system found at least a grade I improvement in 74% of the 58 patients treated, 4 months after two sessions of Pelleve using 3D photography for evaluation; 85% of patients noted an overall improvement in their skin appearance while 81% rated their skin laxity as improved. The degree of improvement was mild for 55% patients and moderate for 18% patients. Initial protocols with this device required weekly sessions for 6-8 weeks but now most practitioner's favor monthly sessions for 3-6 months. Results (Stampar M) can last for more than 1.5 years in many patients depending on age and indications, with some wrinkle results showing persistent improvement beyond 1.5 years.

Accent (Alma Lasers, IL, USA)

Alma Accent is a *combined unipolar and bipolar RF* device and is unique in the way it delivers RF energy into the skin. The word unipolar is a source of much confusion. It means that unlike a monopolar probe no separate grounding plate is required for its functioning—the grounding or patient return electrode in this case is built into the unipolar tip itself. The principle of this device is that bipolar RF is used for superficial heating while unipolar RF is used for deep dermal heating. Several published studies show the effectiveness of this system for tissue tightening and reducing cellulite—this device in particular seems more effective than many other RF machines in treating *cellulite* (Emilia DP) with consistent mild-moderate improvement noted by many authors. The Accent XL is an updated version of this machine. Treatment protocols vary from 4 weekly sessions to two sessions spaced a 2-4 weeks apart; one interesting observation was better cellulite improvement when combining Accent RF with a topical cellulite reduction serum. Facial results (Jaffary F) are moderate at best in accord with other RF machines.

Aluma (Lumenis Inc, CA, USA)

The Aluma is a *bipolar RF* device, which combines bipolar RF with a *vacuum* apparatus. The principle here is that by using suction tissue is pulled into the probe—this allows the normally superficial bipolar RF energy to be delivered deeper into the dermis. This is also called "FACES" (functional aspiration controlled electrothermal stimulation). Nontarget structures such as muscle, fascia, and bone are avoided. The vacuum also diminishes the pain of the procedure—most patients feel no pain at all. Gold et al. treated 46 patients with the device and found a 2-point reduction in the elastosis scale with an excellent safety profile.

Regen TriPolar Radiofrequency (Pollogen Ltd, Jerusalem, Israel)

This is a *three electrode RF* system introduced in the last few years and is indicated for the treatment of *skin laxity* as well as *body contouring* and reduction of c*ellulite* and localized fat pockets. The device comes with a separate facial and body probe and does not require surface cooling. It delivers RF energy at 1 MHz and has a maximum power of 30 W. The depth of heat penetration is approximately the average distance between the three electrodes and depth of penetration is up till the subcutaneous layer. Multiple sessions are required for benefit. Tripolar technology (Mlosek RK, McKnight B) has shown excellent cellulite reduction potential (up to 90% reduction in one study) as well as improvement in body laxity. Sessions are typically done weekly for 6–8 weeks. There is a home use device called STOP available, which is based on the TriPolar RF system. Another TriPolar system is the Viora Reaction.

Venus Freeze (Venus Concepts, AZ, USA)

The Venus Freeze uses *eight poles of RF* energy combined with pulsed magnetic fields to achieve skin tightening and body contouring. There are no published studies on this device as of this writing. The Venus Viora is another product from the same company utilizing a new concept called *nanofractional RF*; again experience with the device so far is limited (This is discussed in the next sections).

Combination Systems

There are numerous devices, which attempt to combine two or more different technologies to enhance clinical benefit and possibly treat more indications. The Aurora SR system (Syneron-Candela, CA, USA), now called the **Elos** system, combines light energies in the 400–900 nm range along with the RF energy up to 25 J/cm^2 to allow a penetration depth of 4 mm below the skin. A second system based on the same principle is the **eMatrix** (Syneron-Candela, CA, USA)—this combines a full-fledged IPL and RF energy into one device. Polaris and ReFirme (Syneron, Yokneam, Israel) combine bipolar RF energy with 780–910 nm diode for the Polaris and 700–1,200 nm infrared light for the ReFirme to deliver even deeper energies into the skin.

These devices have the theoretical advantage of using two technologies acting synergistically to generate heat. When target structures have been prewarmed with optical energy they will conduct RF energy better and thereby get heated better.

These combination systems have been used for indications other than just skin tightening—acne, unwanted hair, as well as some vascular and pigmented lesions can be covered as indications.

The promise of these combination systems still need to translate into better clinical results. A study by Doshi and Alster found only modest improvement in facial wrinkles in 20 patients treated with the Polaris WR system.

Fractional Radiofrequency Systems

Similar in concept to fractional lasers, fractional RF devices split an RF pulse into numerous columns leaving untreated tissue for faster recovery—at least in theory. The first such system was the Matrix which utilized bipolar fractional RF energy (Table 7.4). The eMatrix is similar to the Matrix RF but in smaller delivery system.

Skin rejuvenation and the treatment of acne scars are the primary indications for these devices. These devices have limited skin tightening benefit due to the superficial nature of the energy delivery system—less than 1 mm deep thermal injuries are caused by the patterned fractional array of electrodes.

Microneedling Radiofrequency Systems

Minimally invasive RF treatment recently has gained popularity based on the patient's desire to obtain a more dramatic treatment result after a single treatment. Microneedle RF treats the skin in a minimally invasive manner (Figs. 7.6 to 7.8). These systems *overcome impedance issues* by having physical needles, which puncture the skin and then deliver RF energy at a precise, adjustable, and depth. There are various devices on the market and the two types of needles are insulated and noninsulated (Table 7.5).

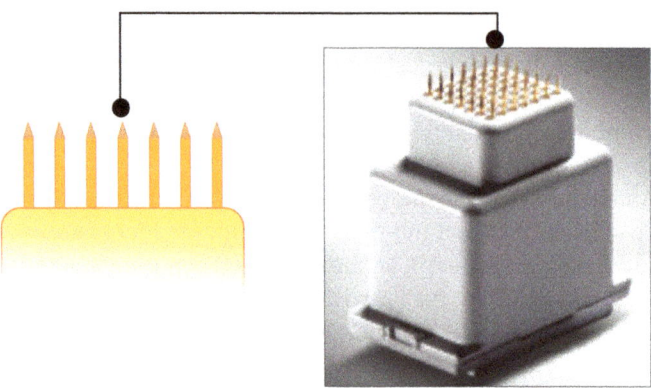

Fig. 7.6: INTRAcel (Jeisys) handpiece.

CHAPTER 7: Cosmetic Use of Radiofrequency in Dermatology

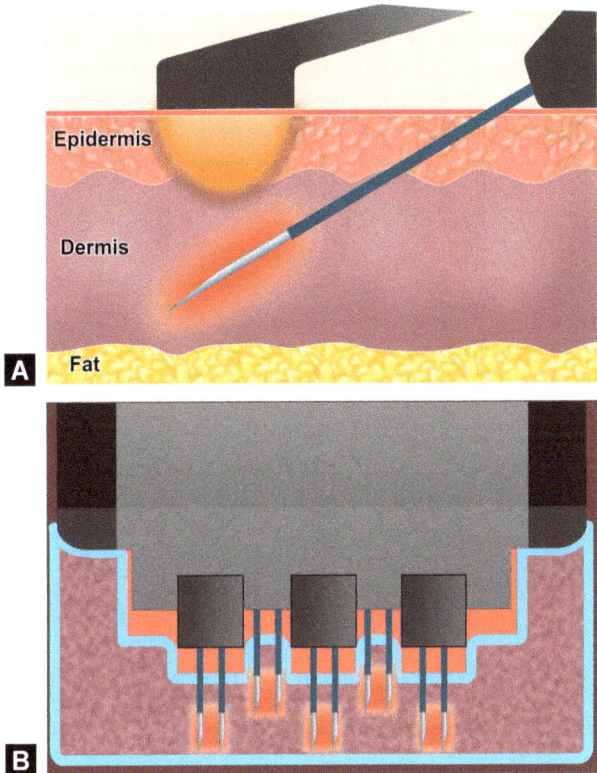

Figs. 7.7A and B: Schematic depiction of microneedle bipolar radiofrequency (RF) and single-use microneedle cartridge: ePrime (Syneron–Candela).

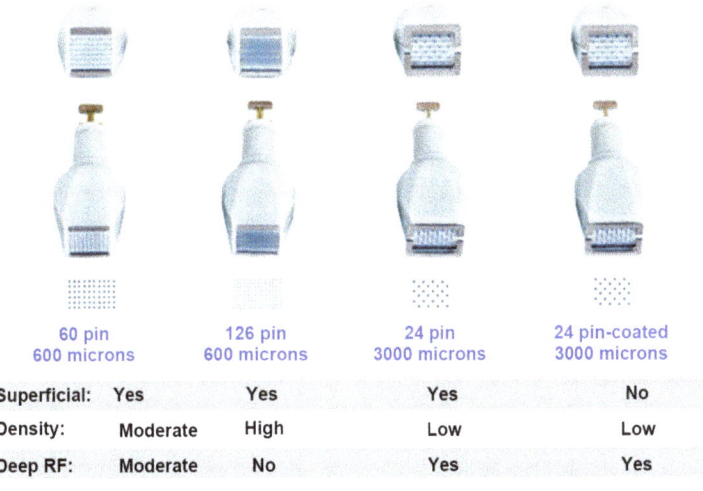

Fig. 7.8: A depiction of variable histological depths achieved by various handpieces.

Table 7.5: Microneedling radiofrequency (RF) devices.

	Secret (Ilooda Co. Ltd, Korea)	Scarlet-S (Viol Co. Ltd, Korea)	Infini (Lutronic Corp, Korea)	Vivace (Sung Hwan E&B, Korea)	INTRAcel (Jeisys Co. Ltd, Korea)
Power	50 W	50 W	50 W	70 W	60 W
Type of RF	Bipolar	Bipolar	Bipolar	Bipolar	Bipolar
Frequency	2 MHz	2 MHz	1 MHz	1 MHz and 2 MHz	1 MHz
Needles	Insulated and noninsulated	Insulated and noninsulated	Insulated	Insulated and non-insulated	Insulated
Tip array	Various tips • 5 × 5 array (25 needles) • 4 × 4 array (16 needles) • Insulated single row of 6 or noninsulated row of 10 needles	5 × 5 array	Various tips MFR tips—ablative bipolar RF • 7 × 7 array • 4 × 4 array SFR tips—nonablative bipolar RF • 12 × 12 array • 8 × 8 array	6 × 6 array	Various tips • 7 × 7 array • SRR (superficial RF resurfacing) tip—nonablative bipolar RF
RF pulse duration	50–950 ms	100–800 ms	10–1,000 ms	NA	NA
Needle depth	0.5–3.5 mm in gradations of 0.1 mm	0.5–3.5 mm in gradations of 0.1 mm	0.5–3.5 mm in gradations of 0.1 mm	0.5–3.5 mm in gradations of 0.1 mm	NA
Shot count per tip	1,000 shots	2,000 shots	NA	2,000 shots	NA

Dielectric coated needles have become popular in delivering aggressive heating to the reticular dermis without thermal damage to the skin's surface. By heating deep dermal collagen at a higher temperature than could be safely used at the epidermal level, a much stronger collagen contraction effect can be achieved in order to improve deep wrinkles and enhance skin tightening. The combination of deep dermal treatment with superficial fractional treatment has a high potential for complete skin improvement while avoiding skin excision.

Insulated needles (Fig. 7.4) have a coating, which only allows the RF energy to exit at the tip—this has the theoretical advantage of lesser epidermal side effects, however in practice *noninsulated* needles also concentrate RF energy at their tips due to the sharp tapering profile of the needle and have minimal epidermal RF energy delivery. They also have the advantage of lesser bleeding during the procedure due to cauterization of superficial vessels in the papillary dermis as the needles go in. Most of these devices come from Asia with Korea producing three very popular brands—Infini (Lutronic Corp), Secret (Ilooda Co. Ltd.), and Scarlet (Viol Co. Ltd.)

Scarlet was the first to be cleared for clinical use in 2007. *Infini* comes with *insulated needles*, *Secret* with *uninsulated needles*, and *Scarlet* with *uninsulated* needles. There is a newer Scarlet-S system, which has the option of insulated needles as well. The technology with insulated needles has been termed **high-intensity focused radiofrequency (HiFR)**, since the insulated microneedles deliver high-intensity energy focused around the active tip.

The major use for these devices is for acne scarring and stretch marks. They do offer skin tightening benefit as well. The maximum epidermal temperature reached with these devices is between 36°C and 37°C. Literature from the devices claims dermal temperatures of 55–60°C.

The *ePrime* (Syneron-Candela, CA, USA) also uses actual needles, which penetrate the skin. This applies RF current between five pairs of needles, where each pair of needles is an electrode pair. This device has five pairs of needles delivering **bipolar RF** energy at 460 kHz with built-in temperature monitoring. Each shot lasts 3–5 seconds targeting a dermal temperature of 65–75°. The needles are inserted at a 25° angle to reach the deep dermis unlike the Korean MNRF systems, which have a 90° insertion. The operator inputs the desired dermal temperature (e.g. 65°C) and duration (e.g. 4 s); the device delivers RF energy until the temperature is reached and then maintains that temperature for the time entered.

While treatment with the ePrime is longer than that of other microneedle devices, it offers greater control of tissue temperature and is likely able to achieve higher sustained temperatures than the rapid delivery devices. This dermal temperature control is not currently available with noninvasive or other minimally invasive FRF devices.

Fractora is another FRF device with a wide array of treatment tips. These are categorized by tip density, with a high-density or low-density epidermal impact, or by depth of the needle and hence ablative injury and RF penetration, from 600 μm to 3,000 μm (Fig. 7.8).

All these MNRF devices have disposable tips with a preset number of shots (1,000-2,000) and these tips are intended for single use. The cost of these tips ($40-70) is much lower than for systems like Thermage making treatments more affordable.

Summary

The MNRF treatments need the application of topical anesthesia as treatments are painful. The concept in MNRF treatment is to perform multiple passes starting at a deeper depth (2.5-3.5 mm depending on what is being treated) and then decreasing the depth as well as the energy delivered with ease successive pass. The pain becomes worse with each successive pass and by the 3rd or 4th pass can become unbearable unless the skin has been numbed properly. On bony areas the depth of the needles should not exceed 1-1.5 mm. Ice packs can be used for patient comfort if required. Unlike the noninvasive RF systems detailed above recovery from an MNRF procedure can take up to 2-3 days and the face can stay sensitive to heat and sunlight for 5-7 days. Patient should be instructed sun protection during this time.

MONOPOLAR RADIOFREQUENCY PROCEDURE

Patient Selection and Periprocedural Preparation

1. The ideal patient for RF skin tightening is one in the fourth or fifth decade of life or younger, with a healthy lifestyle, close to median body weight for height, with a face that shows maintained facial contours and does not have excessive facial fat.
2. Patients with Glogau grade I and II photoaging, i.e. mild and moderate cases of rhytids and skin laxity are the good candidates for RF skin tightening.
3. Patients with grade III photoaging or those with marked laxity of the superficial muscular aponeurotic system do not do as well and usually require surgical intervention for satisfactory improvement. That said even these patients can be treated after detailed counseling about the limited improvement that will be achieved.
4. Patients with increased facial fat, or heavy cheeks and jowls, improve less.
5. Patients must understand that some RF treatments like Thermage need only one session (with a second 6 months later if required) while others like Exilis, Pelleve, etc. need 4-6 sessions spaced a month apart for best results. The modality chosen will depend on the patient's pain tolerating ability, expected downtime, financial status, comorbid conditions if any, as well as response to treatments done in the past.

6. No special precautions are required in the days leading up to the patient's first treatment. On the day of treatment, a numbing cream may be required depending on the treatment being done. In general, the microneedling RF treatments require numbing cream while the noninvasive ones do not.

The author's personal experience is with Pelleve and the Secret Microneedling RF system and the steps for both are detailed here.

Technique

Pelleve Device

Pelleve comes with variously sized probes ranging from 7.5 mm to 20 mm. The 15 mm probe is commonly used for the face with the 10 mm being used around the eyes.

- The face is treated in cosmetic units beginning with the cheeks followed by the forehead, temples, and the periocular area. The cheek is divided into four equal zones for treatment and any can be treated first. The author likes to start medially near the nose and proceed laterally and downward treating the chin area last.
- The patient return electrode is placed on the upper back of the patient and it is important to make sure it is in firm contact with the skin. It is preferable to use the disposable adhesive type patient return electrode versus the common contact plate one.
- A chilled cooling gel is applied on the treatment area with the help of a spatula. The treatment probe (Figs. 7.9A and B) is then placed on the skin and activated by the push button on the handle or via footswitch.
- It is then moved in quick circular motions tracing out four quadrants in each treatment zone—horizontal, vertical, and then the two diagonals. After this, the skin temperature is checked with an infrared temperature gun. The target temperature is between 39°C and 42°C. One pass (Stampar M) is defined as bringing the skin up to the target temperature. Additional passes as needed are given according to the age of the patient and degree of laxity—roughly one pass for each decade is recommended by some authors.
- Cooling may be required in between multiple passes to decrease the chances of tissue edema.
- The power of the machine is adjusted with 25–35 J being used for areas with high impedance (temples, forehead, and Crow's-feet area) and 35–45 J for areas with low impedance (e.g. the masseter area and around the prejowl sulcus)—Figures 7.9A and B show typical treatment parameters for the mid and lower face. The area around the eye can only tolerate between 12 J and 15 J due to the smaller probe being used there and hence more current concentration. Values higher than this are uncomfortable for the patient and risk causing skin burns.

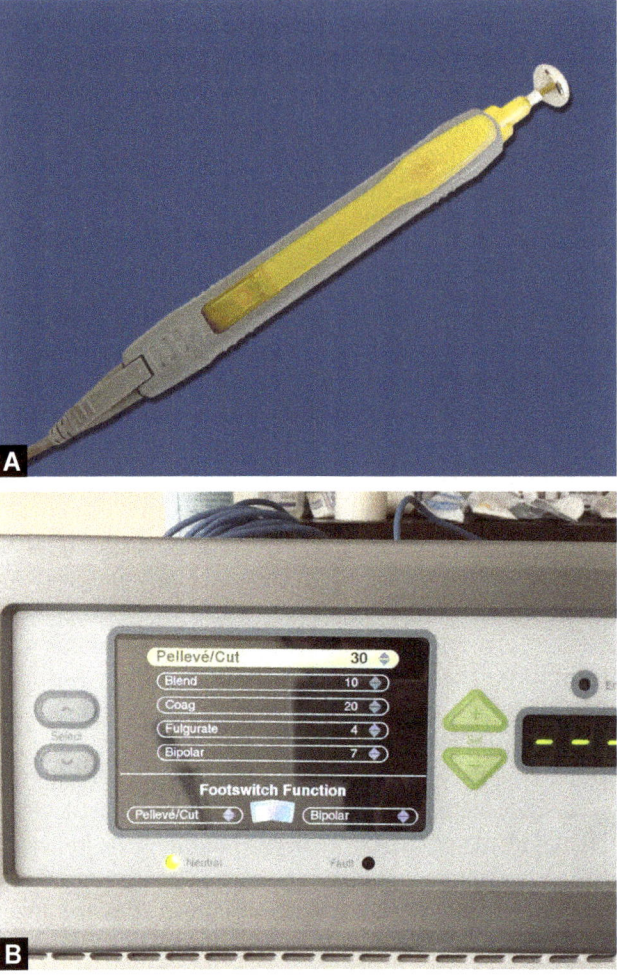

Figs. 7.9A and B: (A) Pelleve treatment probe; and (B) Pelleve user interface showing typical power settings for treating the mid and lower face.

- The patient should feel only a warm heating sensation during treatment. There can be mild skin erythema after completing the passes but this usually fades within 5-10 minutes. There is usually some immediate tightening of the skin after the procedure.
- After the treatment, the gel is wiped off and the patient is sent home with a moisturizer and sunscreen applied. The procedure has no downtime and patients can even have the treatments done in their lunch breaks and go back to work.
- The next session is usually done after 4 weeks and 4-6 sessions are required for optimum results.
- Results after the primary protocol can last 18 months or more—these can be maintained with sessions taken once or twice a year thereafter.

Figures 7.10 to 7.13 showcase some of the results achieved using Pelleve for indications ranging from full face to neck to just periorbital rejuvenation.

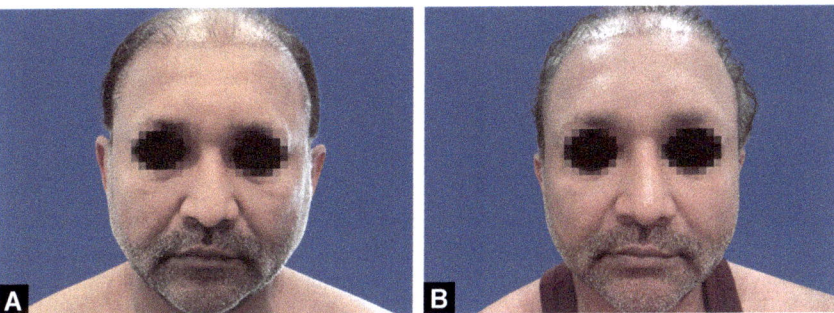

Figs. 7.10A and B: Full face improvement after four sessions of Pelleve spaced 4–6 weeks apart. Note the overall facial tightening, smoothening of forehead wrinkles, and decreased nasolabial and nasojugal grooves. The patient also felt the skin texture had improved feeling smoother and tighter.

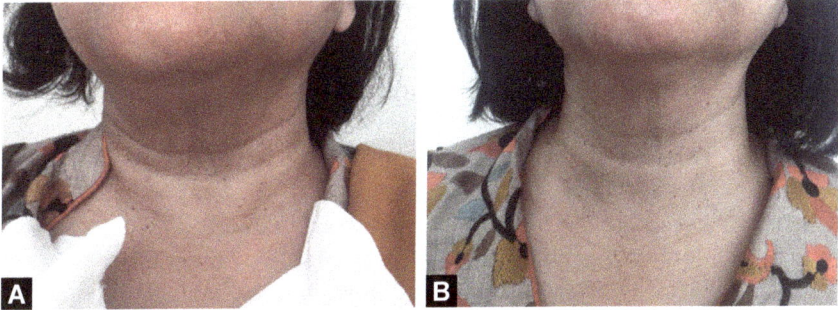

Figs. 7.11A and B: Neck line improvement after one session—immediate postprocedure picture. This improvement is attributed to the immediate contraction of collagen fibers due to increased temperature. This effect lasts a few days after which the wrinkles begin to show again followed by gradual improvement over the next 3–6 months as collagen remodeling takes place.

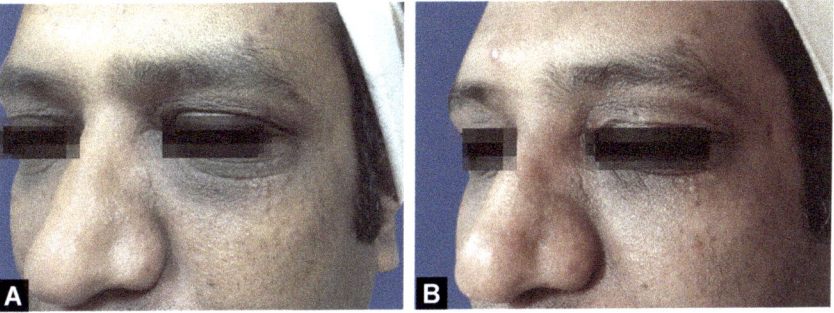

Figs. 7.12A and B: Under eye wrinkle improvement after three sessions of Pelleve spaced 4 weeks apart. The reduction in wrinkles smoothens out the periorbital skin thereby making it appear less dark. Specially designed probes are required for working in this delicate area.

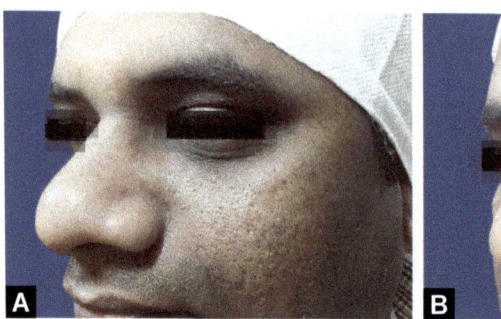 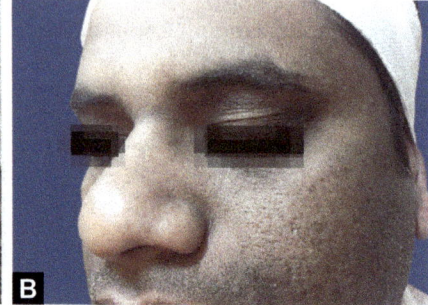

Figs. 7.13A and B: Under eye wrinkle improvement after three sessions of Pelleve spaced 4 weeks apart. Another case showing improvement in under eye darkening and wrinkles with just three sessions.

MICRONEEDLING RADIOFREQUENCY PROCEDURE

Secret Microneedling Radiofrequency

The standard treatment probe with the Secret Microneedling system has gold plated *noninsulated* needles in a 5 × 5 array, i.e. 25 needles per tip (Fig. 7.14). This tip is disposable and should only be used for one patient. It can deliver 1,000 shots before it starts emitting a warning beep but will keep working for a few hundred shots more.

- The treatment is painful and the skin must be numbed with a topical anesthetic for 2 hours before treatment if using lidocaine + prilocaine and 1 hour if using lidocaine + tetracaine. These must be applied under occlusion for maximum pain relief. In patients with very low pain threshold infraorbital and supraorbital nerve blocks can be given in addition since these are usually the most painful areas to treat.
- After this, the skin is cleansed using povidone-iodine solution followed by spirit. Spirit fumes can irritate the patient so good ventilation is important. Treatment is then commenced.
- The authors like to start in the lower face and cover the cheeks with 2–3 passes—horizontal, vertical, and diagonal. The first pass is the deepest and has the longest RF exposure time as well as power. With each pass, all of these parameters are decreased since the amount of pain increases significantly as the needles fire closer the epidermis and there are chances of pinpoint burns with excess power used superficially.
- The end point of treatment is erythema and edema (Fig. 7.15).

With noninsulated needles, there is minimal pinpoint bleeding in some areas; insulated needles can have more bleeding as the papillary dermal vessels are not coagulated at points of needle puncture, since the RF energy is only located at the tip in the mid-dermis.

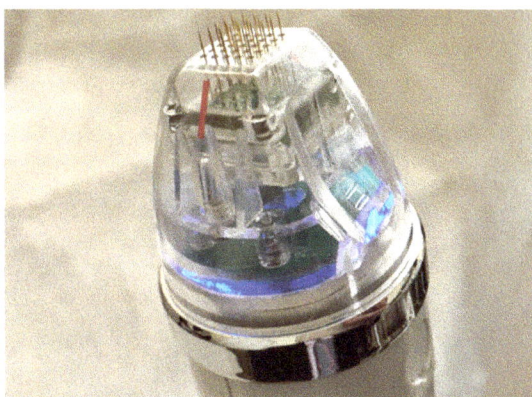

Fig. 7.14: Standard microneedle radiofrequency (MNRF) tip showing noninsulated needles in a 5 × 5 array.

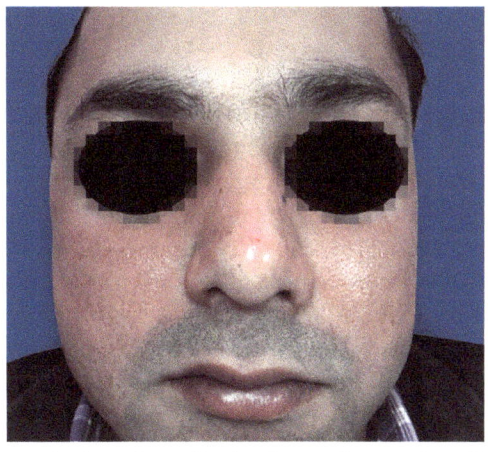

Fig. 7.15: Erythema and edema immediately after a microneedle radiofrequency (MNRF) session to treat centrofacial pores and acne scarring.

- The patients usually have an intense sensation of heat in their face after the procedure and benefit from applying an ice pack for the next 2–4 hours intermittently.
- A mild steroid-antibiotic cream is then applied followed by sunscreen and the patient is asked to avoid sunlight exposure strictly for 5–7 days after treatment. Postprocedure erythema usually lasts only 2–3 days for most patients.

Adverse Events

Adverse effects are very rare with Pelleve. Skin burns at the return electrode because of faulty contact (decreasing surface area of attachment) is possible,

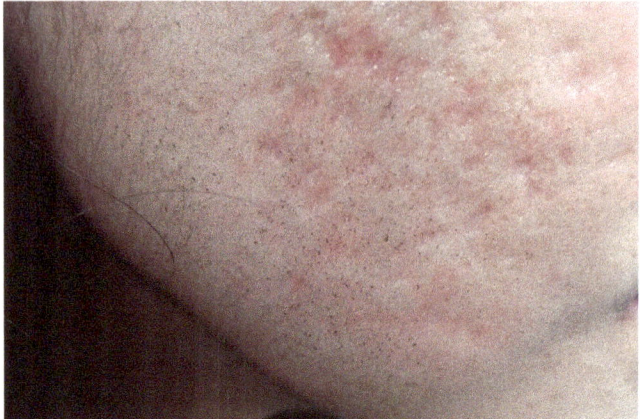

Fig. 7.16: Superficial burns 48 hours after a microneedle radiofrequency (MNRF) session. This is caused by too much radiofrequency (RF) energy being used in the superficial 1.5 mm of the dermis.

as is a skin burn at the site of the active electrode if too much power is used, or if the electrode is held stationary on the skin—it needs to be in constant movement.

Adverse effects with MNRF treatments are again limited to skin burns—these are pinpoint burns though and similar to the crusting seen after fractional CO_2 laser (Fig. 7.16). They clear up in 7-10 days without sequelae in the vast majority of cases. Some patients may have prolonged erythema lasting up to a week. Secondary infection is a possibility since there are hundreds of micropunctures in the skin but the incidence of this is extremely rare with proper after care.

Postprocedural Care

No significant postprocedure care is needed after Pelleve—the patient goes back to his/her normal skin care regimen the next day. It is a good idea to avoid excessive sweating, heat, and sunlight since the skin can become red with exertion for a few days after the procedure.

After MNRF like the Secret MNRF procedure described above the patient is put on a mild steroid-antibiotic cream for 3 days along with a gentle soap-free cleanser and bland moisturizer. Strict sun avoidance is advised for the first 3-5 days as well as protection from excessive heat and sweating. A single dose of prednisolone 40 mg or methylprednisolone 32 mg can be given after the procedure if there is a marked inflammatory response or the erythema from the previous session lasted longer than 3 days. Liberal sunscreen use is advised and typical MNRF sessions are spaced 4-6 weeks apart for 3-6 sessions.

INDICATIONS

Though there are multiple indications including acne scars that is covered in other chapters a few others are listed here. It must be appreciated that there are very head to head trials with fractional lasers, but these systems tend to be robust, hardy and more cost-effective that lasers.

Stretch Marks (Striae)

In a meta-analysis on prevention and treatment approaches proposed for stretch marks from 1950 to 2013, only 13 out of 46 trials were randomized and controlled (including only six evaluating a treatment approach) (Al-Himdani S). The findings demonstrate that **mature** lesions usually show **poor response** compared to immature ones. This is one indication where a control arm is needed to compare the effect of therapy with the intervention.

Bipolar RF, potentiated with infrared (IR) light, can heat the dermis up to 4 mm in depth and stimulates the actin and elastin fibers. A study by Harmelin et al. compared treatment with bipolar RF potentiated with IR light (Sublime 1 applicator) and treatment with fractional bipolar RF (Sublative 1 applicator). Interestingly, this approach is effective on both immature and mature striae. But the addition of IR light was not better than conventional fractional RF.

This has important therapeutic implications, as the best results are usually achieved in immature striae, treated generally by topical tretinoin, while mature striae remained highly challenging (Kang S). The mean improvement in depth after the three sessions was 21% with results ranging from 15% to 35% improvement.

Of course, the improvement may not mirror the satisfaction of the patients who may not be happy with 3D imagery but are more concerned by the visual improvement which may not be marked.

Lower Face and Neck Rejuvenation

Laser rejuvenation has been tried but even with the fractional CO_2 does not achieve sufficient dermal effects to deliver clinically useful results. The use of microneedle electrodes helps to localize the energy in the dermis. The sheathed configuration of the needle and exclusive tip delivery of energy helps to bypass most pain receptors, which are localized within the first 200 mm of the skin. This technology termed HiFR, helps in enhancing the degraded ECM, as well as encourages epidermal renewal through mechanical microneedling. By bypassing thermal injury to the epidermis and dermoepidermal junction (DEJ), the approach was designed to minimize post-treatment downtime and the risk of prolonged erythema and post-inflammatory pigmentation.

The HiFR system delivered 1 MHz RF energy via a bipolar array of microneedles embodied in a single-use disposable tip (INFINI™), Lutronic Corp, Goyang, South Korea. A study by Dr Girish Munavalli found a reasonable skin lifting effect in three sessions.

Noninvasive Labia Tissue Tightening and Orgasmic Dysfunction

Vaginal laxity remains usually underreported, although the majority of women patients consider this condition as bothersome with significant impact on their relationship. The visual aspect and functionality of introitus is marked most often as being responsible for sexual disorder and reduced quality of life (QoL) (Pauls RN). Following the recent recommendations "cosmetic vaginal/vulvar surgery" include labiaplasty, labia minora reduction, excess or redundant clitoral prepuce reduction, labia majora reduction or augmentation, labia majora divergence repair, perineal skin reduction, and mons pubis reduction (McDaniel D). RF has been employed widely in many protocols for skin laxity treatment. A 2010 study by Millheiser et al. of introital/transvaginal monopolar RF (with cryogen cooling) for vaginal laxity after vaginal childbirth reported statistically significant improvement in vaginal laxity in 87% of subjects. Perceived improvement of sexual function (a secondary study end point) was noted in all patients originally reporting reduced sexual function. An investigation by Sekiguchi et al. applied low-energy RF for vaginal introital laxity in premenopausal women, revealing significant improvements in vaginal laxity and sexual function maintained through 12-month follow-up with no reported adverse events.

This topic is discussed in detail in **Chapter 15: Why, When, and How to Buy a Laser?**.

CONCLUSION AND REALISTIC EXPECTATIONS

Regardless of the manner in which the energy is delivered, all RF devices will essentially do the same thing. Some systems are better than others when it comes to treating a specific body part. Combining two or more of these systems is a useful practice. A few principles are reinforced here (Abraham MT, Bogle M, Weiss RA).

- Radiofrequency is ideal for patients with *mild to moderate* facial and neck rhytids and who have *mild* structural ptosis, if they have realistic expectations from this type of procedure.
- When treating loose skin on the body or cellulite the same rules apply. In the best of situations, there is only *a moderate* likelihood that the patient will be very satisfied with change they see in their contour.
- When a patient has photodamage, is in poor health, or smokes, the probability of getting a noticeable result decreases.

- Though collagen production decreases with age, good results can be achieved with RF in older patients if their skin is in good condition.

Long-lasting, predictable skin tightening results with RF can be obtained in the majority of patients by using a technique that allows the use of multiple passes at lower energies, individualizing the treatments based on a patient's feedback on heat sensation, and by treating to a clinical end point.

Some basic practice points are listed in Box 7.1, though various different devices are available though we have discussed the practical application of just two representative devices in the chapter the basic caveats are true for most RF technologies.

Box 7.1: Practice points while using radiofrequency (RF) in aesthetic practice.

- Use test spots in less visible areas to determine how the skin will react to treatment
- Begin with lower settings and gradually increase energy to optimal/advanced parameters
- Use low settings on (a) Small zones, (b) Bone prominences, and (c) Areas with high curvature. Always observe the immediate skin reaction
- Stop energy and treatment when there is any indication for concern and reassess continuation of treatment
- Do not rush treatment
- For both loose skin on the body or cellulite, there is only a 20–25% likelihood that the patient will be very satisfied with change they see in their contour
- When a patient has photodamage, is in poor health, or smokes, the probability of getting a noticeable result decreases
- Determine if patient has realistic expectations
- Show examples of results other patients have achieved in your hands; if the patient cannot see any difference in the photos, this is not someone who will be happy with radiofrequency
- Contraindications to the use of radiofrequency
  - Pacemaker
  - Insulin pump
  - Pregnancy
  - Careful if using over metallic implants such as braces, root canals, tattoos

BIBLIOGRAPHY

1. Abraham MT, Ross EV. Current concepts in nonablative radiofrequency rejuvenation of the lower face and neck. Facial Plastic Surg. 2005;21:65-73.
2. Al-Himdani S, Ud-Din S, Gilmore S, et al. Striae distensae: A comprehensive review and evidence-based evaluation of prophylaxis and treatment. Br J Dermatol. 2014;170:527-47.
3. Alster TS, Tanzi E. Improvement of neck and cheek laxity with a nonablative radiofrequency device: a lifting experience. Dermatologic Surgery. 2004;30:503-7.
4. Bogle M, Ubelhoer N, Weiss RA, et al. Evaluation of the multiple pass, low fluence algorithm for radiofrequency tightening of the lower face. Lasers Surg Med. 2007;39:210-7.
5. Chipps LK, Bentow J, Prather HB, et al. Novel nonablative radio-frequency rejuvenation device applied to the neck and jowls: Clinical evaluation and 3-dimensional image analysis. J Drugs Dermatol. 2013;12:1215-8.

6. Clark Z. Labial tissue rejuvenation and sexual function improvement using a novel noninvasive focused monopolar radiofrequency device. J Cosmet Laser Ther. 2018;20:66-70.
7. Clementoni MT, Munavalli GS. Fractional high intensity focused radiofrequency in the treatment of mild to Moderate laxity of the lower face and neck: A pilot study. Lasers Surg Med. 2016;48:461-70.
8. DiBernardo B. The best of hot topics—lipo-transfer and SmartLipo. ASAPS; 2008.
9. Doshi SN, Alster TS. Combination radiofrequency and diode laser for treatment of facial rhytids and skin laxity. J Cosmet Laser Ther. 2005;7:11-5.
10. Emilia del Pino M, Rosado RH, Azuela A, et al. Effect of controlled volumetric tissue heating with radiofrequency on cellulite and the subcutaneous tissue of the buttocks and thighs. J Drugs Dermatol. 2006;5:714-22.
11. Fisher GH, Jacobson LG, Bernstein LJ, et al. Nonablative radiofrequency treatment of facial laxity. Dermatol Surg. 2005;31:1237-41.
12. Fistonić I, Sorta Bilajac Turina I, et al. Short time efficacy and safety of focused monopolar radiofrequency device for labial laxity improvement-noninvasive labia tissue tightening. A prospective cohort study. Lasers Surg Med. 2016;48:254-9.
13. Fitzpatrick R, Geronemus R, Goldberg D, et al. Multicenter study of noninvasive radiofrequency for periorbital tissue tightening. Lasers Surg Med. 2003;33:232-42.
14. Friedman DJ, Gilead LT. The use of hybrid radiofrequency device for the treatment of rhytids and lax skin. Dermatol Surg. 2007;33:543-51.
15. Fritz K, Bernardy J, Tiplica GS, et al. Efficacy of monopolar radiofrequency on skin collagen remodeling: A veterinary study. Dermatol Ther. 2015;28:122-5.
16. Geronemus R, Goldberg D, Kaminer M, et al. Multicenter study of noninvasive radiofrequency for periorbital tissue tightening. Lasers Surg Med. 2003;33:232-42.
17. Gold MH. Update on tissue tightening. J Clin Aesthet Dermatol. 2010;3:36-41.
18. Goldberg DJ, Yatskayer M, Raab S, et al. Complementary clinical effects of topical tightening treatment in conjunction with a radiofrequency procedure. J Cosmet Laser Ther. 2014;16:236-40.
19. Harmelin Y, Boineau D, Cardot-Leccia N, et al. Fractionated bipolar radiofrequency and bipolar radiofrequency potentiated by infrared light for treating striae: A prospective randomized, comparative trial with objective evaluation. Lasers Surg Med. 2016;48:245-53.
20. Harth Y, Lischinsky D. A novel method for real-time skin impedance measurement during radiofrequency skin tightening treatments. J Cosmet Dermatol. 2011;10:24-9.
21. Jaffary F, Nilforoushzadeh MA, Zarkoob H. Patient satisfaction and efficacy of accent radiofrequency for facial skin wrinkle reduction. J Res Med Sci. 2013;18:970-5.
22. Kang S. Topical tretinoin therapy for management of early striae. J Am Acad Dermatol. 1998;39:S90-2.
23. Lapidoth M, Halachmi S. Radiofrequency in Cosmetic Dermatology. Basel, Switzerland: Karger Publishers; 2015.
24. Lolis MS, Goldberg DJ. Radiofrequency in cosmetic dermatology: A review. Dermatol Surg. 2012;38:1765-76.
25. McDaniel D, Weiss R, Weiss M, et al. Two-treatment protocol for skin laxity using 90-Watt dynamic monopolar radiofrequency device with real-time impedance intelligence monitoring. J Drugs Dermatol. 2014;13:1112-7.
26. McKnight B, Tobin R, Kabir Y, et al. Improving upper arm skin laxity using a tripollar radiofrequency device. J Drugs Dermatol. 2015;14:1463-6.

27. Millheiser LS, Pauls RN, Herbst SJ, et al. Radiofrequency treatment of vaginal laxity after vaginal delivery: nonsurgical vaginal tightening. J Sex Med. 2010;7:3088-95.
28. Mlosek RK, Woźniak W, Malinowska S, et al. The effectiveness of anticellulite treatment using tripolar radiofrequency monitored by classic and high-frequency ultrasound. J Eur Acad Dermatol Venereol. 2012;26:696-703.
29. Mulholland RS, Ahn DH, Kreindel M, et al. Fractional ablative radiofrequency resurfacing in Asian and Caucasian skin: a novel method for deep radiofrequency fractional skin rejuvenation. J Cosmet Dermatol Sci Appl. 2012;2:144-50.
30. Nelson AA, Beynet D, Lask GP. A novel non-invasive radiofrequency dermal heating device for skin tightening of the face and neck. J Cosmet Laser Ther. 2015;17:307-12.
31. Pauls RN, Fellner AN, Davila GW. Vaginal laxity: A poorly understood quality of life problem; a survey of physician members of the International Urogynecological Association (IUGA). Int Urogynecol J. 2012;23:1435-48.
32. Rusciani A, Curinga G, Menichini G, et al. Nonsurgical tightening of skin laxity: A new radiofrequency approach. J Drugs Dermatol. 2007;6:381-6.
33. Sadick NS, Alexiades-Armenakas M, Bitter Jr P, et al. Enhanced full-face skin rejuvenation using synchronous intense pulsed optical and conducted bipolar radiofrequency energy (ELOS): Introducing selective radiophotothermolysis. J Drugs Dermatol. 2004;4:181-6.
34. Sadick NS, Makino Y. Selective electro-thermolysis in aesthetic medicine: A review. Lasers Surg Med. 2004;34:91-7.
35. Stampar M. The Pelleve procedure: An effective method for facial wrinkle reduction and skin tightening. Facial Plast Surg Clin North Am. 2011;19:335-45.
36. Taub AF, Tucker RD, Palange A. Facial tightening with an advanced 4-MHz monopolar radiofrequency device. J Drugs Dermatol. 2012;11:1288-94.
37. Vega JM, Bucay VW, Mayoral FA. Prospective, multicenter study to determine the safety and efficacy of a unique radiofrequency device for moderate to severe hand wrinkles. J Drugs Dermatol. 2013;12:24-6.
38. Weiss RA, Weiss MA, Munavalli G, et al. Monopolar radiofrequency facial tightening: a retrospective analysis of efficacy and safety in over 600 treatments. J Drugs Dermatol. 2006;5:707-12.

NANOFRACTIONAL RADIOFREQUENCY: A PERSPECTIVE

INTRODUCTION

The demand for development of new resurfacing and rejuvenation procedures are on the rise in last decade. In the quest for technologies, which can deliver maximum results with a minimal downtime, gave way to a number of new techniques, machines, and specific treatment protocols to ensure the efficacy of treatment with less side effects.

The introduction of these technologies is providing opportunities for clinicians to experiment and broaden their spectrum of studies in treating patients with different skin conditions, all skin types with effective safety measures.

BACKGROUND

Treatment of skin disorders using laser technologies dates back to the early 1960s, and quickly became a popular method for improving facial wrinkles, scars, skin growths, and blemishes.[1] In the 1980s, continuous wave carbon dioxide (CO_2) lasers became available for more effective esthetic resurfacing, but resulted in mixed outcomes that included many anticipated side effects following resurfacing treatment.[2]

Early CO_2 resurfacing lasers generated a high rate of dyspigmentation, scarring, erythema, skin eruptions, and infections as well as increased pain, discomfort, and downtime. The enhanced thermal injury was due to the continuous wave nature of these early CO_2 lasers that left a wide zone of thermal damage and ablation.[3]

Later, pulsed and scanned CO_2 laser systems, along with erbium-doped yttrium aluminum garnet (Er:YAG) lasers were developed to lessen the thermal damage to treated skin tissue. The reduction in thermal injury was a result of better precision with ablation to the intended target depths, and imparting minimal thermal injury to uninvolved skin. Currently, the erbium:yttrium scandium gallium garnet (YSGG) laser has furthered this ablative laser evolution with technology that better enables a balance of depth and thermal impact not achievable with either of the other ablative wavelengths.[4]

In the early 2000s, further laser development made available the ablative fractional laser (AFL) that enabled delivery of skin treatments with a grid of vertical columns known as microthermal treatment zones (MTZs), which penetrated the epidermis and dermis.[5]

These MTZs have a diameter and depth that are dependent upon the settings of the fractional laser being used. What makes this method unique is that the undamaged skin adjacent to the MTZ provides a reservoir of viable tissue that allows for repopulation of the thermally destroyed and missing epidermis and dermis.[6]

Also, the dermal penetration by the fractional lasers leads to new and remodeled collagen formation by the surrounding fibroblasts, as well as the tightening of existing collagen that contributes to the filling of wrinkles, reduced facial rhytids, and improved skin tone.[7]

The last few years have seen the introduction of a number of new technologies including radiofrequency which could either be insulated or noninsulated. The insulated radiofrequency is preferred as it penetrates deeper and causes dermal injury and thereby causing neocollagenesis and sparing the epidermis.

One of the radiofrequency technologies, which soon became the new technology best suited for resurfacing of skin is microneedling fractional radiofrequency (MFR).

Microneedling fractional radiofrequency, which was considered as the next step beyond CO_2 lasers.

Microneedling fractional radiofrequency device works by creating radiofrequency thermal zones without epidermal injury. After damage to the reticular dermis, long-term dermal remodeling, neoelastogenesis, and neocollagenogenesis results in dermal thickening.[8] The duration of each energy pulse can be set from 10 ms to 1,000 ms. The ability to set multiple needle depths per pass is an advantage, allowing discrete electrothermal coagulation at different layers of the dermis. The insulated needles prevent electrothermal damage from occurring anywhere in the dermis but at the very tip of the needle and never in the epidermis. The mechanisms involved are neocollagenogenesis by needle penetration stimulating the release of growth factors and relative sparing of epidermis and adnexal structures, which contribute to rapid healing.[9]

The new kid on the block replacing all other technologies is nanofractional radiofrequency.

SCIENCE AND RATIONALE

Venus Viva is the first nanofractional radiofrequency device, which delivers a combination of nanofractional radiofrequency with a SmartScan technology along with an MP2, i.e. Magnetic Pulse technology which is used for skin resurfacing.

It is an aesthetically designed, light weight, Food and Drug Administration (FDA) approved, and revolutionary technology for facial remodeling and resurfacing. It is a technology, which allows you to control the ablation coagulation ratio.

Basis of Nanofractional Radiofrequency

State-of-the-art patented tip technology with 700 pulses and a phenomenal depth of penetration (up to 500 µ), provides varying energy density enabling both ablation of the epidermis and coagulation of the dermis area resulting in skin resurfacing with minimal discomfort (Fig. 7.17). It also includes the Magnetic Pulse technology, which is a Multipolar Radiofrequency technology used to heat up the collagen under the skin to achieve better results (Fig. 7.18).

It features a revolutionary new pin design for creating microdermal wounds, which expedites the coagulation process compared to other traditional fractional treatments. It also utilizes the SmartScan feature for nanofractional radiofrequency delivery, which reduces patient discomfort and allows for multiple pattern selections using 160 micropins in a consecutive sequence for faster, less complex treatments.

It has a light handpiece on which fits the consumable 160 micropins tip. There is also a special 80 pin tip which is used specially for acne scars.

The end result is safer, improved energy delivery, flexible treatment sizes, and varied levels of ablation with improved efficacy and reduced downtime.

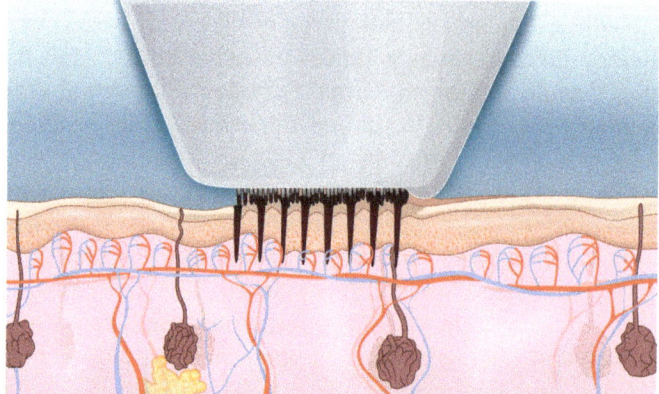

Fig. 7.17: Depth of penetration of the nanofractional radiofrequency (Venus Viva).

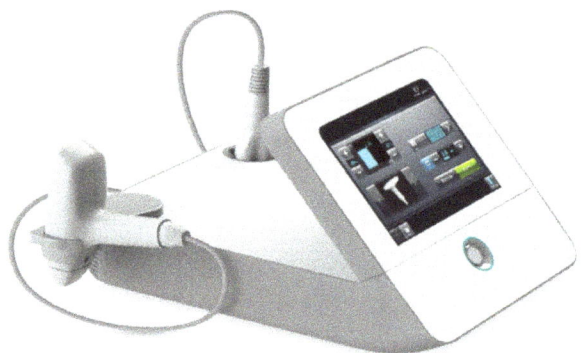

Fig. 7.18: Nanofractional technology (Venus Viva).

Mechanism of Action

It creates vertical microwounds into the skin through which the radiofrequency travels into the skin and stimulates neocollagenesis. The vertical microwounds facilitate rapid release of growth factors leading to reduced downtime and faster healing. The thermal energy generated from nanofractional radiofrequency is created by an oscillating electric current, which causes the charged ions and molecules to collide against each other to generate heat energy in the tissue. Depending upon the intensity, the thermal energy can be used to stimulate or ablate the target tissue in the body.[10]

Using this technique, intended dermal injury is induced with targeted thermal energy while preserving the integrity of the overlying epidermis. While comparing with other technologies in aesthetic medicine, Venus Viva has the highest heat capacity, which can lead to superior contraction of collagen, as well as collagen synthesis and quick healing.

Machine and Its Details

Nanofractional Radiofrequency

- Superior heat conduction
- Largest spot size for radiofrequency to penetrate
- Phenomenal depth of penetration (up to 500 µ)
- Contraction of collagen
- Synthesis of collagen.

Parameters

- *Power:* It ranges from 180V to 280V, which denotes the depth of ablation of the tissue. The deeper the acne scars or pigmentation, the higher would be the power.
- *Pulse width:* It is the amount of coagulation to be induced. To make the treatment stronger, we need to increase the pulse width.
  Hence, this technology allows us to control the amount of ablation and coagulation.
- It has a tip technology with 700 pulses.
- Smaller footprint per pin (150 × 20 µ) creating microwounds for shorter downtime.
- Maximum coverage with minimal discomfort (160 pins per tip with 62 MJ per pin).
- It can generate various patterns to deliver radiofrequency (Fig. 7.19) in order to cover even a small treatment area sparing the surrounding normal skin.
- Pattern generator through unique algorithm enables maximum flexibility during treatment.
- Energy delivered to each pin individually.
- Uniform post-treatment tissue appearance and minimal downtime.
  160 pins tip which can be used for indications like rejuvenation, fine lines, wrinkle, melasma, pigmentation, etc. (Figs. 7.20 to 7.22).

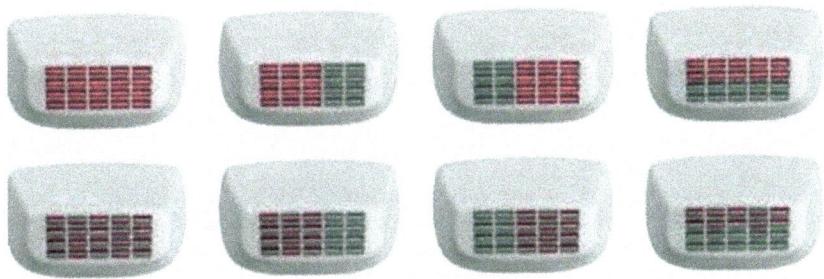

Fig. 7.19: Various patterns of radiofrequency delivered by the tip.

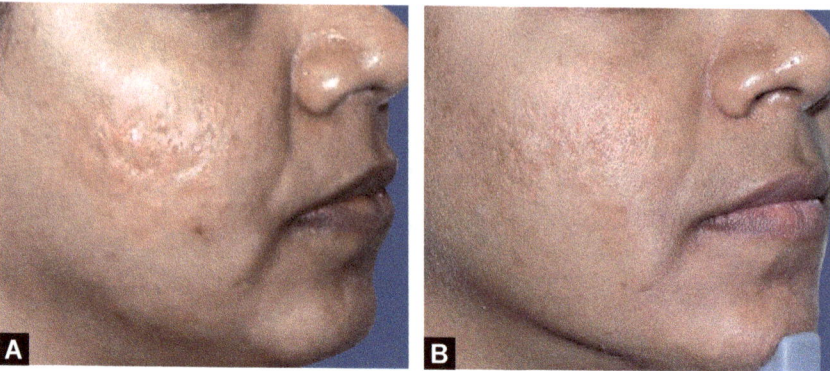

Figs. 7.20A and B: Results after five sessions of nanofractional radiofrequency done for acne scars. Parameters used were between power—240–280V, pulse width—18–25 ms with 160 pins, and continuous pattern. Improvement was seen in box and rolling scars.

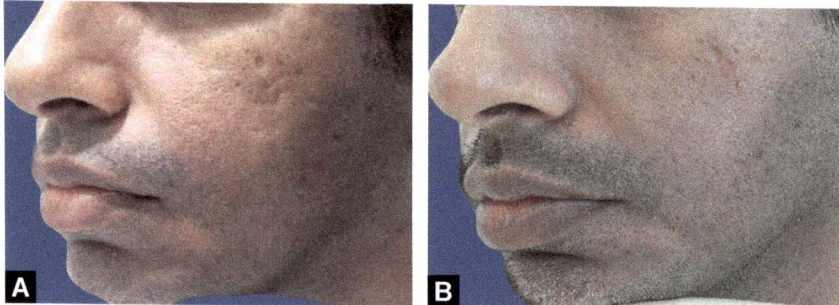

Figs. 7.21A and B: Results after three sessions of nanofractional radiofrequency done for acne scars mainly. Parameters used were between power—250–280V, pulse width—20–28 ms with 160 pins, and continuous pattern. Improvement was seen in box scars.

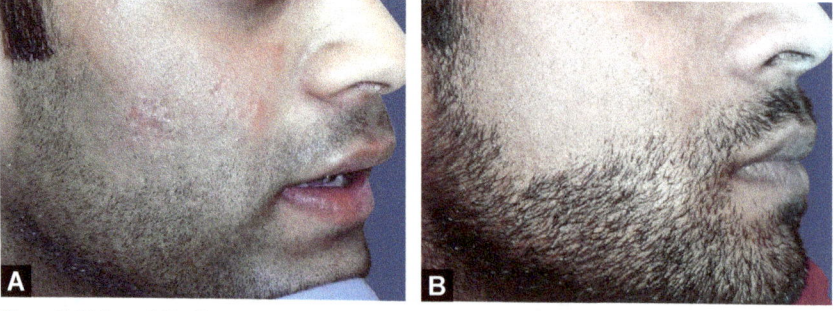

Figs. 7.22A and B: Results after two sessions of nanofractional radiofrequency done for acne scars and open pores. Parameters used were between power—230–260V, pulse width—15–20 ms with 160 pins, and continuous pattern. Improvement was seen in rolling scars and open pores along with textural improvement.

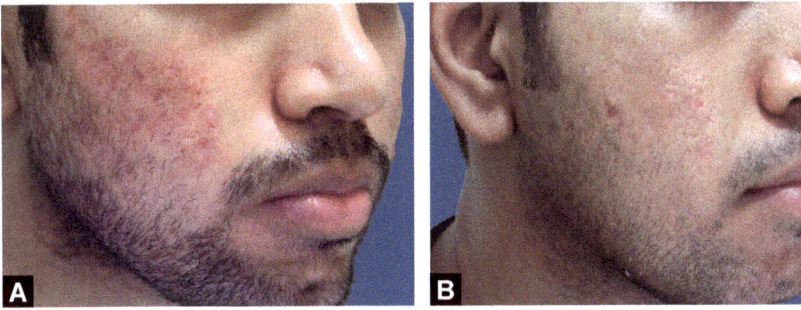

Figs. 7.23A and B: Results after four sessions of nanofractional radiofrequency done for acne scars. Parameters used were between power—260–280V, pulse width—16–25 ms with 80 pins, and continuous pattern. Improvement was seen more in box and rolling scars.

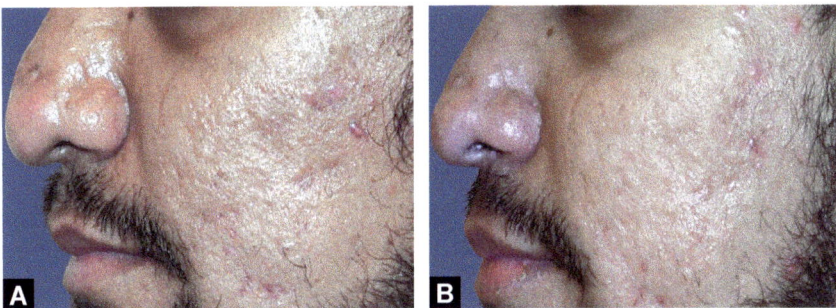

Figs. 7.24A and B: Results after two sessions of nanofractional radiofrequency done for pitted acne scars, open pores. Parameters used were between power—270–280V, pulse width—20–28 ms with 80 pins, and continuous pattern. Improvements were seen in box and rolling atrophic scars, open pores, smoothening of the scars, and improvement in skin texture.

80 pins tip is used specifically for open pores and pitted scars as this forms a bigger loop of radiofrequency under the skin and penetrates deeper to stimulate the collagen under the skin and give better results. Parameters depend upon the indication for which it is used and depth of the condition (Figs. 7.23 and 7.24).

INDICATIONS (TABLE 7.6)

- Dilated open pores
- Reduce signs of aging
- Textural irregularities
- Acne scars
- Diminish deep lines and folds
- Pigmentation (melasma)
- Rosacea.

Table 7.6: Parameters used for treating various indications.

Indications	Power (V)	Pulse width (ms)	Pattern
Rejuvenation/dry skin	220.0	12.0	Alternate
Rejuvenation/oily skin	230–235	14.0	Alternate
Wrinkles—Grade 0–3	220.0	18.0	Alternate
Wrinkles—Grade 4–6	220.0	20–25	Continuous
Stretch marks—Atrophic	260–270	14.0	Continuous
Stretch marks—Nonatrophic	240.0	14.0	Continuous
Postburns scalding	220.0	14.0	Alternate
Hypertrophic scars	260–270	20–30	Continuous
Mild acne scars	230.0	13.0	Continuous
Moderate acne scars	240.0	17.0	Continuous
Deep acne scars	260–280	20–30	Continuous
Open pores/nose	220.0	14.0	Continuous
PIH	220.0	13.0	Alternate
Epidermal pigmentation	220.0	10.0	Alternate
Dermal pigmentation	220.0	5.0	Continuous
PRP—Vitiligo	230–235	30.0	Continuous
PRP—Periorbital	220–230	20.0	Continuous

(PIH: postinflammatory hyperpigmentation; PRP: platelet-rich plasma)

STEP-BY-STEP APPROACH

Patient Selection

- Patient having realistic expectations.
- Age from 15 years to 65 years.
- Patients having all types of pitted scars including box, rolling, or ice pick.
- Patients with the above-mentioned indications.
- Patients should not have any metal or dental implants.
- Rule out any active infections or allergies.

Preoperative Evaluation

- Proper history of the patient is mandatory to assess the type of treatment to be done and the outcome.
- Physical examination of the patient in sufficient light should be done to assess their concern.
- Patient should be counseled about what treatment is being done, what it will do, its downtime, possible complications, number of sessions, and the expected outcome.
- Consent form should be signed prior to doing any treatment.

- Prepictures of the patient in proper lighting should be taken.
- The area to be treated should be cleansed with povidone-iodine or spirit swab.
- The treatment area should be marked.
- Local anesthetic cream should be applied to the treatment area preferably under occlusion for approximately 45 minutes.

Procedure

Using glide gel for smooth movements of the probe, we first employ the MP2 magnetic pulse, a multipolar radiofrequency magnetic pulse to heat up the skin (20–30° for 10 minutes on each side), enabling a deeper penetration of the nanofractional radiofrequency for enhanced outcomes. The targeted skin area is then cleaned from glide gel with warm water and then thoroughly dried to ensure optimal penetration of the radiofrequency energy.

It is important to choose the correct tips, power, pulse duration, and pattern, depending upon the indication.

After choosing the correct tip and parameters, passes are given in a medially downward in cheeks area in a uniform pattern and from brow upward on the forehead with 10% overlap between each pass. This is done by gently touching the tip on the skin surface after stretching the skin.

Postprocedure

There will be redness and swelling immediate postprocedure for which icing is to be done over the treated area for 5–10 minutes. Patients are told to avoid make-up for 24–48 hours post-treatment and apply sunscreen when they go out.

They can be prescribed a mild topical steroid in case the redness persists long. It usually lasts for 2–3 days depending upon the sensitivity of the skin and the parameters used. Avoid use of any creams or products for another 2–3 days to avoid irritation to the treated area. During the initial healing phase of the treatment, minute epidermal crusts are visible which are naturally exfoliated in few days, which then lead to epidermal resurfacing.

Contraindications

- Metal or dental implants
- Active infection
- Keloidal tendency
- Unrealistic expectations.

Side Effects

There are no side effects though few patients can have a downtime, which can last for 5–10 days with lot of swelling and erythema.

Conclusion

Nanofractional radiofrequency can be used to treat a variety of indications ranging from skin rejuvenation to acne scars and pigmentation with minimal side effects and no risk of postinflammatory pigmentation since it is a color blind technology. Nanofractional radiofrequency is currently being used to treat a plethora of cosmetic indications including traumatic and acne scar lesions. The technology has been proven in previous clinical trials to be an effective and safe aesthetic skin rejuvenation treatment modality (Hongcharu et al.).[11]

Considered a milestone in aesthetic treatments, fractional radiofrequency technology has been proven time and again to be a very safe and effective treatment alternative for the gamut of cosmetic indications commonly seen in the aesthetic practice. Radiofrequency-based fractional ablation has several advantages over laser-based fractional ablation including color blind energy [i.e. low risk of postinflammatory hyperpigmentation (PIH)], significantly more coagulation in the tissue surrounding the ablated zones, less downtime, as well as a higher safety profile associated with a lower risk of complications. Nanofractional radiofrequency technology appears to be the natural step in the evolution of radiofrequency energy-based cosmetic treatment solutions. Fractionated radiofrequency energy delivered to the skin modifies the connective tissue through a controlled thermal impact, which in turn activates a physiologic wound healing response (i.e. re-epithelialization and remodeling of the extracellular matrix) to promote a full recovery of the targeted tissue.

The increased efficacy, due to its improved control of both power and pulse duration, results in improved control of tissue ablation or coagulation ratio. This allows for more aggressive treatments, which helps to achieve result in fewer treatments to reach cosmetic goals. The smaller pin footprint allows for the creation of microwounds in the targeted skin, resulting in decreased side effects and shorter downtime. The ability to control these parameters using nanofractional radiofrequency technology enables customizable treatments for each individual case.

Nanofractional radiofrequency technology is an excellent treatment modality for the improvement in the appearance and texture of skin, resurfacing, and acne scars particularly box and rolling type scars. The favorable safety profile associated with treatment underscores the safety of nanofractional radiofrequency technology in cosmetic facial treatments including those patients with darker Fitzpatrick skin types.

REFERENCES

1. Lipozenčić J, Bukvić Mokos Z. Dermatologic lasers in the treatment of aging skin. Acta Dermatovenerol Croat. 2010;18(3):176-80.
2. Airan LE, Hruza G. Current lasers in skin resurfacing. Facial Plast Surg Clin North Am. 2005;13(1):127-39.

3. Tanzi EL, Lupton JR, Alster TS. Lasers in dermatology: four decades of progress. J Am Acad Dermatol. 2003;49(1):1-31.
4. Smith KC, Schachter GD. YSGG 2790-nm superficial ablative and fractional ablative laser treatment. Facial Plast Surg Clin North Am. 2011;19(2):253-60.
5. Alexiades-Armenakas MR, Dover JS, Arndt KA. Fractional laser skin resurfacing. J Drugs Dermatol. 2012;11(11):1274-87.
6. Saedi N, Jalian HR, Petelin A, et al. Fractionation: Past, present, future. Semin Cutan Med Surg. 2012;31(2):105-9.
7. Saedi N, Petelin A, Zachary C. Fractionation: a new era in laser resurfacing. Clin Plast Surg. 2011;38(3):449-61.
8. Hruza G, Taub AF, Collier SL, et al. Skin rejuvenation and wrinkle reduction using a fractional radiofrequency system. J Drugs Dermatol. 2009;8(3):259-65.
9. Calderhead RG, Goo BL, Lauro F, et al. (2013). The clinical efficacy and safety of microneedling fractional radiofrequency in the treatment of facial wrinkles: a multicenter study with the INFINI system in 499 patients. [online] Available from www.westcoastlaser.com/files/pdfs/lutronic-infini/INFINI%20499study.pdf. [Accessed March, 2018].
10. Alster TS, Lupton JR. Nonablative cutaneous remodeling using radiofrequency devices. Clin Dermatol. 2007;25(5):487-91.
11. Hongcharu W, Gold M. Expanding the clinical application of fractional radiofrequency treatment: findings on rhytides, hyperpigmentation, rosacea, and acne redness. J Drugs Dermatol. 2015;14(11):1298-304.

CHAPTER 8

High Intensity and/or Microfocused Ultrasound with/without Visualization

Apratim Goel, Vallari Gatne, Preeti Kothari

INTRODUCTION

With the ever increasing demand for nonsurgical, no downtime skin tightening procedures from patients, physicians are always on a lookout for safe and effective technologies. In the past decade, radiofrequency (RF), ultrasound, and infrared light-based devices have been very popular owing to their ability to deliver precise controlled heat to the dermis. This in turn causes neocollagenesis with some skin tightening. However, the need for multiple sessions usually becomes a limitation with these devices. Recently, high intensity focused ultrasound (HIFU) and microfocused ultrasound (MIFU) with/without visualization was explored in the cosmetic industry as a new treatment modality for skin tightening and rejuvenation (Lee HJ et al.). Owing to lesser number of sessions needed, long lasting effect, minimal downtime and their noninvasive nature, these treatments have gained much importance in the recent past.

HISTORY

Traditional ablative laser skin resurfacing with carbon dioxide or erbium:yttrium-aluminum-garnet devices selectively ablates the epidermis while delivering significant thermal injury of up to 35–45° to the dermis sufficient to stimulate robust wound healing response with subsequent collagen remodeling and contraction (Ross EV et al.; Fitzpatrick RE et al.). However, traditional ablative laser skin resurfacing was associated with extensive postoperative recovery and risk of delayed dyspigmentation (Tanzi EL et al.).

Modest skin tightening can also be induced by RF devices that rely on heat delivery up to 2–4 mm into the dermis to stimulate the wound healing cascade and neocollagenesis without epidermal injury and associated clinical recovery (Alster TS et al.; Zelickson BD et al.; Arnoczky SP et al.).

Thermage was the first RF device approved by United States Food and Drug Administration (US FDA) in 2004 for periorbital wrinkle reduction and subsequently for body contouring in 2006. Since then, many other RF devices using monopolar, bipolar, or multipolar technologies have been developed and combined with other light and laser technologies (Beasley KL et al.).

The latest technologies with minimal number of sessions and downtime which have revolutionized the field of nonsurgical skin tightening are HIFU and MIFU with/without visualization. The first investigations of HIFU were started by Lynn et al. in the early 1940s (Lynn JG et al.).

The first commercial HIFU machine, called the Sonablate 200, was developed by the American Company Focus Surgery, Inc. (Milpitas, CA) and launched in Europe in 1994 after receiving CE approval, bringing a first medical validation of the technology for benign prostatic hyperplasia (BPH). In 2008, HIFU was approved for dermatologic aesthetic uses with advent of commercial machines like ultraformer (Park H).

The Ulthera® Microfocused Ultrasound with Visualization (MFU-V) technology system **(Ultherapy®)** was approved by the US FDA in 2009 initially for brow lift and then later-on skin lifting of the complete face *(upper face, periorbital, lower face, perioral)*, neck and décolleté nonabrasive eyebrow elevation but is routinely used for panfacial and submental treatments (Gutowski KA et al.).

HIGH INTENSITY AND MICROFOCUSED ULTRASOUND WITH/WITHOUT VISUALIZATION

High intensity and microfocused ultrasound with/without visualization have created a benchmark in the field of nonsurgical facelifts. They have an acoustic energy, known to propagate much deeper through tissue than laser or RF energy and have been recently adapted for subcutaneous lipolysis (Fatemi A et al.).

These focused ultrasound technologies can produce small, microthermal lesions by heating the tissues at 65° at precise depths in the dermis up to the fibromuscular layer, causing thermally-induced contraction of collagen and tissue coagulation with subsequent collagenesis, while sparing the epidermis (Alam M et al.; Suh DH et al.; Lee HS et al.)

Introduction of focused ultrasound for skin tightening could help achieve better clinical results owing to the precise thermal zones at various depths, which further can achieve higher tissue temperature, cause stronger tissue remodeling, and produce longer lasting results in lesser number of sessions.

Ultherapy® is one such treatment which has microfocused ultrasound with visualization for precise and accurate skin lifts at different depths of 1.5 mm, 3.0 mm, 4.5 mm (Fig. 8.1). Each line of Ultherapy® that is transmitted through the transmitter, creates 17–23 thermal coagulation points (TCPs).

The parameters and variables of Ulthera® that we use are given here in Figure 8.1.

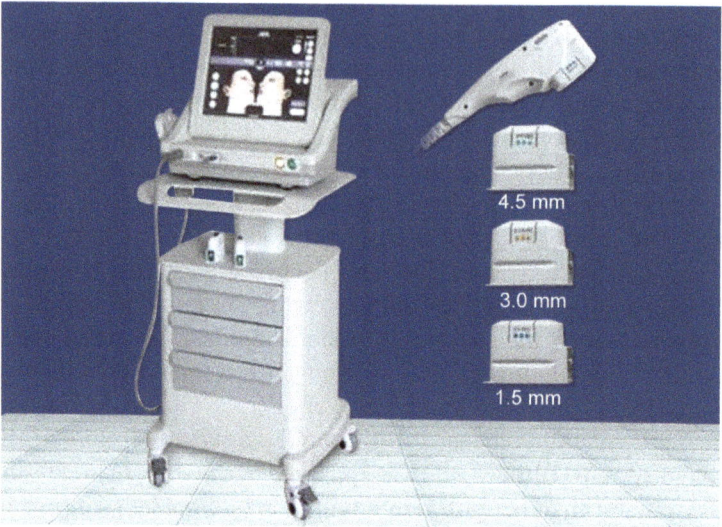

Fig. 8.1: A photograph of the Ulthera® control unit (CU).

There are three transducers used in Ulthera® for different depths as mentioned below:
1. 4.5 mm depth (for lower face, upper and lower neck)
2. 3.0 mm depth (for upper face, lower face, upper and lower neck)
3. 1.5 mm depth (for upper face, lower face, upper and lower neck).

Energy ranges are from 0.1 Joule to 1.2 Joules which can be adjusted as per the clinician's discretion based on patient's BMI and tolerance level.

Length of the treatment area on the transducer is marked as 25 mm which can be adjusted on the touch screen of the Ulthera® monitor.

Mechanism of Action

These ultrasound waves penetrate deeper into the tissues without affecting the epidermis and focus at a single point in the adipose tissue and cause thermal injury. Each treated area is tightly focused at a given depth and heated precisely using shorter pulses to produce small zones of coagulative necrosis at the site with surrounding tissue and superficial layers essentially unaffected (White WM et al.; White WM et al.). The epidermal surface remains unaffected as long as the energy delivered is not excessive for the given focal depth and frequency ranging from 4 MHz to 7 MHz emitted by a given transducer, eliminating the need for superficial cooling, and speeding the recovery process, as healing occurs rapidly from untreated adjacent tissue (Alam M et al.; Har-Shai Y et al.). The device is able to penetrate deeper into tissue than its nonsurgical predecessors in an effort to affect superior tissue

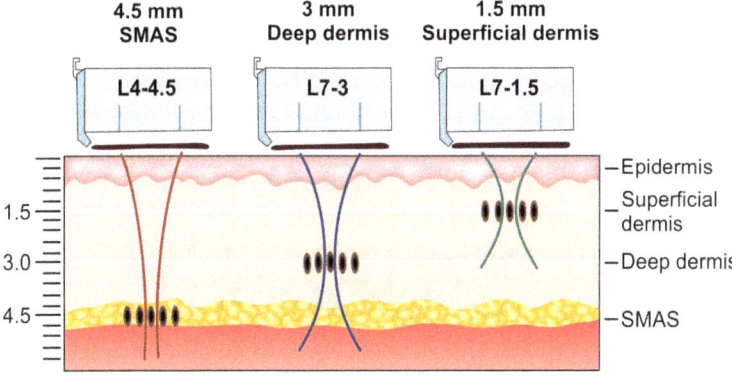

Fig. 8.2: Depiction of the depth of penetration into the skin using various probes. (SMAS: superficial musculoaponeurotic system).

tightening and longevity of results by selectively targeting the superficial musculoaponeurotic system (SMAS) (Fig. 8.2).

The SMAS lies deep to the subcutaneous fat, envelops the muscles of facial expression, and extends superficially to connect with the dermis (Suh DH et al.). The SMAS layer is composed of collagen and elastic fibers similar to the dermal layer of the skin, however, it has more durable holding property and less delayed relaxation after lifting procedures than skin alone (Sasaki GH et al.). Thus, SMAS is a desirable target for noninvasive skin tightening procedures.

Unlike lasers, which penetrate the skin from the outside in, the focused ultrasound procedure bypasses the surface of the skin, and delivers targeted energy specifically into the deep, structural tissues and SMAS targeting the collagen and connective tissue. HIFU and MIFU with/without visualization involve penetrating ultrasound energy to stimulate collagen production in the deeper dermal and subdermal levels, which results in microinjury to that tissue. As the tissue heals, it causes neocollagenesis and as the collagen fibers organize and shorten, a tightening effect is seen on the tissues. The mechanism is depicted in Figure 8.3. The process of wound healing is depicted here in the Table 8.1.

Ultherapy® Mechanism of Action: The Ulthera System uses microfocused ultrasound with visualization (MFU-V) to lift and tighten the skin through specific mechanisms. The initial lift seen immediately after an Ultherapy treatment arises from thermally induced collagen coagulation, denaturation and contraction within precise, well-defined lesions. The creation of these lesions leads to an inflammatory wound-healing response which stimulates long-term tissue remodeling and leads to further lifting and tightening.

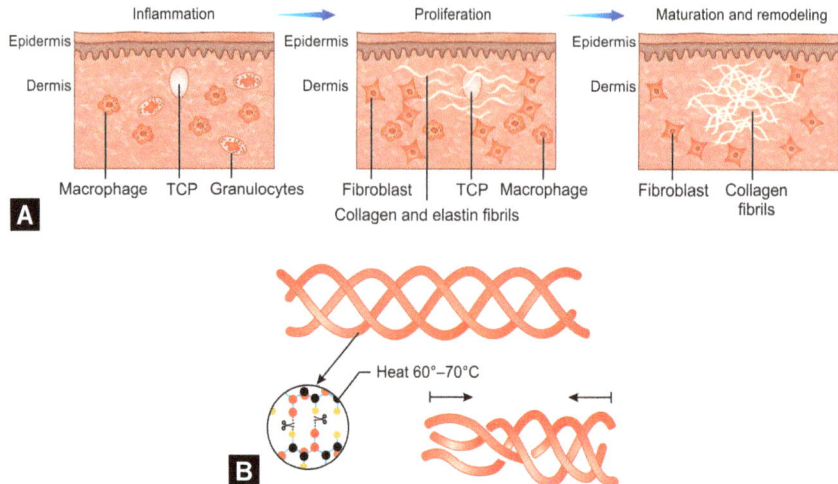

Figs. 8.3A and B: The application of heat at specific temperatures to tissue disrupts and breaks the hydrogen bonds holding the collagen fibrils together, resulting in contraction of the collagen structures.

Table 8.1: Wound healing process with the high intensity focused ultrasound (HIFU).

Clinically	Pathologically
• *Inflammation phase*—Mild tenderness, 0–48 hours. Edema, erythema, bruise, and nerve coagulation, and damage	• *Inflammation phase*—Hemostasis, skin cell migration
• *Proliferative phase*—Tightness, tenderness extended, start seeing reduction, and contouring	• *Proliferative phase*—2–6 weeks. Granulation tissue, wound contraction, and collagen synthesis
• *Remodeling phase*—Main contour 3 weeks to 6 and lipolysis seen here	• *Remodeling phase*—Maximum 3–6 months. Collagen rearrangement, strength increase, and skin lifting effect

Indications

The Ulthera® system is indicated for use as a noninvasive dermatological aesthetic treatment to:
- Lift the eyebrow
- Lift lax submental (beneath the chin) and neck tissue
- Improve lines and wrinkles of the décolleté.

The Ulthera System, in conjunction with the Ulthera DeepSEE transducer, allows for ultrasonic visualization of depths up to 8 mm below the surface of the skin. The indicated use of the imaging is to visualize the dermal and subdermal layers of tissue to:
- Ensure proper coupling of the transducer to the skin
- Confirm appropriate depth of treatment such as to avoid bone.

Contraindications

- Open facial wounds or lesions
- Active infection or open skin at the treatment site
- Cystic acne
- Metal stents/implants in the face or neck (dental implants OK)
- Implantable electrical devices
- Within 2 weeks after the botulinum toxin A
- Pregnant or breastfeeding woman
- Permanent dermal implants
- Antithrombosis therapy
- Active systematic or skin disease which may hinder regeneration
- Hemorrhagic disorders or dysfunctions
- Unrealistic expectations of treatment.

Patient Evaluation

- *History:* Taking proper history of the patient is mandatory to decide the plan of treatment. Knowledge of medical and drug history of the patient helps us in avoiding a number of complications.
- *Assessment:* Proper physical examination is essential to decide the type of technology to be used, the number of sessions needed, and the outcome. Patients with sagging skin on jowls, wrinkles, and fine lines with thin skin would require only one session as compared to patients with a bulky face who would require around 2–3 sessions.
- *Photographs:* Photographs of the patient in adequate lighting and in different angles are essential to assess the response to treatment. There should be a documentation of pictures taken in similar lighting and angle in each follow-up visit for ease of assessment.
- *Expectations:* It is very important to know what is in the mind of the patient. Only the candidates with realistic expectations should be selected to avoid unhappy patients.
- *Counseling:* It forms a major part of any doctors practice. Explaining to the patient what the treatment would do, how it works, the number of sessions needed, and the final result helps not only to build confidence in the patient but also makes the patient aware of what to expect post-treatment.
- *Consent form:* It is an essential prerequisite before starting any treatment as it gives you a written proof of all the above mentioned points and saves you in difficult situations and keeps a transparency in the treatments.

Prerequisites

- Choosing the right candidate is very important for satisfactory results. The ideal patient for nonsurgical tissue tightening displays mild to moderate

skin and soft tissue laxity. Severe skin laxity, marked platysmal banding, severe jowling, and low cervicomental angle are problems best addressed by surgical interventions.
- Younger patients are more likely to have a good outcome, as the wound healing response to thermal injury is vigorous.
- Patients with excessively photodamaged skin or a history of smoking are less favorable candidates, as their ability to create collagen in response to thermal injury may be inadequate.

Preprocedure

After taking the consent, measurements, photographs of the patient, and making sure that all the indications are met, the procedure can be commenced.
- Face is cleansed with povidone-iodine and saline or alcohol swab.
- Marking is done with a different color on the face to denote the areas to be targeted and those to be avoided.
- Proper positioning of the patient like stretching the neck of the patient making sure that the patient is comfortable is important to cover all the areas and ensures ease of the treatment.

Procedure

- Gel is applied on the face, and initially shots with 4.5 mm cartridge are given on neck and lower face only. The direction of the shots is always antigravity, pulling the tissues upward. Firm pressure is applied perpendicular to the skin surface making sure that the entire surface of the probe is in contact with the skin along with the transducer.
- *Upper face contouring*: 1.5 mm and 3 mm cartridge only is used for *upper face* as the skin is thinner compared to lower face (Figs. 8.4 and 8.5).
- Again, the parameters are adjusted as per the need and tolerability of the patient.
- The number of shots to be given depends upon the bulk of the adipose tissue. On an average, 50–250 shots of 4.5 mm and 50–150 shots of 3.5 mm are given on each side. Spot treatment can also be given to the problem area restricting the number of shots.
- Then, the skin is cleaned, gel is removed, and icing is done. In case of too much redness, oral anti-inflammatory and mild topical steroid can be given.

Postprocedure

Patients can resume their routine activities immediately after treatment. There may be redness, which settles in about an hour.

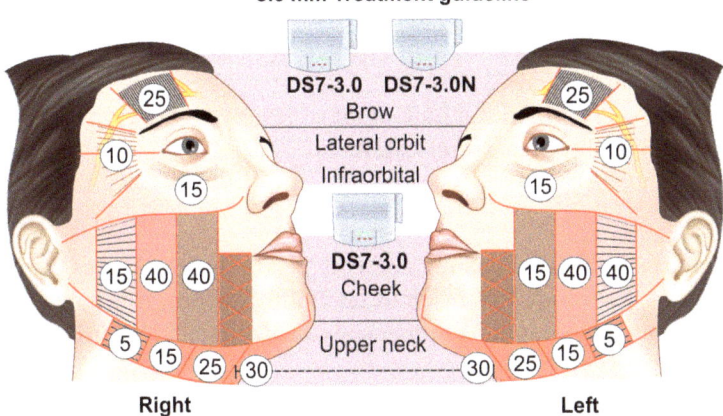

Fig. 8.4: Figure depicts the number of shots to be delivered in each area with 3 mm cartridge.

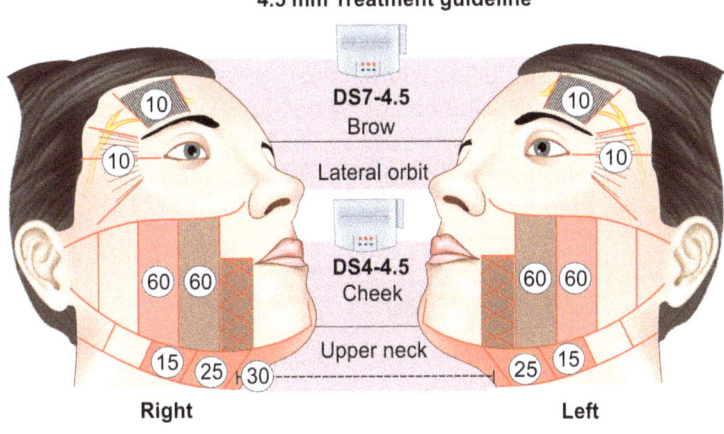

Fig. 8.5: Figure shows the number of shots to be delivered with 4 mm cartridge.

The patient is advised to avoid excessive movements that night which helps in immobilization of the tissues, thereby ensuring adequate healing. The patient may feel little soreness on the face, which lasts for around 1–2 weeks.

Protocol

- The number of sessions is decided by the bulk of adipose tissue, the extent of sagging skin, and the desired result. The sessions are to be spaced at an interval of 3 months.
- Maintenance should be once a year for patients above 60 years.

- Need for neuromodulator like botulinum toxin in masseter and lower face can be assessed after 3 months of first session.
- In author's experience, there has been a need to inject neuromodulators after 3 months of HIFU.
- This is because, when the bulk of fat is destroyed, the facial asymmetry due to inequality of masseters shows up.

Results

As the process of wound healing and collagen remodeling takes 2–3 weeks, the patient will see only 10% result in 1st month, another 10% in 2nd month, and 80% result in 3rd month. Some results are depicted in Figures 8.6 to 8.10.

Final Outcomes

- Tighter, better skin, including forehead, eyes, mouth, neck, and décolleté
- Reduced fine to deep wrinkles
- Under eye troughs, bags, and dark circles
- Skin lifting
- Slows down the development of aging signs
- Lifts and tightens the cheeks without the surgery
- Slows down the development of aging signs on the face, neck, and décolleté
- Improves skin elasticity and shaping of the face contour
- Improves jaw line.

Prevention of Complications from High Intensity Focused Ultrasound

- *Motor nerve paresis*: Ask patient to report any facial muscle twitching during treatment near superficial motor nerves and apply ice to any red or inflamed areas after treatment.
- *Nodules*: Use appropriate treatment density and technique as confirmed by corresponding ultrasound image on monitor.
- *Bruising*: Avoid treating patients on blood thinning medications and administering pulse directly to a visible vessel on the ultrasound image.
- *White striations or geometrical wheals:* Typically occur with superficial transducer—ensure proper coupling with corresponding ultrasound image before each pulse delivery.

Small areas of *purpura* may develop and are expected to resolve over 1–2 weeks.

Linear or geometrical striations seen after treatment with the superficial transducer are treated with topical corticosteroids and followed for rapid resolution (Suh DH et al.; Sasaki GH et al.; Alam M et al.). No permanent textural changes from these lesions have been reported. Lingering mild to

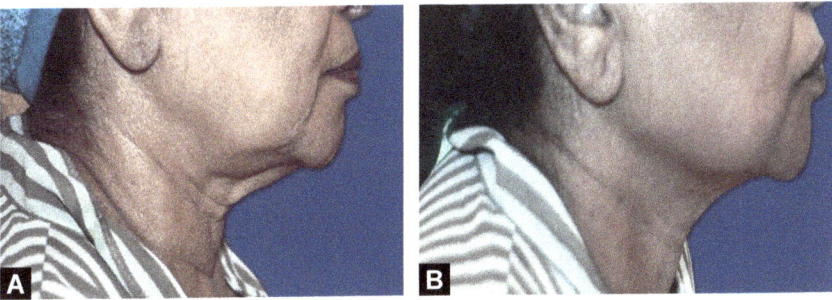

Figs. 8.6A and B: Figures showing the results immediately after high intensity focused ultrasound (HIFU) for sagging jowls and loose skin. Total 600 shots were given. Parameters used—4.5 mm–200 shots on each side, power–1 J, and pitch–1.4 mm; 3 mm–100 shots on each side, power–0.9 J, and pitch–1.5 mm. Improvement noticed was an instant skin lift with clear demarcation of the mandibular angle and reduction in the wrinkles and sagging skin on the neck.

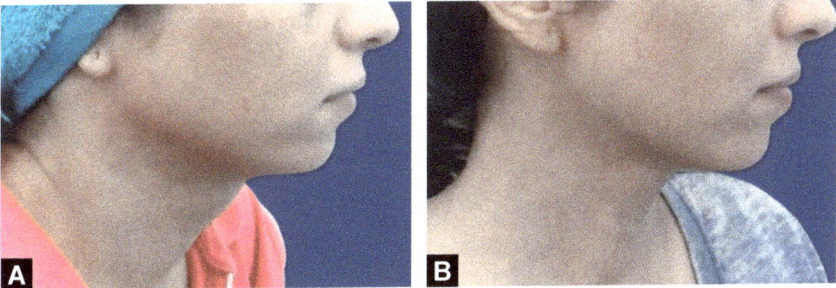

Figs. 8.7A and B: Figures showing the results after 3 months of high intensity focused ultrasound (HIFU) mainly done for sagging jowls. Total shots were given—500. Parameters used—4.5 mm–150 shots on each side, power–1 J, and pitch–1.5 mm; 3 mm–100 shots on each side, power–0.9 J, and pitch–1.5 mm. Improvement was seen in the lower face mainly with a more sharp jawline.

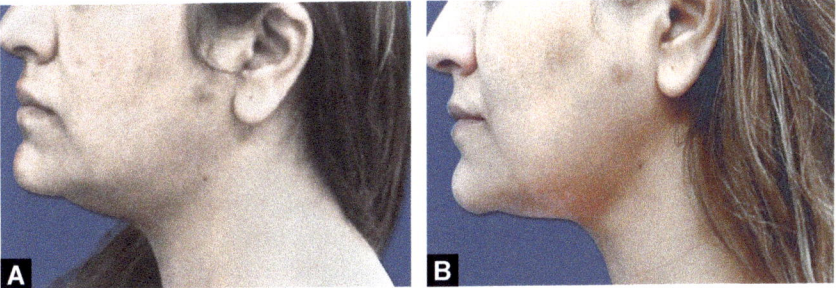

Figs. 8.8A and B: Figures showing the results of high intensity focused ultrasound (HIFU) after 3 months mainly for double chin. Spot HIFU was done where 200 shots were given on double chin. Parameters used—4.5 mm–100 shots on each side, power–1 J, and pitch–1.5 mm; 3 mm–100 shots on each side, power–0.9 J, and pitch–1.5 mm. Improvement was seen with reduction in double chin and a sharper jawline.

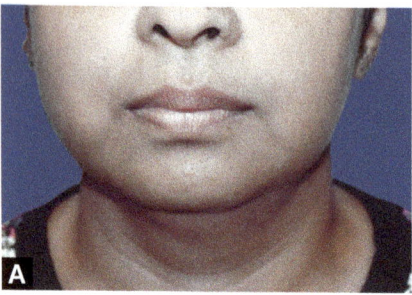
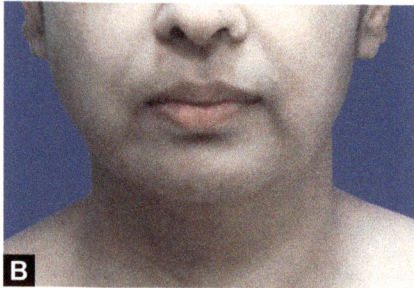

Figs. 8.9A and B: Figures showing the results of high intensity focused ultrasound (HIFU) after 3 months done mainly for skin tightening and contouring along with facial debulking. Total shots were given—700. Parameters used—4.5 mm–200 shots on each side, power–1 J, and pitch–1.5 mm; 3 mm–100 shots on each side, power–0.9 J, and pitch–1.5 mm; and 1.5 mm–50 shots on each side, power–0.9 J, and pitch–1.5 mm. Improvement was seen with volume reduction, a more firmer and tighter skin, and a contoured jowl.

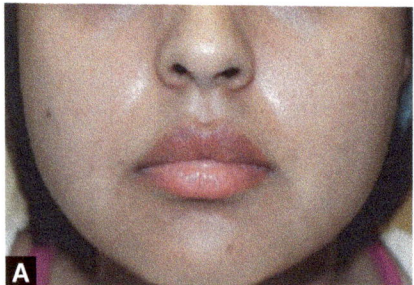
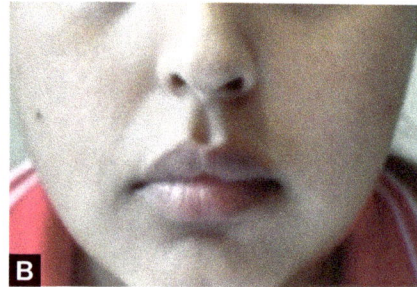

Figs. 8.10A and B: Figures showing the results of high intensity focused ultrasound (HIFU) after 3 months done mainly for facial debulking. Total shots were given—800. Parameters used—4.5 mm–250 shots on each side, power–1 J, and pitch–1.5 mm; 3 mm–150 shots on each side, power–1 J, and pitch–1.5 mm. Improvement was seen with reduction of fat and face looking slimmer. It was combined with neuromodulator for masseters after 3 months.

moderate skin tenderness and edema in the first 1–4 weeks after treatment is common (Chan NP et al.; Alster TS et al.).

Although uncommon, more serious complications after HIFU or MIFU skin tightening can occur, including the development of palpable subcutaneous nodules and/or motor nerve paresis. Fortunately, these effects are temporary and can be avoided with proper operative technique.

Motor nerve paresis is the most concerning potential complication in the immediate post-treatment period, and its incidence is limited to case reports. The areas at the greatest risk for injury are the temporal branch of the trigeminal nerve as well as the marginal mandibular nerve, where the course of the nerve becomes relatively superficial. The affected patient will present with an inability to contract the frontalis muscle or perioral asymmetry. Symptoms usually occur within the first 1–12 hours after treatment and are likely related to nerve inflammation. Resolution is expected in 2-6 weeks, and no permanent nerve injury has been reported to date.

For patients who notice facial muscle twitching during treatment near "danger zone" regions, ice should be immediately applied and anti-inflammatory medication considered.

CONCLUSION

The increased use of noninvasive ultrasound, as an alternative body contouring technique is directly linked to the patient preference for noninvasive procedures. Early devices for fat reduction with ultrasound appear to show some promise but the degree of consequent improvement remains to be substantiated by better controlled, unbiased studies. Newer refinement of these devices may offer further efficacy while maintaining a good safety profile and continuing to meet the patient's needs for comfort during the procedure.

The HIFU/MIFU is soon about to replace a number of surgical as well as nonsurgical technologies used for skin tightening. It is truly a remarkable breakthrough in technology, offering a noninvasive alternative to a surgical facelift, a must have treatment option, and the only FDA approved treatment with a specific intent for improvement of lines and wrinkles on the face and décolleté, penetrating to depths only previously possible with surgery.

As it is easy to perform, less time consuming, and almost painless technology, it is the technology at the top of the list of various skin tightening treatments. Since, it is a gradual process and takes 3 months to show full result, it gives the patients a natural looking and desired youthful look.

BIBLIOGRAPHY

1. Alam M, White LE, Marin N, et al. Ultrasound tightening of facial and neck skin: A rater-blinded prospective cohort study. J Am Acad Dermatol. 2010;62:262-9.
2. Alster TS, Tanzi E. Improvement of neck and cheek laxity with a nonablative radiofrequency device: a lifting experience. Dermatol Surg. 2004;30:503-7.
3. Alster TS, Tanzi EL. Noninvasive lifting of arm, thigh, and knee skin with transcutaneous intense focused ultrasound. Dermatol Surg. 2012;38:754-9.
4. Arnoczky SP, Aksan A. Thermal modification of connective tissues: basic science considerations and clinical implications. J Am Acad Orthop Surg. 2000;8:305-13.
5. Beasley KL, Weiss RA. Radiofrequency in cosmetic dermatology. Dermatol Clin. 2014;32(1):79-90.
6. Chan NP, Shek SY, Yu CS, et al. Safety study of transcutaneous focused ultrasound for non-invasive skin tightening in Asians. Lasers Surg Med. 2011;43(5):366-75.
7. Fatemi A. High-intensity focused ultrasound effectively reduces adipose tissue. Semin Cutan Med Surg. 2009;28:257-62.
8. Fitzpatrick RE, Rostan EF, Marchell N. Collagen tightening induced by carbon dioxide laser versus erbium:YAG laser. Lasers Surg Med. 2000;27:395-403.

9. Gutowski KA. Microfocused ultrasound for skin tightening. Clin Plast Surg. 2016;43(3):577-82.
10. Har-Shai Y, Bodner SR, Egozy-Golan D, et al. Mechanical properties and microstructure of the superficial musculoaponeurotic system. Plast Reconstr Surg. 1996;98:59-70.
11. Lee HJ, Lee KR, Park JY, et al. The efficacy and safety of intense focused ultrasound in the treatment of enlarged facial pores in Asian skin. J Dermatolog Treat. 2015;26:73-7.
12. Lee HS, Jang WS, Cha YJ, et al. Multiple pass ultrasound tightening of skin laxity of the lower face and neck. Dermatol Surg. 2012;38:20-7.
13. Lynn JG, Zwemer RL, Chick AJ, et al. A new method for the generation and use of focused ultrasound in experimental biology. J Gen Physiol. 1942;26:179-93.
14. Park H, Kim E, Kim J, et al. High-intensity focused ultrasound for the treatment of wrinkles and skin laxity in seven different facial areas. Ann Dermatol. 2015;27(6): 688-93.
15. Ross EV, McKinlay JR, Anderson RR. Why does carbon dioxide resurfacing work? A review. Arch Dermatol. 1999;135:444-54.
16. Ross EV, Naseef GS, McKinlay JR, et al. Comparison of carbon dioxide laser, erbium:YAG laser, dermabrasion and dermatome: a study of thermal damage, wound contraction and wound healing in a live pig model: implications for skin resurfacing. J Am Acad Dermatol. 2000;42:92-105.
17. Sasaki GH, Tevez A. Clinical efficacy and safety of focused-image ultrasonography: a 2-year experience. Aesthet Surg J. 2012;32:601-12.
18. Suh DH, Shin MK, Lee SJ, et al. Intense focused ultrasound tightening in Asian skin: clinical and pathologic results. Dermatol Surg. 2011;37:1595-602.
19. Tanzi EL, Lupton JR, Alster TS. Lasers in dermatology: four decades of progress. J Am Acad Dermatol. 2003;49:1-31.
20. White WM, Makin IR, Barthe PG, et al. Selective creation of thermal injury zones in the superficial musculoaponeurotic system using intense ultrasound therapy: a new target for noninvasive facial rejuvenation. Arch Facial Plast Surg. 2007;9:229.
21. White WM, Makin IR, Slayton MH, et al. Selective transcutaneous delivery of energy to porcine soft tissues using intense ultrasound (IUS). Lasers Surg Med. 2008;40:67-75.
22. Zelickson BD, Kist D, Bernstein E, et al. Histological and ultrastructural evaluation of the effects of a radiofrequency-based nonablative dermal remodeling device: a pilot study. Arch Dermatol. 2004;140:204-9.

CHAPTER 9

Noninvasive Body Contouring and Lipolysis

Shruti Dewan, Vivek Nair, Kabir Sardana

INTRODUCTION

Noninvasive body contouring is an ever-expanding field that has seen exciting research and development over the last decade. Beginning with suction-massage machines over 20 years ago, the technology has progressed to involve sophisticated laser and radiofrequency (RF) devices. The commonly practiced laser lipolysis is one component of the array of devices.

The ability to alter the three-dimensional (3D) aspects of the face with optical, ultrasonic, and/or electromagnetic technology has led physicians, scientists, and engineers to develop new ways to alter the topography of the human body—especially as it relates to pockets of fat deposition, irregular contours or laxity of skin, cellulite reduction, and circumferential reduction of legs, arms, abdomen, and buttocks.

As per the revised nomenclature (Alam et al. 2013) the devices for body contouring can be divided into three categories (Box 9.1).

This classification may seem daunting for someone getting into body shaping platforms. However, the picture becomes clearer if the machines are classified according to the *energy* used for transepidermal delivery to the adipocyte; in which case there are *four primary modalities*:

1. Suction/massage machines
2. Radiofrequency (RF) machines
3. Ultrasound machines
4. Laser machines.

There are **four components** to be addressed when approaching *body contouring*:

1. Excess fat
2. Skin laxity
3. Cellulite
4. Irregular contours.

The suggested therapeutic interventions are listed here in Table 9.1.

Box 9.1: Body contouring devices (as per revised nomenclature by Alam et al. 2013).

- *Nonsurgical body contouring and fat reduction:*
  - *Ultrasound:*
    - High intensity (e.g. Liposonix, Ultrashape)
    - Low intensity
    - Focused
    - Nonfocused (e.g. Bella contour)
  - Cryolipolysis (e.g. Zeltiq)
  - Low-level light therapy (LLLT) (e.g. Zerona)
  - Massage
  - Electric field (e.g. Bella contour)
- *Energy device-assisted liposuction:*
  - Laser lipolysis with liposuction (e.g. CoolLipo, ProLipo, SmartLipo, LipoLite)
  - Ultrasound-assisted liposuction
  - Water-assisted liposuction (e.g. Body-Jet)
  - Power-assisted liposuction (e.g. MicroAire)
- *Radiofrequency and ultrasound skin tightening:*
  - *Noninvasive radiofrequency:*
    - Monopolar radiofrequency (e.g. Thermage, Exilis)
    - Unipolar radiofrequency
    - Bipolar radiofrequency (e.g. Alma Accent, Syneron eMax)
    - Tripolar radiofrequency (e.g. Pollogen RegenXL)
    - Multipolar radiofrequency
  - *Minimally invasive radiofrequency:* Needle insertion array
  - Fractional radiofrequency (by any radiofrequency delivery method listed earlier)
  - Focused, high-intensity ultrasound (synonym: ultrasound skin tightening) (e.g. Ulthera, Ultherapy).

Table 9.1: Categorization of methods of body contouring according to components addressed by modality.

	Cellulite	Laxity	Excess adiposity	Irregular contour
Suction massage (endermologie)	+	–	–	+
Liposuction	–	+/–	+*	+
Chemical lipolysis (mesotherapy)	–	–	+*	+
Laser lipectomy (Smart Lipo, Cool Lipo)	–	+	+*	+
Combo suction, rollers, IR light, bipolar radiofrequency (VelaSmooth)	+	+/–	–	+
Diode laser + suction massage (Triactive)	+	+/–	–	+
VelaShape	+	+	+†	+
Focused ultrasound (Ultrashape)	–	+/–	+*	+
Tissue tightening (Thermage, Titan, Lux IR, ReFirme, Accent)	–	+	–	+

*Physical reduction of fat quantity; †Redistribution of fat quantity.

This chapter mainly deals with noninvasive body contouring technologies focusing on fat reduction as well as a brief discussion on the minimally invasive liposuction techniques that have become possible because of the use of lasers and adjunctive technologies, like RF and ultrasound. The first part of the chapter will address cellulite reduction while the second half will focus on subcutaneous fat reduction.

SKIN TIGHTENING CONCEPTS AND TIPS

There appears to be a unifying principle underlying all of the tissue tightening devices. Each type of technology produces heat in the dermis in a range of 1-3 mm, except those that are focused on fat, which aim for a greater depth, more like 5-7 mm.

With **RF**, there is no specific chromophore as there is with photothermolysis, but it is an effective way of producing bulk thermal heating via capacitance coupling, tissue resistance, or induction of molecular bipole motion. The geometry of the tip, and the pattern of cooling (duration and timing) governs the depth of the heating.

With **broadband light**, there is a chromophore (water), although some of the strongest water-absorbing wavelengths have been blocked in the Titan handpiece; this is due to the fact that the heating with these wavelengths could be too great, yielding coagulation rather than stimulation. Since this chromophore does not yield specific tissue effects because all cells contain water, it is another method of achieving bulk dermal heating. The target depth here is a bit *shallower* than that of Thermage. This may yield a better performance with wrinkles, which may be why Thermage came out with a dual tip.

Finally, **ultrasound** is another modality that can achieve bulk dermal heating with absorption of sound waves into tissue generating heat.

Principle

Most of the current understanding revolves around the fact that the stimulation of collagen requires the temperature of the dermis to be in the 40-60°C range for a period of time. A look at the Arrhenius rate equation (Fig. 9.1), which is at best an approximation of collagen stimulation dynamics, shows that at *any point* along this curve the effect is *equal*. The application of this (Fig. 9.1) is that although nobody knows what the ideal time is, it has been established that having *lower fluences* (temperatures) for a *longer period* of time is more effective at collagen stimulation than high temperature and shorter time. In addition, the Thermage story has demonstrated that this method also yields less complications and better results.

A reasonable inference from multiple studies and devices is that the dermis needs to be kept at an elevated temperature, preferably in the 40-60° range to stay comfortably away from the coagulation threshold (enough for stimulation but less than coagulation), for a few minutes. This is consistent with the fact that multiple passes/pulses are used with all of these machines,

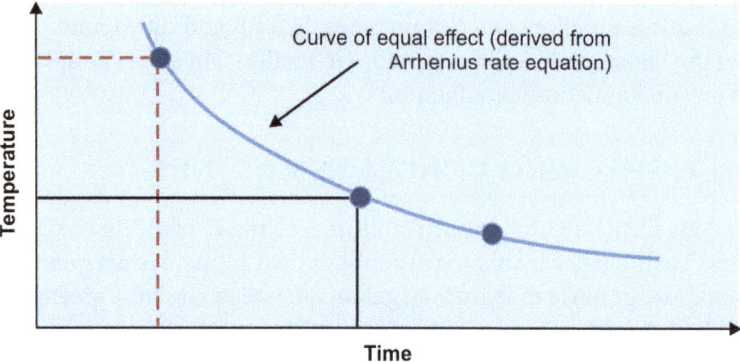

Fig. 9.1: Schematic drawing of the Arrhenius rate equation.

to achieve endpoints of both visible tightening as well as remaining below the threshold of significant discomfort.

It is more efficient to treat a palm-sized area than treating large cosmetic units in one go. This area should be repeatedly treated and kept at a higher energy for a period of minutes before moving on to the next area. Treating a small area like this allows it to reach the key temperature faster, and less energy is needed to keep it there for a few minutes, than treating a larger area, which allows the first area treated to cool somewhat before it is treated again. The latter is less efficient as you have to spend some time getting back to the target temperature after it has cooled.

With *fat*, it appears that tissue tightening devices reduce the appearance of cellulite and also improve contour via strengthening the *fibrous bands* that restrain the fat underneath them. It is much less clear if there are any direct effects on the fat via transferred heat that might alter the metabolism, distribution, or number of fat cells.

FAT AND CELLULITE

The areas of fat deposition are essentially localized to certain areas (e.g. love handles, lower abdomen, bulges, and thighs). *Tumescent liposuction* using suction cannulas is a time-tested technique with about 300,000–400,000 procedures performed in the US annually. Though overall a safe procedure, complications like prolonged swelling, areas of numbness, bruising, persistent erythema, thrombophlebitis, and pulmonary embolism can occur. Given the fact that many patients do not want to undergo surgery of any kind to remove excess fat, the market for the noninvasive devices is expected to grow at an exponential rate.

The number of men who underwent noninvasive body contouring treatments in the US increased from 14,598 in 2012 to 26,902 by 2015, an annual increase of 22.6%. India has joined a list of 15 countries where

Targeted reduction of subcutaneous fat with nonablative laser devices and focused ultrasound is also being tried. Anderson et al. recently showed that the *1,210 nm* and *1,720 nm* wavelengths, are ideal as the absorption coefficient of human fat is greater than that of water, and allow selective heating of adipose tissue with minimal damage to surrounding structures. **There are no commercially available devices utilizing these wavelengths as yet.**

Though most of the devices listed (Table 9.3) can be used for cellulite, as the pathogenesis has multiple factors including fibrosis, circulatory failure, and an underlying metabolic failure, no single therapy is effective. Of the available devices on the market, those based on the principle energy source of radiofrequency seem to have the most effect. Even so, these devices do not yield more than a 50% improvement in most subjects. Most studies do not employ clearly objective means of proving clinical efficacy, casting doubt on the true efficacy of these devices. Altzadeh Z et al. in their recent review found that only 73 articles of the 2,024 available through a database search (using keywords such as body contouring, fat reduction, etc.) were of sufficient quality for analysis. Of these 66 were original articles with the maximum being for cryolipolysis followed by RF and then low-level light therapy (LLLT), high intensity focused ultrasound (HIFU), EST, and WBV in that order.

Summary

The best option for your patient is dependent on their clinical presentation, treatment goal, and most importantly, their preferences. It is important to emphasize that *none* of these treatments provides more than a *modest, local contouring* benefit in most instances.

SUBCUTANEOUS FAT REDUCTION

To understand how noninvasive body shaping works, it is important to understand how fat is metabolized and stored in the human body. Whenever the caloric intake exceeds demand, the excess energy is stored in the form of triglycerides in specialized cells called adipocytes. Such cells are present in various body areas, but for the purpose of noninvasive body shaping, we will concentrate our attention on the adipocytes in the skin which make up the subcutaneous fat layer.

The adipocyte is a cell with a large amount of cytoplasm capable of storing a large amount of triglycerides. These form the energy reserve of the body. The number of adipocytes is regarded to be fixed as explained earlier, but their size can show great variability. When enlarged, they disrupt the natural body contours resulting in local fat collection, and in extreme cases, obesity.

So, how does one go about decreasing fat in the subcutaneous layer? There are only *two ways*:
1. Either decrease the cell number or
2. Decrease their size.

The former is accomplished by methods, which either mechanically removes fat cells, such as liposuction or by methods which cause adipocyte death through one mechanism or the other. The latter involves getting the adipocyte to give up its triglyceride content through membrane manipulation. The released triacylglycerol (TAG) is transported from the interstitial space to the lymphatic channels from where it is metabolized in the liver. Numerous studies have shown the safety of these techniques, and there have been no reports of fatty liver/liver dysfunction or increased serum triglycerides following noninvasive fat reduction techniques.

The first mechanism, adipocyte removal or death, offers longer-lasting results than adipocyte fat removal. However, since the remaining adipocytes can increase greatly in size to compensate for the numbers lost, it is essential that lifestyle modifications (i.e. diet, exercise) are done on a sustained basis by the patient to maintain desired results. This is even more important with the more temporary method of fat removal from a viable adipocyte.

There are three mechanisms of removal of fat (TAG) from the adipocytes:
1. Thermal augmentation of normal metabolic processes of the fat cell.
2. Thermal or cavitational destruction of fat cells.
3. Creation of a temporary pore in the fat cell membrane.

A significant barrier to noninvasive treatments is the issue of fat localization after treatment. As explained above, adipose tissue stores triglycerides. Unlike cholesterol, which can be excreted, triglycerides are not excreted by the body; in fact, they are stored and used for synthesizing such molecules as plasma lipoproteins. Thus, the removal of large deposits of subcutaneous fat may yield redistribution to other sites in the body. Since increased visceral fat has been linked to increased cardiovascular disease, noninvasive therapies should be approached cautiously, and their use may be limited to treatment of small deposits of fat.

Indications and Contraindications of NonInvasive Body Contouring

Indications

- *Realistic expectations* of a modest reduction of *localized fat*—generally only soft tissue deformities with at least **1.5 cm** of fat thickness should be treated.
- Patient opposed to a surgical procedure for fat reduction.
- Compliance with *multiple visits* for procedures.

Contraindications

- Pregnancy.
- Patients with a pacemaker.

- Patient with a serious or debilitating medical illness.
- Patients with a large BMI.
- Unrealistic expectations.

Treatment Devices

Table 9.3 had summarized the main body contouring technologies available in the market today. They are discussed here briefly.

Suction/Massage Devices

These are among the oldest machines available for noninvasive fat loss. Endermologie® (LPG Systems, Valence, France) is a Food and Drug Administration (FDA)-cleared device that massages and kneads the skin to improve the appearance of cellulite. It originated nearly 3 decades ago in France and uses paddles coupling suction and a roller to stimulate fatty areas. The concept is that lymphatic circulation in the treated area is stimulated resulting in mild fat loss from adipocytes. In selected patients, particularly, those with edematous type of fatty deposits, the procedure can result in measurable circumference reduction. For most people, the improvement is very mild. Endermologie® is mostly confined to use in spa settings now since other more effective devices are available for medical use.

Newer machines take the earlier concept further by coupling the suction with transepidermal thermal energy delivery. This thermal energy is generated with the help of diode arrays or nonfocused ultrasound (NFU) around the probe head. TriActive™ (Cynosure Inc., Westford, MA, USA) and SmoothShapes™ (Cynosure Inc., Westford, MA, USA) are two such devices. Again results are modest and these machines are often used as adjuncts to other fat removal methods (e.g. for smoothening out results and tightening skin after surgical liposuction).

Bruising is a common side effect of laser and light source treatments for fat. Most commonly, the bruising is related to the vacuum pressure and physical manipulation of the device, rather than the actual laser.

Radiofrequency Energy Devices

These are the most popular noninvasive fat loss devices in the world. RF devices can be classified into multiple types (Box 9.2), and unipolar, bipolar, or multipolar devices have all shown some degree of cellulite and/or subcutaneous fat reduction in numerous studies—most studies show that cellulite improves more than subcutaneous fat. In addition, RF devices are very efficient for skin tightening so a global improvement in appearance of the treated area is possible as compared to HIFU and cryolipolysis, which do not contract skin as well; albeit being better at targeting subcutaneous fat.

Box 9.2: Body contouring devices.

- *Suction:* Massage devices
  - Endermologie® (LPG Systems, Valence, France)
- *Suction massage:* Thermal devices
  - TriActive™ (Cynosure Inc., Westford, MA, USA)
  - SmoothShapes™ (Cynosure Inc., Westford, MA, USA)
- *Radiofrequency energy devices:*
  - VelaSmooth™, VelaShape™ (Syneron, Inc., Irvine, CA, USA)
  - Thermage™ (Solta Medical, Hayward, CA, USA)
  - Accent™ (Alma Lasers Inc., Buffalo Grove, IL, USA)
  - TriPollar™ (Pollogen, Tel Aviv, Israel)
  - Freeze™ (Venus Concepts, Karmiel, Israel)
  - TiteFX™ (Invasix, Inc., Yokneam, Israel)
- *High-frequency focused ultrasound energy devices:*
  - UltraShape™ (UltraShape Ltd., Yokneam, Israel)
  - LipoSonix™ (Medicis, Scottsdale, AZ, USA)
- *Nonfocused ultrasound devices:*
  - Medcontour™ (General Project, Florence, Italy)
  - Ultracontour™ (Medixsysteme, Nimes, Florence)
  - Proslimelt™ (Medical Care Consulting, Murten, Switzerland)
  - Novashape™ (UltraMed, Milton, Canada)
  - Accent Ultra™ (Alma, Buffalo Grove, USA)
  - Vaser Shape™ (Sound Surgical Technologies, Louisville, USA)
- *Cryolipolysis energy devices:*
  - Zeltiq™ (Zeltiq Aesthetics, Pleasanton, CA, USA)
- *Low-level light laser therapy devices:*
  - Zerona™ (Erchonia Medical, McKinney, TX, USA)
- *Microwave thermolysis.*

How Do They Work?

Bipolar RF devices are based on the principle of heat generation as a result of poor electrical conductance, as the RF waves pass through fat. The resulting heat is strong enough to cause thermal damage to the adipocytes and connective tissue septae. Adipose tissue has high tissue resistance and a relatively low heat transfer coefficient; thus, adipose tissue can be readily heated, and the heat will be predominantly confined to the adipocytes.

Bipolar RF devices have *a limited penetration depth* and, therefore, are of not much use in adipose tissue alteration when used on in isolation; however, as seen later when bipolar RF is *combined* with suction or another source of energy like infrared light its fat reduction property improves. *Unipolar devices* utilize high frequency electromagnetic radiation (EMR) which penetrates *deeper*. High frequency EMR induces high frequency rotational oscillations in water molecules, which in turn produce heat, i.e. greater the presence of water, greater is the tissue heat generation. The depth and breadth of thermal damage is greater and in a rather diffuse pattern, with little control as compared to bipolar RF devices.

Effects: The end result is the creation of dermal fibrosis through neocollagenesis or so-called "appearance-enhancing scarring" that leads to long-term improvement after a few treatments. The heat generated increases adipocyte fat turnover but does not kill the adipocyte.

Unipolar and bipolar RF technologies also exist as combination in the Accent device (Alma Lasers™, Buffalo Groove, IL). Both the Accent and ThermaCool® (Thermage®, Hayward, CA) are FDA approved for the treatment of wrinkles and rhytids. The ThermaCool® is a unipolar RF, while the Accent system is a unipolar and bipolar RF device. Of the two devices, only *Accent system* has been evaluated for the treatment of localized adiposities (Table 9.3).

VelaSmooth™ and VelaShape™ (Fig. 9.5)

VelaSmooth™ was the *first RF-based device* approved for cellulite reduction by the FDA in 2005. This was followed 2 years later by the higher powered VelaShape™ which has since then undergone three revisions. VelaShape™ is FDA approved for both cellulite and circumference reduction.

Both VelaSmooth™ and VelaShape™ systems combine infrared light (700–2,000 nm) with suction coupled bipolar RF (1 MHz) and mechanical manipulation, the difference being that VelaSmooth™ is rated at 25W while VelaShape™ is rated at 50W and is thus more powerful.

During treatment, *suction* is used to pull the skin into the handpiece where the skin is exposed to *IR* and *RF* while its surface temperature is being monitored. **IR** mainly targets dermal **water** while **RF** targets the deeper **dermis and subcutaneous** fat layer. The resulting heat stress causes dermal contraction and stimulates increased vascular flow and neocollagenesis and in the subcutaneous layer increases the metabolism of the adipocyte resulting

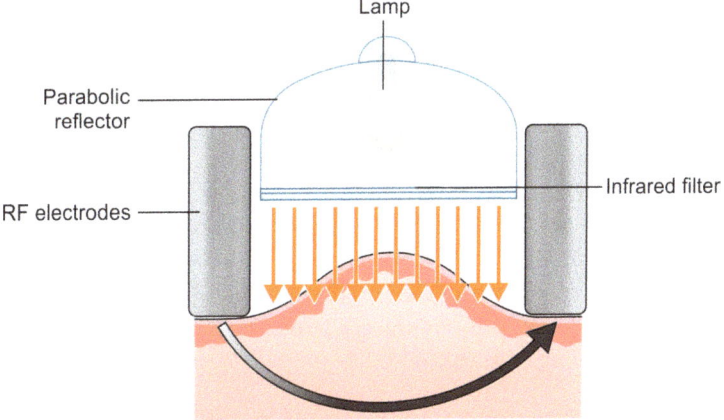

Fig. 9.5: Schematic diagram of VelaSmooth™ handpiece (RF: Radiofrequency).
Courtesy: Syneron Medical, Irvine, CA, USA.

in TAG removal from the cell. The suction and mechanical massage from the probe stimulate lymphatic flow further enhancing fat removal.

Results: In the largest study of VelaSmooth™, Sadick evaluated 35 patients who completed either 8 or 16 treatments with VelaSmooth™. A blinded dermatologist evaluated the photographs and found 40% improvement on average in cellulite appearance, and there was a circumference reduction in all. Numerous studies have repeatedly shown the efficacy of VelaSmooth™ in improving cellulite, and a few studies have shown circumference reduction as well ranging from 1.25 cm to 3.5 cm on the abdomen and thighs, and 0.5–0.75 cm on the arms.

A more recent study of VelaSmooth™ found a statistically significant decrease in thigh circumference at 4 weeks, but no immediate change or a persistent decrease at 8 weeks. Visual improvement of less than 50% was noted in the majority of subjects and 31% of the subjects experienced bruising.

Hence, it seems that cellulite reduction remains the main application of the machine. Sessions vary from weekly to biweekly with total number of sessions ranging from 4 to 16. Benefit is seen as early as 1 month, and in one Asian study was sustained over 1 year.

Unipolar Radiofrequency Devices

Thermage® and Accent® are two prominent unipolar (monopolar) RF devices employing pure RF *without* adjunctive IR or suction coupling. The limitation of RF is that the energy is *not specific*, unlike ultrasound waves, and their depth of penetration into the skin is *limited* unless very high levels are used. Hence, both treatments are more suited to nonsurgical skin tightening than fat reduction. Cellulite is superficial fat as compared to the subcutaneous fat layer, and hence may improve as well. Both machines can be associated with significant discomfort during the procedure.

Results: Studies have assessed Thermage® in the treatment of cellulite with improvement scores ranging from 30% to 70%, 6 months post-treatment.

Goldberg et al. studied the use of the Accent® unipolar RF device for cellulite treatment. Their study included subjects with higher grade cellulite of upper thighs. They were treated every other week for a total of six treatments. Results obtained 6 months after the last treatment showed an average of 2.45 cm reduction in thigh circumference with minimal side effects, and no serum lipid abnormalities. They attribute their longer-lasting effects to the formation of dermal fibrosis in the upper dermis and increased contraction between the dermis and Camper's fascia, which has been previously reported in ultrasound imaging studies.

Multipolar Radiofrequency Devices

TriPollar® (Pollogen, Tel Aviv, Israel) and Freeze® (Venus Concepts) are some other RF machines—the former uses three poles while the latter uses eight poles to generate RF energy. TiteFx™ is a variation of the RF concept and uses suction coupled RF to heat the dermis and first 1.5–2 cm of fat. When the epidermal temperature reaches 43–45°C, a high-voltage, electroporation pulse is generated through the adipose tissue resulting in damage to the adipocyte membrane and resultant apoptosis over the following week. The device is much quicker than Thermage® making the treatments more tolerable.

Conclusion: Though most of these RF devices have been used for skin tightening, some have a potential for use in cellulite. However, significant statistical outcomes using RF devices for cellulite and fat reduction are low and limited, so patient alignment is essential for a satisfactory outcome.

High Intensity Focused Ultrasound

Ultrasound devices for fat reduction can be divided into those using nonfocused (NFU) versus focused high frequency ultrasound (HIFU). *NFU devices (also called ultracavitators) just have a dermal heating effect with no rigorous evidence of fat reduction.* External nonfocused ultrasound (NFU) has been applied to body contouring but was found to be effective only as an adjunct to tumescent liposuction, improving tissue hydration, and distribution of the tumescent solution.

How Does It Work?

In a conducive setting, ultrasonic energy affects tissue destruction through three mechanisms:
1. Cavitation,
2. Micromechanical disruption, and
3. Thermal damage.

It is thought that *cavitation* is predominantly responsible for tissue destruction in internal ultrasound-assisted liposculpting (UAL). NFU devices lack the ability to cause cavitation, and hence, are not effective for fat loss. It is postulated that external ultrasound prior to liposuction works either through thermal or micromechanical effects.

In the market, there are two types of ultrasound devices. The thermal effects of HIFU rapidly raise the temperature of adipose tissue to above 55°C causing thermal coagulative necrosis and secondary mechanical effects due to acoustic pressure. Low-frequency focused ultrasound is a nonthermal ultrasound which causes ablation of adipocytes through mechanical disruption. The difference with HIFU is that it uses high-frequency acoustic energy such as 2 MHz, at more than 1,000 W/cm^2 causing thermal and mechanical damage, whereas low frequency focused ultrasound uses 200 kHz, 17.5 W/cm^2, with a focal depth of 1.5 cm, causing mechanical damage and cavitation.

UltraShape™

Transdermally focused contour I UltraShape™ (Tel Aviv, Israel) uses focused ultrasound to deliver a finite amount of acoustic energy at a controlled distance from the ultrasound transducer to achieve noninvasive body contouring.

Ultrasound energy is emitted from a hemispherical transducer (Fig. 9.6). The energy is low near the transducer surface and is concentrated in an additive manner at a distant focus. The transducer is placed directly on the skin and focuses the energy at the depth of the subcutaneous fat. As a result, the energy can be delivered through the skin, with low energy density at the epidermis and dermis, and with a high energy density in the subcutaneous fat. The ultrasound energy is delivered in pulses, using parameters that provide a nonthermal effect. High levels of ultrasound energy within the subcutaneous fat can disrupt adipose tissue safely and effectively, as has been demonstrated in ultrasound-assisted liposuction. Tissue selection is achieved partly due to the pulsed nature of the pulses and partly due to the differential susceptibility of different tissues to mechanical (nonthermal) stress.

Results: A prospective, nonrandomized, and controlled trial (n = 164 patients) conducted by Teitelbaum et al. found that after one ultrasound treatment to the abdomen, thighs, or flanks, there was a mean circumference reductions of 2.3 cm (abdomen), 1.8 cm (thighs), and 1.6 cm (flanks) after 12 weeks. The majority (77%) of the improvement in circumference was noted to occur within the first 14 days following the treatment.

Interestingly, one Asian study *failed* to demonstrate much improvement—53 patients were treated with three sessions spaced a month

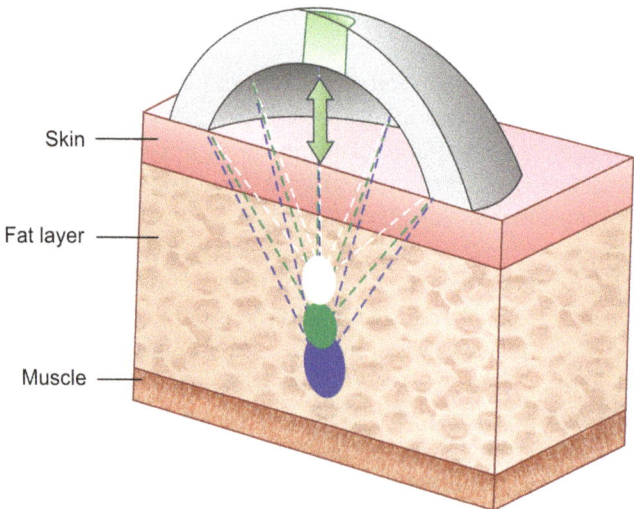

Fig. 9.6: A figurative depiction of focused USG used for fat reduction.

apart and there was no significant difference in the pre- and post-treatment parameters, such as circumference reduction, ultrasound fat thickness, and skin caliper fat thickness. This has been hypothesized to be because of *body habitus* difference between Asians and Caucasians.

Since then the UltraShape™ has undergone two revisions—the so-called second- and third-generation UltraShape™—with software upgrades and better transducers. The third-generation UltraShape™ also has two additional technologies built into it—(1) Advanced nonthermal selective focused ultrasound and (2) Vacuum-assisted RF. These two technologies allow same session combination therapy, facilitating a synergistic treatment protocol, thus providing a complete body-contouring solution.

Over 200,000 UltraShape™, treatments have been performed worldwide with no reports of any significant adverse event. The procedure is comfortable and patients start seeing a difference within a month. In general, an average of 2-4 cm of circumferential fat reduction can be achieved over three sessions spaced 2 weeks apart from the abdominal and hip regions, and about 2-3 cm from the inner and outer thighs. With the third-generation machine, it is anticipated that this can occur after a single treatment.

LipoSonix™

LipoSonix™ is the other main HIFU system; however, it differs significantly from UltraShape™ in several parameters.

LipoSonix™ uses two HIFU rays to focus on a very localized area causing rapid heating (>56°C) of the tissue, with a variable focal depth of 1.1-1.8 cm. This causes coagulative necrosis of the fat cell and instantaneous cell death. So, the effect is thermal as opposed to the nonthermal effect of UltraShape™. This also makes the procedure quite painful and sedation is required in contrast to UltraShape™, which requires none. Distilled water needs to be used as a coupling agent to prevent acoustic reflection of the high frequency ultrasound waves from air pockets in between the transducer–skin interface. Adverse events seen include swelling, ecchymoses, dysesthesia, and pain on treatment, unlike UltraShape™ which has virtually no side effects. Fewer sessions are required with the LipoSonix™ with studies showing 2-5 cm circumferential reductions after a single sitting.

Doublo-S

This is an advanced HIFU technology and is considered as a second-generation HIFU system (Fig. 9.7A). It can be used in both facial and body contouring with no downtime. There are different cartridges targeting different treatment depths (Fig. 9.7B). It has a double effect of:
- Collagen remodeling
- Superficial musculoaponeurotic system (SMAS) contraction.

It is approved by FDA and CE. Some results are as shown in Figures 9.7C and D.

SECTION 1: Laser and Energy-based Technologies

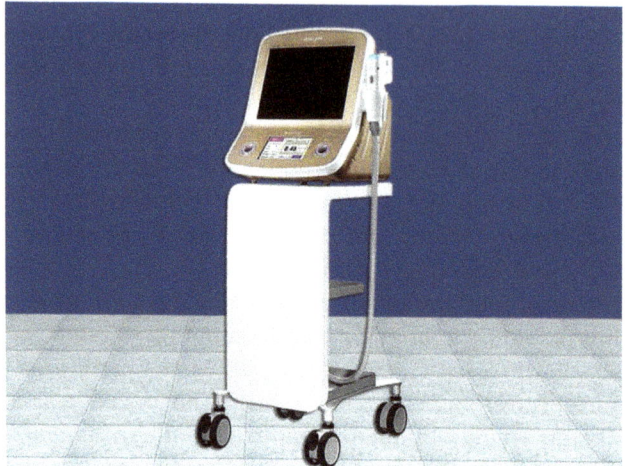

Fig. 9.7A: The second-generation liposculpting DOUBLO-S.

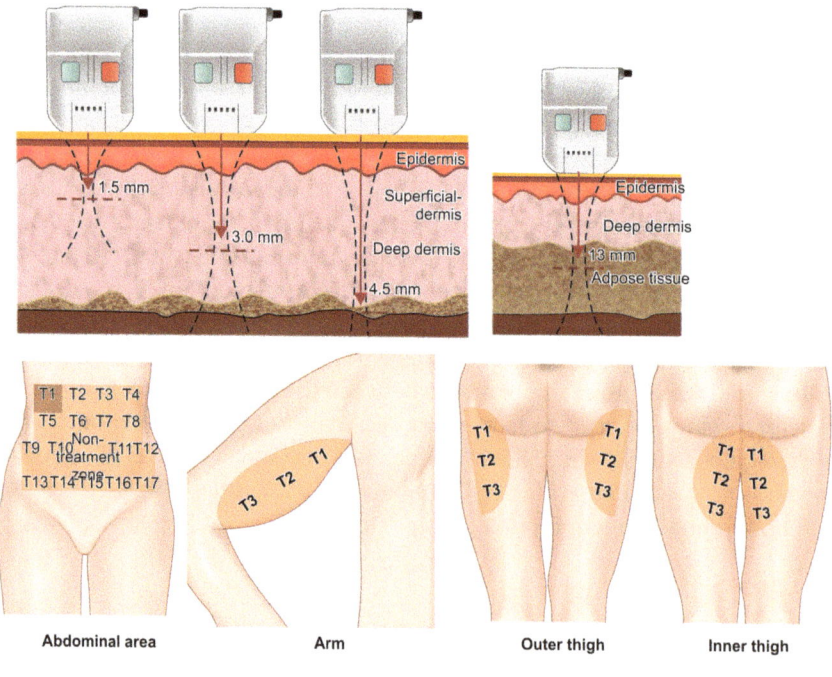

Fig. 9.7B: Application of cartridges in second-generation high intensity focused ultrasound (HIFU).

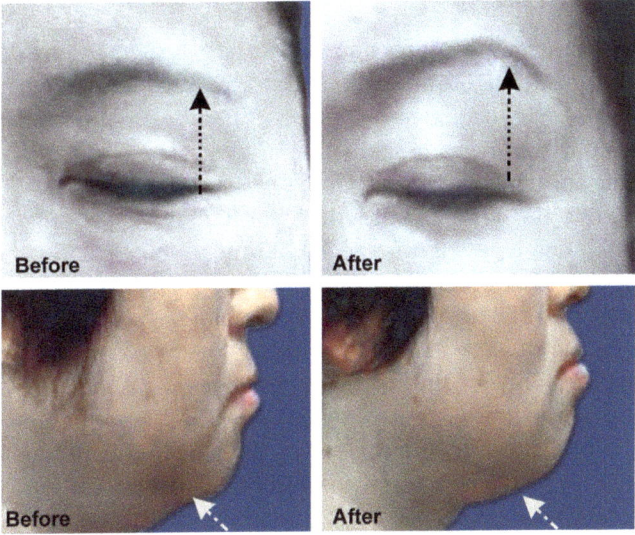

Fig. 9.7C: Before and after pictures 4 weeks after the session.

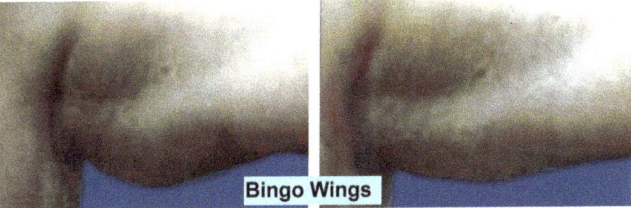

Fig. 9.7D: Before and after one session.

Summary

Although contour I UltraShape™ is widely used for noninvasive body contouring, data regarding the long-term efficacy and persistence of satisfactory results is still lacking. Whether the treated patients will require regular treatments for maintenance of achieved results indefinitely, is still unanswered. A recent study combined RF with USG in Asian patients to maximize results (Shek SY).

Light-based Devices and Laser-assisted Lipolysis

Laser lipoplasty with pulsed neodymium-doped yttrium aluminum garnet (Nd:YAG) laser, also called interstitial laser lipolysis was first described in 1994. This technique is widely used in Europe and Latin America and has recently been introduced in Japan and the United States. Less trauma, bleeding, and pain have been the main advantages of this technique (*see* Table 9.3).

How Does It Work?

The mechanisms leading to laser lipolysis are largely temperature dependent. At low-energy settings, tumescent adipocytes were observed. At higher energy settings, cytoplasmic retraction, disruption of membranes, and heat-coagulated collagen fibers are seen.

The ideal wavelength used for laser lipolysis, as the table shows, can vary, even though, in the Table 9.4 the ideal wavelength seems to be *1,440 nm*. Wavelengths, such as 1,210 nm and 1,720 nm, are highly specific for lipids, but there are no devices at present with these wavelengths.

Some authors (Parlette EC) believe that *924 nm* wavelength has the highest *selectivity for fat melting*, but may not be as effective for skin tightening as other modalities unless combined with another wavelength. They continue by stating that the *1,064 nm* wavelength has good tissue penetration, but relatively *low-fat absorption*. The lower fat absorption of the 1,064 nm wavelength may be tempered by its superior heat distribution, and therefore, skin-tightening effect. Finally, the *1,320 nm* wavelength demonstrates greater fat absorption with less tissue penetration and scatter, and therefore, may be safer for treatment around more *fragile areas*, such as the neck, inner thighs, and arms.

Devices Used

Pure laser devices:
- The *Nd:YAG laser* was first used in laser lipolysis, because of the penetration depth of its wavelength (*1,064 nm*). The Nd:YAG laser has been used alone or in combination with suction liposuction. SmartLipo™ (Cynosure, USA), a 300-µm fiber encased in a microcannula, is an example of this type of device. The cannula is inserted subcutaneously to destroy lipid membranes and release lipids. Adipocytes appear to swell at lower energies and lyse at higher energies. This process is termed as "laser lipolysis" (Ichikawa K). The laser heat also coagulates collagen fibers.
- *Diode lasers*, which can typically emit at *810, 940, and 980* nm, is another alternative. Their wavelengths are in the same spectral region as 1,064 nm, and they offer the advantages of higher efficiency (usually 30%) and

Table 9.4: Adipocyte absorption spectrum of various wavelengths.

Wavelength	Fatty tissue/water absorption
924 nm (diode)	2.8/1.4
980 nm (diode)	1.7/3.6
1,064 nm neodymium-doped yttrium aluminum garnet (Nd:YAG)	1/1
1,320 nm (Nd:YAG)	5.9/11.5
1,440 nm (Nd:YAG)	127/252

higher power (25 W or more). The absorption spectrum of mammalian fat obtained by VanVeen et al. using three independent methods show that the absorption coefficient obtained with a wavelength of 980 nm is very similar to that obtained with a wavelength of 1,064 nm.

- *1,440 nm lasers:* Based on the absorption spectrum as given in Table 9.4, the ideal wavelength for fat absorption is 1,440 nm. The 1,440 nm wavelength is highly absorbed in adipose tissue, which is composed of 75% fat, 20% water, and 5% proteins. This is as the 1,440 nm wavelength is absorbed by adipose tissue 127 times greater and absorbed by water 252 times greater than the 1,064 nm wavelength.

    Cellulaze (Cynosure™) is a laser device that uses a 1,440 nm Nd:YAG fiber with a novel delivery system to target the structural components of cellulite. The technology incorporates a unique SideLight side-firing fiber as well as a ThermaGuide thermal sensing system for safer treatments. A recent study safely treated cellulite and lipodystrophy in a single stage by using the Nd:YAG 1,440 nm side-firing fiberoptic laser system for cellulite and lipodystrophy. The combined laser treatment was associated with a high degree of both patient and physician satisfaction but requires skills and practice and should be left to surgeons (Petti C).

- *635 nm laser and liposuction:* Neira has combined low level 635 nm laser and liposuction in a technique labeled the "Neira 4 L technique". Patients are irradiated with a low level 635 nm laser after tumescent anesthesia. Following irradiation, removal of fat is accomplished with a cannula or other technique. Neira postulated that low level laser creates a pore in the adipocyte membrane, causing leakage of lipid into the interstitial space. He studied 12 patients and found that after 6 minutes of low level laser, fat was completely removed from the cell.

Combined Devices (For cellulite and deeper subcutaneous fat)

- The *SmoothShapes*™ (Eleme Medical, Merrimack, NH, USA) device for the treatment of cellulite is a dual wavelength, *915 nm and 650 nm*, laser device that is combined with a *vacuum-assisted* mechanical massage.

    The basis of these wavelength selections is based on adipose samples treated with a 635 nm light from a 10 mW diode laser, which showed emptying of fat from these cells (Neira R). Then the 915 nm wavelength penetrates into the tissue and is preferentially absorbed by lipids, causing a thermal effect. The temperature inside the adipocyte is elevated by up to 60°C.

    The 650 nm wavelength is thought to modify the permeability of the fat cell membranes, allowing expressed fat to move into the interstitial space, without destroying the adipocyte cell membrane. The fat is moved into the interstitial space and lymphatic system for elimination with the aid of mechanical rollers and mild suction. Without the use of rollers and suction, the fat would return into the adipocyte within 45 minutes.

- The *TriActive*™ *device* (Cynosure Inc., Bedford, MA) combines deep tissue massage and suction, similar to Endermologie®, with contact cooling and a low-intensity diode laser *808 nm*. It has been shown that the diode laser component significantly contributes to clinical improvement.

  Work done by Nootheti PK et al. compared the efficacy of treatment of cellulite using TriActive™ versus VelaSmooth™. Patients were treated twice weekly for 6 weeks with either VelaSmooth™ or TriActive™. They calculated a 28% versus a 30% improvement rate, respectively, in the upper thigh circumference measurements, while a 56% versus a 37% improvement rate was observed, respectively, in lower thigh circumference measurements. Statistical significance of these results was p more than 0.05. Incidence and extent of bruising was higher in VelaSmooth™ than in TriActive™ system, which may be attributed to mechanical manipulation.

- The *VelaSmooth*™ *and VelaShape*™ (Syneron Medical Ltd, Irvine, CA) devices, as discussed previously, combine physical manipulation with RF energy, as well as infrared energy, to facilitate a multimodality approach to fat and cellulite treatment.

- *Obesity platform* (Fig. 9.8A) which has all in one technology RF/vacuum/roller/IR/cavitation (Fig. 9.8A)—is an innovative nonsurgical RF that enhances the penetrating depth.

  The vacuum therapy optimizes heat penetration and improves blood supply, stimulate lymphatic drainage, and shrinking of fat cell volume.

  The IR heats up tissue to **5 mm** depth and RF heats tissue from **2–20 mm** depth (Figs. 9.8B to D). Before and after pictures are as shown after 8–10 sessions done twice a week (Fig. 9.8E). The machine has been used in

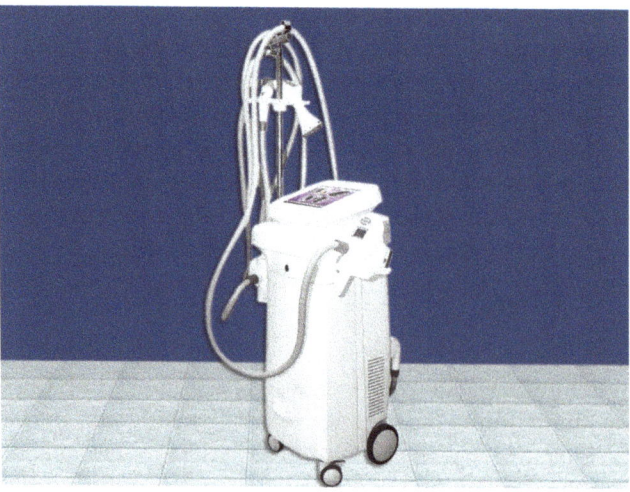

Fig. 9.8A: The obesity platform machine.

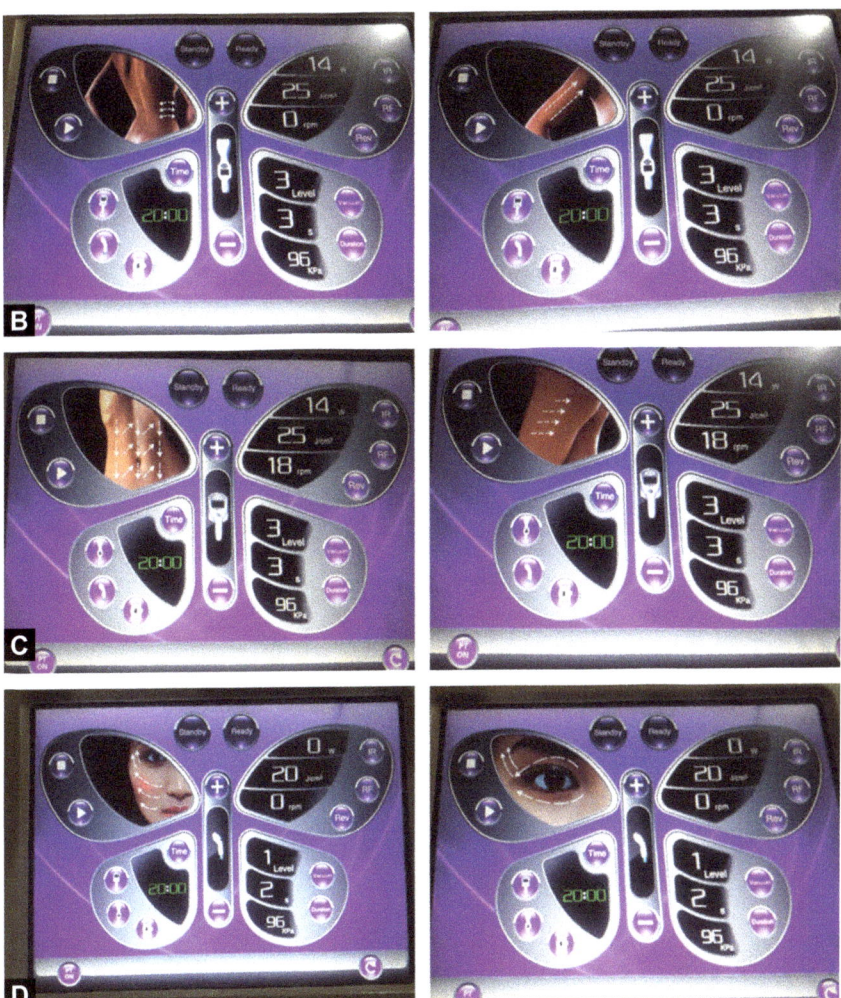

Figs. 9.8B to D: Various settings of the obesity platform depending on the site of treatment.

some patients as a postliposuction maintenance therapy to improve laxity and texture of skin and has shown good improvement over sessions done two times per week for 1 month starting after 4 weeks of the surgery (Figs. 9.8F to H).

Summary

Laser lipolysis is a new technique still under development. The use of 1,064 nm Nd:YAG and the 980 nm diode laser as an auxiliary tool has refined the traditional liposuction technique. For any given energy settings, 1,064 nm and 980 nm wavelengths gave similar histologic results (Figs. 9.9A and B).

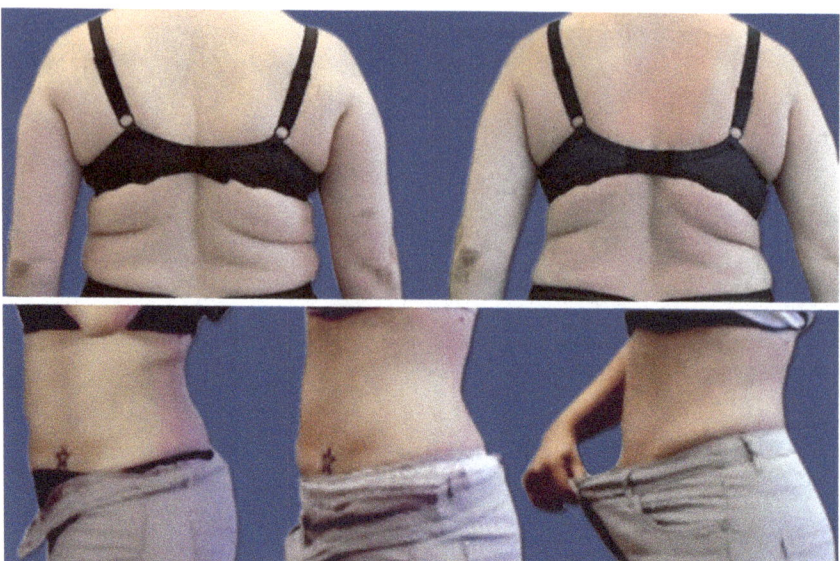

Fig. 9.8E: Before and after pictures after eight sessions (obesity platform).

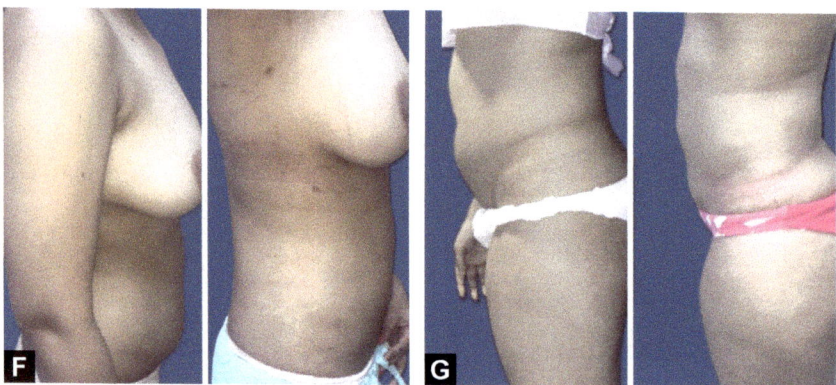

Figs. 9.8F and G: Results after six sessions postliposuction.
Courtesy: Dr Ashutosh Mishra, plastic surgeon in NCR.

Recently DiBernardo reported that the use of a 1,440-nm laser subdermally could disrupt and reduce herniated fat in the dermis, through a process of tissue coagulation. They demonstrated ultrasound evidence of a 25% increase in skin thickness and a 29% decrease in skin laxity, which was maintained at 1 year.

We are particularly impressed with the study of Katz et al. where a single treatment with the Nd:YAG 1,440 nm wavelength laser was analyzed by objective two-dimensional (2D) and 3D photography (Vectra). Of patients, 62% showed improvement at 3 months and 66% showed improvement at 6 months.

CHAPTER 9: Noninvasive Body Contouring and Lipolysis

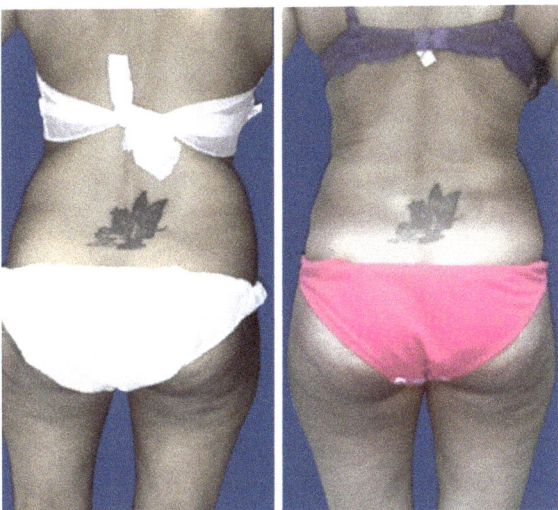

Fig. 9.8H: Before and after pictures six sessions after liposuction.
Courtesy: Dr Ashutosh Mishra, plastic surgeon in NCR.

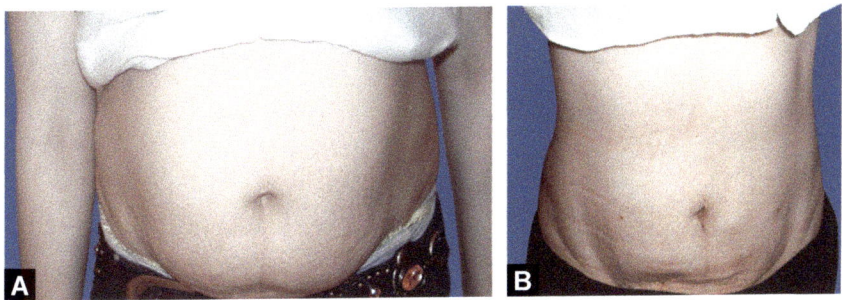

Figs. 9.9A and B: (A) A 28-year-old female with localized adiposity in the lower anterior abdomen and flanks; and (B) Same patient 10 days after laser-assisted liposuction demonstrating a 3.5-inch circumference loss with minimal skin laxity and no bruising. The access ports are visible on either side of the umbilicus and will gradually fade over 3–6 months. The abdominal skin will also tighten with time.

There are numerous advantages of laser-assisted lipolysis (LAL) and it is a useful **adjunct** to tumescent liposuction. But the smaller size of cannulas limits the ability of this technology to be used on areas other than face, medial arms, knees, periumbilical, and perhaps medial thighs as a sole treatment.

Selective Cryolipolysis

There is evidence that adipose tissue is selectively sensitive to cold injury. This is akin to cold-induced fat necrosis of the newborns and infants called "popsicle panniculitis" and are the basis of this therapy (*see* Box 9.1).

How Does It Work?

Cryolysis of fatty tissue is possible due to this biological selectivity. Biological selectivity refers to a specific response (e.g. inflammation) that is confined to a certain tissue (e.g. fat) on account of a stimulus (Fig. 9.10).

Studies have revealed that a delayed, cold-induced lobular panniculitis is involved. The adipose tissue loss continues for many weeks following a single, local exposure to cold, reaching an apparent maximum at 4 weeks after and resolving about 3 months after cold exposure.

Temperature and time of application are both important to induce selective cryolipolysis of fatty tissue (Fig. 9.11). A skin surface temperature as high as 1°C can induce a mild panniculitis within the various tested anatomical locations. The anatomic depth of panniculitis and of fat loss are increased when lower temperatures are applied. The most effective temperature for fat reduction is a subject of debate—the lowest studied in a porcine model is –7°C. Most commonly treated areas are as shown in Figure 9.12.

Results and Summary

Work done by Anderson et al. has suggested that lipid crystallization is perhaps responsible for lipoatrophy seen in their Yucatan pig models.

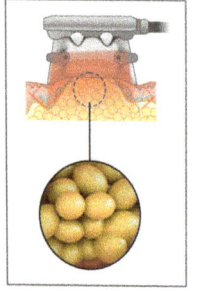

1. Start of Cryolipolysis™
Applicator is placed on the treatment area and the cooling is started

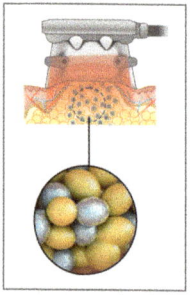

2. Immediate reaction
The fat cells in the treatment area react to the cooling

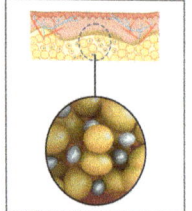

3. Elimination of fat cells
After the treatment the fat cells are eliminated naturally

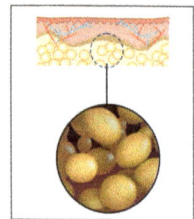

4. The result
After 8–12 weeks the final result can be observed

Fig. 9.10: Mechanism of cryolipolysis.

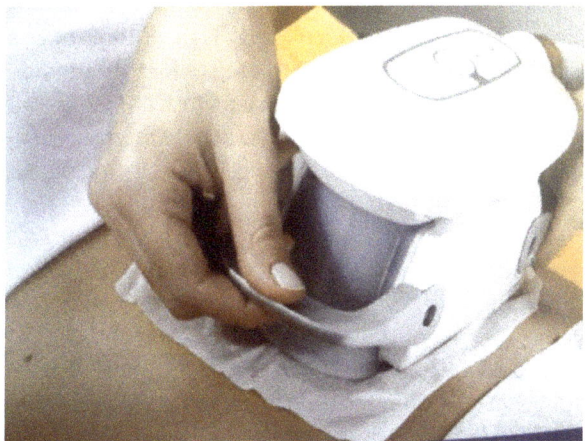

Fig. 9.11: Application of cryoprobe.

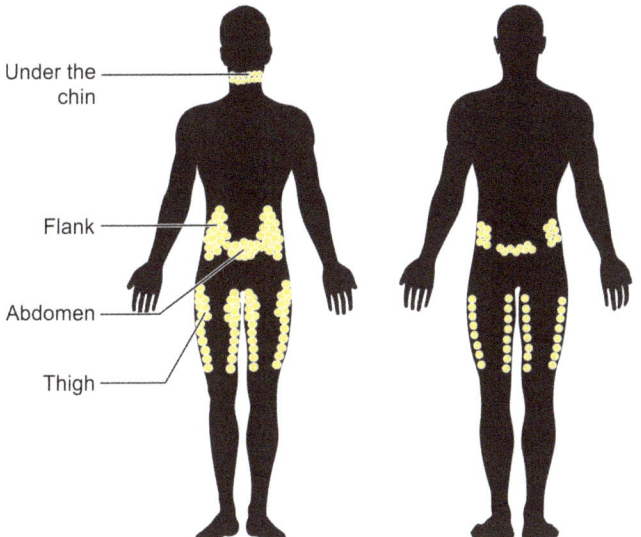

Fig. 9.12: Common areas chosen for cryolipolysis.

This mechanism will pose challenges to the development of selective cryolipolysis for clinical use, as pigs have a higher content of saturated fatty acids compared to unsaturated ones. Additionally, it is not apparent that the intracellular crystals seen in adipocytes were large enough to elicit the inflammatory panniculitis, largely responsible for producing the effects.

Zeltiq CoolSculpt (Zeltiq Aesthetics, Pleasanton, CA, USA) is the main cryolipolysis device available in the market and is FDA approved for treating the abdominal flanks (love handles). The part to be treated is sucked into the probe with mild suction and then held between the panels for 30–60 minutes at a subzero temperature. Once the probes are removed, the area is red and feels frozen solid and numb. This numbness can persist for 2–3 months but there are no reports of permanent nerve damage. Studies have shown a 25% reduction in the fat content of the treated areas. No systemic side effects have been seen. The machine does not require a technician to operate but has the disadvantage of long treatment time and a high disposable cost.

Following a CoolSculpting treatment, gentle massage of the treated area should be performed to break up crystallized adipocytes and improve the efficacy of the treatment.

A recent study has tried to change the probe to ensure a shorter duration of treatment. The medium cryolipolysis cup was designed to maximize tissue contact with the cooling surface. The cup allowed the tissue to seat fully against the entire surface, thus reducing the significant vacuum tension on the skin. The reduced skin tension resulted in an enhanced treatment experience with significantly lower procedural pain scores and lower incidence of post-treatment bruising and numbness. Area of 122 cm^2, whereas the CoolCore standard parallel plate applicator has a typical treatment area of 110 cm^2; thus, treatment area is increased by approximately 10% while treatment time is decreased by over 40% with the cup applicator (Kilmer SL).

Conclusion

Cryolipolysis represents a novel, noninvasive treatment option for fat. Patients can undergo a safe, effective, and simple procedure, which will gradually reduce the appearance of unwanted fat over the following *2–4 months*. It should be noted that the device works best for *localized, discrete fat bulges* and is not intended for the treatment of obesity or as a substitute for large-volume liposuction.

The procedure is *not* suitable for obese patients or patients with considerable skin laxity. A major *advantage* is that there is minimal operator involvement once the suction cup is in place and hence results are not operator dependent.

Cryolipolysis is the *best studied* among all the fat reduction technologies. Future modifications will need to address certain issues, however, in particular a way to treat larger body areas as well as combine technologies for skin tightening. There are two case reports of men who maintained their result for 2 years and 5 years, respectively after the cryolipolysis—more data is required on the longevity of results.

STEP-BY-STEP APPROACH

Procedure of Laser-assisted Lipolysis

Patient Selection

This is a crucial part of delivering results with LAL. The ideal patient should be thin with localized pockets of fat that need treatment. The patient should be in good health. The need for maintaining a healthy lifestyle (diet, exercise) after the procedure should be emphasized, and there should preferably not be a history of frequent or rapid weight gain and weight loss in the past. The patient should have realistic expectations from the procedure, and it must be clearly explained beforehand that LAL is not a method of weight loss but of body contouring.

Any areas with unwanted adiposity can be treated with LAL. Commonly treated areas are the abdomen, flanks, submental region, upper arms, buttocks, and thighs. Other areas like the knees, calves, ankle, breast, lipomas, and localized adiposities left from previous liposuctions can also be treated.

Contraindications

Absolute

- Pregnancy
- Bleeding diathesis
- Lignocaine allergy
- Serious debilitating illness of any kind.

Relative

- Compromised liver function
- Age over 65 years
- Hypertension
- Diabetes
- Cardiovascular problems.

Preoperative Workup

Standard preoperative investigations that must be done in every patient include complete blood count (CBC), liver function tests, blood sugar, kidney function tests, lipid profile, human immunodeficiency virus (HIV), HBsAg, anti-HCV, bleeding parameters, and in the case of women, a urinary pregnancy test, if applicable.

Surgeons differ in their use of preoperative medications, and the experts do not recommend any routine medications.

Techniques

- The part to be treated is clearly marked out in a standing position. This is important because once the patient is lying down and tumescent anesthesia has been administered the contours can change dramatically.
- There should be at least 1.5 cm of fat in the pinch test in the area to be treated (Fig. 9.13).

The decision must be made whether suction will be employed after laser lipolysis. In smaller areas like the submental region and inner thighs suction is not required while larger areas like the abdomen usually benefit from suction.

- The procedure is performed under tumescent anesthesia. For this, a tumescent solution is prepared using lignocaine with epinephrine, sodium bicarbonate, and normal saline. The concentration of the lignocaine is between 0.05% and 0.1% depending the region being treated and that of 1:1,000,000 epinephrine is usually 0.05–0.75 mg/L. 10 mEq of sodium bicarbonate is added to each liter of the tumescent solution to raise its pH and thus prevent stinging (lignocaine is acidic in nature). The maximum safe dose of lignocaine in tumescent anesthesia is 55 mg/kg; however, experts recommend keeping the concentrations at a more conservative 35–45 mg/kg for additional safety.
- The next step is to make access ports around the area to be treated. These can be made as small stab incisions with a No. 11 blade or with a 1.5 mm punch, after infiltrating 1 mL of 1–2% lignocaine with 1:100,000 epinephrine at each site. The number of ports depends on the area being treated and a typical number for the abdomen is 4–6. The tumescent

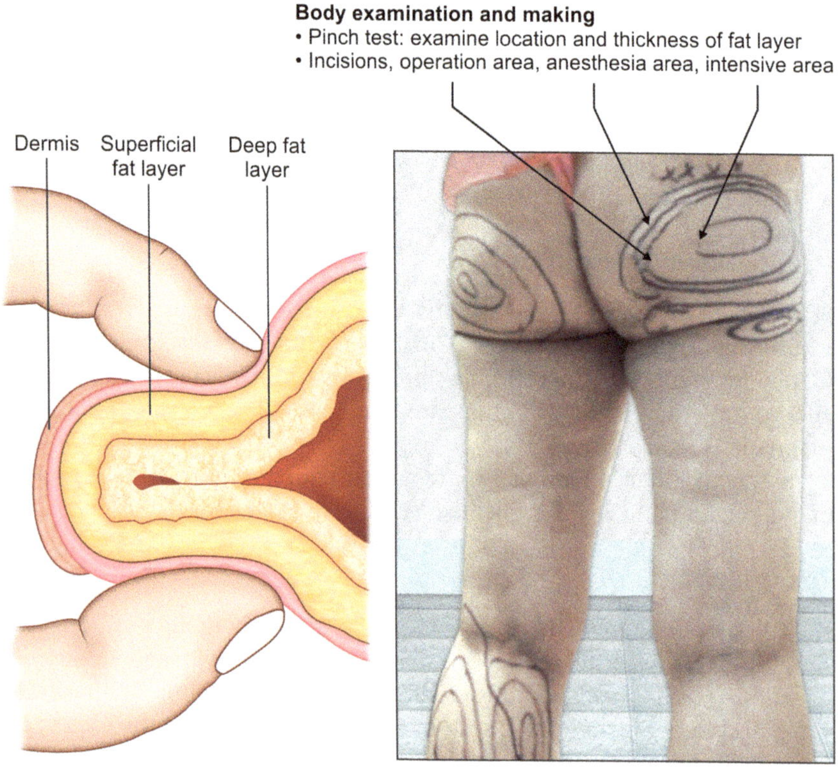

Fig. 9.13: Preoperative preparation for laser-assisted liposuction [QuadroStar+ 980 (diode laser)].

solution is then infiltrated gradually into the entire area to be treated. This can be done using large syringes (50 mL) or with specialized devices, such as infiltration pressure cuffs. Because of the large volume required in areas, such as the abdomen (2-3 L), this step can take 45-60 minutes or more. About 30 minutes must be given after all the solution has been infiltrated to allow proper diffusion and adequate anesthesia before commencing the procedure.

- After this, the fiberoptic cable carrying the laser is inserted through stainless steel cannulas and then introduced in the subcutaneous plane. The cannulas can be inserted empty to begin with and a tunneling to and fro motion used to create an easier path, once the laser is introduced. The laser cable extends 2 mm beyond the steel tip of the cannula and is visible as a bright red light shining through the skin. As the laser is fired, the cannula is moved slowly to cover the treatment field. On an average 10 passes are required to adequate laser lipolysis. There is a reduction in volume of the treated area, felt with the finger pinch test, and this serves as a tactile marker of the endpoint for lasing (Fig. 9.14).
- Once this is done, the suction apparatus is attached to the stainless steel cannulas and the liquefied fat from the laser treated areas is aspirated. Typically 2-5 L of fat can be removed from areas, such as the abdomen. This step takes 1.5-2 hours to complete.
- In the end, the ports are dressed (not sutured) and a compression garment is applied to support the treated area. The patient is then sent home on antibiotics and painkillers.

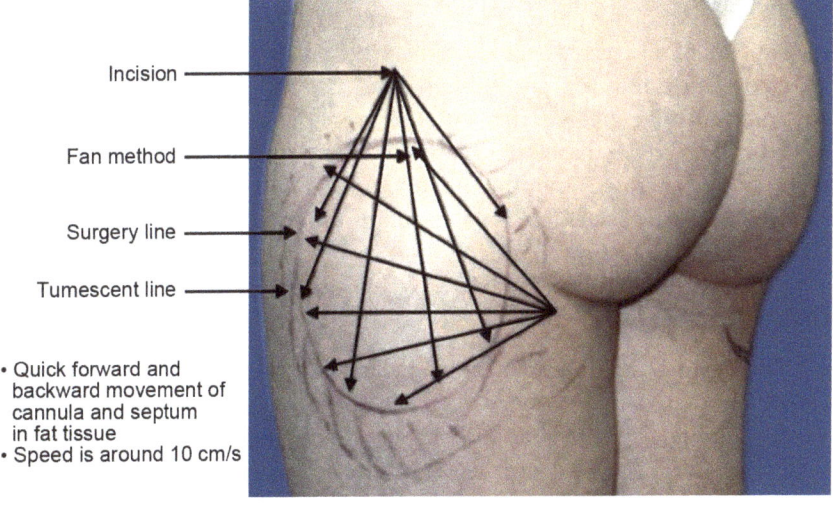

Fig. 9.14: A depiction of the procedure planes in laser-assisted liposuction.

Advantages of Laser-assisted Liposuction

- Shorter recovery time. Most patients able to go back to work within 2–3 days.
- Less bruising and edema and hence, less postprocedure pain.
- Less trauma during the procedure due to smaller size of the cannula used.
- Skin tightening is perhaps the most important benefit of LAL as compared to suction-assisted liposuction (SAL).
- More uniform fat reduction and hence smoother external appearance.
- Lower rate of revision surgeries (3.5% as compared to 12–13% with SAL).
- Limited role in improving cellulite as compared to SAL, which is ineffective for this indication.

Limitations of Laser-assisted Liposuction

- High cost of the laser machine.
- Increased procedure time as compared to SAL.
- Risk of thermal injury (skin burns).
- Unsuitable to treat large areas.
- Steeper learning curve as compared to SAL.

CRYOLIPOLYSIS

Cryolipolysis is performed in an outpatient setting. This has been mentioned in the text and a generic overview is given here.

Preoperative Counseling

- These devices are reduction of localized areas of fat accumulation. It is not ideal for obese patients or those with significant skin laxity.
- Patients should be screened for a history of cryoglobulinemia, paroxysmal cold hemoglobinuria, and cold urticaria.
- There are mild adverse effects such as immediate but transient erythema, bruising, and decreased pain sensation for several weeks.
- Results require 2–3 months to reach full potential, and patients should not expect to see immediate results nor should they anticipate large volume fat reduction.

Procedure

- The device contains a control unit and a cup-shaped applicator into which tissue is drawn.
- A coupling gel sheet is applied to the intended treatment site, then the applicator is placed over it using moderate vacuum suction to position the tissue between two cooling panels. Suction decreases the blood flow in the treated area and thereby allows for more efficient skin cooling.

- A cooling intensity factor (CIF) is then selected using the control console, which allows the operator to control the rate of heat flux into and out of the tissue, and treatment begins for a cycle of up to 60 minutes. During this time, no further operator intervention is required, as the energy extraction rate is monitored by the device, using thermoelectric cooling cells.
- The device automatically ceases the cooling exposure when the cycle time expires.
- The applicator is then removed and may be placed on other treatments sites, repeating the process for more thorough results.

ISSUES AND CONTROVERSIES WITH NONSURGICAL SCULPTING

Cellulite is a well-documented condition, and although many treatment options have been used, few have lasting clinical results. This historically notorious problem will always be the focus of device technologies, but considering the multiple mechanism involved in cellulite, we feel that technology may not by itself help in this condition.

Depending on the grade and severity, some cellulite patients may see a lesser degree of improvement. It is important in the consultation to address patient expectations. Noninvasive treatments require multiple treatments as well as possible interval maintenance treatments. Resistant cases could be due to severity of the case or undertreatment of the area. When using laser, RF, or ultrasound devices, it is important not to deliver excessive fluences, as this could lead to unwarranted treatment, complications, and/or thermal damage.

There are other issues, which have to be ironed out. It is important to see all patients in follow-up. Measurements to be taken include *dimple severity*, *circumference*, and *overall laxity*. Patient satisfaction should also be assessed. The use of traditional 2D imaging as well as 3D imaging can augment follow-up visits giving an objective comparison from baseline.

The controversies and unanswered questions with regard to laser lipolysis are many and include lack of standardized treatment protocols and the amount of the tumescent fluid to be used in laser-assisted liposuction. If too little fluid is used, the anesthesia is incomplete. If a proper "supertumescence" is applied, much of the laser energy is absorbed by the infiltrated fluid instead of the tissue. The most effective energy that can be delivered with the fewest side effects has not been determined. Lastly, the best way to move the handpiece through the subcutaneous tissue: release of the laser energy only when pulling back or during a back and forth movement; moving slowly and evenly or faster and in a more random way is another vexing issue. Thus at present, laser lipolysis is to be used mostly in conjunction with tumescent liposuction. Because the same risks and side effects apply, the surgeon should be well trained and experienced in liposuction surgery and untrained dermatologists should not venture into the invasive procedures. As fat reduction is a cosmetic and commercial necessity, a lot of refinements are needed, and thus, this will continue to be a topic of active future research.

To *conclude,* at present with little direct comparisons between the various methods, it is difficult to decide which is the ideal device for noninvasive body contouring, fat, and cellulite reduction. Further, *none* of these devices should be thought of as "weight loss" devices; rather, *modest contouring* is typically the most realistic outcome. Cryolipolysis is considered safe and effective, with a high patient satisfaction rate of up to 73% after one treatment. This rate is comparable with that of HIFU and acoustic wave therapy (62.3% and 64%, respectively). Cryolipolysis is safe for all skin types, with no reported pigmentary changes, and is safe for repeated application. But if a substantial end result is the aim, laser-assisted liposuction seems to be the best bet at present in our opinion.

Even though the technology mentioned earlier might seem path breaking these methods are meant for localized adiposities and cannot change the contour of the body fat substantially. Hence, objective analysis of the data and patient results might not always justify the costs of the interventions employed. Surgical and invasive liposuction is the gold standard and the noninterventionist approaches can help modify local fat deposits and are at best addendum's to the treatment of fat.

BIBLIOGRAPHY

1. Alam M, Dover JS, ASDS Dermatologic Surgery Lexicon Task Force. American Society for Dermatologic Surgery dermatologic surgery drug and device nomenclature recommendations. Dermatol Surg. 2013;39(8):1158-66.
2. Alizadeh Z, Halabchi F, Mazaheri R, et al. Review of the mechanisms and effects of noninvasive body contouring devices on cellulite and subcutaneous fat. Int J Endocrinol Metab. 2016;14(4):e36727.
3. Anderson RR, Farinelli W, Laubach H, et al. Selective photothermolysis of lipid-rich tissues: a free electron laser study. Lasers Surg Med. 2006;38(10):913-9.
4. Christ C, Brenke R, Sattler G, et al. Improvement in skin elasticity in the treatment of cellulite and connective tissue weakness by means of extracorporeal pulse activation therapy. Aesthet Surg J. 2008;28(5):538-44.
5. DiBernardo BE. Treatment of cellulite using a 1440-nm pulsed laser with one-year follow-up. Aesthet Surg J. 2011;31(3):328-41.
6. Goldberg D, Fazeli A, Berlin A. Clinical, laboratory and MRI analysis of cellulite treatment with a unipolar radiofrequency device. J Dermatol Surg. 2008;34(2):204-9.
7. Ichikawa K, Miyasaka M, Tanaka R, et al. Histologic evaluation of the pulsed Nd:YAG laser for laser lipolysis. Lasers Surg Med. 2005;36(1):43-6.
8. Katz BE. Quantitative and qualitative evaluation of the efficacy of a 1440 nm Nd:YAG laser with novel bidirectional optical fiber in the treatment of

cellulite as measured by 3-dimensional surface imaging. J Drugs Dermatol. 2013;12(11):1224-30.
9. Kilmer SL. Prototype CoolCup cryolipolysis applicator with over 40% reduced treatment time demonstrates equivalent safety and efficacy with greater patient preference. Lasers Surg Med. 2017;49(1):63-8.
10. Manstein D, Laubach H, Watanabe K, et al. Selective cryolysis: a novel method of non-invasive fat removal. Lasers Surg Med. 2008;40(9):595-604.
11. Mathew AM. Fat Removal: Invasive and Non-invasive Body Contouring. New York: John Wiley & Sons Ltd; 2015.
12. Mulholland RS, Paul MD, Chalfoun C. Non-invasive body contouring with radiofrequency, ultrasound, cryolipolysis, and low-level laser therapy. Clin Plast Surg. 2011;38(3):503-20.
13. Neira R, Ortiz C. Low-level laser-assisted liposculpture: clinical report of 700 cases. Aesthet Surg J. 2002;22(5):451-55.
14. Neira R, Toledo L, Arroyave J, et al. Low-level laser-assisted liposuction: The Neira 4 L technique. Clin Plast Surg. 2006;33(1):117-27.
15. Nootheti PK, Magpantay A, Yosowitz G, et al. A single center, randomized, comparative, prospective clinical study to determine the efficacy of the VelaSmooth system versus the Triactive system for the treatment of cellulite. Lasers Surg Med. 2003;38(10):908-12.
16. Nürnberger F, Müller G. So-called cellulite: An invented disease. J Dermatol Surg Oncol. 1978;4(3):221-9.
17. Parlette EC, Kaminer ME. Laser-assisted liposuction: Here's the skinny. Semin Cutan Med Surg. 2008;27(4):259-63.
18. Petti C, Stoneburner J, McLaughlin L. Laser cellulite treatment and laser-assisted lipoplasty of the thighs and buttocks: Combined modalities for single stage contouring of the lower body. Lasers Surg Med. 2016;48(1):14-22.
19. Rossi AM, Katz BE. A modern approach to the treatment of cellulite. Dermatol Clin. 2014;32(1):51-9.
20. Russe-Wilflingseder K, Russe E, Vester JC, et al. Placebo controlled, prospectively randomized, double-blinded study for the investigation of the effectiveness and safety of the acoustic wave therapy (AWT) for cellulite treatment. J Cosmet Laser Ther. 2013;15(3):155-62.
21. Sadick NS, Mulholland RS. A prospective clinical study to evaluate the efficacy and safety of cellulite treatment using the combination of optical and RF energies for subcutaneous tissue heating. J Cosmet Laser Ther. 2004;6(4):187-90.
22. Shek SY, Yeung CK, Chan JC, et al. The efficacy of a combination non-thermal focused ultrasound and radiofrequency device for noninvasive body contouring in Asians. Lasers Surg Med. 2016;48(2):203-7.
23. Sommer B, Bergfeld D. Laser-assisted liposuction. In: Raulin C, Karsai S (Eds). Laser and IPL Technology in Dermatology and Aesthetic Medicine. Berlin Heidelberg: Springer-Verlag; 2011.
24. Teitelbaum SA, Burns JL, Kubota J, et al. Non-invasive body contouring by focused ultrasound: Safety and efficacy of the Contour I device in a multicenter, controlled, clinical study. Plast Reconstr Surg. 2007;120(3):779-89.
25. van Veen RL, Sterenborg HJ, Pifferi A, et al. Determination of visible near-IR absorption coefficients of mammalian fat using time- and spatially resolved diffuse reflectance and transmission spectroscopy. J Biomed Opt. 2005;10(5):054004.

CHAPTER 10

Combination Laser Therapy: Rationale and Indications

Kabir Sardana

INTRODUCTION

Though some of us are "purists", most clinicians often combine procedures including lasers for various indications. There is a notable medical rule that applies to therapies for common cold, wherein if a "multitudes of therapies are needed for a disorder—there probably is no real cure". This would apply to the concept of combination lasers as if a disorder does not respond to a single laser, based on the principles of lasers physics, rarely would they respond to a combination of lasers.

Here it is important to distinguish between combining *nonlaser procedures* with laser procedures which is a valid concept and combining *various lasers* in the same session. A classic example of the former is carbon dioxide (CO_2) laser resurfacing combined with facial rejuvenation surgery including blepharoplasty, rhytidectomy, forehead lift, and neck rejuvenation surgery to enhance the appearance of the skin.

But here we will focus on combining laser devices which should have a logic and a rationale and both of these prerequisites are satisfied in the following scenarios:
1. If the disorder does not respond to a single laser procedure and is *not* a dynamic disorder (never in melasma, but possible in tattoos).
2. A disorder that has multiple components and causative factors, like photoaging.
3. If the two laser systems do not contradict the principles of laser physics. Like say combining fractional lasers with a Q-switched (QS) laser. They have different chromophores and the heat produced by a fractional laser would mitigate the effects of a QS laser if used simultaneously.
4. If the same class of lasers is used, like various QS pigment-specific lasers in nevus of Ota. Using the Active Fx and Deep Fx can be used in the same session for acne scars, as the laser physics are similar.

One aspect (point 3) is important as remember the dynamics of single laser are defined considering the skin as an optical window, which it is not in pigmented skin (Sardana K). Modulating the skin with a laser and then simultaneously using another laser may be counterproductive. A classic example is combining fractional ablative and QS 1,064 nm lasers for nevus of Ota in the same session. The use of an ablative system changes the tissue pathology and the QS laser if used concurrently may actually have a differential response as the optical properties of the tissue change. The concept that a fractional device can create microcraters and help in penetration of a QS laser is an illogical concept as the QS 1,064 nm laser is a deeply penetrating laser and does not need a microchannel on the skin. And to believe that the QS laser will penetrate only through those channels is a highly improbable concept. On the contrary sequentially using different wavelengths (like multiple QS lasers for nevus of Ota) has a logic as the nevus cells are at different depths of the tissue.

Here it may be pointed out that combination devices do exist but they usually combine radiofrequency (RF) with lasers as the former is "blind" to a target, unlike lasers and may not interact with laser physics. The combination of a superficial fractional treatment (sublative), improving epidermis and collagen remodeling in the upper dermis, with deep dermal remodeling produced by the microneedle device, represents a high potential for a complete skin improvement with minimal adverse effects and recovery time. There are other devices that combine optical energy to electrical energy, in general, the association of RF with laser (Laser Diode—Polaris WR system) or light source (LIP—Aurora˙ SR, Syneron) and allow the treatment of vascular injuries and pigmented hair removal and treatment of rhytides addition and sagging (Lanigan, 2008). The combination of the two types of energy has a synergistic effect, allowing the use of lower doses of both, with less risk of adverse effects (Sadick, 2007). In combined systems, in which the optimal energy used is lower than that usually required, there is the possibility of use in patients with higher phototypes with less risk of adverse effects (Alster and Lupton, 2007).

Except possibly in photoaging, any decision to combine should be done *sequentially* and not concurrently. Here, we will highlight some of the combination procedures and highlight their advantages.

AGED SKIN

There are several different aspects of photoaging—lentigines, erythema and telangiectasia, and wrinkles or skin texture changes (Table 10.1). This is a classic scenario where different lasers would be needed as different pathology needs to be targeted.

It has been known that facial rejuvenation via ablative resurfacing has the potential to achieve excellent outcomes but the adverse events and downtime can be significant. This lead to the invention of nonablative modalities where the morbidity is considerably less, but the clinical efficacy is often also substantially reduced. The fractional photothermolysis—first nonablative,

Table 10.1: Classification of photodamage skin.

Grade	Classification	Age	Wrinkles	Clinical findings	Cosmetic camouflage
I	Mild	20s or 30s	No wrinkles	Early photoaging: • Mild pigmentary change • No keratoses • Minimal wrinkles	Minimal or no makeup
II	Moderate	30s or 40s	Wrinkles in motion	Early to moderate photoaging: Early solar lentigines, keratoses palpable but not visible Parallel smile lines begin to appear	Wears some foundation
III	Advanced	50s	Wrinkles at rest	Advanced photoaging: Dyschromia Visible telangiectasias Visible keratoses	Always wears heavy foundation
IV	Severe	60s and older	Only wrinkles	Severe photoaging: Yellow-gray skin color Wrinkles throughout	Makeup 'cakes and cracks'

then ablative—is a compromise between achieving satisfactory clinical results while also minimizing associated adverse reactions. If these are used in isolation the results achieved are not marked as there are multiple aspects of an aging face (Table 10.1). The combinations can vary from pulsed light and nonablative fractional lasers to aggressive use of combination modalities (*see* **Chapter 12E: Facial Rejuvenation**).

Devices Used and Classification

A classification of lasers and light sources utilized for photorejuvenation are outlined in Table 10.2 but we admit that it is arbitrary as many devices are capable of delivering multiple wavelengths.

The first category is visible light lasers or light sources that have more absorption by *hemoglobin* and *melanin*. These visible light sources and lasers have more influence on the telangiectatic and melanocytic components of photoaging. These sources can be subdivided into coherent, single wavelength, broadband (flashlamps), or narrow band such as light-emitting diodes (LEDs). Intense pulsed light (IPL) is a broadband light source with filters used to limit the lower end of the emitted spectrum.

The next category is infrared with absorption predominantly by *water*. Infrared wavelengths with primarily water absorption are used to create

Table 10.2: Lasers and energy devices used for aging skin.

Visible laser light sources	• Frequency doubled Nd:YAG, KTP (green 532 nm) • Pulsed dye (yellow 585–595 nm): Long pulse versus short PDL
Visible nonlaser light sources	• Intense pulsed light (IPL)—broadband filtered light of various organs: Visible infrared • Light-emitting diodes (LEDs)—narrowband: UV, visible, and infrared
Infrared lasers (target pigment, hemoglobin, and water)	• *Q-switched and millisecond domain Nd:YAG 1,064 nm:* Infrared lasers (target is water only) • 1,320 nm Nd:YAG laser • 1,450 nm diode laser • 1,540 nm erbium glass laser
Others	Fractional lasers, radiofrequency (RF), microwave, and ultrasound

(KTP: potassium titanyl phosphate; Nd:YAG: neodymium-doped yttrium aluminum garnet; PDL: pulsed dye laser; UV: ultraviolet)

thermal, dermal, and collagen injury. The most commonly employed devices are 1,320 nm, 1,450 nm, and 1,540 nm lasers. The 1,927 nm thulium laser can be used alone or in combination with a deeper (1,550 nm) nonablative fractionated device (Fraxel® Restore Dual, Solta Medical). Posttreatment recovery involves epidermal necrosis and reepithelialization manifested clinically as mild erythema and edema, followed by skin bronzing and sandpapery surface texture during the desquamation process that lasts for several days.

Another category is the near-infrared lasers or light sources, which are absorbed by a combination of *melanin, hemoglobin*, and *water*. The tradeoff is that these wavelengths are absorbed at a lesser intensity but cover more targets. The 1,064 nm neodymium-doped yttrium aluminum garnet (Nd:YAG) laser is the most commonly used example. Lee compared the efficacy of the 532 nm, millisecond potassium titanyl phosphate (KTP) laser alone and the 1,064 nm, millisecond Nd:YAG laser alone as well as in combination for the treatment of skin changes of photoaging. The combination of the two wavelengths gave slightly better results than either alone.

The broadband flashlamp pumped light sources also have a number of effects for structural photorejuvenation in that they emit not only wavelengths absorbed by melanin and hemoglobin, but wavelengths absorbed by water as well. IPL broadband sources emit 515–1,200 nm with high energy available for thermal absorption although the output is nonlinear and is stronger in the visible light spectrum than the infrared. Here, it must be remembered that the *IPL* is best used for mild changes of sun damage, maintenance of results achieved from other procedures, or for those who desire a treatment with less downtime as, the energy is spread over a range of wavelengths, no single wavelength is particularly focused or powerful. Chan et al. demonstrated the safety of combination IPL and nonablative fractional treatment on the same treatment day (either before or after nonablative fractional treatment).

Berlin et al. reported successful combination of very light erbium followed sequentially by IPL.

Other devices on the market use RF to heat tissue. Depending on the delivery system and frequency, deep or superficial heating can be produced. Monopolar RF has a very different and deeper penetration (as the result of the patient being grounded) than bipolar RF devices, in which the RF travels from one electrode to another over relatively short distances. RF energy has been combined in several devices with IPL and diode lasers. The goal of the combination of technology is to achieve skin tightening and improvement in the visible changes of sun damage in the skin, or enhancement of the improvement seen with the light-based device alone. Electro-optical synergy (ELOS) that combines RF and IPL energy in a single pulse and RF with a diode laser have both been studied for aging skin. This combination is often used to treat cellulite/fat where a combination of bipolar RF vacuum and ultrasound (Syneron Candela VelaShape˚) is used. Of course, the fractional lasers remain the most commonly used devices.

When selecting a thermal photorejuvenation system it is, therefore, critical to understand the physics behind the wavelength and the method of delivery rather than exaggerated manufacturer's claims. Having knowledge of the *output* of a device, understanding whether the *target* is hemoglobin, melanin, or water (or all three) and understanding *spot size* and method of delivery, the physician may be better able to choose the correct system for the correct application. For example, photorejuvenation of pigmented lesions would not be possible with a unit emitting 1,450 nm, for which the target is water and not melanin. This knowledge is also vital if the clinician is to minimize possible adverse clinical events in darker ethnic skin types. Visible light, more strongly absorbed by melanin, must, therefore, be used with greater caution in darker skin.

Component-wise Therapy

A summary of the various devices needed to treat aspects of photodamage skin are given in Table 10.3 and discussed here.

Vascular Component

The pulsed dye laser (PDL) is an excellent choice for reducing redness and very fine telangiectasias. Larger telangiectasias are more effectively treated with a 1,064 nm Nd:YAG laser. The longer wavelength of 1,064 nm can penetrate more deeply to better reach the deeper vessels, and longer pulse widths can be matched to larger vessel sizes.

For the persistent redness the *1,064 nm wavelength* is first used to treat the more visible and larger telangiectasias which is followed by the *PDL* is used to treat the finer vessels and diffuse erythema.

Table 10.3: Suggested laser and energy devices for aged skin.

Morphology	Devices
Telangiectasias	• IPL • PDL (LP) • Nd:YAG (LP 532 nm)
Diffuse redness (nonvisible telangiectasia)	• IPL • PDL • LED photomodulation
Mottled pigmentation	• IPL • Nd:YAG (LP) 532 nm • LED
Mild rhytides	• Fractional lasers • LED photomodulation • IPL • PDL
Moderate rhytides	• Infrared lasers • Fractional lasers • RF

(IPL: intense pulsed light; LED: light-emitting diode; Nd:YAG: neodymium-doped yttrium aluminum garnet; PDL: pulsed dye laser; RF: radiofrequency)

Pigmented Component

The long-pulsed (LP) alexandrite and QS lasers—including QS 532 nm Nd:YAG, QS ruby, and QS alexandrite—can target specific pigmented lesions such as freckles or lentigines. A thumb rule is, that **lighter** the lesion, the **more** energy is required to have an effect on the target. For **darker** lesions, **lower** energy is needed to achieve a clinical effect and to minimize side effects. Hence, lower energies should be used in pigmented skin.

In the case of a light-skinned patient with darker lentigines that are either diffusely spread over a large area or just a few larger lesions, most prefer the LP 755 nm alexandrite laser. Typically, a spot size of 12 mm and an energy setting of 16–30 J/cm^2 are used, depending on patient skin type and darkness of the lesion. The *efficacy* of this treatment is best when the contrast between skin color and pigmented target is great (very fair skin and very dark spots are the most ideal situation).

If there are lighter lentigines, darker skin types, treatment location of arms or legs, or very little contrast between skin color and lesion color, the ideal laser is the *QS 532 nm* laser spot treatment *or* a *nonablative fractional laser* alone *or* in combination with an LP alexandrite or a QS laser.

Desired endpoints of treatment with the QS laser are varying degrees of whitening or an ashy appearance—in lighter skin types, a larger degree of whitening is appropriate and more effective; however, in darker skin types, a very slight whitening or only slight ashy appearance is preferred in order to minimize size effects of hypopigmentation and postinflammatory hyperpigmentation (PIH).

Scenarios

Melasma with aging: A nonablative fractional laser (1,550 nm or 1,927 nm) is used either alone or in combination with low energy LP alexandrite laser *prior* to the fractional laser. If there is any erythema or telangiectasia, it is treated with one or both of the vascular lasers *prior* to treatment with the nonablative fractional laser. Here the logic is that different aspects of the skin pathology are taken care of by various devices. The fractional laser can have a high energy impact and tissue heat production and can thus change the tissue dynamics that may impede with the laser physics of the vascular and pigmented lasers, hence the classic *sequence* is:

"*V*ascular lasers *first*, then *P*igment lasers LP alexandrite or QS 532 nm Nd:YAG laser, then *F*ractional nonablative laser."

Textural changes with pigmentation: Here the ideal would be a nonablative fractional device. But it would be better to treat the skin first with an LP alexandrite laser prior to the fractional laser on the same day. Similarly, erythema and telangiectasias are pretreated with a vascular laser before the fractional treatment. Though the fractional nonablative lasers do effectively treat pigment, but this is more in patients with a high contrast (fair individuals).

Severe textural changes with aging: Here a fractional CO_2 is the choice of device. This can be preceded by treatment of lentigines with the LP alexandrite and occasionally treatment of vascular lesions with the PDL or Nd:YAG laser. The nonspecific heat of the fractional CO_2 laser can reduce telangiectasias so that often the treatment of the telangiectasias, especially smaller diameter ones, is not needed.

Lipolysis with skin tightening: In recent years, laser-assisted lipolysis has been used not only to remove fat, but also to induce skin tightening. Many lasers ranging from 924 nm to 1,320 nm have been employed (McBean JC and Weiss RA). More recently, combined lasers have been used to improve clinical outcome with the intention of utilizing one laser for lipolysis and another for skin tightening. The intention is to use such lasers to disrupt the adipocytes by a combination of photothermal and photoacoustic effects. After draining fat, further heating of the dermis can lead to skin tightening.

A recent study examining the role of a sequentially firing of 1,064 nm and 1,320 nm Nd:YAG lasers for laser-assisted lipolysis indicated skin tightening of 18% 1 month after a single treatment. Another study examining the use of a combined 924/975 nm diode laser revealed skin tightening to be excellent with retraction of up to 25% in a subject with a pretreatment umbilical tattoo.

SCARS

Pulsed dye laser may be applied alone for small hypertrophic scars, but is often combined with fractional laser therapy in either concurrent or alternating treatment sessions. A conference study presentation of

100 patients with keloid scars (Aldana G, Viera M, ELSD conference), combined 595 nm PDL and fractional CO_2 during the same session. Three sessions were given in 45 days interval. There was an improvement in thickness, erythema, appearance, and pliability, with no recurrence of 1 year later.

Atrophic acne scars can be treated in a single session with the combined deep and superficial modes of an ablative CO_2 fractional laser. Hyaluronic acid (HA) fillers may improve the appearance of atrophic acne scars alone or they can be combined with subcision. Disadvantages of using HA fillers include the need for frequent treatments, and HA fillers may only improve the appearance of mildly atrophic scars. Fat grafting and subcision have also been combined simultaneously. The combination approach to acne scars is detailed in **Chapter 12A: Acne Scars**. The treatment of acne scars has received additional attention with the development of deep fractional CO_2 lasers. The combination of both a deep fractional treatment with a more superficial fully ablative treatment has good results in fair skin patients but is ill advised in pigmented skin.

ACNE AND ROSACEA

A combination of blue and red light has also been used for acne. Goldberg and Russel used a combination of blue and red LED therapy to treat acne in 24 subjects. The study showed that this combination appears to have excellent potential in the treatment of mild to severe acne; it is side effect free and with no pain.

Laser Genesis (Cutera), which is an Nd:YAG 1,064 nm wavelength with a patented 300 μs technology, has been combined with the use of IPL. Laser Genesis alone has been shown to reduce erythema and induce new collagen production in the papillary dermis to improve the appearance of wrinkles after three treatment sessions at 1 month and 3 months. When combined with IPL, the two lasers have yielded excellent results in reducing facial erythema and flushing.

PIGMENTED DISORDERS

The combination of QS lasers—532 nm followed by 1,064 nm—was shown to be significantly more effective in the treatment of Hori's nevus than the 1,064 nm alone (Ee HL et al.). Here is a classic example of combination where both the systems have the same laser principles. Here the combination treatments appear to allow more effective eradication of dermal pigmentation by eliminating epidermal pigmentation, and thereby allowing better dermal penetration of laser. The treatment of Hori's macules remains challenging in some patients, since the condition often coexists with other dyschromia, such as melasma, and the postlaser PIH risk is higher than in nevus of Ota. In Indian skin though, this may not be a preferred option.

Recent case reports have shown a potential benefit from a combined therapeutic approach employing both QS and fractional CO_2 ablative laser technology for tattoo removal compared to QS laser therapy alone (Ibrahimi OA). The application of a fractional CO_2 laser over a tattooed region provides additional direct escape routes for transepidermal ink-particle efflux, as well as a potentially more robust inflammatory response for immune-mediated particle clearance. In addition, the dermal micropunctures achieved with the fractional ablative laser modality assist in preventing the formation of postprocedure blisters and may thereby shorten the healing time. We have published a series of studies (Sardana K) combining up CO_2 or erbium-doped yttrium aluminum garnet (Er:YAG) with QS lasers for tattoos with rapid reduction in turnaround time in patients (*see* **Chapter 3: Pigmented Lesions and Tattoos**) referred to as the rapid tattoo removal (RTR) technique (Figs. 10.1A to C). This is a low cost option and this technique can achieve rapid results without the need for PICO lasers.

This author has always maintained that dermal pigmented disorders are decidedly difficult to treat, especially in pigmented skin. The pigment in the epidermis and dermis in our skin can scatter and dissipate the wavelength thus, reducing the end effect markedly and nevus of Ota is one such disorder. The conferences either dwell on the "best" results or showcase results of our colleagues from Southeast Asia, where the skin is not as pigmented as our skin. Here, a study by Park SH et al. is instructive where for dermal pigmentations, like nevus of Ota and congenital nevus, a combined therapy of a resurfacing laser (CO_2) and a selective photothermolytic laser [the Q-switched ruby laser (QSRL)] was tried, and the results were compared with those treated with the QSRL alone. The results with the combined mode were better and hence in certain indications epidermal ablation may be of value.

In Indian skin, the Er:YAG would be better than the CO_2 due to the better tissue dynamics of the former. Here, it is important to understand that in dermal disorders, a combination does not always mean, complete clearance. A study of Hori nevus found that, epidermal ablation using the scanned CO_2 laser before QSRL, assessed by 3- and 16-month posttreatment melanin index, found that "the percentage of reduction in melanin index", was significantly higher on the sides treated with scanned CO_2 laser followed by QSRL, compared with the sides irradiated with QSRL alone at both follow-up visit. Note that the authors did not claim complete clearance, which goes to prove how difficult dermal disorders can be to treat (Manuskiatti W).

VASCULAR INDICATIONS

Leg Vein Treatment

Sadick and Trelles et al. reported better results in leg vein treatment (blue veins and veins > 1 mm responded best) using a laser that combined a pulsed

CHAPTER 10: Combination Laser Therapy: Rationale and Indications

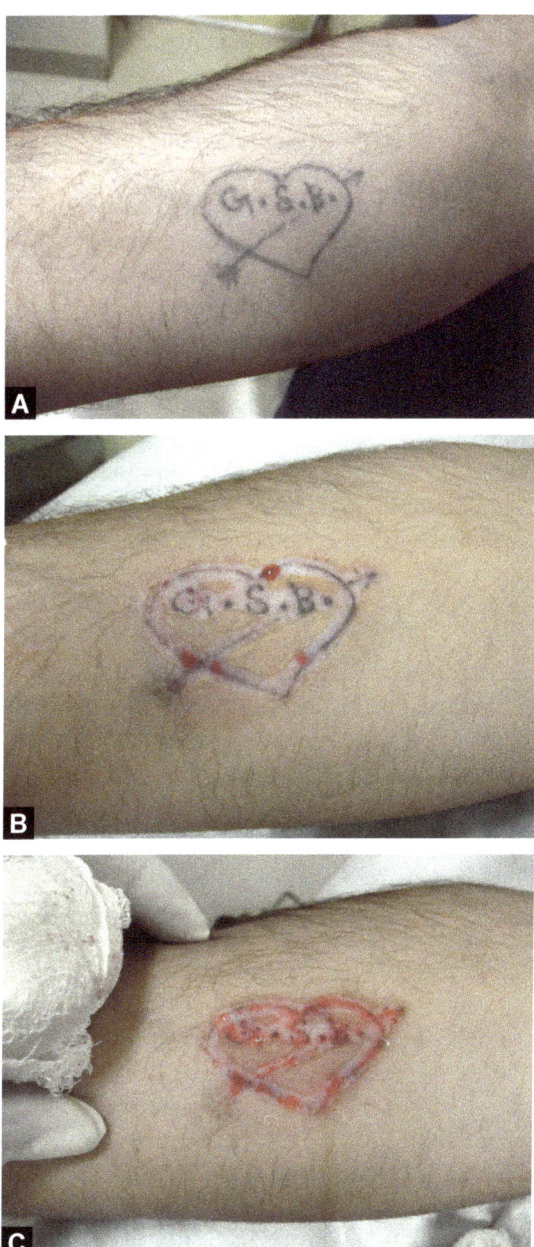

Figs. 10.1A to C: (A) The RTR technique. First pass is with the Er:YAG laser. A setting of 5 J/cm² is sufficient. Note the clean pass with the perfect removal of the epidermis; (B) The pinpoint bleeding is classic of upper papillary dermis. This is enough for tattoo removal; and (C) This is followed by a quick pass of the QS Nd:YAG 1,064 nm. Note the heightened bleeding as with the destruction of the tattoo, the concomitant heat damage leads to bleeding. Most patients respond to 1–2 sessions. The repeat session does not require ablation. (Er:YAG: erbium-doped yttrium aluminum garnet; QS Nd:YAG: Q-switched neodymium-doped yttrium aluminum garnet; RTR: rapid tattoo removal)

dye and Nd:YAG laser sequentially in the same pulse. The sequential pulsed dye 1,064 nm Nd:YAG laser has also been reported to be an effective and safe treatment for venous malformation. In the armamentarium of lasers available for leg vein treatment, the KTP laser, PDL, alexandrite laser, and diode lasers have all been utilized successfully, but the higher wavelength technologies are rapidly becoming the leaders in treatment of telangiectasias. Further novel approaches include combination of diode laser plus RF technology for treating lower extremity telangiectasias. When combined, the RF energy heats the outer vein thereby destroying it while the laser targets the endoluminal hemoglobin. Histopathological findings indicate that no matter which laser is utilized in treatment of lower extremity telangiectasias, some degree of intravascular thrombosis associated with vessel fragmentation will be seen.

A simple and effective concept in fair skin patients is to combine LP 1,064 nm Nd:YAG laser with PDL in the same session for more effective clearance of vascular conditions. If there is a pigment involved like lentigines or freckles with telangiectasias, it would be better to first treat the lentigines with a QS laser.

Laser Therapy for Extrafacial Port-wine Stain

These can be particularly difficult to treat. A protocol suggested (Cretu S et al. ELSD conference), is to treat the nodules with LP Nd:YAG, PDL for the rest of the lesion, and additional tacrolimus 0.1% ointment. The settings used were for the LP Nd:YAG: 10-40 ms, 3-7 mm spot diameter, and 120-140 J/cm^2; for the PDL 595 nm: 0.45-3 ms, 7 mm (7.25-10 J/cm^2), 10 mm (5-12 J/cm^2), or 3 × 10 mm (10-14 J/cm^2) spot size. Clearance of vascular nodules was obtained after an average of four sessions. More than 50% clearance can be achieved after an average of eight sessions for the rest of the lesions. No scarring was observed.

The difficult to treat port-wine stain (PWS) located in acral areas, have two problems: (1) one the stratum corneum is thicker compared to the face and (2) secondly they tend to have a pink or purple color. It is believed that in distal extremities vessels are placed more deeply. The logic of adding tacrolimus ointment 0.1% was to inhibit angiogenesis and hence may prevent formation of new vessels.

The LP alexandrite has selective absorption of deoxyhemoglobin and 50-75% deeper tissue penetration than PDL. The 755 nm wavelength may be used alone or in combination with PDL for improved efficacy of treatment-resistant PWS or hypertrophic lesions without an increase in complications.

ABLATIVE LASERS

A decade back, this would have been possibly the only indication of any practical use, but today in pigmented skin, these lasers are almost never used for full face resurfacing. The idea of discussing this here is to emphasize that there are situations where Er:YAG and CO_2 can be combined with better results, using their different tissue dynamics.

Combination Carbon Dioxide and Erbium-doped Yttrium Aluminum Garnet Laser Treatment

Necrotic tissue directly dysregulates wound healing, induces proteases, and inflammation. Many experts believe that the thermally-induced zone of necrosis left behind by the CO_2 laser is one of the main factors contributing to its adverse sequelae including prolonged postoperative erythema, pain, delayed healing, and scarring. Therefore, some authors have investigated the effect of removal of this residual zone of thermally damaged tissue after CO_2 laser resurfacing.

Goldman and colleagues (1999) studied the effect of Er:YAG laser resurfacing aimed to remove the residual zone of thermal damage left behind after CO_2 laser resurfacing. They employed the 950 ms pulsed CO_2 laser (three passes, 300 mJ, CPG settings of 596, 595, and 584) and resurfaced the other side of the face with two passes of the same CO_2 laser at the same settings followed by two passes with a short pulse Er:YAG laser (4 mm spot, 1.7 J, and 14 J/cm^2). They found that both reepithelialization time and the duration of erythema were significantly less for the side treated with the combination CO_2-Er:YAG as compared to the side treated with CO_2 laser alone. Moreover, this beneficial effect on postoperative healing was accomplished without compromising clinical efficacy.

McDaniel et al. (1999) compared resurfacing of the upper lip using a CO_2 laser alone (UltraPulse 5,000 C, two passes, 300 mJ, 95 W, CPG density 6, and spot diameter 2.25 mm, 7.5 J/cm^2) with the combination of the same CO_2 laser treatment followed by three passes with a short-pulsed Er:YAG laser (7 mm spot, 2J, and 5.2 J/cm^2). Medium to deep (class III) rhytides were improved with both techniques. However, the duration of postoperative crusting, swelling, and pruritus was significantly reduced at the sites treated with the CO_2-Er:YAG laser combination.

Protocol for Combination Carbon Dioxide-Erbium-doped Yttrium Aluminum Garnet Laser Treatment

Both the CO_2 laser and the Er:YAG laser have unique qualities that can be exploited during resurfacing. The CO_2 laser is unique in the following ways:
- Hemostasis is achieved.
- A plateau of ablation is reached, limiting resurfacing depth if proper treatment protocols are followed.
- Collagen (skin) tightening occurs as a heat-related phenomenon, resulting in correction of loose tissue and atrophic scars.
- The first pass causes an epidermal/dermal split that allows easy and complete removal of the epidermis with a single pass.

The Er:YAG laser is unique in the following ways:
- Minimal residual thermal damage or tissue heating occurs.
- This pure ablation laser continues to ablate with each pass and does not reach an ablation plateau with depth.
- Only minimal tissue water is required for laser–tissue interaction.

The most successful use of lasers for resurfacing would utilize each laser to take advantage of its unique benefit and to eliminate the disadvantages of each as much as possible.

Various protocols have been described for early photodamage and for moderate to advanced photodamage. These may not be used nowadays but if the two ablative devices are available, the CO_2 can be followed by the Er:YAG which enables the latter to finely ablate dermal pathologies after the CO_2 has removed the epidermis, with minimal thermal damage as Er:YAG has minimal thermal impact.

FRACTIONAL ENERGY DEVICES AND THEIR COMBINATION

To study and understand the effect of fractional lasers, it would be pertinent to first understand that the various settings used have been studied first in histological specimens, using in vivo or ex vivo models. Thus, the settings used are based on this template and then extrapolated to human scenarios (Sardana K, 2012). Of the many parameters, the "aspect ratio" of fractional lasers is of fundamental importance, which is detailed in **Chapter 4: Fractional Photothermolysis**, and in essence is the width and depth of a microthermal zone (MTZ). It has been accepted that even though fractional lasers have less downtime, there is a need to increase the efficacy by combining various fractional lasers.

Combination Devices—Acne Scar

Cho et al. reported treating acne scars with a combined fractional laser treatment using 1,550 nm Er:Glass and CO_2 lasers. Mittelman et al. reported increased patient satisfaction for facial rejuvenation with combined fractionated CO_2 and low-power Er:YAG laser treatments. Tenna et al. treated acne scars with a combined simultaneous emission of CO_2 laser and RF waves, which resulted in a resurfacing effect from epidermal coagulation and a deeper remodeling due to dermal denaturation.

Rationale of Combination

The basis of these combinations is based on histological comparison of data where it has been shown that when epidermal and dermal change was compared, Er:YAG showed more superficial ablation of the epidermis with little dermal change, whereas Er:Glass showed more dermal-thermal change with little epidermal change (Figs. 10.2A and B) (Shin MR et al.).

It is accepted that while Er:YAG creates the clear "punched-out" ablation craters without any identifiable surrounding cellular injury, fractional CO_2 laser causes collateral thermal injury, which correlates with collagen remodeling. Fractional RF caused stronger ablation and collateral thermal damage than Er:YAG.

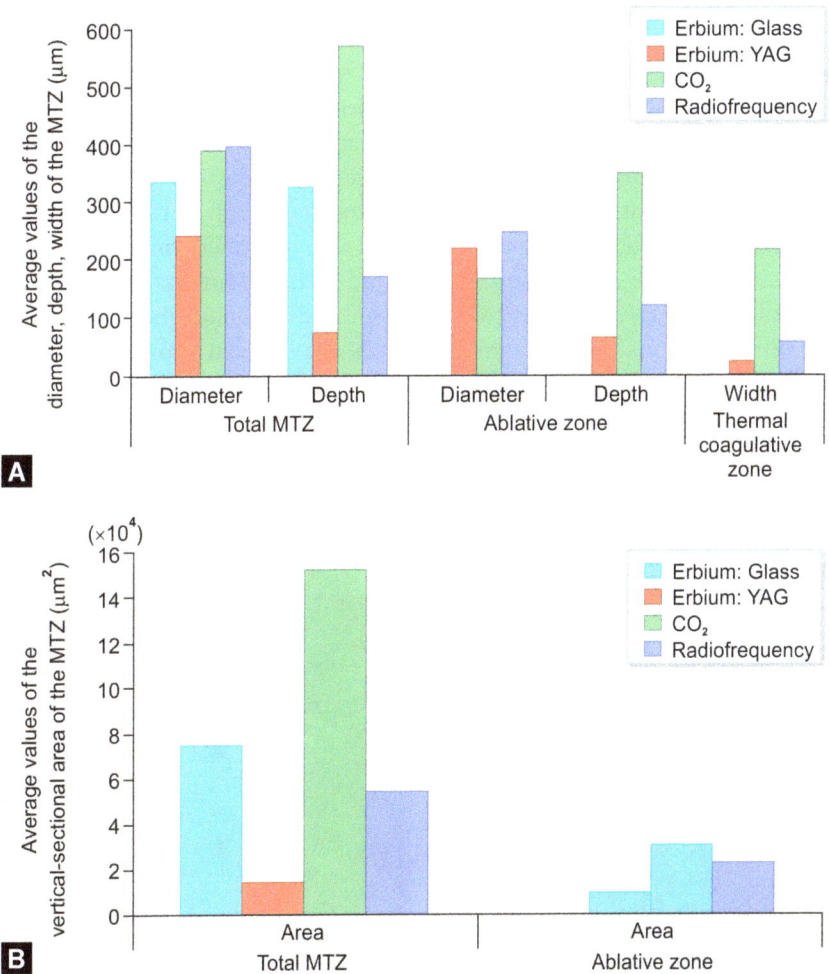

Figs. 10.2A and B: An artistic depiction of the various aspects of the dimensions of an MTZ with various energy devices. (CO_2: carbon dioxide; Er:YAG: erbium-doped yttrium aluminum garnet; MTZ: microthermal zone)

While using the fractional CO_2, the *depth* of the total MTZ, rather than the diameter, tended to increase according to the increase in energy. With the Er:Glass or RF higher energy levels increased the *diameter* of MTZ, rather than the depth. The *widest diameter* values of ablation were observed with fractional Er:YAG. In fractional CO_2 and RF, relatively deep ablative zones were observed, and fractional RF displayed superficial and broad "crater"-like microchannels; fractional CO_2 displayed narrow and deep "cone"-like microchannels (Figs. 10.3A and B).

So, in essence, the salient features of each energy devices are as follows:
- If a **superficial** ablation and minimal coagulation is needed, the fractional Er:YAG is ideal.
- If a **dermal** collagen remodeling is needed, the Er:Glass is an ideal tool.
- If a **deeper** and **narrow** channel is needed, the fractional CO_2 is ideal.
- If a **superficial** and **broad** channel is needed, the fractional RF is ideal.

But considering the downtime, one can combine lasers to optimize results. Hence, for rolled up acne scar, the fractional Er:YAG, fractional Er:Glass, and fractional RF are equally good with less downtime and PIH. For deep ice pick scar, the fractional CO_2 would be ideal. For box car scars, the fractional Er:Glass and the fractional RF would also be enough.

Thus, a rational combination of devices can be used depending on the type of scars. For a patient with largely superficial scars, a fractional Er:Glass or fractional RF would suffice. The fractional CO_2 can be used for the deeper scars. Here as the tissue chromophore is the same a combination of these devices makes scientific sense.

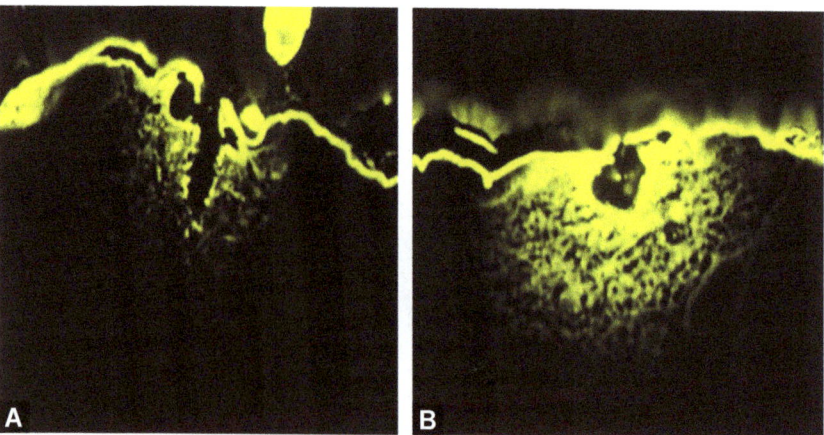

Figs. 10.3A and B: Comparison of the MTZ and aspect ratio of fractional CO_2 and fractional RF. (CO_2: carbon dioxide; MTZ: microthermal zone; RF: radiofrequency)

BIBLIOGRAPHY

1. Goldman MP, Manuskiatti W. Combined laser resurfacing with the 950-microsec pulsed CO_2+ Er:YAG lasers. Dermatol Surg. 1999;25:160-3.
2. McDaniel DH, Lord J, Ash K, et al. Combined CO_2/Erbium:YAG laser resurfacing of perioral rhytides and side-by-side comparison with CO_2 laser alone. Dermatol Surg. 1999;25:285-93.

DRAWBACKS OF COMBINATION LASERS THERAPY

Lasers deliver significant amounts of heat to the tissue. When different lasers are combined in the same session, there is a definite risk of heat damage. This is especially truer for fractional ablative lasers. In Indian skin, I would not advise the concurrent therapy with this laser as most do not use the correct settings and give too many passes with little regard to the aspect ratio **(Chapter 4: Fractional Photothermolysis and Chapter 17: Complications and their Management)**. Thus, if a high thermal impact laser is used, it is better not to use another lasers concurrently. A simple way is to feel the tissue by touching the skin, if the skin feels very hot, then the procedure should be paused until the skin cools to the touch. Using a vascular lasers or a fractional laser can lead to edema and crusting and thus, combining it with another laser is of little use in the same setting.

The classic indication of combination is the treatment of aging and photodamage skin, it is treated by addressing different aspects of the aging face including treating laxity of skin and facial structures, addressing loss of volume in the face, and relaxing lines of muscle movement as well as addressing the visible changes of sun damage and aging in the skin.

CONCLUSION

The text earlier delineates the various aspects of combining lasers but it is a point of active debate whether the same will be followed by most clinicians. The idea here is to understand the logic of combining lasers and to understand the risks especially in Indian and other richly pigmented skin. But it is my view and experience buffeted by existing data that combining multiple lasers in one sessions, except in some disorders, makes little sense, except adding some color and complexity to conference proceedings, which never correlate with objective improvement over conventional measures.

BIBLIOGRAPHY

1. Alexiades-Armenakas M. Rhytides, laxity, and photoaging treated with a combination of radiofrequency, diode laser, and pulsed light and assessed with a comprehensive grading scale. J Drugs Dermatol. 2006;5:731-8.
2. Alster TS, Lupton JR. Nonablative cutaneous remodeling using radiofrequency devices. Clin Dermatol. 2007;25:487-91.

3. Bagazgoitia L, Boixeda P, Lopez-Caballero C, et al. Venous malformation of the eyelid treated with pulsed-dye-1064-nm neodymium yttrium aluminum garnet sequential laser: an effective and safe treatment. Ophthal Plast Reconstr Surg. 2008;24:488-90.
4. Berlin AL, Hussain M, Phelps R, et al. Treatment of photoaging with a very superficial Er:YAG laser in combination with a broadband light source. J Drugs Dermatol. 2007;6:1114-8.
5. Cho SB, Lee SJ, Kang JM, et al. Combined fractional laser treatment with 1550-nm erbium glass and 10600-nm carbon dioxide lasers. J Dermatolog Treat. 2010;21:221-3.
6. Ee HL, Goh CL, Khoo LS, et al. Treatment of acquired bilateral nevus of ota-like macules (Hori's nevus) with a combination of the 532 nm Q-Switched Nd:YAG laser followed by the 1,064 nm Q-switched Nd:YAG is more effective: prospective study. Dermatol Surg. 2006;32:34-40.
7. Goldberg DJ, Russel BA. Combination blue (415 nm) and red (633 nm) LED phototherapy in the treatment of mild to severe acne vulgaris. J Cosmet Laser Ther. 2006;8:71-5.
8. Ibrahimi OA, Syed Z, Sakamoto FH, et al. Treatment of tattoo allergy with ablative fractional resurfacing: a novel paradigm for tattoo removal. J Am Acad Dermatol. 2011;64:1111-4.
9. Lanigan SW. Lasers in dermatology. Med Laser Appl. 2008;23:51-4.
10. Lee MW. Combination 532-nm and 1064-nm lasers for noninvasive skin rejuvenation and toning. Arch Dermatol. 2003;139:1265-76.
11. Manuskiatti W, Sivayathorn A, Leelaudomlipi P, et al. Treatment of acquired bilateral nevus of Ota-like macules (Hori's nevus) using a combination of scanned carbon dioxide laser followed by Q-switched ruby laser. J Am Acad Dermatol. 2003;48:584-91.
12. Mittelman H, Furr M, Lay PC. Combined fractionated CO_2 and low-power erbium:YAG laser treatments. Facial Plast Surg Clin North Am. 2012;20:135-43.
13. McBean JC, Katz BE. A pilot study of the efficacy of a 1,064 and 1,320 nm sequentially firing Nd:YAG laser device for lipolysis and skin tightening. Lasers Surg Med. 2009;41:779-84.
14. Park SH, Koo SH, Choi EO. Combined laser therapy for difficult dermal pigmentation: resurfacing and selective photothermolysis. Ann Plast Surg. 2001;47:31-6.
15. Sadick NS, Trelles MA. A clinical, histological, and computer-based assessment of the Polaris LV, combination diode, and radiofrequency system, for leg vein treatment. Lasers Surg Med. 2005;36:98-104.
16. Sadick N. Bipolar radiofrequency for facial rejuvenation. Facial Plast Surg Clin North Am. 2007;15:161-7.
17. Sadick NS, Alexiades-Armenakas M, Bitter P, et al. Enhanced full-face skin rejuvenation using synchronous intense pulsed optical and conducted bipolar radiofrequency energy (ELOS): introducing selective radiophotothermolysis. J Drugs Dermatol. 2005;4:181-6.

18. Sardana K, Chugh S, Garg VK. Are Q-switched lasers for Nevus of Ota really effective in pigmented skin? Indian J Dermatol Venereol Leprol. 2012;78:187-9.
19. Sardana K, Garg VK, Bansal S, et al. A promising split-lesion technique for rapid tattoo removal using a novel sequential approach of a single sitting of pulsed CO_2 followed by Q-switched Nd:YAG laser (1064 nm). J Cosmet Dermatol. 2013;12:296-305.
20. Sardana K, Ranjan R, Ghunawat S. Optimising laser tattoo removal. J Cutan Aesthet Surg. 2015;8:16-24.
21. Sardana K, Ranjan R, Kochhar AM, et al. A rapid tattoo removal technique using a combination of pulsed Er:YAG and Q-Switched Nd:YAG in a split lesion protocol. J Cosmet Laser Ther. 2015;17:177-83.
22. Sardana K, Garg VK, Arora P, et al. Histological validity and clinical evidence for use of fractional lasers for acne scars. J Cutan Aesthet Surg. 2012;5:75-90.
23. Shin MK, Choi JH, Ahn SB, et al. Histologic comparison of microscopic treatment zones induced by fractional lasers and radiofrequency. J Cosmet Laser Ther. 2014;16:317-23.
24. Tenna S, Cogliandro A, Piombino L, et al. Combined use of fractional CO_2 laser and radiofrequency waves to treat acne scars: A pilot study on 15 patients. J Cosmet Laser Ther. 2012;14:166-71.
25. Wang CC, Huang CL, Sue YM, et al. Treatment of cosmetic tattoos using carbon dioxide ablative fractional resurfacing in an animal model: A novel method confirmed histopathologically. Dermatol Surg. 2013;39:571-7.
26. Weiss RA, Beasley K. Laser-assisted liposuction using a novel blend of lipid- and water-selective wavelengths. Lasers Surg Med. 2009;41:760-6.
27. Weiss ET, Geronemus RG. Combining fractional resurfacing and Q-switched ruby laser for tattoo removal. Dermatol Surg. 2011;37:97-9.
28. Wu DC, Friedman DP, Fabi SG, et al. Comparison of intense pulsed light with 1,927-nm fractionated thulium fiber laser for the rejuvenation of the chest. Dermatol Surg. 2014;40:129-33.

CHAPTER 11

Laser Toning in Dermatology

Vivek Mehta, Kabir Sardana

INTRODUCTION

The efficacy of high-peak powers and ultrashort pulse width of the 5-ns Q-switched laser with low fluence was demonstrated first in zebrafish and then in melasma patients. Laser toning is essentially defined as the process of targeting melanin in the melanophores in keratinocytes, melanocytes, and dermal melanophores through the ultrashort-acting radiant heat effect, which is also known as subcellular selective photothermolysis.

In study by Mun JY et al., the three-dimensional (3D) structure of melanocytes in the epidermis was analyzed using serial images acquired by a 3View surface block face scanning electron microscope to understand the mode of action. In the epidermis, after laser treatment, fewer dendrites in the melanocytes were observed compared with pretreatment. In addition, ultrastructural changes in the melanosome were studied using transmission electron microscopy, which showed that laser treatment caused selective photothermolysis of stage IV melanosome.

After subcellular selective photothermolysis, human melanocytes were shown through 3D tomography and high-voltage electron microscopy to be melanosome-free but alive, and looked as if they had undergone a "dendrectomy". Furthermore, levels of protease-activated receptor 2 (PAR-2), an essential substance mediating the transfer of melanin from melanocyte to daughter keratinocyte was decreased.

BIBLIOGRAPHY

1. Mun JY, Jeong SY, Kim JH, et al. A low fluence Q-switched Nd:YAG laser modifies the 3D structure of melanocyte and ultrastructure of melanosome by subcellular-selective photothermolysis. J Electron Microsc (Tokyo). 2011;60(1):11-8.

Types of Laser Toning

The three types of laser toning are:
1. Conventional laser toning
2. Dual pulse laser toning or photoacoustic toning pulse (PTP) mode
3. Dual laser toning.

1. Conventional Laser Toning

A collimated low-fluence 1,064 nm Q-switched neodymium-doped yttrium aluminum garnet (Nd:YAG) laser with a pulse width of less than 7 ns is applied using top-hat beam mode. Fluence used is between 1.2 J/cm^2 and 1.8 J/cm^2.

2. Dual Pulse Laser Toning or PTP Mode

Dual pulse at half fluence and 140 μs intervals is a unique laser emitting mode in which double pulses are delivered within one Q-switching cycle. Each pulse has relatively weak energy compared to the standard single Q-switched beam.

- This pulse-to-pulse mode can transfer higher peak energy (up to 60% more) to the target melanosome than a single beam because double beams are successively irradiated at very short intervals (100–130 μs) and their energy can be accumulated.
- As a result, the high-peak energy instantly increases the temperature of the chromophore, leading to pressure changes and vibration, which then effectively destroys the chromophore through the form of a shock wave (photoacoustic effect).
- There are some drawbacks to the laser toning as this delivers a subthreshold dose and therefore, this treatment modality requires many treatment sessions to obtain satisfactory clinical improvement.

3. Dual Laser Toning

It is a combination of conventional mode and genesis mode (300 μs pulse width). While Q-switched laser toning affects the epidermis and very superficial dermis, when this mode is combined with the micropulsed 300 μs mode of the Nd:YAG with multiple passes and pulse stacking, a deep-reaching tissue heating is additionally achieved.

The micropulsed mode delivers a controlled photothermal effect into the deep dermis, which is enhanced by the pulse stacking and induces the wound-healing process together with heat shock proteins, reduction of proinflammatory interleukin (IL)-8 and the induction of wound-healing mediator transforming growth factor (TGF)-β.

Active collagenesis results, followed by the remodeling process, so the dual toning technique not only improves the pigmentation, but also skin tone.

BIBLIOGRAPHY

1. Choi M, Choi JW, Lee SY, et al. Low-dose 1064-nm Q-switched Nd:YAG laser for the treatment of melasma. J Dermatolog Treat. 2010;21:224-8.
2. Kim BW, Lee MH, Chang SE, et al. Clinical efficacy of the dual-pulsed Q-switched neodymium:yttrium-aluminum-garnet laser: Comparison with conservative mode. J Cosmet Laser Ther. 2013;15(6):340-1.

3. Lee MC, Hu S, Chen MC, et al. Skin rejuvenation with 1,064-nm Q-switched Nd:YAG laser in Asian patients. Dermatol Surg. 2009;35(6):929-32.
4. Na SY, Cho S, Lee JH. Intense pulsed light and low-fluence Q-switched Nd:YAG laser treatment in melasma patients. Ann Dermatol. 2012;24:267-73.

Laser Machine Settings

The machine that this author (Dr Vivek Mehta) uses is the United State Food and Drug Administration (US FDA)-approved Tribeam from Jeisys Medical Inc. (Fig. 11.1).

Following are the features of Tribeam machine:
- High-peak power of 1.6 J in PTP mode and 1.2 J in top hat (TH) mode
- Pulse width of Q-switched mode is 5–10 ns and genesis mode is 300 µs
- Rich-PTP™ for subcellular selective photothermolysis
- Dual power supply
- True flat-top hat beam
- Comfortable user interface
- Handpiece in three types—(1) collimated (6-mm spot size), (2) zoom handpiece (1–10-mm spot size), and (3) fractional handpiece (81 dots in 5 by 5-mm spot size)
- Stable energy and system optimization.

Genesis or 300 µs mode settings used in dual laser toning has a fluence of 6.4–7.1 J/cm^2 using collimated handpiece (Fig. 11.2) and TH mode settings used in dual laser toning are 1.2–1.8 J/cm^2 using collimated handpiece (Fig. 11.3). In dual laser toning, single pass of genesis mode is followed by double pass of TH mode on whole face.

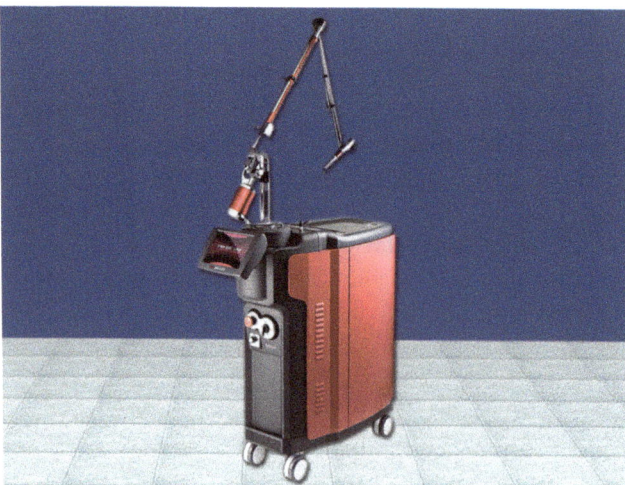

Fig. 11.1: Tribeam machine.

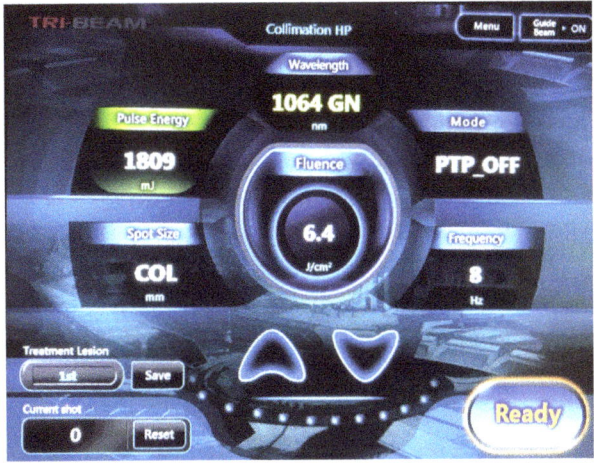

Fig. 11.2: Genesis (GN) mode settings 6.4–7.1 J/cm².

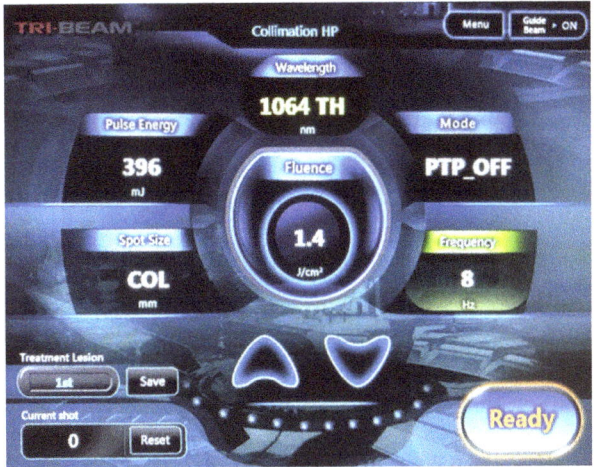

Fig. 11.3: Top hat (TH) mode settings 1.2–1.8 J/cm².

LASER TONING FOR REJUVENATION

Lee MC et al. evaluated the efficacy of Q-switched Nd:YAG laser (QSNYL) in improvement of pore size, sebaceous secretion, skin texture, and skin tone of Asian patients and found QSNYL as a safe and effective rejuvenation modality in Asian patients.

Dual laser toning has advantage, as it not only lightens the skin but also tones and refreshes the skin. It has advantage of improving the open pores alone though topical carbon suspension as photoenhancer improves the efficacy. In study of 25 female subjects by Chung HJ et al., authors were able to prove both subjectively and objectively that use of combination of micropulsed and Q switch modes of the ND:YAG was useful in reducing pore size and photoenhancer improved the efficacy.

Another benefit is subtle skin tightening that has been observed in patients who underwent dual laser toning as genesis or microsecond mode as microsecond mode can produce new collagen in papillary dermis. In study by Schmults CD et al., younger patients showed more collagen formation as compared with older patients with photodamage after microsecond mode. Photographic evaluation showed that those patients with pre-existing erythema showed improvement in erythema along with an associated improvement in skin quality.

BIBLIOGRAPHY

1. Chung H, Goo B, Lee H, et al. Enlarged pores treated with a combination of Q-switched and micropulsed 1064 nm Nd:YAG laser with and without topical carbon suspension: A simultaneous split-face trial. Laser Ther. 2011;20(3):181-8.
2. Kang HY, Kim JH, Goo BC. The dual toning technique for melasma treatment with the 1064 nm Nd:YAG laser: A preliminary study. Laser Ther. 2011;20(3):189-94.
3. Lee MC, Hu S, Chen MC, et al. Skin rejuvenation with 1,064-nm Q-switched Nd:YAG laser in Asian patients. Dermatol Surg. 2009;35(6):929-32.
4. Schmults CD, Phelps R, Goldberg DJ. Nonablative facial remodeling: Erythema reduction and histologic evidence of new collagen formation using a 300-microsecond 1064-nm Nd:YAG laser. Arch Dermatol. 2004;140(11):1373-6.

MELASMA

Melasma is a common pigmentation lesion of the skin and it predominantly affects women with darker complexions. Among various etiologic factors including genetic predisposition and hormonal influences, exposure to ultraviolet (UV) light plays key role in pathogenesis of melasma. Melasma is often refractory to chemical peels, topical therapy with hydroquinone, retinoids, azelaic, or kojic acids due to resistance to the agent and rapid recurrence of the lesion.

Several laser systems such as carbon dioxide or Q-switched alexandrite (755 nm) are reported to improve hyperpigmentation. However, high rates of postinflammatory hyperpigmentation and/or long-downtime rates were commonly observed, as well as melasma recurrence. Q-switched frequency doubled the Nd:YAG (1,064/532 nm) and the Q-switched ruby (694 nm) lasers failed in treating melasma, as they used the high-fluence modus.

Laser Toning in Melasma

Laser toning has been found to be safe and effective modality to treat melasma in Asian skin. Laser toning in melasma leads to fragmentation of melanin granules and dispersion into the cytoplasm without cellular destruction by repetitive laser energy with a subphotothermolytic fluence (<5 J/cm^2) over large spot size. The volume of the melanocytes, the number of melanosomes, and connecting melanocytic dendrites considerably reduced in epidermis after the laser treatment.

In a study by Sim JH et al., low-fluence 1,064-nm QSNYL has found to be safe and effective treatment of melasma in Asian Skin. In Indian Study by Kar HK et al., authors compared the therapeutic efficacy of low-fluence QSNYL, high-fluence QSNYL, and glycolic acid peel in melasma in three study groups of 25 patients each and found low-fluence QSNYL and glycolic acid peel in melasma to be effective options as compared to high-fluence QSNYL and other conventional methods for the treatment of melasma.

Omi T et al. investigated the efficacy of QSNYL toning for melasma, with a histopathological comparison with the Q-switched ruby laser. Authors concluded that QSNYL toning and Q-switched ruby laser treatment achieved good melasma pigment removal in the Japanese skin immediately after treatment, the former gave better short-term and long-term results for melasma in the Asian skin type III female patients.

We usually suggest low-fluence laser toning to treat melasma (1.0–1.6 J/cm^2), as it is safe and effective at low fluence (Figs. 11.4A to F). In study by Wattanakrai P et al., high incidence of hypopigmentation and rebound hyperpigmentation as author was using high fluence between 3.0 J/cm^2 and 3.8 J/cm^2.

Dual laser toning (combination of micropulsed and Q-switch modes of the ND:YAG) has also been used in melasma by Kang H et al. and it was found to be safe, effective, and well tolerated in Asian patients. The dual toning technique offers both bleaching and whitening of the skin together with skin rejuvenation to restore a youthful appearance and well-organized architecture to both the dermis and very importantly, the epidermis. The approach is effective, side effect free, well tolerated, and minimally invasive with practically no downtime for the patient. The efficacy may be improved even further with adjunctive techniques such as peels, creams, or light-emitting diode (LED) phototherapy.

Choi CP et al. assessed the effectiveness and safety of combination therapy using low-fluence QSNYL and long-pulse Nd:YAG laser (LPNYL) (dual toning) in patients with rebound melasma. It was found that dual toning may be a safe and effective salvage treatment for patients with aggravated melasma after previous treatment. LPNYL may stabilize melasma activity to prevent rebound hyperpigmentation via dermal remodeling.

In another study by Choi CP et al., the effectiveness and safety of combination therapy using low-fluence QSNYL and LPNYL (dual toning) was compared with low-fluence QSNY monotherapy (QS toning), in Asian melasma patients. Mottled hypopigmentation or rebound hyperpigmentation was significantly lower and the treatment efficacy was improved in the dual toning group compared with the QS toning group. Periorbital melasma showed distinctively high rates of adverse events in the QS toning group (23.9% vs 5.7%), which were significantly reduced in the dual toning group (2.9%).

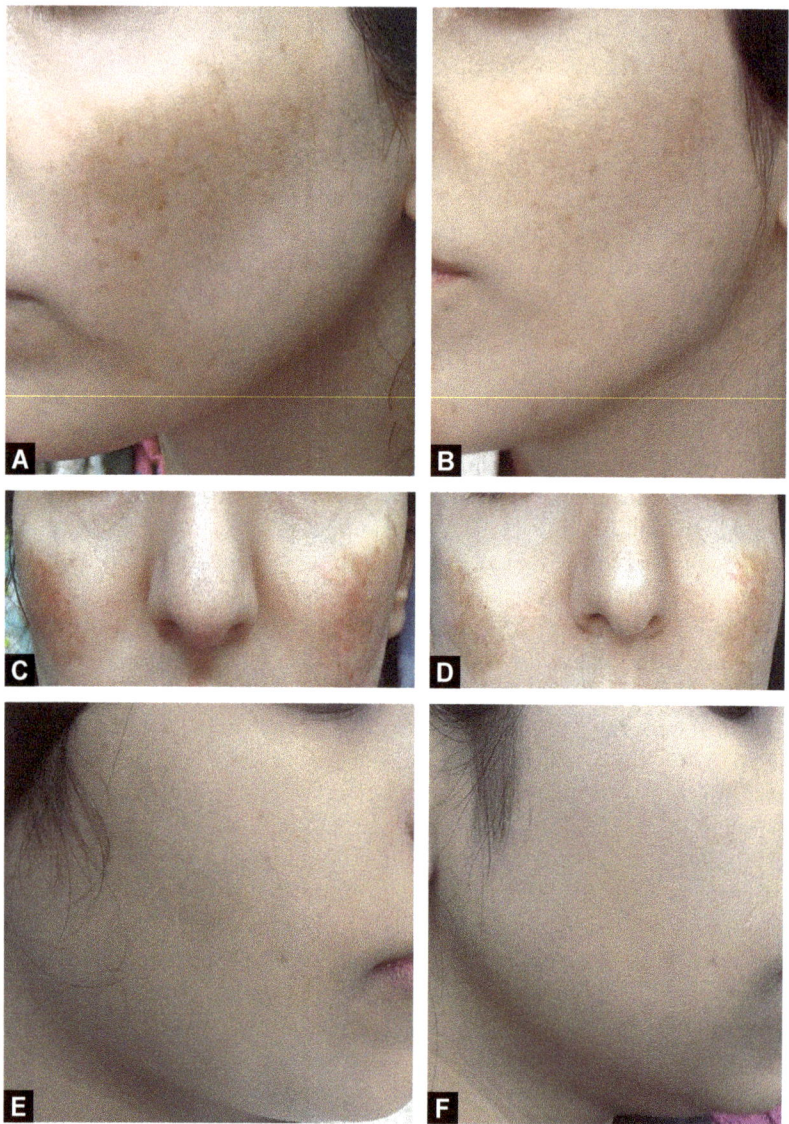

Figs. 11.4A to F: (A to D) Melasma with dual laser toning after 3 sessions. (E and F) Dual laser toning skin rejuvenation after 6 sessions.

Dual toning could represent a safe and effective treatment for Asian melasma patients, as it is associated with minimal adverse events and improved treatment efficacy compared with QS toning monotherapy.

BIBLIOGRAPHY

1. Choi CP, Yim SM, Seo SH, et al. Retreatment using a dual mode of low-fluence Q-switched and long-pulse Nd:YAG laser in patients with melasma aggravation after previous therapy. J Cosmet Laser Ther. 2015;17(3):129-34.

2. Choi CP, Yim SM, Seo SH, et al. Retrospective analysis of melasma treatment using a dual mode of low-fluence Q-switched and long-pulse Nd:YAG laser vs. low-fluence Q-switched Nd:YAG laser monotherapy. J Cosmet Laser Ther. 2015;17(1):2-8.
3. Gupta AK, Gover MD, Nouri K, et al. The treatment of melasma: A review of clinical trials. J Am Acad Dermatol. 2006;55:1048-65.
4. Hurley ME, Guevara IL, Gonzales RM, et al. Efficacy of glycolic acid peels in the treatment of melasma. Arch Dermatol. 2002;138:1578-82.
5. Kang HY, Kim JH, Goo BC. The dual toning technique for melasma treatment with the 1064 nm Nd: YAG laser: A preliminary study. Laser Ther. 2011;20(3): 189-94.
6. Kar HK, Gupta L, Chauhan A. A comparative study on efficacy of high and low fluence Q-switched Nd:YAG laser and glycolic acid peel in melasma. Indian J Dermatol Venereol Leprol. 2012;78(2):165-71.
7. Khunger N, Sarkar R, Jain RK. Tretinoin peels versus glycolic acid peels in the treatment of melasma in dark-skinned patients. Dermatol Surg. 2004;30:756-60.
8. Omi T, Yamashita R, Kawana S, et al. Low fluence Q-Switched Nd:YAG laser toning and Q-switched ruby laser in the treatment of melasma: A comparative split-face ultrastructural study. Laser Ther. 2012;21(1):15-21.
9. Sarkar R, Kaur C, Bhalla M, et al. The combination of glycolic acid peels with a topical regimen in the treatment of melasma in dark skinned patients: A comparative study. Dermatol Surg. 2002;28:828-32.
10. Sim JH, Park YL, Lee JS, et al. Treatment of melasma by low-fluence 1064 nm Q-switched Nd:YAG laser. J Dermatol Treat. 2014;25:212-7.

SIDE EFFECTS OF LASER TONING

Side effects of laser toning are divided into two subheads:
1. Those because of sublethal damage or stimulation of hyperactive melanocytes:
    - Recurrence or darkening of melasma and rebound hyperpigmentation
    - Unmasking of previously subclinical melasma
    - Leukoderma
    - Mottled hypopigmentation.
2. Others:
    - Physical urticaria
    - Acneiform eruption
    - Minute petechiae
    - Whitening of fine facial hair
    - Herpes simplex reactivation.

All the side effects because of sublethal damage or stimulation of hyperactive melanocytes can be prevented by using low fluence of QSNYL between 1 J/cm^2 and 1.8 J/cm^2.

Most dreaded complication, which is difficult to treat, is mottled hypopigmentation. In study by Jang YH et al. it was demonstrated that histological features of laser toning-induced hypopigmentation are characterized by almost destroyed melanosome pigments and preserved the number of melanocyte. Melanocytes survived but were functionally downregulated such that they did not produce fully matured melanosomes. Thus, early intervention aiming to restore melanocyte function would be required.

The cumulative dose of repetitive laser treatment may affect melanocyte function, resulting in the development of hypopigmentation.

Laser toning with Nd:YAG 1,064-nm laser for the treatment of melasma should be used with caution. Following are practical tips to avoid hypomelanosis:

- Laser toning treatment should be limited to not more than once every fortnight, and the total number of treatment sessions should be limited to prevent the development of hypopigmented macules.
- The appearance of hypopigmented macules should alert the physician to stop the laser treatment.
- Use low-energy parameters—personal experience.
- Use PTP or dual pulse toning mode.

As treatment of mottled hypopigmentation is difficult, it is better to prevent rather than to treat. Treatment with focused narrowband UV-B therapy has been used with some success.

BIBLIOGRAPHY

1. Jang YH, Park JY, Park YJ, et al. Changes in melanin and melanocytes in mottled hypopigmentation after low-fluence 1,064-nm Q-Switched Nd:YAG laser treatment for melasma. Ann Dermatol. 2015;27(3):340-2.
2. Sim JH, Park YL, Lee JS, et al. Treatment of melasma by low-fluence 1064 nm Q-switched Nd:YAG laser. J Dermatol Treat. 2014;25:212-7.

OTHER CLINICAL INDICATIONS FOR LASER TONING

- Skin rejuvenation—dual laser toning (Figs. 11.5A and B)
- Open pores—dual laser toning (Figs. 11.6A and B)
- Melasma—dual laser toning (Figs. 11.4 and 11.7)
- Seborrheic melanosis—dual laser toning (Figs. 11.8A and B)
- Acanthosis—dual laser toning (Figs. 11.9A and B)
- Lichen planus pigmentosus—conventional laser toning after disease is inactive
- Postinflammatory pigmentation—conventional laser toning (Figs. 11.10 and 11.11)
- Postburn scarring and pigmentation—dual laser toning (Figs. 11.12A to D)
- Telangiectatic rosacea—dual laser toning (Figs. 11.13A and B)
- Frictional melanosis (Figs. 11.14A and B).

CHAPTER 11: Laser Toning in Dermatology

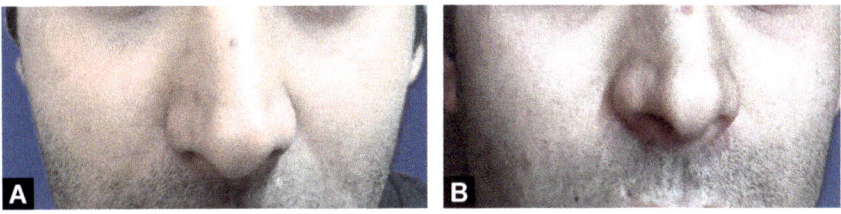

Figs. 11.5A and B: Skin rejuvenation dual laser toning after 6 sessions.

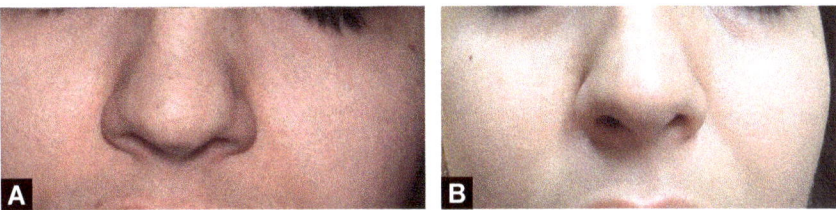

Figs. 11.6A and B: Open pores dual laser toning after 6 sessions.

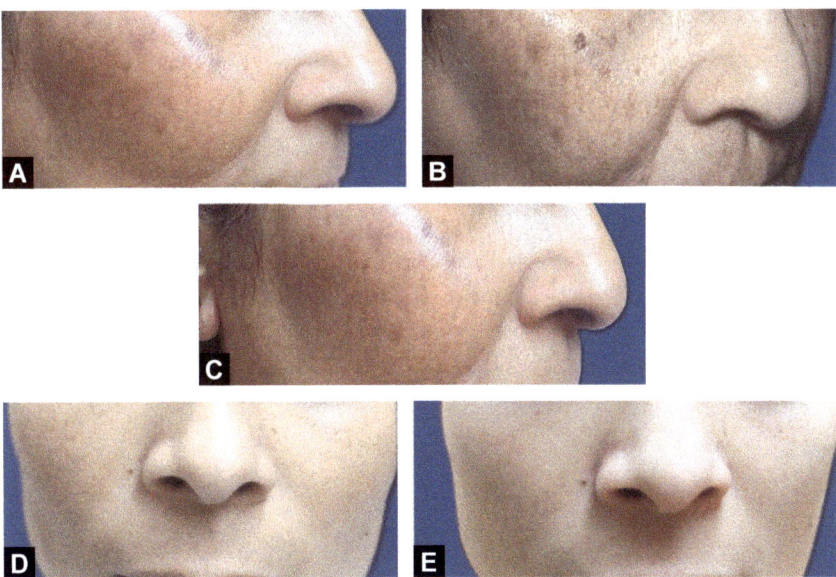

Figs. 11.7A to E: Melasma dual laser toning after 6 sessions.

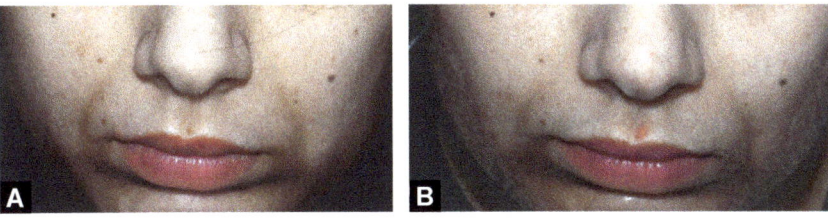

Figs. 11.8A and B: Seborrheic melanosis dual laser toning after 6 sessions.

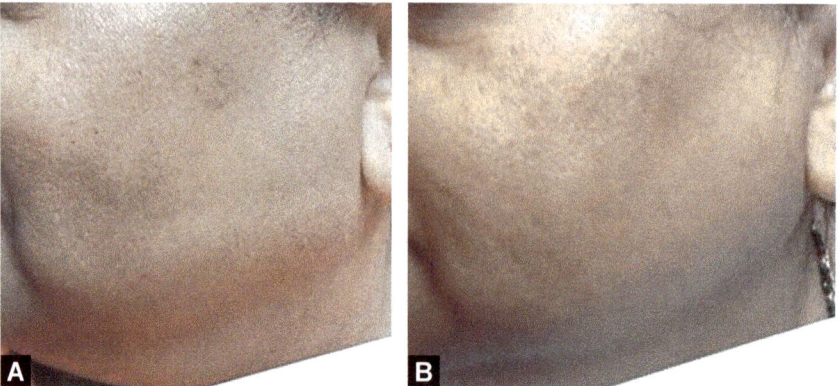

Figs. 11.9A and B: Acanthosis dual laser toning after 6 sessions.

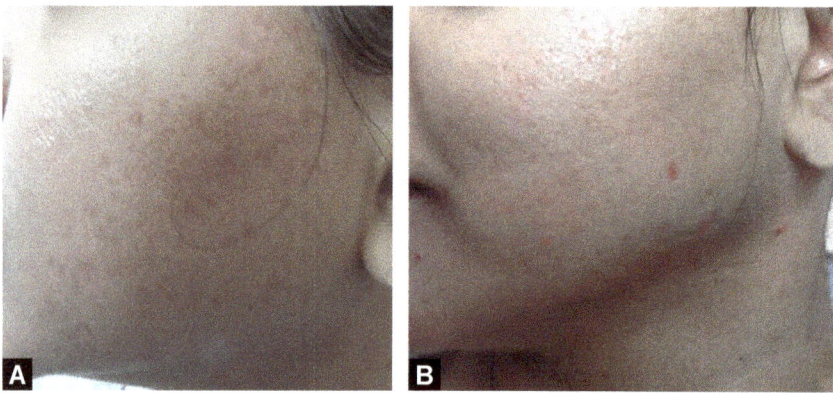

Figs. 11.10A and B: Post-acne hyperpigmented macules and rolling scars dual laser toning after 6 sessions.

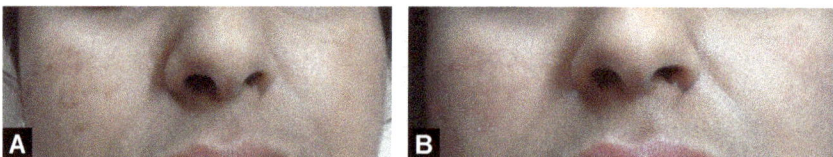

Figs. 11.11A and B: Post-acne hyperpigmented macules dual laser toning after 6 sessions.

CONCLUSION

Laser toning is one of the many means to treat melasma and in pigmented skin, it is not particularly successful or consistent. One problem is trying to translate extraneous data to Indian skin types. One common cause of side effects including leukoderma is the frequency of sessions and a session

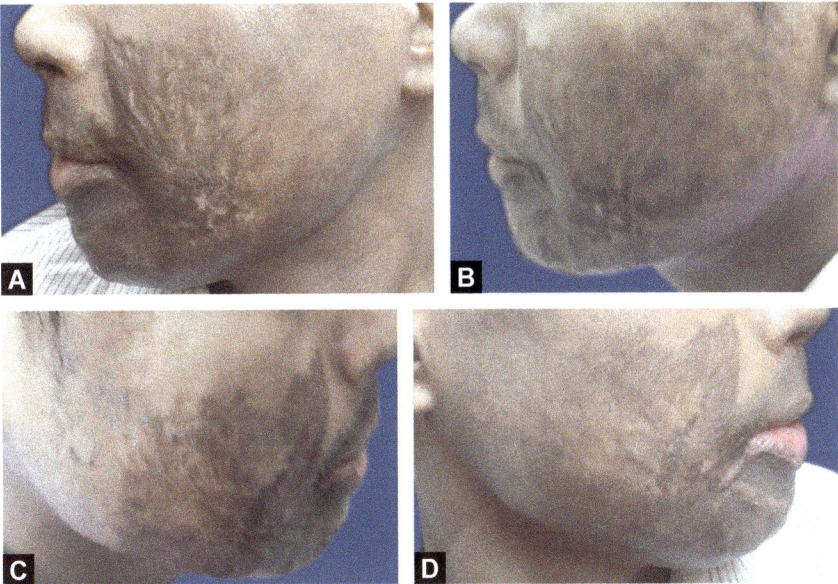

Figs. 11.12A to D: Post-burn scarring and hyperpigmentation dual laser toning after 6 sessions.

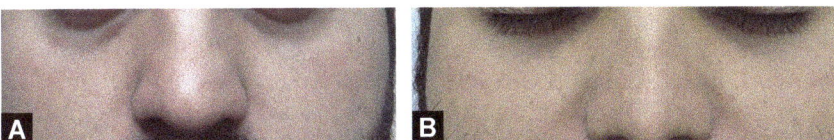

Figs. 11.13A and B: Rosacea dual laser toning after 6 sessions.

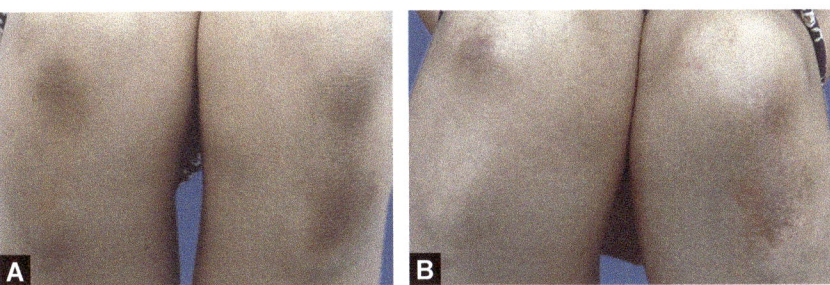

Figs. 11.14A and B: Frictional melanosis dual laser toning after 5 sessions.

once in 2 weeks or once a month is better than three times a week. The loss of pigment is prolonged and can be a source of concern (Cahn NP). The leukoderma can be of 2 types, type 1 leukoderma, which seems to be related to the cumulative laser energy delivered, and type 2 leukoderma, which may be due to direct phototoxicity (Sugawara J).

A large study (Tian B) using the Revlite system, reported that 56.3% had a fair improvement, 22.3% had good improvement and only 5.1% had excellent improvement. Though the pico Alex has also been used with low power settings, there is overwhelming data that shows that this technique does not lead to consistent results. This is evidenced by a study (Kim JH) using the zebrafish model, which clearly demonstrated that laser toning does not prevent melanosome regeneration. Though it is believed that dual toning is a good option for treating melasma, if the correct parameters and machine are employed, it is my (Dr Kabir Sardana) concerted view that, apart from selective results exhibited in dedicated and focused conference talks, laser toning is an ill-advised concept in Indian and other richly pigmented skin types, with side effects that are commonly seen but rarely reported.

BIBLIOGRAPHY

1. Chan NP, Ho SG, Shek SY, et al. A case series of facial depigmentation associated with low fluence Q-swithced 1,064nm Nd:YAG laser for skin rejuvenation and melasma. Lasers Surg Med. 2010;42(8):712-9.
2. Kim DH, Kim JH, Lee SG, et al. Recovery of pigmentation following selective photothermolysis in adult zebrafish skin: Clinical implications for laser toning treatment of melasma. J Cosmet Laser Ther. 2012;14(6):277-85.
3. Saluja R. Evaluation of the safety and efficacy of a low fluence, picopulsed, alexandrite laser in a pico-toning technique with a diffractive lens optic for the treatment of photodamage and textural improvement in "Off the Face" Applications. J Drugs Dermatol. 2016;15(11):1398-401.
4. Sugawara J, Kou S, Kou S, et al. Influence of the frequency of laser toning for melasma on occurrence of leukoderma and its early detection by ultraviolet imaging. Lasers Surg Med. 2015;47(2):161-7.
5. Tian B. Laser toning for melasma: A single-centre experience with 38 970 cases. J Cosmet Laser Ther. 2017;19(3):140-2.

Section 2
Therapeutic Indications

CHAPTER 12

Clinical Indications

Shilpa Garg, Kabir Sardana, Niteen V Dhepe, Ashraf Badawi, Aastha Gupta,
Ananta Khurana, Sidharth Tandon, Khushbu Goel, Red Alinsod,
Avitus John Raakesh Prasad, Ajay Deshpande, Surabhi Sinha

The application of lasers is an intrinsically more endearing and practical aspect of lasers and energy devices. Here we detail the various indications with a different approach of various clinicians.

While reading the same, the reader is encouraged to first understand the logic behind the use and then to assimilate the settings. This is as the settings are highly device dependent.

Various parts of this section have been contributed by numerous contributors and the sequence of names does not do justice to their contributions.

Dr Shilpa Garg and Dr Niteen V Dhepe have co-written the section on Acne Scars.

The sections on Scars and Body Shaping again have been contributed by two doctors, from Pune, Dr Niteen V Dhepe and Dr Ajay Deshpande.

Similarly the various clinical disorders have a host of contributors with Dr Red Alinsod contributing on Vulval Rejuvenation.

The vascular section has been co-written by Dr Ajay Deshpande and Dr Avitus.

The team at RML Hospital, Dr Ananta Khurana, Dr Surabhi Sinha, Dr Aastha Gupta, and Dr Sidharth Tandon have filled in the rest. Dr Khushbu, a former colleague at MAMC has contributed on Xanthelasma.

Thus, this section is like the string of pearls, with the pearls being the contributor and my role was to put them together like the invisible thread.

I, for one, am a conventional ablative, fractional, intense pulsed light (IPL) and pigment laser person and therein lies the "men and women behind the machines" that are discussed in the following sections.

12A. ACNE SCARS

Shilpa Garg, Kabir Sardana, Niteen V Dhepe

INTRODUCTION

There are numerous ways to classify acne scars and the heterogeneity in their classification makes clinical trial comparisons difficult.

A simple way of classifying scars is to divide them into hypertrophic and atrophic. By far the commoner is the atrophic scar, wherein there is loss or damage of soft tissue (Fig. 12.1). These acne scars result from collagen destruction in the dermis and soft tissue atrophy. Scar contraction results in the indentation of the skin. Atrophic acne scars are often erythematous initially and can become hypopigmented or hyperpigmented with time. In 2001, Jacob et al. proposed a classification of atrophic acne scars into three types: ice pick, rolling, and boxcar scars. Ice pick scars are narrow (less than 2 mm), V-shaped epithelial tracts that extend deep into the dermis. Rolling scars are wider (4-5 mm) and are tethered to the subcutaneous tissue, resulting in an undulating appearance. Boxcar scars are sharply delineated round or oval depressions that can be shallow or deep and range in diameters of 1.5-4 mm. There is another variety of atrophic acne scars known as the papular scars. Papular scars are 3-4 mm sized soft elevated skin colored papules, which are mostly present on the chin, nose, and back. These are

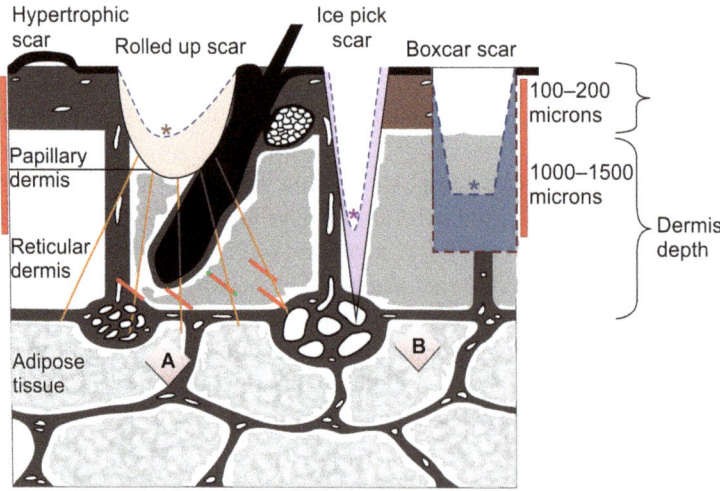

* Post laser depiction of scar, red line indicated depth of laser beam

Fig. 12.1: An overview of acne scars and the effect of fractional lasers. (A) Rolling scars respond due to snapping of dermal bands; (B) Deep ice pick scars and boxcar scars need collagen remodeling to "fill" the tissue defect which may *not completely* eliminate the scars.

often mistakenly diagnosed as acne. However, stretching the skin of the affected area makes the papules flat. Histologically dermal fibrosis is seen in these scars.

Goodman and Baron proposed a new qualitative grading system for acne scarring with suggested therapies for each scar type (Tables 12.1 and 12.2). This grading system has four levels of acne scarring: (1) macular, (2) mild, (3) moderate, and (4) severe.

The subdivisions for level 1 macular disease include erythematous, hypopigmented or hyperpigmented. Grades 2 to 4, mild to severe disease, are classified as being atrophic or hypertrophic. Grade 3, moderate acne scars can be *flattened* by manually stretching the skin, and include *rolling or shallow boxcar scars*. Grade 4 scars are *not distensible* and include—ice pick, *deep boxcar*, and *significant hypertrophic*, and keloid acne scars.

For practical purposes, a simple classification is based on the morphology, i.e. rolling, boxcar, ice pick, and hypertrophic scars is ideal as this enables a simple interventional protocol as given in Table 12.2. We will give an overview of the medical and surgical aspects of the treatment of scars. Then we will focus on 3 approaches to treatment, the 3-step approach using frcational lasers, the minimally invasive approach (Dr Shilpa Garg) and the 5-step approach by Dr Niteen Dhepe.

Medical Therapy for Acne Scars

- *Topical retinoids* are recommended as part of a combination treatment for inflammatory acne disease. Topical retinoids stimulate collagen formation, increase dermal collagen synthesis, and improve elastic fibers. Use of a 0.05% topical tretinoin for 4 months was reported to improve the appearance of facial ice pick scars.

Table 12.1: Classification of acne scars (Goodman).

Grade	Level of disease	Characteristic
1	Macular	Erythematous, hyperpigmented or hypopigmented flat marks visible to patient or observe at any distance
2	Mild	Mild atrophy or hypertrophy that may not be obvious at social distances of 50 cm or more, and may be covered adequately by make-up or the normal shadow of shaved beard hair in men or normal body hair if extrafacial
3	Moderate	Moderate atrophic or hypertrophic scarring that is obvious at social distances of 50 cm or more, and is not covered easily by make-up or the normal shadow of shaved beard hair in men or body hair if extrafacial, but is still able to be flattened by manual stretching of the skin (if atrophic)
4	Severe	Severe atrophic or hypertrophic scarring that is obvious at social distances greater than 50 cm, and is not covered easily by make-up or the normal shadow of shaved beard hair in men or body hair if extrafacial and is not able to be flattened by manual stretching of the skin.

Table 12.2: A practical intervention based on morphological type of scars (Goodman GJ, 2007).

Scar	Treatment modality
Ice pick scars	Punch excision, CROSS lasers Ablative and nonablative fractional lasers are largely ineffective against ice pick scars
Boxcar scars	
(i) Shallow boxcar scars	• Dermabrasion, subcision, dermaroller lasers • Fractional lasers are useful

(ii) Deep boxcar scars	• With regular base
	  – Punch floatation if diameter <3.5 mm, elliptical excision and suturing if diameter >3.5 mm
	• With irregular base
	  – Punch excision with primary closure or graft replacement if diameter <3.5 mm
	  – Elliptical excision and suturing if diameter >3.5 mm
	• Fractional lasers
	  – The volumizing effect is not sufficient for most deep scars

Rolling scars	• Subcision, dermal fillers • Fractional lasers – They consistently respond and are an ideal indication for this technology
Papular scar (Lee SJ, 2017)	Pinhole method using 2,940 nm erbium: YAG laser
Hypertrophic scars	Intralesional steroid, cryosurgery

(CROSS: chemical reconstruction of skin scars; YAG: yttrium-aluminum-garnet)

    Other agents include retinoic acid, hydroquinone, azelaic acid, and kojic acid useful for decreasing postinflammatory hyperpigmentation (PIH).
- Options for treatment of hypertrophic and keloid scars include the glucocorticoids (triamcinolone, hydrocortisone, methylprednisolone, and dexamethasone).
    i. Serial intralesional injections spaced 4-6 weeks apart can result in flattening and softening of hypertrophic and keloid scars. Injection of cystic, inflammatory acne lesions with steroids may help to prevent scarring by decreasing the inflammatory response.
    ii. *5-fluorouracil (5-FU)* has been shown to inhibit wound healing. This compound has an inhibitory effect on human fibroblast by inhibiting proliferation and myofibroblast differentiation. Fluorouracil is usually used at a concentration of 50 mg/mL with a total dose between 50 mg and 150 mg per session. Fluorouracil can be used alone or mixed at a ratio of 80:20 with a low-strength steroid. In a 2002 study by Gupta and Kalra, more than 50% of patients showed significant flattening of keloids as a result of intralesional injections with 5-FU.

iii. Additionally, *bleomycin* has been shown to flatten hypertrophic scars by inhibiting collagen synthesis through its cytotoxic effects on dividing fibroblasts. We use a combination of bleomycin (15 U/mL) with a ratio of 3:7 with triamcinolone acetonide once in 3 weeks with heartening results in difficult cases.
iv. Silicone gel sheeting is recommended as a safe and effective management option for keloid and hypertrophic scars. Several studies report that silicone gels and silicone sheets are equal inefficacy in improvement of scar redness, elevation, pain, and pruritus. Research suggests that the possible mechanism of action of silicone products is not only a result of occlusion but also the magnitude of the occlusion may be an important component in the mechanism of action of silicone. In addition, the decrease in transepidermal water loss and resulting increase in hydration from the occlusion provided by the silicone product may modulate the signaling cascade initiated by the epidermis that stimulates the collagen production by dermal fibroblasts. The use of silicone gels may be better accepted by patients than the silicone sheets due to the decreased visibility of the applied gel on the scar (Mustoe TA).

Surgical and Procedural Measures

A multitude of diverse methods have been tried and some are temporary like fillers and botox, others rarely treat the scar like chemical peels and some are not as useful as claimed, like chemical reconstruction of skin scars (CROSS). In fact we have seen cases of badly done CROSS with PIH that lasts for months and accentuated the scars. The Table 12.2 delineates a scar-specific protocol and three different protocols are given here. Fundamentally surgical interventions are more useful, with peeling being used to primarily even out the skin.

Depressed scars or atrophic scars are divided in *distensible scars*, which disappear when the skin is stretched, and *nondistensible scars*, which do not disappear when the skin is stretched. In distensible scars, fibrous attachments tether the epidermis and dermis to the subcutis.

- *Undulated scars or rolling scars* are distensible and show good responses to the filler techniques.
- *Distensible retraction scars* respond better with subcision before filler techniques.
- *Nondistensible scars* normally accumulate make-up and sunscreen lotion in the depressed area and are divided into superficial scars, ice pick scars, and deep scars. Superficial scars are shallow depressions and should be treated with ablative techniques. Ice pick scars are small but deep, and normally respond well with complementary techniques like punch elevation, and punch grafting. Deep scars (crater-like) can be treated with block excision.

Fractional Lasers in Acne Scars (Three-step Approach)

Fractional lasers are used for non-distensible superficial scars or to supplement the localized scar techniques used. Except for ice pick other atrophic scars respond to lasers (Sardana K) (Figs. 12.2A to E). The standard approach is a *3-stage approach*. Though two different approaches used are given here (Shilpa Garg and Niteen Dhepe), this 3-step approach tackles all the scars seen in clinical practice (Kadunc BV et al., Fulton JE et al.).

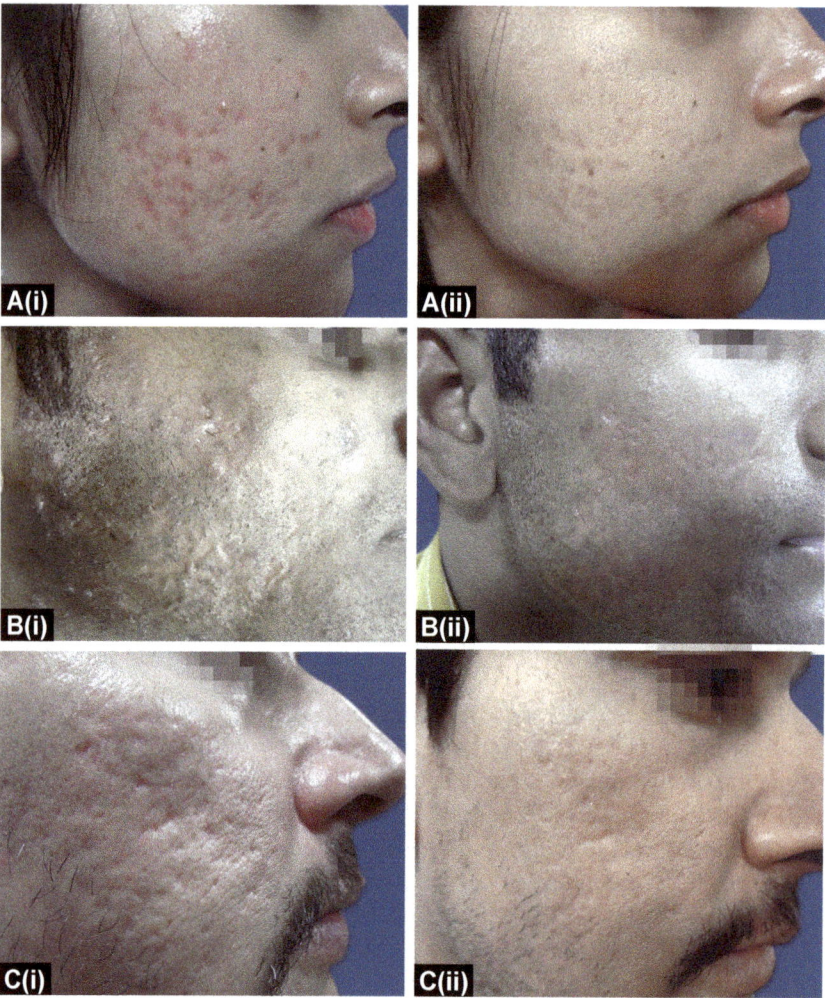

Fig. 12.2A to C: A(i) Mild scar with erythematous shallow boxcar scars. A(ii) After treatment with Er:Glass (Lux Palomar) 70 mJ; 4 passes; 5 sessions marked improvement. B(i) The images depict boxcar and hypertrophic scar. B(ii) Intralesional corticosteroids (ILC) followed by Er:YAG (Fr) Dermablate, Ascepelion. For nondistensible scars like this ILC is a useful adjunct. C(i) A patient with a mixture of rolling and superficial boxcar scars (distensible). C(ii) This case is amenable to treatment by laser monotherapy. Here we treated using the Fr Er:YAG (Dermablate) with marked improvement.

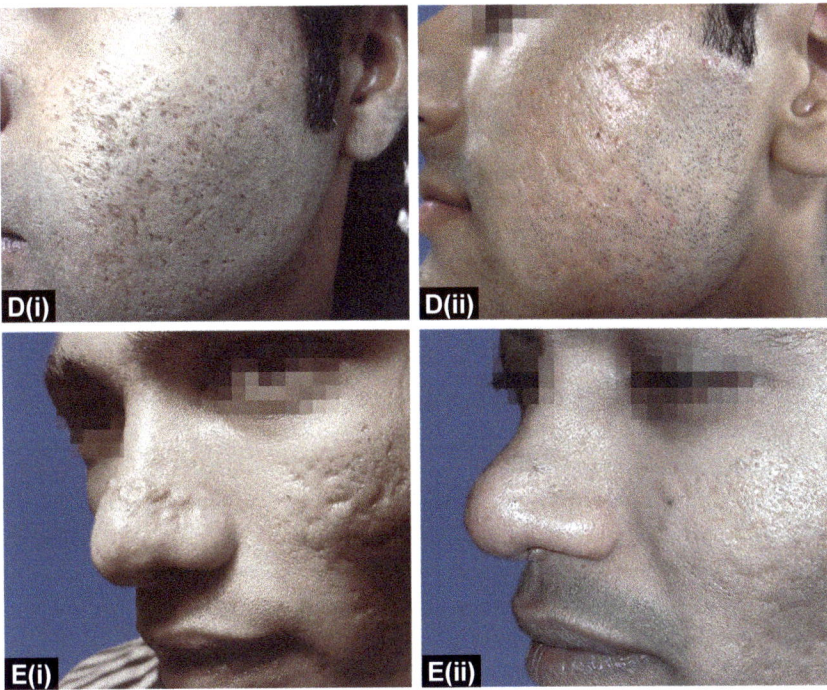

Figs. 12.2D and E: D(i) A patient with deep boxcar and ice pick scars. These are largely nondistensible scars. D(ii) Here aggressive settings with variation in the aspect ratio enabled heartening results. E(i) and E(ii) Papular scars, treated by the pinhole technique, using the ablative CO_2 laser followed by the fractional CO_2 laser. (*Courtesy:* Dr Nina Madnani, Mumbai).

1. *Step 1*: Therapy for individual scars (Box 12.1). Several modalities may be needed in tune with the type of scar and several sessions may be necessary. Papular scars can also be managed with the fractional laser (Fig. 12.2E).
2. *Step 2*: Fractional lasers for the whole face and nondistensible scars (Figs. 12.2A to D).
3. *Step 3*: Fillers: Used to complement the techniques in stages I and II, and to correct distensible scars Hyaluronic acid injections are recommended to treat superficial (dermal) tissue loss and microlipoinjections or polylactic acid injections to treat subcutaneous tissue.

Minimally Invasive Approach for Treatment of Atrophic Acne Scars

Three important aspects in the management of atrophic acne scars are:
1. Combining the right procedures that would broadly address all types of scars.

Box 12.1: Therapy for individual scars.

Papular scars, bridge scars	Tangential excision/scissor excision
Distensible scars	Subcision
Keloidal scar	Intralesional (steroids, bleomycin, fluorouracil) injection Excision
Ice pick scars*	Deep scars smaller than 3 mm size (punch elevation) pigmented deep scars smaller than 3 mm (punch grafting)

*CROSS technique essentially creates a scar within a scar, but the TCA can cause marked PIH which becomes an issue in our skin type. Hence, we do not favor its use.
(CROSS: chemical reconstruction of skin scars; TCA: trichloroacetic acid; PIH: post-inflammatory hyperpigmentation)

2. Ideal time interval between these procedures so as to maximize the results and minimize the side effects.
3. Choosing procedures that cause minimal epidermal damage or abrasion so as to prevent or minimize postinflammatory dyspigmentation.

Acne scars are best addressed with combination of procedures, which would address the following aspects of the scar:
1. *Releasing* the scars from their underlying adhesions.
2. Promoting *collagen synthesis* to correct volume loss.
3. Addressing the *surface and textural damage* seen with scarring.

The author (Shilpa Garg) prefers to combine minimally invasive procedures to address scars especially in Indian skin type, as it is melanin-rich and tends to heal with hyperpigmentation after any epidermal damage which may not be easy to address. Thus, it is important to choose procedures that cause minimal epidermal damage. Since in majority of the patients we see a mix of almost all types of scars (ice pick, rolling, and boxcar), the combination of procedures used should be able to address all types of scars to a large extend.

We (Garg S and Baveja S, 2014) have reported a series of 50 patients with atrophic acne scars, which were treated with combination therapy of subcision, dermaroller, and chemical peel with good results in patients with severe scars, minimum downtime and side effects (Figs. 12.3 to 12.5). I recommend adding platelet-rich plasma (PRP) to this combination to further increase the improvement in acne scars.

Protocol

1. *Priming*: In this method, the skin of the patient is primed with tretinoin cream 0.05% along with sun protection 15 days prior to starting the treatment.
   - Skin is primed using tretinoin cream 0.05% at night along with sunscreen for 2 weeks prior to starting the procedure.

CHAPTER 12: Clinical Indications **523**

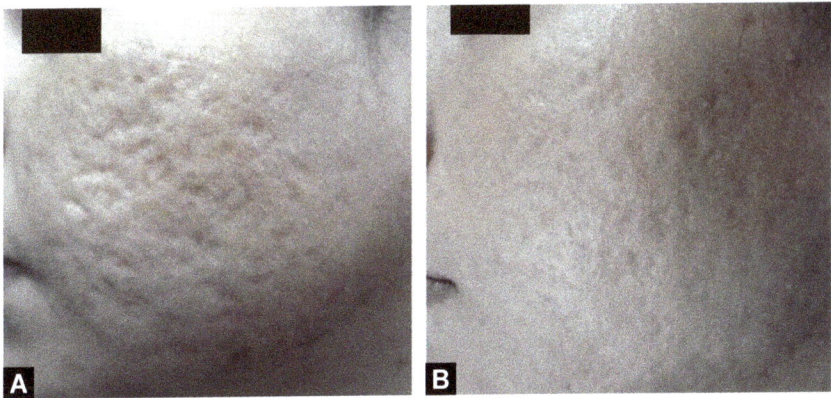

Figs. 12.3A and B: Improvement in acne scar from Grade 4 to Grade 2 (Goodman Baron Scale) after combination therapy (subcision, dermaroller, and trichloroacetic acid peel).

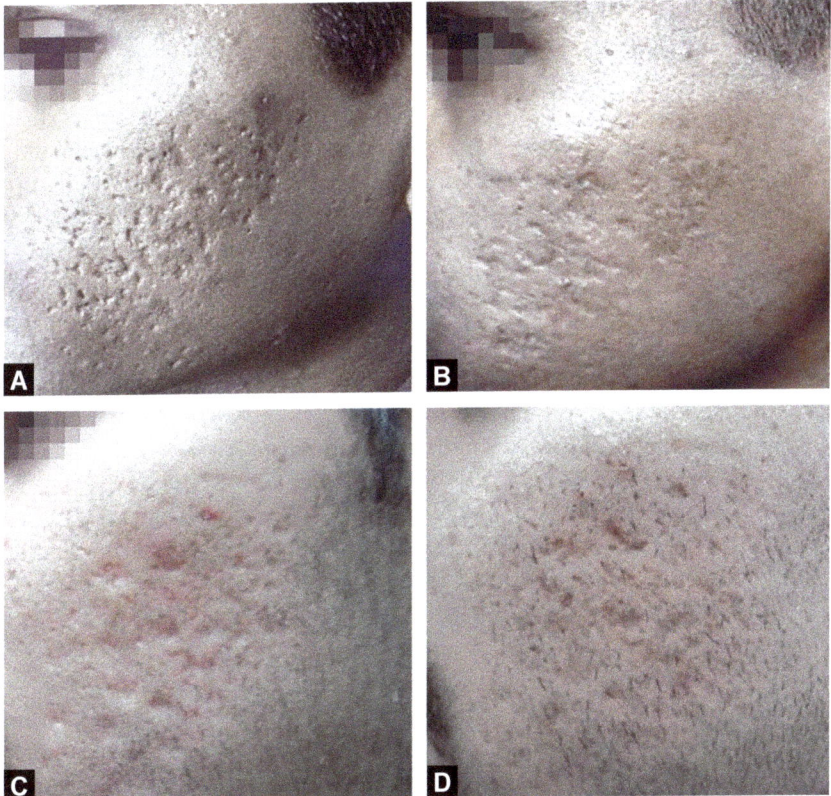

Figs. 12.4A to D: Improvement in acne scar from Grade 4 to Grade 3 (Goodman Baron Scale) after combination therapy (subcision, dermaroller, and trichloroacetic acid peel).

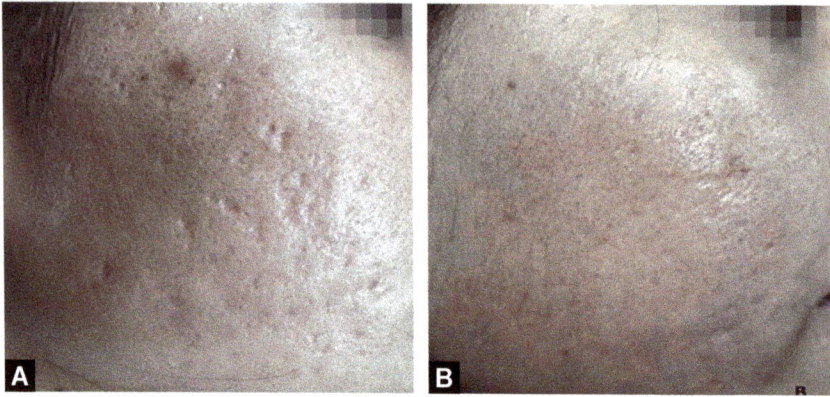

Figs. 12.5A and B: Improvement in acne scar from Grade 3 to Grade 2 (Goodman Baron Scale) after combination therapy (subcision, dermaroller, and trichloroacetic acid peel).

- Tretinoin cream is discontinued 5 days before each procedure (dermaroller-PRP and peel) and till 4 days post dermaroller-PRP therapy, 4 days after trichloroacetic acid (TCA) peel, and till 2 days after glycolic acid (GCA) peel.
- Also patient is instructed to avoid facial waxing, threading, facials, abrasive face wash, and hair dyes 7 days before and after procedure.

2. *First visit*: In the first visit, subcision is done under topical anesthesia using a 23–24 gauge needle. [Avoid *subcision* on scars on forehead (chances of hematoma formation is more) and nose (not very easy area to subcise)].
   - At the beginning of treatment, subcision of scars is done under topical anesthesia.
   - Patient is asked to wash his face with soap and water. A thick layer of eutectic mixture of lidocaine and prilocaine is applied on the affected area of cheeks under occlusion for 75 minutes. The anesthetic cream is removed with a gauze and area is cleaned with saline soaked gauze.
   - Choose a fine needle (23G or 24G needle) for subcision as it minimizes the risk of hematoma formation. If the number of scars is less, then each can be subcised individually. However, if the number of scars are more, then one entry point can be used for subcising a bunch of scars which can be accessed with a single entry point (Figs. 12.6 to 12.10).
   - Since the most common complication seen after subcision is hematoma formation, it is very important to apply pressure for at least 15 minutes post subcision and thereafter apply ice pack for another 5 minutes in order to reduce the risk of hematoma formation, which takes weeks to resolve. Antibiotic cream is applied post subcision.

3. *Second day*: If the patient does *not experience any side effects* from subcision, then the following day after subcision, dermaroller (1.5 mm size

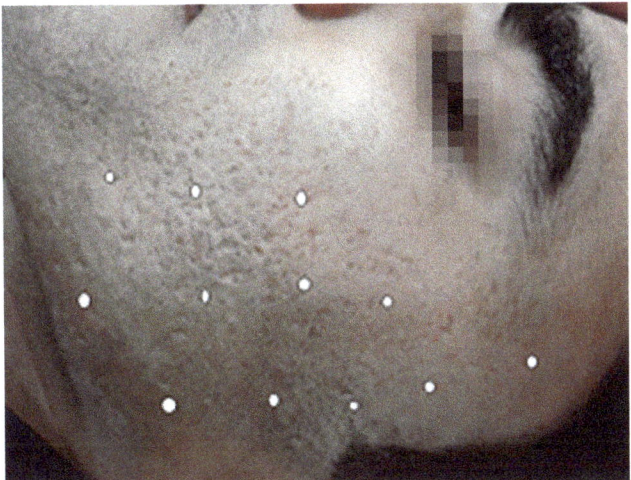

Fig. 12.6: Points of entry of needle to cover the entire area affected by acne scars.

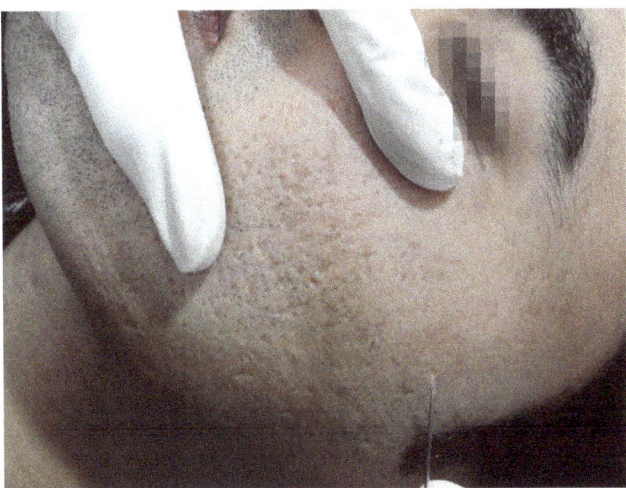

Fig. 12.7: Skin should be stretched and inferior orbital margin should be guarded with finger in order to avoid injury. Fine needle (23 G) is used for subcision.

needles) along with PRP therapy is performed. The next day *microneedling* is done with dermaroller (1.5 mm size needles). Tretinoin cream 0.05% is applied just before doing dermaroller and immediately after the dermaroller and massaged and kept for 5–10 minutes.

In the same sitting, PRP is also injected in the area of scarring.

- After washing the face with soap and water, skin is anesthetized by application of thick layer of eutectic mixture of lidocaine and prilocaine kept

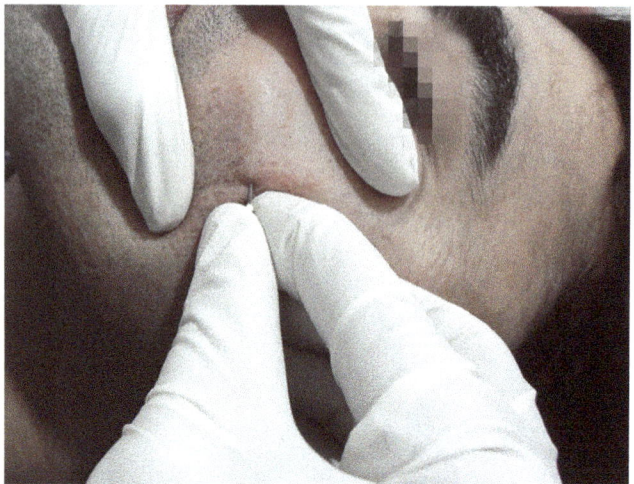
Fig. 12.8: After entering, the needle is slightly lifted up to see its movements.

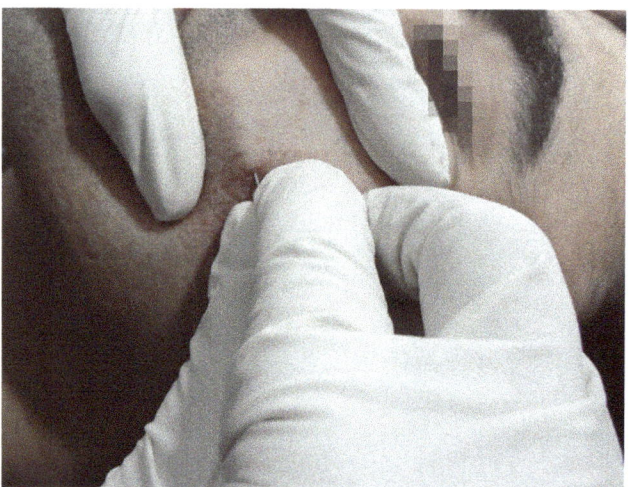
Fig. 12.9: The needle is directed toward the left side to cover the scars in that area.

under occlusion for 75 minutes. This is removed with normal saline soaked gauze and a very thin layer of tretinoin cream 0.05% is applied on the scars.
- Skin is stretched well and dermaroller is rolled in vertical, horizontal, and diagonal directions in the affected area of scars (on cheeks, forehead, nose, and chin) until appearance of fine, uniform, pinpoint bleeding is seen which is the end point of treatment with dermaroller (Fig. 12.11). Then the area is wiped with saline soaked gauze and pressure is applied for 1 minute to stop the bleeding.

CHAPTER 12: Clinical Indications 527

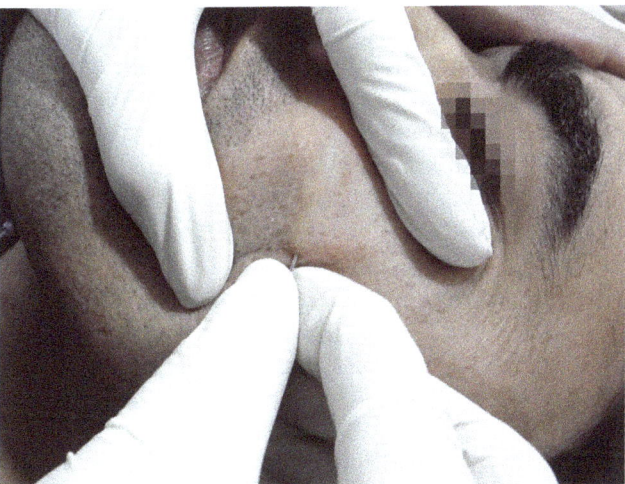

Fig. 12.10: And then toward the right side to cover the scars in that area.

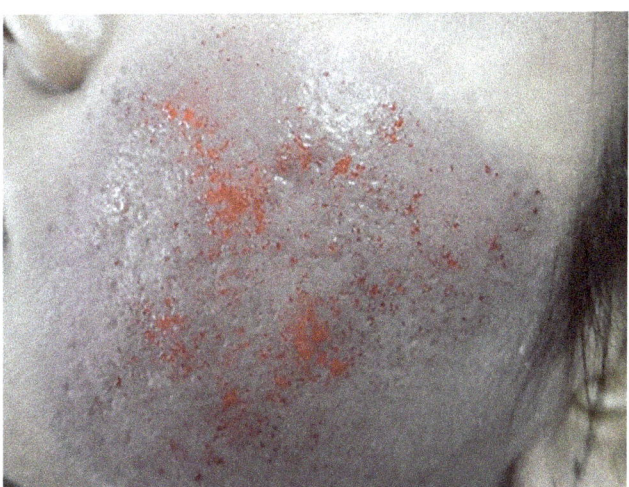

Fig. 12.11: Pinpoint uniform fine bleeding is the end point of treatment with dermaroller.

- A very thin layer of tretinoin cream 0.05% is applied again on the area of scars where dermaroller was done, gently massaged into the skin, and left for 5 minutes.
- After 5 minutes tretinoin cream is wiped away with saline soaked gauze and PRP is injected in the scars with approximately 0.1 mL of plasma injected at each point at a distance of 0.5 cm apart to cover the entire area of scars. After the PRP is injected in the scars, platelet poor plasma is applied over the scars and gently massaged into the skin for 3 minutes in order to absorb it. Apply firm pressure for 1 minute after injection of PRP in order to avoid the pinpoint bruising at the injection site.

- Post-procedure, ice packs are kept for 10 minutes on the treated area to reduce the redness and edema seen after dermaroller and PRP therapy.
- After this procedure, patient is instructed to apply mometasone furoate cream 0.1% twice daily for 2–4 days (till erythema exists) along with sunscreen, after which sunscreen is continued and tretinoin cream 0.05% is restarted at night. Patient discontinues tretinoin cream application 5 days prior to peeling which is scheduled after 2 weeks of dermaroller-PRP session.

4. *Day 15*: After 15 days, peeling of the whole face is done with superficial peel (either 35% to 50% GCA or 15% TCA).

   After washing the face with soap and water, skin is degreased using acetone only if it is oily. Peeling is done on full face while stretching the skin using either 15% TCA peel or 35–50% GCA peel.

   Appearance of speckled white frost is the end point of 15% TCA peel (Fig. 12.12) and 3–5 minutes is the end point for GCA peel. GCA peel needs to be neutralized with sodium bicarbonate solution. No neutralization is required post-TCA peel. Post-peeling, face is splashed with cool water and ice pack applied for 3–5 minutes to cool the skin off to minimize chances of PIH.

   Patient is instructed to apply mometasone furoate cream 0.1% only once after GCA peel and for twice a day for 3–4 days after TCA peel along with sunscreen, after which sunscreen is continued and tretinoin cream 0.05% is restarted at night.

5. Thereafter, dermaroller-PRP and peel are repeated alternately after every 2 weeks of each other for a total of six sessions of each. Sunscreen and tretinoin cream 0.05% are continued for 1–2 years after completing the procedures in order to continue resurfacing the scars.

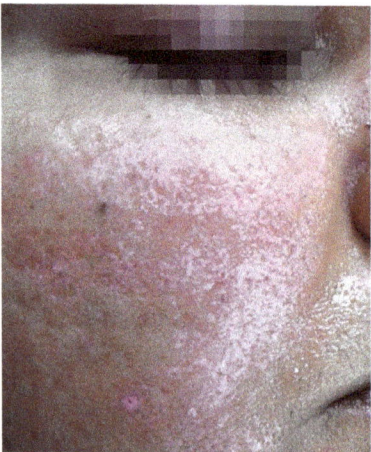

Fig. 12.12: Presence of speckled white frost (net-like pattern) is the end point of treatment with 15% trichloroacetic acid peel.

The rationale of this combination is as follows:
- *Subcision as the first step to treatment*: This should be the first step as it releases the scar from their underlying attachments so that they can be resurfaced. Also using a fine needle (23–24 gauge) minimizes the complication of hematoma formation and pain.
- *Dermaroller and PRP therapy*: Helps in collagen induction and resurfacing the scars. The holes created by dermaroller are used to introduce tretinoin cream to enhance its penetration.
- *Tretinoin cream*: Helps in collagen remodeling and enhances the effect of superficial peel by exfoliating the stratum corneum.
- *Chemical peel*: Helps to improve textural irregularity and hyperpigmentation seen in scars and also helps to resurface the scars.

FIVE-STEP APPROACH TO TREATING ACNE SCARS

This is an approach where except for subcision, most of the scar remodeling procedures are performed by a fractional CO_2 laser. This enables use of a single modality to tackle acne scars, but would be useful for atrophic scars and not for hypertrophic scars (Figs. 12.13A and B), and would be costly and device dependent.

CONCLUSION

Though lasers are used, it has been the recurring experience that they are good for superficial boxcar and rolling scars and not always for ice pick scars. Any procedure that causes PIH, including CROSS should be avoided in our skin. The reader may adopt two methods; one is detailed in Box 12.1 and encapsulates the **3-step approach**. Another approach is the **five-step approach**.

A non-device approach is also elucidated where the combination of subcision, dermaroller, and peeling with priming, helps to target therapy

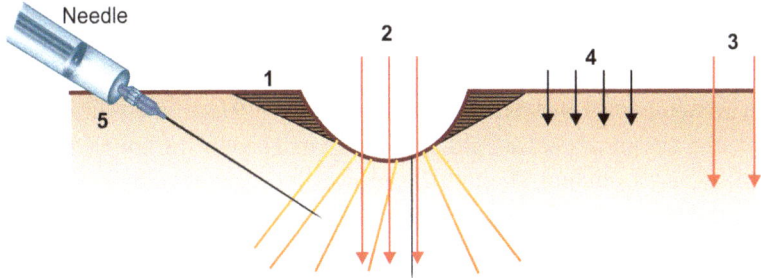

Fig. 12.13A: Overview of the steps of the 5-tier technique of acne scar reduction. (1) Scar shouldering, (2) Vertical subcision with very high dose low density Deep FX, (3) Deep narrow fractional with Deep FX, (4) Superficial resurfacing for color match with active FX, (5) Horizontal subcision with needle tip.

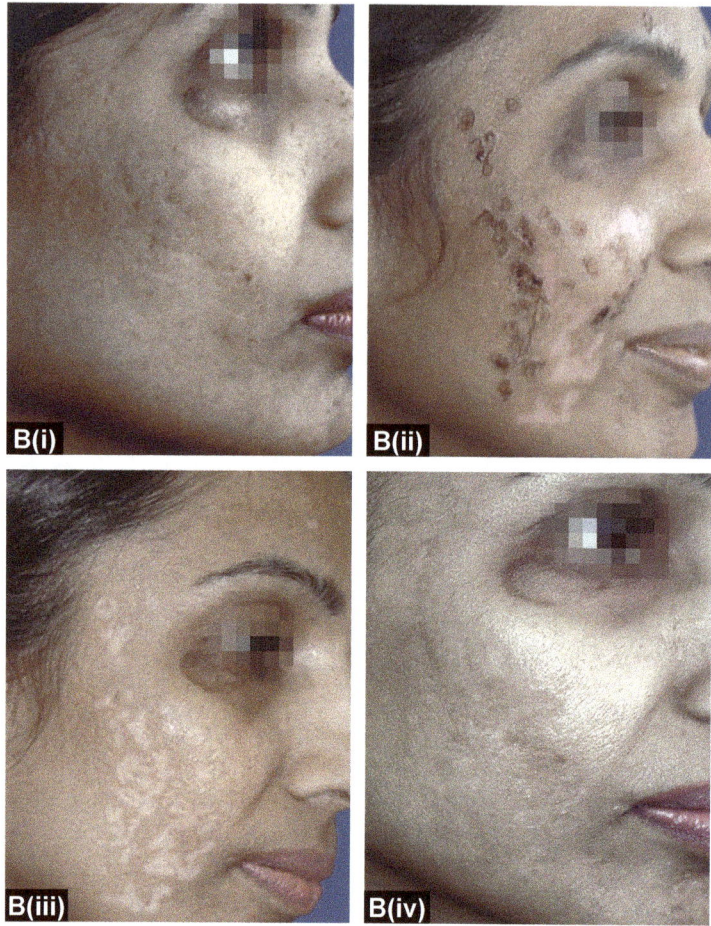

Figs. 12.13B(i) to (iv): Scar shouldering with Ultrapulse Active FX fractional CO_2 laser. Spot size 2 mm 60 W 200 mJ used as surgical knife. (B1) Pretreatment image; (B2) Treatment of the scars by the 5-tier technique; (B3) There would be PIH (hypopigmentation) due to the aggressive settings; (B4) Heartening results at the end of therapy.

toward different aspects and levels of the skin (subcision at deep dermal/subcutaneous level, dermaroller at dermal level, PRP at dermal/subcutaneous level, and chemical peel at epidermal to dermal level). The combination also results scar remodeling. Keeping the interval between procedures to 15 days is ideal as it keeps the skin tissues in continuous stimulation and alternating the procedure addressing different layers (epidermis to very superficial dermis by chemical peeling and superficial dermis to deep dermis/subcutaneous tissue by dermaroller and PRP), thus preventing excessive injury to that particular section of skin (Goodman GJ, 2014). As the demand for minimally invasive, highly effective cosmetic procedures is growing, combining these procedures for the treatment for acne scars might be more cost effective than lasers for acne scars. It is well-tolerated in Indian skin type (Fitzpatric skin types III, IV, and V), has low morbidity with minimal downtime, high level of patient satisfaction, and is cost-effective to the patient. Since Indian skin type is very prone for dyspigmentation, this low morbidity but highly effective procedure is ideal for addressing postacne scarring.

There is no fixed approach to treating scars but if the basic principles targeting the varied scar morphology are addressed (Fig. 12.1), heartening results can be achieved immaterial of what approach is followed as the basic principles of the surgical, laser and nonlaser approaches are similar.

12B. LASERS FOR SCARS, KELOIDS, AND STRETCH MARKS

Kabir Sardana, Niteen V Dhepe

INTRODUCTION

The psychosocial impact of cutaneous scarring can be profound. The multifaceted causes of scars include traumatic incidents, surgical procedures, and severe acne and can profoundly affect the quality of life of patients. We will largely focus on the role of laser in nonacne scars in this chapter. Acne scars have been discussed in the chapter of fractional lasers.

ETIOPATHOGENESIS

Scars are the result of a deviation in the orderly pattern of healing and can be caused by a variety of factors, such as excessive wound tension, improper surgical repair, delayed reepithelialization, or a history of radiation to the affected area. An excessive tissue response can create a raised nodule of fibrotic tissue, whereas "pitted" and atrophic scars may result from inadequate replacement of deleted collagen fibers. There are several currently available scar reducing medical therapies, but we will largely focus on lasers.

Types of Scars

In medical literature, scars are often analyzed by their etiology, the most common sources being surgery, trauma, burns, and acne or inflammatory processes. While analyzing literature, the important parameters to assess improvement include reduction of the redness and height of the scar, improvement of pliability, and symptomatic relief of pruritus.

Hypertrophic Scars

They are erythematous, raised, firm nodular growths that occur more commonly in areas subject to increased pressure or movement or in body sites that exhibit slow wound healing. The growth of hypertrophic scars is limited to the site of original tissue injury, unlike keloids, which proliferate beyond the boundaries of the initial wound and often continue to grow without regression.

Keloids

Keloids present as deep reddish-purple papules and nodules, often on the earlobes, anterior chest, shoulders, and upper back. These lesions are more common in darker-skinned persons and, like hypertrophic scars, may be pruritic, dysesthetic, and cosmetically disfiguring. Whereas the histology of hypertrophic scars is indistinguishable from that of other scarring processes, keloidal histology may be recognized by thickened bundles of hyalinized acellular collagen haphazardly arranged in whorls and nodules with an increased amount of hyaluronidase.

There are a few salient differences between these two scars that are as follows:
- Hypertrophic scars are generally white to pink scars that remain within the borders of the original wound.
- These generally occur within 1 month of the injury and tend to improve over time.
- Keloids are composed of disorganized, thick, collagen fibers with a prominent mucoid matrix. Hypertrophic scars contain more organized collagen fibers within a scant mucoid matrix.

Atrophic Scars

These are dermal depressions that result from an acute inflammatory process affecting the skin, such as cystic acne or varicella. The inflammation associated with atrophic scars leads to collagen destruction with dermal atrophy. Surgery or other forms of skin trauma may also result in atrophic scars, which are initially erythematous and become increasingly hypopigmented and fibrotic over time. Based on their width, depth, and 3-dimensional architecture, acne scars are sometimes further subclassified into icepick, rolling, and boxcar scars. They are discussed in the chapter on fractional lasers.

Prescars

These are early wounds in scar-prone skin. Prophylactic or early laser treatment of traumatized skin concomitant with or shortly after cutaneous wounding has been shown to reduce or even prevent scar formation in patients at high-risk for scarring.

APPROACH TO THERAPY

The scars should be treated depending on the *type*, *stage*, *duration*, *color*, and taking into consideration *patient characteristics*. Thus, an algorithmic approach can be used (Flowchart 12.1) to first decide which laser to use, which can then be tweaked depending on patient characteristics (Table 12.3). But, it must be appreciated that hypertrophic scars, if left alone, tend to improve with time, and most of the studies published may have inadvertently overlooked this fact.

Most of the hypertrophic scars have an average of 50–80% improvement after two laser treatments. Keloids, however, usually require more treatments and/or other ancillary treatments, including surgical excision, to achieve acceptable results.

Flowchart 12.1: An overview of management of scars by lasers.

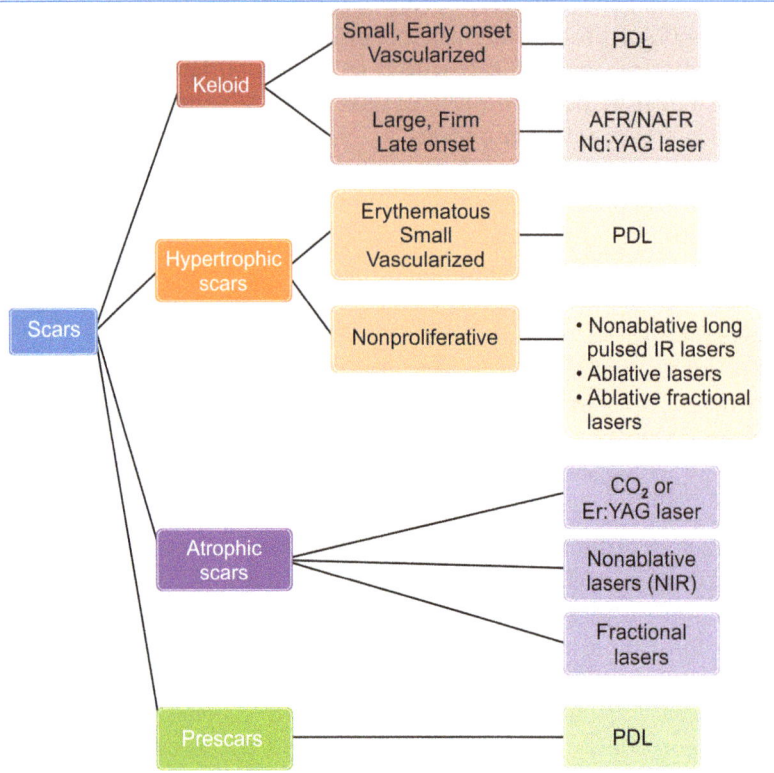

(PDL: pulsed dye laser; AFR: ablative fractional resurfacing; NAFR: nonablative fractional resurfacing; Nd:YAG: neodymium-doped yttrium aluminum garnet)

Table 12.3: Parameters that determine laser therapy for scars.

Characteristics	Variables	First-line	Second-line
Severity	Mild	Nonablative lasers	Ablative lasers
	Moderate	Ablative lasers	Fractional (NAFR)
	Severe	Ablative lasers	Fractional (AFR)
Skin type	Type 1–3	All are equally good	
	Type 4–6	Fractional lasers	
Etiology	Burn scar	PDL	Fractional lasers
	Surgical scar	Fractional lasers	PDL/ablative
	Acne scar	Fractional lasers	
Patient choice	Minimum downtime	Nonablative lasers	
	Some downtime	Fractional (NAFR)	
	Can tolerate downtime	Ablative lasers	

Ablative (CO_2/Er:YAG), Fractional (NAFR/AFR)
(PDL: pulsed dye laser; AFR: ablative fractional resurfacing; NAFR: nonablative fractional resurfacing; Er:YAG: erbium-doped yttrium aluminum garnet)

Some factors to consider before choosing the parameters of a laser device include:
- *Thickness* of the scar (thicker scars need increased depth)
- *Age* of the scar (younger scars decreased depth and density)
- *Location* of the scar (off-face decreased depth and density)
- *Skin type* of the patient (darker skin types decreased density) and comorbid medical conditions
- Scar type determine if a scar is hypertrophic, keloid, contracture or atrophic. Also dyschromia of a scar should be evaluated for erythema, hyperpigmentation, and hypopigmentation.

Here, it is important to remember that for most scar lasers may not always be the ideal intervention modality. The next section details the use of lasers in treatment of scars. The history of lasers is summarized in the Table 12.4.

When to Treat a Scar with Fractional Lasers?

As a general rule, there should be a healed and intact epidermis prior to laser treatment. Treatment of freshly healing wounds with unstable epidermal coverage in the first 1 to 3 months after injury may lead to unpredictable and potentially harmful outcomes. Younger, less mature scars are less tolerant of aggressive processes and should be treated more judiciously in terms of laser settings and combination procedures than more mature scars (years after injury). Mature scars, whether 1 year old or 60 years old, all respond well to laser therapy. A minimum treatment interval of 1 month to 3 months between fractional laser treatments is recommended to give time to heal to the scar tissue that is compromised. Even after just one therapy session, a patient may continue to have improvement for many months up to 1 year.

Table 12.4: An overview of lasers in scar management.

First laser studied	1060 nm neodymium: yttrium aluminum garnet (Nd:YAG)
Avoid these lasers	CO_2 and argon lasers
The PDL era	• Improves scar texture, redness, and pliability • Can prevent hypertrophic scars • Can be used postscar surgery also
Fractional lasers RF	Not very effective in hypertrophic scars Effective in atrophic scars
Settings	• Be flexible and select pulse energies proportional to the scar thickness as estimated by palpation and desired treatment depth without extending beyond the depth of the scar • Aggressive pulse energy settings require a concomitant reduction in procedure density • Low-density fractional treatment is favored to reduce the risk of complications when treating scars • The treatment area includes the entire scar sheet and a 1–2 mm rim of normal skin • Procedure parameters should be lowered when treating off-face scars

(PDL: pulsed dye laser; RF: radiofrequency).

Hypertrophic Scars and Keloids

Laser used: Pulsed dye laser (PDL), fractional laser, light emitting diode (LED), photodynamic therapy (PDT).

Initial studies used 1064 nm neodymium:yttrium-aluminum-garnet (Nd:YAG) laser, argon, and carbon dioxide (CO_2) which showed promising results, but high recurrence rates were observed. Thus, the most commonly recommended system is the PDL, though it makes more sense to stratify therapy according to the type of scars. A recent study examined the combined approach of using the dual-wave-length PDL and Nd:YAG in treatment of hypertrophic scars with sessions at 4–6 weeks intervals was found to produce good results (Lin L). We are detailing results with the IPL but we reiterate that the results depend on the device (Figs. 12.14A to D).

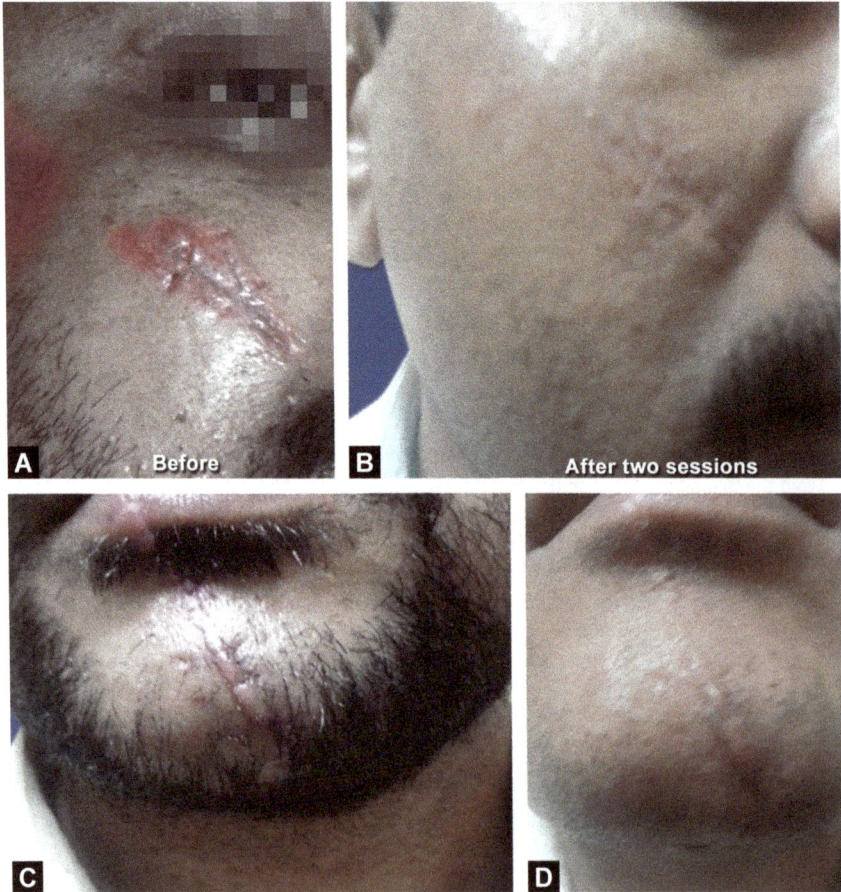

Figs. 12.14A to D: Hypertrophic scar. 550–1,100 nm filter 16.5 mJ/cm² six passes in single pulse mode weekly.

Pulsed Dye Laser

(Brewin MP, 2014; Mamalis AD, 2013)
Pulsed dye lasers have been shown to help in improving scar size, erythema, pliability, pruritus, and texture and are used for all forms of hypertrophic scarring and keloids, regardless of etiology.

Indications: Burn scars, sternotomy scars, acne scars, and facial scars resulting from cutaneous surgery.

Mechanism of action:
- Reduce expression of transforming growth factor beta, fibroblast proliferation, and collagen type III deposition.
- Selective photothermolysis of vasculature.
- Modulation of released mast cell constituents (such as histamine and interleukins) that could affect collagen metabolism.
- Heating of collagen fibers and breaking of disulfide bonds with subsequent collagen realignment.

Procedure:
Patient characteristics: History of the scar or keloid in terms of age, evolution, and previous treatments.
- *Preoperative:* If topical anesthesia is desired, a lidocaine-containing cream or gel can be applied to the treatment areas 30–60 minutes before laser irradiation. Wear protective goggles.
- *Intraoperative*
  - Skin should be cleansed with soap and water to remove residual makeup, powder, or creams. Flammable solutions, such as alcohol, should be avoided in skin preparation.
  - Wet gauze may be used to protect hair-bearing areas during treatment and to avoid unnecessary thermal injury to nontargeted skin.
  - A test spot should be employed and if there is postoperative crusting or vesiculation, the fluence applied on subsequent visits should be decreased and retreatment postponed until the skin has completely healed. The fluence and pulse duration can be adjusted if scar proliferation continues despite laser irradiation. Generally speaking, higher fluences and shorter pulse durations result in improved scar size and pliability.
  Dose: In general, hypertrophic scars and keloids are treated with moderately low energy densities ranging from 6.0 J/cm^2 to 7.5 J/cm^2 (5 or 7 mm) or 4.5–5.5 J/cm^2 (10 mm spot size). Pulse durations ranging from 0.45 to 1.5 milliseconds are commonly used.
  Energy densities should be lowered by at least 0.5 J/cm^2 in patients with darker skin and for scars in delicate or thin-skinned locations (e.g. eyelids, neck, and chest). The entire surface of the scar is treated with adjacent, nonoverlapping laser pulses.
  - Laser treatments are typically repeated at 6–8 weeks' time interval.

- *Postoperative:* A topical healing ointment under a nonstick bandage can be applied for the first few postoperative days to protect the skin. Treated areas should be gently cleansed daily with water and mild soap. Strict sun avoidance and photoprotection should be advocated between treatment sessions to reduce the risk of pigment alteration. Topical bleaching agents (such as hydroquinone or kojic acid) may be applied to hasten pigment resolution.

Pearls/Pitfalls:
- It is ideal to treat hypertrophic scars early, possibly within the first few months of appearance.
- Previous treatments, such as cryotherapy, may cause increased fibrosis, and thus adjustments of laser parameters and treatment sessions may need to be made.
- Location of the scar is also important to note. Dierickx et al. have found that facial scars respond better to treatment. Nouri et al. have also found that facial, shoulder, and arm scars respond better than those on the anterior chest wall.
- Laser treatment may be used alone or in combination therapy with intralesional corticosteroids or fluorouracil (5-FU). Alster (2003) compared PDL treatment alone with laser therapy combined with intralesional corticosteroid treatment and found that both were similarly effective with no significant difference.
- The use of concomitant intralesional corticosteroids or 5-fluorouracil has been shown to provide additional benefit in proliferative scars. Intralesional injections of corticosteroids (20 mg/mL triamcinolone) are more easily delivered immediately *after* (rather than before) PDL irradiation because the laser-irradiated scar becomes edematous (making needle penetration easier). An additional consideration is that when steroid injection is performed before laser irradiation the skin blanches, rendering the skin a potentially less amenable target for vascular-specific irradiation.

Results: The appearance of most hypertrophic scars will improve by approximately 50% after two treatments. Keloids often require additional treatment sessions to achieve significant improvement, but some may prove unresponsive.

Side effects:
- The most common side effect of treatment with the PDL is postoperative purpura, which often persists for several days. Pulse durations shorter than 6 milliseconds are almost certain to bruise the skin.
- Edema of treated skin may also occur but usually subsides within 48 hours.
- Hyperpigmentation has been reported with varying frequencies. If skin darkening occurs, further laser treatment should be suspended until resolution of the dyspigmentation has occurred in order to reduce the risk of cutaneous melanin interference with laser energy penetration.

Fractional Laser

Nonablative fractional photothermolysis with near infrared 1,540 and 1,550 nm erbium-doped fiber lasers is a promising new modality for the treatment of hypertrophic scars. But these may help in *textural* improvement and are *not* likely to affect the scar quality especially in keloids.

Thus, as stated above studies should be analyzed with respect to redness and height of the scar, improvement of pliability, and symptomatic relief of pruritus as these constitute substantial improvement.

Nonablative fractional resurfacing (1,550 nm erbium-doped fiber laser): Niwa AB et al. demonstrated significant improvement after two to three treatments, with improvement in pigmentation in all eight hypertrophic scars evaluated. The dose used was from 35 to 50 mJ, and 8 to 10 passes were applied with treatment levels 6-8. The ultimate evaluation was done by the quartile scoring system.

Haedersdal M et al. used a 1,540 nm nonablative fractional laser (Starlux, Palomar Medical Technologies, Burlington, Mass, USA) in 17 burn scars (five with meshed split-thickness skin grafting) and showed significant textural improvement after three treatments.

Ablative fractional resurfacing lasers
Ablative fractional resurfacing lasers have been used in the treatment of hypertrophic scars especially after burn cases (Haedersdal M). A treatment protocol using the fractional CO_2 is shown in Figures 12.15A and B.

Conclusion

One of the most common indications is in the treatment of burn scars (Hultman CS et al.). Restoration of form and function after burn injury remains challenging, but traditional and emerging laser and light-based technologies may offer new hope for patients with burn scars. Depending upon the constellation of patient symptoms and functional deficits, treatment of the burn scar involves a number of modalities, which may include massage and moisturizing agents, pressure garments, silicone sheeting, topical and intralesional steroids, and experimental therapies, such as interferon. The three different laser and light-based technologies are now increasingly being used in the management of burn scars.
1. Vascular-specific pulsed dye laser (PDL) therapy to reduce *hyperemia* and *hypertrophic scar* formation.
2. Ablative fractional CO_2 laser resurfacing to help correct the *abnormal texture, thickness, and stiffness* of the burn scar.
3. Intense pulsed light (IPL) therapy to improve *burn scar dyschromia* and alleviate chronic folliculitis.

Thus, it must be emphasized that the fractional laser may be *one* tool to help in targeting an aspect of the scar and a multifaceted team approach is needed for significant improvement.

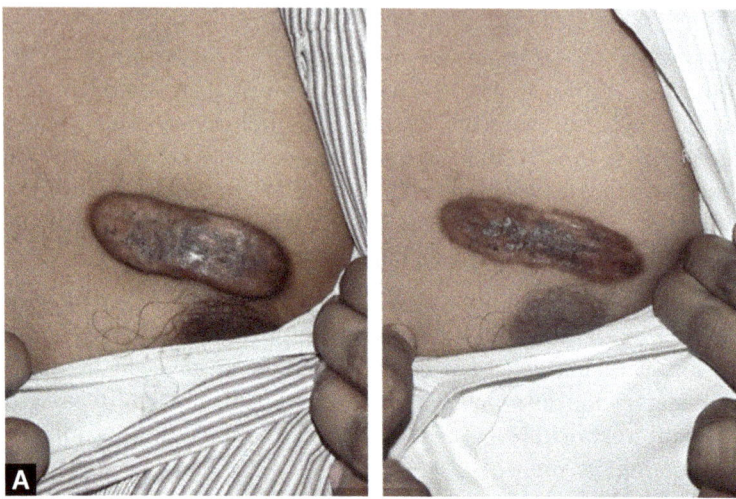

Pretreatment image (Left) and after 1 session (Right)

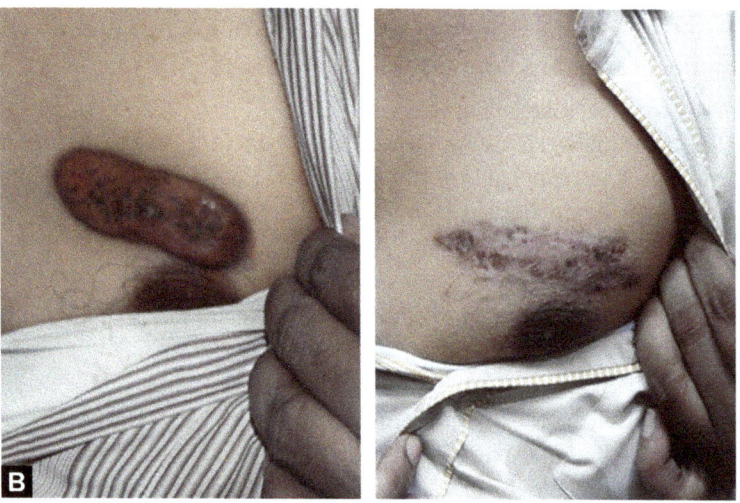

Pretreatment image (Left) and after 5 session (Right)

Figs. 12.15A and B: Keloid treated with Ultrapulse SCAAR FXTM 130 mJ density 5%, power 60 W and fractional drug delivery by topical application of 5-FU and triamcinolone within a minute of the procedure.

Atrophic Scars

Laser used: Ablative lasers, nonablative lasers and fractional lasers.

Atrophic scars resulting from acne, chickenpox, and trauma can be treated with laser therapy, though the results depend on numerous factors. Atrophic scars are initially erythematous and with time become increasingly fibrotic and hypopigmented. It is believed that atrophic scars result from inflammatory destruction of collagen with resultant dermal atrophy. Thus, the tissue defect has to be targeted and explains why methods like subcision are of little use in chickenpox scars.

Newer ablative resurfacing in the "spot" mode is our favored mode of therapy. Nonablative resurfacing is considered safe but is not as effective as ablative resurfacing. Fractional resurfacing offers the effectiveness of ablative resurfacing and the safety of nonablative resurfacing.

Ablative Lasers

Though this has been detailed previously in the chapter of ablative lasers, an overview will be given here. The advantages of this modality include selective and reproducible vaporization of skin with improved operator control and clinical efficacy. This is achieved by the novel devices including, high energy-short pulsed CO_2 laser, the variable pulsed or dual-mode erbium YAG laser and the combined-mode Er:YAG/CO_2 laser system.

Treatment goal: Laser treatment of atrophic scars is aimed at reducing the depth of the scar borders and stimulating neocollagenesis to fill in the depressions.

Mostly spot (or local) vaporization of isolated scars is used as full face resurfacing is not practised nowadays.

Procedure:
- *Preoperative*: Various anesthetic options can be employed, though for spot ablation local anesthesia is used.
- *Intraoperative*: The CO_2 laser is generally used at fluences of 250 to 350 mJ to ablate the epidermis in a single pass. An appropriate scanner can also achieve good results (*see* Fig. 12.1). Short-pulsed erbium-doped yttrium aluminum garnet (Er:YAG) lasers that are operated at 5 to 15 J/cm^2 often require several passes to result in a similar depth of penetration as CO_2, whereas longer-pulsed Er:YAG systems can be operated at higher fluences (22.5 J/cm^2) to achieve comparable results in a single pass.

  Though the details have been discussed previously in the chapter of Ablative Lasers, the basic steps are as follows:
  i. Remove the epidermis over the scar (1-2 passes).
  ii. Focus *around* and *over* the scar *shoulder* and ablate it carefully to the level of the base of the scar.
  iii. Give a pass over the center of the scar.
- *Postoperative*: Postoperative erythema typically lasts several weeks after ablative laser treatment.

Hyperpigmentation is transient and generally appears 3-4 weeks after treatment. Its resolution can be hastened with the use of topical bleaching agents.

Pearls: Ablative Er:YAG lasers may be the preferred treatment for mildly atrophic scars, whereas ablative CO_2 lasers may be preferable for more extensive scarring. But, it is our view that a dual mode Er:YAG can achieve results comparable to that of CO_2.

Nonablative Lasers

As a consequence of the side effects and prolonged postoperative recovery associated with ablative laser treatment, nonablative lasers were subsequently developed to provide a noninvasive option for atrophic scar revision. But it must be emphasized that the results are slower and less dramatic than ablative lasers.

Devices and lasers:
- 1,064 nm Q-switched Nd:YAG laser/1,064 nm long pulse Nd:YAG laser
- 1,320 nm Nd:YAG laser
- 1,450 nm diode laser
- 1,540-nm erbium-doped phosphate glass laser (Er:Glass)
- 585 nm PDL and intense pulse light system.

Although, protocols vary, treatments are generally performed at monthly intervals for three consecutive months. Best results are observable 3–4 months after the last treatment.

Mode of action: These devices deliver concomitant epidermal surface cooling with deeply penetrating infrared wave-lengths that target tissue water and stimulate collagen production via controlled dermal heating without epidermal disruption.

It is possible that the absorption of the 1,064 nm wavelength by the blood vessels in the scar may lead to either conduction to the surrounding dermis to alter the fibrotic collagen within the scar or to significant ischemia within the laser-treated tissue to affect collagen or release collagenase.

Results: A series of 3–5 treatments are typically performed on a monthly basis, with optimal clinical efficacy appreciated several (3–6) months after the final laser treatment session. Sustained clinical improvement of scars by 40–50% has been observed after the series of treatments. The low side effect profile of these nonablative systems (limited to local erythema and edema and, rarely, vesiculation or herpes simplex reactivation) compensates for their reduced clinical efficacy (relative to ablative lasers).

Conclusion: The results of the nonablative resurfacing depend on the patient's own wound-healing capacities and, as stated before, will not equal those obtainable with ablative treatments.

Fractional Lasers

Though this has been discussed in detail previously, our focus is primarily on nonacne scars, namely, chickenpox and smallpox scars. As the thermal coagulation required for ameliorating the tissue defect is more than what is required for acne scars, the dose settings have to be more aggressive than normal, which can be an issue as the side effects are also proportionately more.

Procedure:
- *Preoperative*: The ideal patient for fractional laser skin resurfacing has a fair complexion (skin phototype I, II, or III), but darker skin tones (IV-VI) can also be treated.

  Sun exposure should be avoided prior to treatment in order to decrease the risk of postoperative dyspigmentation.

  For patients with a strong history of herpes labialis, prophylactic oral antiviral medications should be considered when treating the perioral skin. Reactivation of prior herpes simplex infection can occur despite absence of an external wound, due to the intense dermal heat produced by the laser.
- *Intraoperative*
  - The treatment areas should be cleansed of debris (including dirt, makeup, and powder) using a mild cleanser and 70% alcohol (let it dry before attempting the procedure).
  - A topical anesthetic cream is applied to the treatment sites for 60 minutes before treatment.
  - Nonablative fractional resurfacing can be done by using a dose setting of 40-60 mJ (maximum 70 mJ; total 3-5 kJ). Retreatments with gradually higher fluences should be performed at 4-weeks interval until patients are satisfied with clinical outcomes (typically 3-5 sessions are necessary to produce substantial clinical improvement).
  - Ablative fractional resurfacing lasers require 1-2 sessions.

  Fraxel repair: 20-100 mJ with treatment densities of 600-1600 MTZ/cm^2.

  Lumenis system (Total Fx): (Deep FX: 15-25 mJ, active FX: 80-125 mJ) and densities (Deep FX: 10-15%, active RX: 1-3%) depending on the severity of scarring.
- *Postoperative*
  - Patients who receive NAFR treatment should use a mild cleanser and moisturizer several times daily for the first few days after each treatment session (or as long as bronzing/xerosis is apparent).
  - Sun exposure should be avoided during this time.

Conclusion: Both ablative and nonablative fractionated lasers can be used and can help to resolve both textural and pigmentary changes. The latter is important as with most ablative treatments hypopigmentation and even depigmentation is seen.

Prescars

Treatment of potential scars with lasers is a relatively new concept that is gaining in popularity. Two different approaches for scar prevention within prescars have been outlined. Wound edges can be vaporized with either a CO_2 or an Er:YAG laser before primary surgical closure to enhance ultimate cosmesis. Alternatively, a 585 nm PDL system can be used to treat surgical sites, traumatic wounds or ulcerations to improve the quality of scarring and prevent excessive scar formation.

Surgical Scars

All surgical scars improve with fractional ablative laser. First, one must evaluate if the surgical scar is elevated (hypertrophic) or depressed (atrophic). The thicker, hypertrophic scars need deeper treatment depths, whereas more atrophic scars can be dealt with more superficially. Early surgical scars with significant erythema respond to vascular lasers, with or without same-day treatment of fractional lasers.

Erythematous, hypertrophic scars are seen frequently in the first year after injury. Vascular-specific lasers and light devices, especially the 595 nm PDL, are useful and are discussed in two recent reviews. PDL may be applied alone for small hypertrophic scars, but is often combined with fractional laser therapy in either concurrent or alternating treatment sessions.

Burn and Trauma Scars

Hypertrophic burn and traumatic scars are best improved by either ablative or nonablative fractional lasers. Ablative fractional lasers have the capacity to induce a more robust remodeling response than nonablative fractional lasers.

An estimation of scar pliability and thickness through palpation is central to determining appropriate laser pulse energy settings (treatment depth). Treatment depth should not exceed the thickness of the scar. Pigmentary abnormalities (hypopigmentation, hyperpigmentation, dyspigmentation) of scars also improve with fractional therapy.

Though costly, sequential laser use, is a useful and elegant concept wherein 3 lasers are used (Tao J et al.). The PDL targets scar hypervascularity, the 1550 nm erbium:glass stimulates collagen remodeling and the 1927 nm thulium targets epidermal processes, particularly hyperpigmentation. This is useful in patients with a high chance of hyperpigmentation, like Indians with skin of color. Multiple sittings are required with the PDL preceding the other two lasers at a monthly interval with topical tacrolimus usage. The logic of using this is based on their different targets. The 1550-nm wavelength injures the dermis to stimulate collagen remodeling while the 1927 nm wavelength targets dyspigmentation by shuttling melanin into collections of microscopic epidermal necrotic debris just above the MTZs.

Ablative lasers have a significantly greater potential depth of thermal injury compared to nonablative lasers, 1.8 mm compared to 4.0 mm, respectively

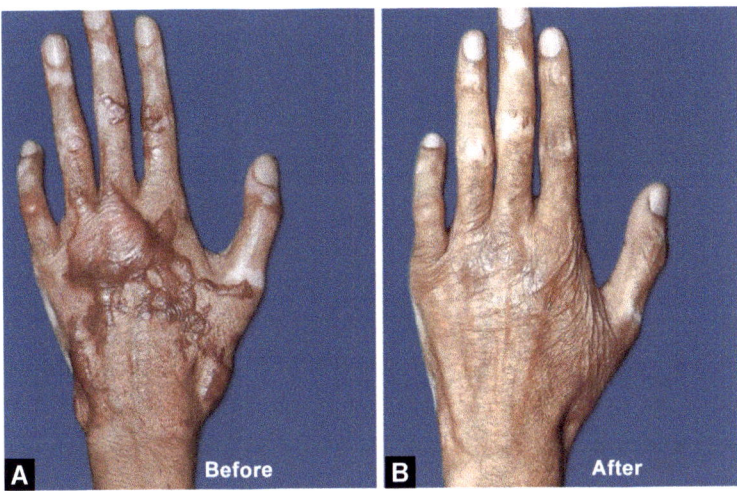

Figs. 12.16A and B: Caustic burn scar treated with very deep and very narrow fractional CO_2 laser, i.e. Ultrapulse SCAAR FXTM (width 110 µ and depth 2,500 µ) 140 mJ density 5%, power 60 W and fractional drug delivery by rubbing in triamcinolone and 5 FU within a minute of the fractional procedure. Six to eight sessions over 18 months are required.

(Lumenis SCAAR FX software). Furthermore, tissue ablation appears to induce a modest immediate photomechanical release of tension in some restrictive scars. An appropriate degree of surrounding thermal coagulation seems to facilitate the subsequent remodeling response (Figs. 12.16A and B).

Flat or atrophic scars from burns and trauma also respond to fractional laser therapy. We have treated such scars using a scanner mode of a superpulsed CO_2 laser (Figs. 12.17A to D). Atrophic scars are dermal depressions that occur due to collagen destruction during an injury. The goal of laser treatment for atrophic scars is to stimulate collagen production within the atrophic areas. Neocollagenesis is stimulated the most from fractional laser therapy, and thus makes it the best choice for flat or thin scars.

CONCLUSION

Though lasers are now being used increasingly for treating scars, it must be emphasized that they are one of the many tools that can be adopted. Except for atrophic scars in most other indications, conventional modalities like intralesional (IL) steroids/fluorouracil (FU) can and should be combined with lasers. The cost, time, and effort required for results with lasers, do not justify their use in all cases. In burn cases, the use of PDL ± fractional lasers can be at best an adjunct to traditional modes of therapy. Thus, we favor using laser in additions to standard modalities.

The issue of dermal fillers in the area to be treated is important. Studies have been done to determine the effect of different laser devices on skin

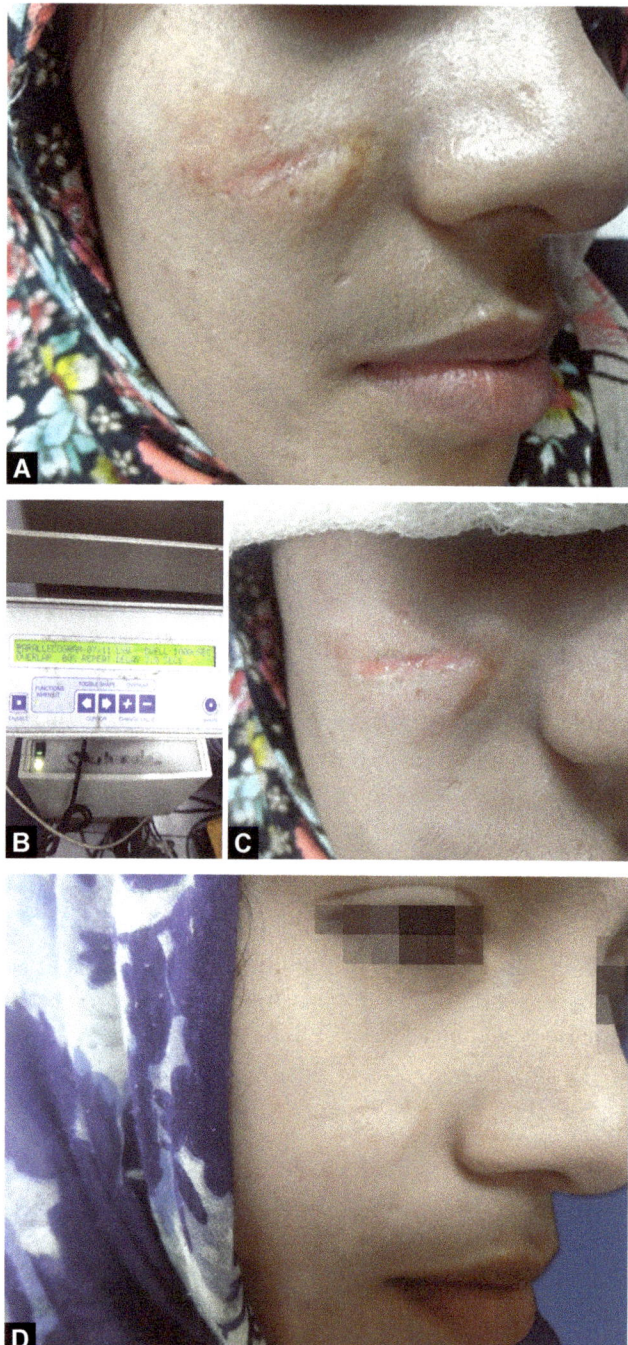

Figs. 12.17A to D: (A) A case of post-traumatic scar; (B) The scanner mode is used with a scan aligning with the scar. The ultrapulse setting is used with a fluence of 4 J/cm^2; (C) Immediate postoperative; (D) Postoperative result after 4 months. Patient was asked to apply tretinoin 0.025% after the lesion healed, which adds to the ultimate therapy results.

previously treated with hyaluronic acid fillers (Farkas JP). Although the injected material was unaffected by the nonablative laser and intense pulsed light treatments, deeper laser treatments did demonstrate laser-filler interaction. The effect of this interaction is not yet known. Also, newer ablative and nonablative fractional lasers have the ability to penetrate deep into the dermis and, again, the effects this may have on the fillers is not yet known. Thus, care must be taken when planning to use lasers in combination with soft tissue fillers for the treatment of scars.

A few principles are given in the Box 12.2, and a guide to dosimetry is given in Table 12.5, which can help guide the clinician to plan a therapeutic intervention.

There is growing trend of using the fractional ablative tunnel for *laser-assisted delivery systems (LADS)* of a variety of drugs, topical agents, and other living tissue. Laser-assisted drug delivery may allow for greater precise depth of penetration by existing topical medications, more efficient transcutaneous delivery of large drug molecules, and even systemic drug administration via a transcutaneous route (Fig. 12.16). This concept is exemplified by a study with the combined use of fractional CO_2 laser with topical triamcinolone suspension applied immediately after each laser session followed by clobetasol propionate gel for 1 week after each laser session (Majid I). These zones may be used immediately postoperatively to deliver drugs and other substances to synergistically create an enhanced therapeutic response.

Box 12.2: Principles of laser therapy for scars.

- Keloids may be responsive only in the early stage. In late stage once the keloid becomes firm and hard the PDL is not very useful. Even though various other lasers have been tried the results are not satisfactory
- Hypertrophic scars are easy to treat. A combination of PDL followed by fractional CO_2 can be used
- Atrophic scars are best treated by an ablative laser. Nonablative NIR lasers and fractional lasers are slower in action and incomplete in results
- Traditional medical therapies can be combined with lasers (Waibel JS et al.).

(PDL: pulsed dye laser; NIR: near infrared)

Table 12.5: Dose parameters for scar treatment for lasers.

Condition	Laser	Settings
Hypertrophic scars	585–595 nm PDL	6.0–7.5 J/cm^2 (7 mm spot) or 4.5–5.5 J/cm^2 (10 mm spot) 1.5–3 ms
	CO_2 (10,600 nm)	1 pass, 300 mJ, 60 watts, 5 J/cm^2
	Er:YAG (2940 nm)	2–3 passes, 5 mm spot size, 5–15 J/cm^2
	Fractional CO_2	DeepFX^{TM}: Thick, stiff scar,: density of 15%, frequency 600 Hz, 12.5–17.5 mJ per micropulse ActiveFX^{TM}: Textural: frequency of 150 Hz, 70–90 mJ per micropulse

Contd...

Contd...

Condition	Laser	Settings
Keloids	585–595 nm PDL	6.0–7.5 J/cm² (7 mm spot) 4.5–5.5 J/cm² (10 mm spot) 1.5–3 ms
	CO₂ (10600 nm)	1 pass, 300 mJ, 60 watts, 5 J/cm²
	Er:YAG (2940 nm)	2–3 passes, 5 mm spot size, 5–15 J/cm²
	Nonablative fractional (1540/1550 nm)	15 mm handpiece, 35–50 J/cm²
Atrophic scars (surgical or trauma)	CO₂ (10 600 nm)	1 pass, 300 mJ, 60 watts, 5 J/cm²
	Er:YAG (2940 nm)	2–3 passes, 5 mm spot size, 5–15 J/cm²
	Diode (1450 nm)	8–14 J/cm², 250 ms, 6 mm spot size
	Nd:YAG (1320 nm)	18 J/cm², 200 µs, 6 mm spot size

(PDL: pulsed dye laser; Er:YAG: erbium-doped yttrium aluminum garnet; Nd:YAG: neodymium-doped yttrium-aluminum-garnet)

BIBLIOGRAPHY

1. Alster T, Zaulyanov L. Laser scar revision: a review. Dermatol Surg. 2007;33:131-40.
2. Alster T. Laser scar revision: Comparison study of 585-nm pulsed dye laser with and without intralesional corticosteroids. Dermatol Surg. 2003;29(1):25-9.
3. Brewin MP, Lister TS. Prevention or treatment of hypertrophic burn scarring: A review of when and how to treat with the Pulsed Dye Laser. Burns. 2014;40(5): 797-804.
4. Choi JE, Oh GN, Kim JY, et al. Ablative fractional laser treatment for hypertrophic scars: Comparison between Er:YAG and CO₂ fractional lasers. J Dermatolog Treat. 2014;25(4):299-303.
5. Dierickx C, Goldman MP, Fitzpatrick RE. Laser treatment of erythematous/hypertrophic and pigmented scars in 26 patients. Plast Reconstr Surg. 1995; 95(1):84-90.
6. Haedersdal M, Moreau KE, Beyer DM, et al. Fractional nonablative 1540 nm laser resurfacing for thermal burn scars: A randomized controlled trial. Lasers Surg Med. 2009;41(3):189-95.
7. Haedersdal M. Fractional ablative CO₂ laser resurfacing improves a thermal burn scar. J Eur Acad Dermatol Venereol. 2009;23(11):1340-1.
8. Hultman CS, Edkins RE, Lee CN, et al. Shine on: Review of laser- and light-based therapies for the treatment of burn scars. Dermatol Res Pract. 2012;2012:243651.
9. Khatri KA, Mahoney DL, McCartney MJ. Laser scar revision: A review. J Cosmet Laser Ther. 2011;13(2):54-62.
10. Lin L, Guo P, Wang X, et al. Effective treatment for hypertrophic scar with dual-wave-length PDL and Nd:YAG in Chinese patients. J Cosmet Laser Ther. 2018. pp. 1-6.

11. Majid I, Imran S. Fractional carbon dioxide laser resurfacing in combination with potent topical corticosteroids for hypertrophic burn scars in the pediatric age group: an open label study. Dermatol Surg. 2018;44(8):1102-8.
12. Mamalis AD, Lev-Tov H, Nguyen DH, et al. Laser and light-based treatment of Keloids—a review. J Eur Acad Dermatol Venereol. 2014;28(6):689-99.
13. Niwa AB, Mello AP, Torezan LA, et al. Fractional photothermolysis for the treatment of hypertrophic scars: clinical experience of eight cases. Dermatol Surg. 2009;35(5):773-7.
14. Nouri K, Jimenez GP, Harrison-Balestra C, et al. 585 nm pulsed dye laser in the treatment of surgical scars starting on the suture removal day. Dermatol Surg. 2003;29:65-73.
15. Tao J, Champlain A, Weddington C, et al. Treatment of burn scars in Fitzpatrick phototype III patients with a combination of pulsed dye laser and non-ablative fractional resurfacing 1550 nm erbium:glass/1927 nm thulium laser devices. Scars Burn Heal. 2018;4:2059513118758510.
16. Ud-Din S, Bayat A. Strategic management of keloid disease in ethnic skin: a structured approach supported by the emerging literature. Br J Dermatol. 2013;169(Suppl 3):71-81.
17. Waibel JS, Wulkan AJ, Shumaker PR. Treatment of hypertrophic scars using laser and laser assisted corticosteroid delivery. Lasers Surg Med. 2013;45(3):135-40.
18. Westine JG, Lopez MA, Thomas JR. Scar revision. Facial Plast Surg Clin North Am. 2005;13(2):325-31.

12C. STRIAE DISTENSAE
Kabir Sardana

INTRODUCTION

Striae distensae or stretch marks are a common skin abnormality affecting both sexes and all races. These lesions usually evolve through various stages, which are important to recognize before attempting any intervention (Fig. 12.18A)

Acute: The striae appear red or violaceous and are referred to as striae rubra. During this stage, they may be raised and often irritated.

Chronic: Here the striae become white, atrophied, and depressed. At this stage, they are referred to as striae alba.

Though we are focusing on lasers there is a discussion of the treatment in **Chapters 4 and 7** and the reader is advised to refer to those sections also.

MANAGEMENT

There is no medical indication to treat striae. Of the numerous options there is none that has consistent success, with most treatment doing nothing except rhyming with the natural course of healing. The main aspects that need to be addressed while treating striae include the effect of any therapy on the following parameters:
1. Increased *collagen production and fibroblastic* activity
2. Increase in *elasticity and blood perfusion*
3. Improvement in *cell proliferation*
4. Increased *skin hydration*
5. *Anti-inflammatory properties*.

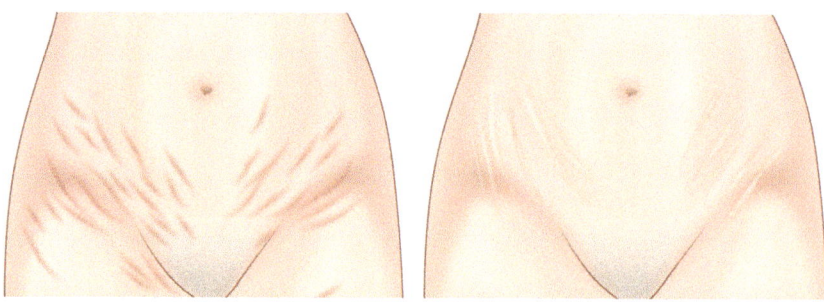

Striae rubrae   Striae albae

Fig. 12.18A: An artistic illustration of striae rubrae and striae albae. Striae rubrae are considered as an early form of striae distensae, which are erythematous, red, and sometimes slightly raised linear lesions. They do not recur and are classified as temporary striae. Striae albae are atrophic, wrinkled, and pale. They also do not recur but are permanent striae.

A summary of the various therapeutic options are listed in Table 12.6. A stage and morphology-specific therapy is given in Table 12.7.

Topical Agents

Although striae are a common cause of concern, highly effective, low-risk treatment modalities are lacking. These lesions are notoriously hard to treat. Many treatments have been tried but rarely tested.

The various topical agents tried include *Trofolastin, Alphastria, cocoa butter, olive oil* and *silicone gel*. With tretinoin, the studies have shown that the use of 0.1% daily for 6 months help in ameliorating both the length and width of SD.

Table 12.6: Overview of the treatments for striae.

Published data	Unpublished data
Topicals • Kelo-Cote • Tretinoin **Procedures** • Laser therapy • light therapy • Acid peels • Collagen injections • Radiofrequency devices • Microdermabrasion	• Apothederm™ • Bio-Oil™ • Clarins™ • Kelo-Stretch™ • RegimA™ • SilDerm™ • Skinception™ • StriVectin-SD™ • Thalgo™

Table 12.7: An overview of therapy for various components of striae (Suh DH et al.).

Target parameters	Interventions	
	Laser, RF and light devices	Medical therapy
Length	Fractional ablative laser (CO_2)	10% l-Ascorbic acid
Width Depth	• Fractional ablative laser (Er: YAG) • Nonablative fractional lasers (1550 nm) • Fractionated microneedle radiofrequency • 1064 nm Nd:YAG laser • RF + PDL • IPL	20% Glycolic acid/ Tretinoin 0.05% Centella asiatica GA peel PRP TCA Peel
Color		Tretinoin 0.1%
Striae rubra Striae alba	• PDL • Excimer laser • IPL • NB: UVB	

(PDL: pulsed dye laser; RF: radiofrequency; IPL: intense pulse light; NB:UVB: narrow band UVB; GA: glycolic acid; PRP: platelet-rich plasma)

The problem is that very few topical treatments have been shown to increase collagen or elastin production within the lesions. A host of agents have been used as a prophylactic measure including, Cussons, Liforma, Kelo-Cote, Thalgo, TriLASTIN-SR, Kelo-Stretch™; Alphastria, cocoa butter, olive oil, almond oil and Trofolastin. In this author's view, except for time and tretinoin no other topical has any marked affect.

Laser Treatment

Lasers Used

The principles of therapy are akin to those given under the section on scars, thus *newer lesions* respond better than old ones.

The laser used include flash-pumped 585 nm PDL, IPL, 308 nm excimer laser, nonablative 1,450 nm diode laser, radiofrequency device, 1,064 nm Nd:YAG laser, nonablative fractional CO_2 resurfacing.

The basic principles are depicted in the Figures 12.18B to C and a stage-wise treatment approach is given below. Lasers should demonstrate clinical improvement in depth and width and histological improvement with increase in the numbers of collagen and elastin fibers (Figs. 12.18D and E).

- *Early stages (Rubra)*: 585 and 595 nm PDLs. The settings used are (585 nm) with a 7- or 10- mm spot size and 2 to 4 J/cm^2. But it works **only** on the **erythema**. A clinical end point of deep erythema or light purpura is optimal. Improvement can be seen even in cases of poor initial response 6 months after treatment.
- *Late Stages (Alba)*: Use subsurface lasers and fractional lasers and radio frequency (RF). There is little data to suggest whether deep depth, high coverage treatments are more effective than lower depth, lower coverage treatments. The results are variable.
- *Pigmentary alteration*: Excimer laser.

i. **Pulsed Dye Laser:** It should be used in striae rubra. In pigmented skin, lower fluencies can lead to hyperpigmentation. One or two treatment sessions are necessary.

ii. **Fractional Lasers:** All the available technologies have been used including Er:Glass laser (1,550 nm), 1,540 nm, 1,505 nm, Er:YAG and CO_2. Fractional photothermolysis creates multiple noncontiguous zones of thermal damage in the epidermis and dermis, sparing the tissue surrounding the wound. This in turn stimulates epidermal turnover and dermal collagen remodeling, which results in improvement of a variety of scar types. As all fractional lasers have water as a chromophore they are safe and we prefer using the 1,540 nm as it has a relatively less absorption spectrum for water and thus can lead to more collagen remodeling. The efficacy of NAF lasers has been

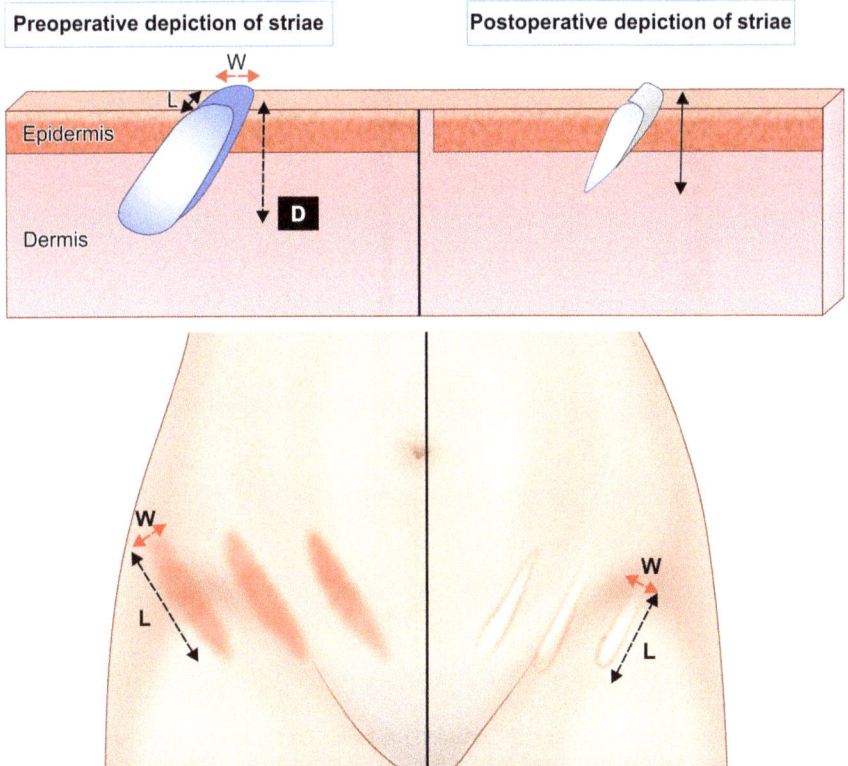

Fig. 12.18B: A diagrammatic three-dimensional depiction of striae distensae, which depicts the pathology akin to an atrophic scar with a depth up to the mid dermis. The laser employed should be able to ameliorate all the dimensions of the scar (L: length, W: width and D: depth).

shown by vivo evaluation of the skin using reflectance confocal microscopy (RCM) (Guida S). After 6 months of sessions every 4 weeks RCM revealed the dissolution of collagen bundles and the appearance of new papillae, as compared to baseline. The problem as always is that it is difficult to quantify the amount of collagen remodeling that can result with the dosimetry used with various laser systems.

Dose: Use a low dose, high density setting spaced at 4-6 weeks.
(Example: Lux Palomar. Treatment parameters included two to three passes with the 1,540 nm laser, with energy settings from 35–55 mJ/mb with the 10 mm optical tip or 12–14 mJ/mb with the 15 mm optical tip).

Comparison: As the depth of the pathology is in the upper dermis, as expected little difference is seen between NAFR and AFR (Yang YJ).

iii. **Other devices:** Intense pulsed light (590 nm), fractional RF, and platelet rich plasma have also been tried.

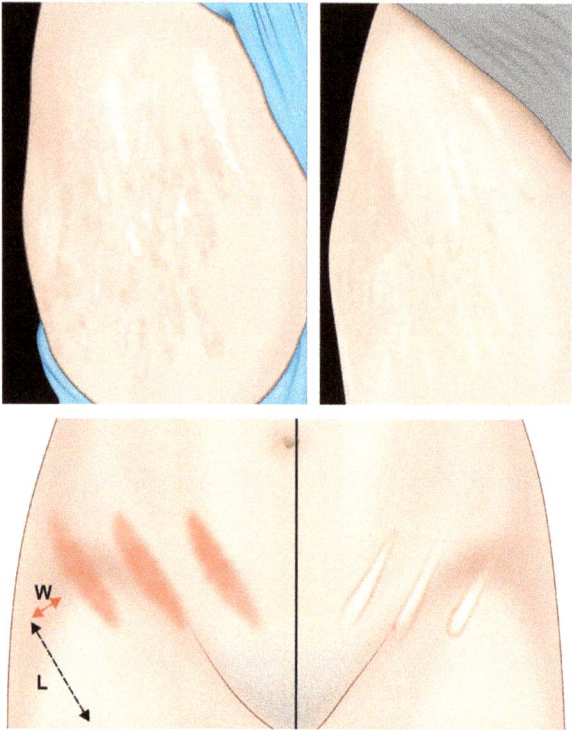

Fig. 12.18C: A surface "topographical" depiction of striae. As striae are linear tissue defects with a length and a width, both need to be addressed in its treatment. The postoperative view depicts a "realistic" partial amelioration of the scar.

Other Treatments

As visible and quantifiable results are difficult to achieve, a combination protocol (Shen J) has been tried in striae distensae alba, where the 2,940-nm Er:YAG AFL was first employed, 6 times at 4-week intervals. After the treatment, rb-BFGF was sprayed for 1 week at home. LED-RL was used once every 7 days for three sessions between the two laser treatments.

A more useful and practical concept is that of *needling* which mirrors the MTZ channels of fractional lasers. An elegant study compared, the fractional laser and microneedling (Soliman M). The laser used was the fractional CO_2 laser (SmartXide DOT™; DEKA, Calenzano, Florence, Italy) at a settings of 12 ~ 15 watt with a lower power, setting, (scanning dwelling time 500 ~ 600 µs, spacing 700 µm). The dermaroller (Mesotech Srl, Italy) had 540 fine titanium microneedles of 2 mm in length. Even though, 55% had a moderate-to-excellent improvement in the dermaroller-treated side compared to 76% with the fractional laser side, the cost and ease of performance of dermaroller cannot be overlooked. This contrast with a previous study where needling was found to be a superior treatment modality (Khater MH).

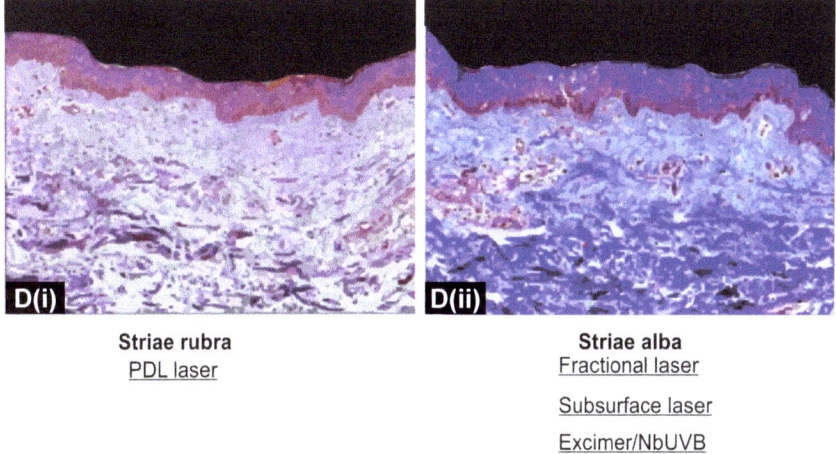

Striae rubra
PDL laser

Striae alba
Fractional laser

Subsurface laser

Excimer/NbUVB

An artistic depiction of histology of striae rubra before and after therapy. The diagram on the left shows increase in the epidermal thickness and the amount of collagen and elastic fibers. The preferred therapies for each stage are depicted above.

Figs. 12.18D(i) and (ii): Overview of lasers and light devices for treating striae. Note that *three* aspects have to be treated the *width, depth, and color of the striae*. (PDL: pulsed dye laser; NbUVB: narrow band UVB).

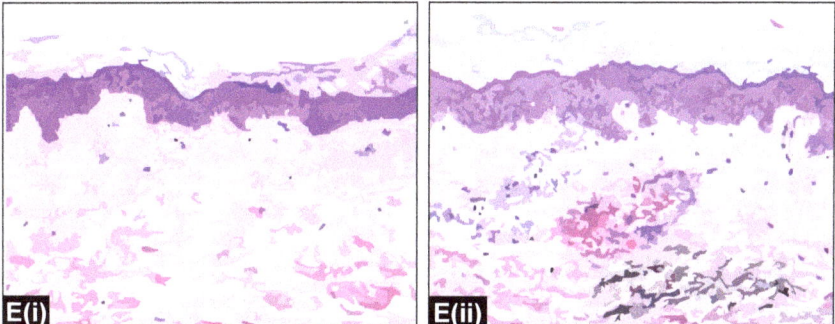

Figs. 12.18E(i) and (ii): A depiction of the histological effect of lasers on striae distensae. Pretreatment shows a thin epidermis while the post-treatment image shows an increase in the thickness of the epidermis with an increase collagen and elastin.

CONCLUSION

It is the author's opinion that the result with most devices has rarely been compared with a placebo group and there is a good chance that the patients may have spontaneous remission (Sardana K). If an intervention is desired any fractional device would suffice, with no advantage of AFR over NAFR.

Conservative fluencies should be used to ensure a mid-dermis depth. As the condition is akin to an atrophic scar, a 30% decrease in fluence from the conventional settings for acne scars can be used. Do not hope for more than a 50% improvement. Proof of cure is histological and that is rarely done in most studies (also *see* **Chapter 7 on Cosmetic Use of Radiofrequency in Dermatology**).

Striae therapies abound (Tables 12.6 and 12.7) and the therapies for this are like those for the common cold where there are many therapies but no cure and thus is largely as, to put it bluntly, nothing really is proven to work. A placebo arm and histological confirmation and clinical comparison with a placebo remain the gold standard and no study has been able to achieve only superiority over simple needling (Khater MH).

BIBLIOGRAPHY

1. Al-Dhalimi MA, Abo Nasyria AA. A comparative study of the effectiveness of intense pulsed light wavelengths (650 nm vs 590 nm) in the treatment of striae distensae. J Cosmet Laser Ther. 2013;15(3):120-5.
2. de Angelis F, Kolesnikova L, Renato F, et al. Fractional nonablative 1540 nm laser treatment of striae distensae in Fitzpatrick skin types II to IV: Clinical and histological results. Aesthet Surg J. 2011;31(4):411-9.
3. Gauglitz GG, Reinholz M, Kaudewitz P, et al. Treatment of striae distensae using an ablative Erbium: YAG fractional laser versus a 585-nm pulsed-dye laser. J Cosmet Laser Ther. 2014;16(3):117-9.
4. Guida S, Galimberti MG, Bencini M, et al. Treatment of striae distensae with non-ablative fractional laser: Clinical and in vivo microscopic documentation of treatment efficacy. Lasers Med Sci. 2018;33(1):75-8.
5. Jiménez GP, Flores F, Berman B, et al. Treatment of striae rubra and striae alba with the 585-nm pulsed-dye laser. Dermatol Surg. 2003;29(4):362-5.
6. Khater MH, Khattab FM, Abdelhaleem MR. Treatment of striae distensae with needling therapy versus CO_2 fractional laser. J Cosmet Laser Ther. 2016;18(2):75-9.
7. Sardana K. Lasers for treating striae: An emergent need for better evidence. Indian J Dermatol Venereol Leprol. 2014;80(5):392-4.
8. Shen J, Lu XG, Jin JJ, et al. Combination of a 2940 nm Er:YAG laser with recombinant bovine basic fibroblast growth factor (rb-bFGF) and light-emittingdiode-red light (LED-RL) for the treatment of striae alba: A pilot study. J Cosmet Dermatol. 2018;17(2):176-83.
9. Soliman M, Mohsen Soliman M, El-Tawdy A, et al. Efficacy of fractional carbon dioxide laser versus microneedling in the treatment of striae distensae. J Cosmet Laser Ther. 2018. pp. 1-8.
10. Suh DH, Lee SJ, Lee JH, et al. Treatment of striae distensae combined enhanced penetration platelet-rich plasma and ultrasound after plasma fractional radiofrequency. J Cosmet Laser Ther. 2012;14(6):272-6.
11. Yang YJ, Lee GY. Treatment of striae distensae with nonablative fractional laser versus ablative CO_2 fractional laser: A randomized controlled trial. Ann Dermatol. 2011;23(4):481-9.

12D. CELLULITE, FAT REDUCTION, LAXITY, AND BODY CONTOURING

Kabir Sardana, Niteen V Dhepe

Though the major aspects of this topic are discussed in Chapter 9, an overview with a focus on the main modalities for its management is given here.

CELLULITE

Cellulite is a topographic and localized alteration of the skin that creates a dimpled or "orange peel" appearance, most commonly found on the posterolateral thighs, buttocks, and abdomen. In 1978, Nürnberger and Müller first described cellulite as a result of sex-related differences in the structure of skin and subcutaneous tissue. This was further confirmed recently where it was shown that other aspects are also important including focally enlarged fibrosclerotic septa that tether the skin in areas of cellulite, or an uneven dermal-hypodermal interface (Hexsel DM). Cellulite is present in over 80–90% of postpubertal women. Given the ubiquitous nature of cellulite, it is more appropriately thought of as a secondary sex characteristic rather than a disease.

Options (Medical/Surgical)

Paradoxically, though cellulite is not a disease with no definition but there are numerous treatment modalities available for the disorder. This includes multiple over-the-counter creams that claim to remove cellulite with little science behind them (Table 12.8).

Currently available medical devices aim to target the structural features of cellulite. In addition to the application of ultrasound and radiofrequency (RF) energy and mechanical manipulation and disruption, laser and light based modalities are one of the latest advances in the treatment of cellulite.

External laser and light emitting diode (LED) irradiation has the capacity to trigger a photobiomodulatory effect in the targeted tissue stimulating several cellular functions such as neocollagenesis or adipocyte lipolysis. Depending on the wavelength, intensity, and total energy (J/cm^2) delivered, the therapeutic benefit may stem from a thermogenic or nonthermogenic effect (Neira R).

There are numerous devices with different actions but a few are being discussed here.

VelaSmooth™

The VelaSmooth™ technology (Syneron Medical Ltd, Yokneam, Israel) is based on the simultaneous application of light energy to the tissue at a

Table 12.8: Herbal creams for the management of cellulite.

Herbal name	Concentration (%)	Parts of the plant	Main constituents	Mechanism of action
Bladderwrack	1	Whole dried thallus		Stimulates vascular flow
Butcher's broom	1–3	Rhizome and flowering tops	Saponins, ruscogenin and neuroruscogenin	Improves microcirculation
Ginkgo biloba	1–3			Improves microcirculation
Cynara scolymus or artichoke		Leaves, flower heads and roots	Enzymes, cynarine, ascorbic acid, caffeoylquinic acid derivatives, and flavonoids	Reduces edema and promotes diruresis
Common ivy	2	Dried leaves, stems	Saponins (especially hederin)	Improves venous and lymphatic drainage, and reduces edema
Ground ivy	2		Flavonoids, triterpenoids, and phenolic acids	Increases microvascular flow
Indian or horse chestnut	1–3	Seeds, shells	Triterpenoid saponins and flavones, coumarins acid tannins	Reduces lysosomic enzyme activity and capillary permeability
Sweet clover	2–5	Flowers and leaves	Coumarin	Reduces lymphatic edema and capillary permeability
Centella asiatica	2–5	Leaves and roots	Asiaticoside, madecassic acid, asiatic acid	Anti-inflammatory and potent healing effects
Red grapes	2–7		Tannins, procyanidins	Contains antioxidants that decrease lipid peroxidation and increase permeability of lymphatic and microarterial vessels
Corynanth yohimbe, Pausinystalia johimbe, and *Rauwolfia serpentine*		Leaves, shells, roots	Yohimbe	Stimulates metabolism of fat cells
Papaya	2–5	Fruits, leaves	Papain and bromelain (proteolytic enzymes)	Anti-inflammatory effects, decreases edema

controlled infrared (IR) wavelength, conducted RF energy, and mechanical manipulations of the skin and fat layer (Sadick NS). It was the *first medical light-based device* to achieve US Food and Drug Administration (FDA) approval.

Bipolar RF (up to 35 W) and infrared light in the wavelength range of 700–2000 nm are used to heat the subcutaneous tissue, while vacuum suction is applied to shape the skin for optimal delivery of RF energy up to a depth of 15 mm.

Mode of action: Proposed tissue reaction is an increase in local blood supply to the subcutaneous tissue promoting an increase in fat metabolism. Eventually, the mechanical action due to suction and massage lead to a collapse of fat cell clusters and fibrous bands smoothing the skin surface.

Further advancements of the VelaSmooth technology are the VelaShape™ II and VelaShape III devices (Table 12.9). Both of these devices use the combined modality treatment of controlled heating and mechanical action (Fig. 12.19) and offer a more powerful RF power of up to 150 W allowing a faster and deeper heat penetration into the tissue. With these alterations, treatment duration is shortened by approximately 30%, and fewer treatment sessions are needed.

Protocol

- A conductive fluid is used immediately before treatment to hydrate the skin surface.
- Using the handheld applicator, the area is treated with 4-6 passes by moving the handpiece back and forth several times. The applicator must be in full contact with the skin surface area to allow the vacuum to be most effective and to ensure that the electrode rollers are fully coupled to the skin. The end point of treatment is achieved when significant erythema and warmth radiating from the treated skin is observed. The average duration of a thigh and buttock treatment lasts about 30–45 minutes.

Table 12.9: Variants of VelaSmooth.

	IR power	IR light spectrum	RF power	RF frequency	Vacuum suction	Massage
VelaSmooth™ Plus	Up to 35 W	700–2000 nm	Up to 35 W	1 MHz	200 mbar	Yes
VelaShape™ II	Up to 35 W	700–2000 nm	Up to 60 W	1 MHz	200 mbar	Yes
VelaShape™ III	Up to 35 W	850 nm	Up to 150 W	1 MHz	350 mbar	Yes

(IR: infrared; RF: radiofrequency)

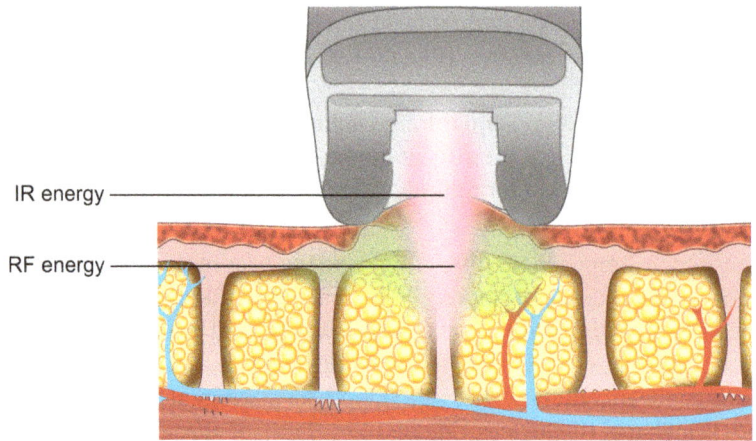

Fig. 12.19: A depiction of the dual mode of action of VelaSmooth.

- The treatment is generally very well tolerated with only minimal to no discomfort. However, heating sensations and pinching as well as transient erythema, bruising and localized swelling have been reported.

SmoothShapes®

The SmoothShapes® (Cynosure Inc., Chelmsford, MA) uses lower-level 915 nm continuous wave laser and 650 nm LED energy in combination with mechanical manipulation of the skin to treat cellulite (Fig. 12.20). This patented technology is called Photomology® and promises targeted treatment of adipose cells.

Mode of action: The infrared 915 nm laser light is known to be among the peak absorption spectra for fat (Anderson RR) while the low-level 650 nm light improves cell membrane permeability due to the creation of temporary 'pores' allowing the fat to escape in the extracellular space (Neira R). Mechanical massage then helps in the movement of the fat into the lymphatic system and promotes lymphatic drainage, subcutaneous blood flow, new collagen deposition, as well as firming and toning of the skin.

A typical treatment session is about 20 minutes for a set of body parts. Thus far, no adverse events have been reported; however, transient side effects occur. Patients may experience pain or tingling during treatment, changes in urinary habits, swelling, and skin redness.

Cellulaze™

Cellulaze™ (Cynosure Inc., Chelmsford, MA) is a minimally invasive modality approved for the treatment of cellulite. A pulsed 1440 nm Nd:YAG

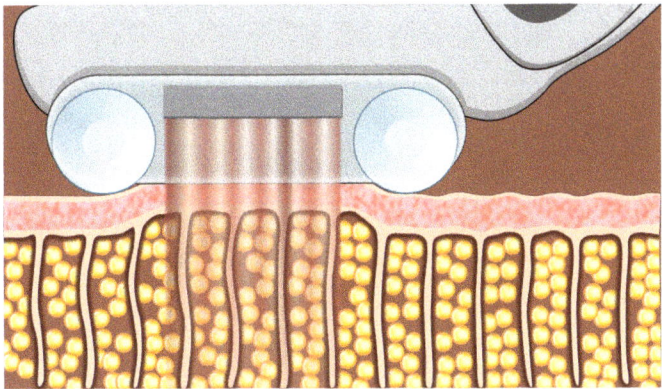

Fig. 12.20: A depiction of the energy flow of SmoothShapes®, the handheld roller glides over the treated area, creating a gentle massage-like sensation. A vacuum component positions the skin more effectively for optimal light and laser penetration. The contoured rollers assist in moving the evacuated fat and fluids from the interstitial space into the lymphatic system. A combination of light and laser energy penetrates into the tissue causing a thermal effect and increasing cell permeability, allowing fat molecules to pass through cells, away from the surface of the skin.

laser delivers energy to the dermal–hypodermal interface with the objective of treating structural features that cause the clinical appearance of cellulite.

Mode of action: The technology is believed to smooth the uneven dermal–hypodermal interface by selectively melting the hypodermal adipocytes that protrude into the dermis. It targets the hypodermal septa connecting the dermal and muscle layers by thermal subcision. Finally, it heats the dermis to increase skin thickness and elasticity by stimulating neocollagenesis and collagen remodeling (DiBernardo BE).

Protocol: The cellulaze system delivers laser energy directly to the subdermal tissue without penetrating the upper skin layer. The target area is therefore infused with tumescent solution to a maximum total volume of 1 L, before a 600 μm "side-firing" fiber enclosed in a 1 mm cannula is introduced through a small incision close to the target area below the skin surface. The cellulaze procedure is divided into following three steps (Figs. 12.21A to C).

1. In the first phase, the cannula, moved in a fanning motion, is placed in the "down" position in order to thermally denature the hypodermal adipocytes (Fig. 12.21A).
2. This is followed by the "horizontal" position that breaks the hypodermal septa by thermal subcision (Fig. 12.21B).
3. In the last position, so called "up", the fiber is positioned 2-3 mm below the skin surface to stimulate collagen remodeling, and to increase skin elasticity by heating the tissue (Fig. 12.21C).

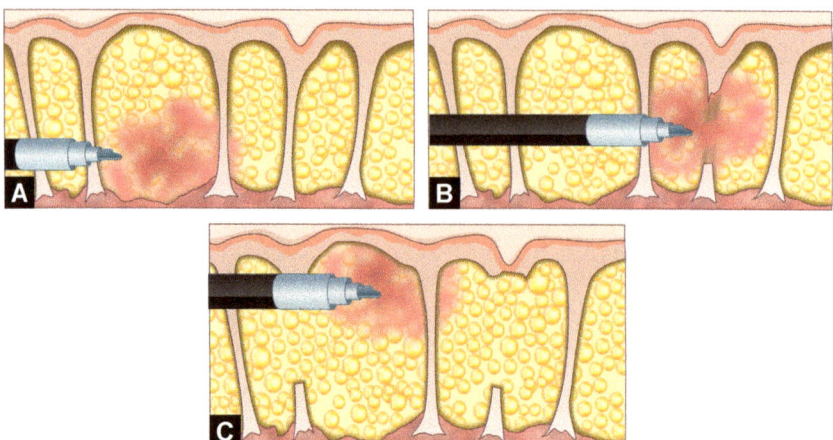

Figs. 12.21A to C: Three steps of action. (A) Denaturation of hypodermal adipocytes; (B) Denaturation of dermal septa; and (C) Stimulation of hypodermal tissue.

Both skin surface and subdermal temperature are monitored during the procedure to prevent thermal burns. Upon completion of the laser procedure, patients should wear a compression garment for up to 3 weeks post-treatment. Generally, the cellulaze procedure is relatively free of any side effects, but mild discomfort, bruising, swelling, itching, and numbness may occur. All side effects resolve within 3 months.

Combination Therapy

The application of a combination of topical and light-based approach in the treatment of cellulite has also been attempted. In one pilot, split-design, randomized study, subjects with lower extremity cellulite applied phosphatidylcholine topical gel combined with light-emitting diode (LED) of red (660 nm) and near-infrared (950 nm) wavelengths to one thigh, with placebo and LED to the contralateral thigh. Greater improvement was observed in the combination phosphatidylcholine/LED-treated thighs as compared with the placebo/LED-treated thighs (Sasaki GH).

Almost all energy devices have been combined this includes lasers, RF and ultrasound guidance USG (Kapoor R), in an attempt to target cellulite.

Future Research

Potential future areas of research employing laser and light-based technology includes the application of near-infrared wavelengths to induce neocollagenesis at the subcuticular junction.

Some novel devices have been used, including a tissue stabilized-guided subsicion system (*TS-GS system*) (Kaminer MS), *extracorporeal shockwaves* (Modena DAO), *intradermal mesotherapy* (Sylwia M) and *carboxytherapy* which is transcutaneous infusion of carbon dioxide into the affected site (Eldsouky F).

Additional areas of future research include facilitated delivery methods and photodynamic therapy as methods of boosting therapeutic efficacy. In the case of facilitated delivery, a fractional resurfacing device may be used to deliver a compound that boosts efficacy with subsequent laser and light-based technologies. Alternatively, a lipophilic photosensitizer may be combined with a laser or light of a deeply penetrating wavelength to boost adipocyte-programmed cell death. Further exploration of combination therapies to enhance efficacy using facilitated delivery, topical application of a fat metabolizer or photosensitizer concomitant with laser or light-based therapy will provide future avenues of exploration in the treatment of cellulite.

FAT

Excess adiposity is usually treated by multiple means but nonsurgical means work only for localized areas. The gold standard remains bariatric surgery. The two most commonly performed operations for obesity are laparoscopic Roux-en-Y gastric bypass and laparoscopic sleeve gastrectomy. The laparoscopic Roux-en-Y gastric bypass resulted in greater weight loss than laparoscopic sleeve gastrectomy at 5 years.

Apart from cryolipolysis, focused ultrasound is used using parameters that provide a nonthermal effect. Earlier investigations showed that the nonthermal effect may be due to mechanical cavitation of fat cells that leave surrounding structures intact. Ultrasound has been used in other areas of medicine for therapeutic indications.

LAXITY

Tissue laxity on the body can be caused by overstretching of the skin as with the postpartum abdomen, loss of collagen and elastin, gravitational forces of aging and/or excess adiposity, or sudden weight loss. Reduction of tissue laxity of the face has been a major force in facial rejuvenation over the past 5 years. It is a natural extension to consider these technologies for body contouring. Body treatments pose a challenge in that there are greater surface areas with concomitant increases in time per procedure as well as different (often greater) depths of the dermal or subdermal structures that are being tightened. Radiofrequency is the most common method used and has been used in the monopolar, bipolar, vacuum-assisted method and in combination with IR and even USG.

Mode of Action

There appears to be a unifying principle underlying all of the tissue tightening devices. Each type of technology produces heat in the dermis in a range of

1-3 mm, except those that are focused on fat, which aim for a greater depth, more like 5-7 mm. With RF, there is no specific chromophore as there is with photothermolysis, but it is an effective way of producing bulk thermal heating via capacitance coupling, tissue resistance, or induction of molecular bipole motion, the geometry of the tip, and the pattern of cooling (duration and timing) governs the depth of the heating.

With broadband light, there is a chromophore (water), although some of the strongest water-absorbing wavelengths have been blocked in the Titan handpiece; this is due to the fact that heating with these wavelengths could be too great, yielding coagulation rather than stimulation. Since this chromophore does not yield specific tissue effects because all cells contain water, it is another method of achieving bulk dermal heating. The target depth here is a bit shallower than that of Thermage®. This may yield a better performance with wrinkles, which may be why Thermage® came out with a dual tip, that contains both superficial and deep heating. Finally, ultrasound is another modality that can achieve bulk dermal heating with absorption of sound waves into tissue generating heat.

Most of the current understanding revolves around the fact that the stimulation of collagen requires the temperature of the dermis to be in the 40-60° range for a period of time. It is established that having lower fluences (temperatures) for a longer period of time is more effective at collagen stimulation than high temperature and shorter time.

Summary

A reasonable inference from multiple studies and devices is that the dermis needs to be kept at an elevated temperature, preferably in the 40-60° range to stay comfortably away from the coagulation threshold (enough for stimulation but less than coagulation), for a few minutes.

Also it is better to repeat the energy on a small area, for a period of minutes before moving on to the next area. Treating a small area like this allows it to reach the key temperature faster, and less energy is needed to keep it there for a few minutes, than treating a larger area, which allows the first area treated to cool somewhat before it is treated again. The latter is less efficient as you have to spend some time getting back to the target temperature after it has cooled.

With fat, it appears that tissue tightening devices reduce the appearance of cellulite and also improve contour via strengthening the fibrous bands that restrain the fat underneath them.

CONTOURING (BODY SHAPING)

Definition

Body contouring is defined as changing the shape and/or topography of the soft tissues of the legs, thighs, arms, and abdomen. It is thus a combination of all the aspects discussed so far. Any device that improves the appearance of cellulite will also have at least some effect on contour. Similarly, most tissue-tightening devices will have an effect on the overall shape with a contraction of the dermis and subcutaneous tissue. Finally, any type of technology that reduces the adipose compartment will change the body shape.

It is difficult to quantify three-dimensional change with current technologies. Photography is based on rendering three-dimensional objects in two dimensions and has limitations in being able to render an accurate perception of three-dimensional change, especially when it comes to the surface of the skin. Using a Vectra system (Canfield Imaging Systems, Fairfield, NJ, USA), which is a three-dimensional photography system, could be helpful in this regard but has limitations in that it is expensive and the digital files are so large that they are difficult to work with. Many of the studies on cellulite, tissue tightening, and fat reduction on the body depend on circumferential reduction as a measure of effectiveness.

Body Shaping in Clinical Practice

There is huge demand in society for loosing weight and getting better shape. Though everybody knows that diet balance and exercise are the healthy ways of achieving good weight and shape, search for a support or "quick fix" is eternal. Many of those genuinely are unable to follow this ideal healthy lifestyle. This pressing demand for slimming and shaping has evolved many scientific, nonscientific, and pseudoscientific modalities in market. A cosmetic dermatologist needs to validate these on sound scientific basis before advocating to his patients.

Weight Management versus Shape Management

Though most of the medical shaping treatments do not aim at weight loss, patient approaches cosmetic physician with expectation of weight loss only. Thorough counseling is necessary to separate weight loss from medical shaping treatments. Various options for weight loss treatments are listed here in Table 12.10.

If we gain weight we loose a good natural shape. You can get back to shape if loose the weight. This is not true every time. If weight gain is too much, tissue looses its elasticity and shape loss or tissue laxity becomes irreversible. It is also worth emphasizing that kilogram is not a correct health parameter. Rather body mass index (BMI) correlates well with health status. Scientifically fat percentage and its proportion to muscle mass and bone mass correlates best with the bodies healthy or unhealthy composition.

Devices for Body Shaping

There are various body shaping devices that are listed in Table 12.11.

Table 12.10: Overview of weight loss treatments.

Therapy options			Complications
Natural	Diet control		
	Exercise		
	Manage depression and stress	Yoga, meditation	
	Dehydration	Some slimming parlor protocols	Unhealthy
Medical	Control fat absorption	Statins	Reduce absorption of fat soluble vitamins like vitamin D3
	Reduce appetite	Metformin, sibutramine	Safe
Surgical	Reduce gastric space	Balloon, gastric stapling	Invasive procedure
	Reduce intestinal space	Intestinal bypass surgeries/anastomosis	Only for morbid obesity
Assisted fat catabolism	Faradic current stimulation of skeletal muscles	Most slimming parlor devices	Safe, may not develop proportionate muscle mass

Status of Medical Shaping Treatments

Medical shaping treatments target only subcutaneous fat and tissue tightening due to collagen remodeling in dermis, subcutaneous tissue, and deeper septae and fascia till fat and muscle layers. Though muscle toning is mostly achieved by voluntary exercises, many devices stimulating muscles by electromagnetic waves are useful. None of these technologies target visceral fat directly.

Number of adipocytes in fat layer remains same throughout life, though they swell up 3–4 times of their original size to store more fat. Most of fat loss after diet and exercise is reversible as only fat content of adipocytes is reduced which eventually get reversed. Adipolysis is a term used for "permanent destruction of fat cells".

Liposuction is the gold standard treatment for adipolysis of subcutaneous fat. Tumescent anesthesia in liposuction coupled with use of microcannula has consistently proven safer option compared to general anesthesia procedure. Many energy-based devices (EBDs) are tried as adjuvant in liposuction including RF, optical fibers emitting lasers like diode, and Nd:YAG of various wavelengths between 900 nm and 1,500 nm (Table 12.12). Most optical bare fibers emit laser energy in forward direction. LipoLife™ has developed radially emit tip of 1,470 nm laser energy with diameter of 600 µ called angel fiber. The RF tips or tip of bare optical fibers had a risk to get

Table 12.11: Overview of medical shaping devices.

Target	Mechanism	Options	Comments
Fat	Fat loss: Lipolysis	Noninvasive	Diet, exercise, muscle stimulation, massage, etc.
	Fat cell destruction: Adipolysis	Surgical	Liposuction with or without general anesthesia, with or without EBD like laser, or RF
		Nonsurgical	Chemical lipolysis, injection lipolysis with PPC/DC
			Cryolipolysis (Figs. 12.22A to C)
			Cavitation ultrasound
			HIFU
Tissue collagen		Noninvasive	• HIFU • RF: Monopolar, bipolar, tripolar, multipolar, MNRF, and IR lasers
		Invasive	ThermiRF™, optical fiber subdermal laser ablation
Muscle tone	Electrical stimulation in muscles		
Cellulite	Lymphatic drainage and microcirculation	Pneumatic pressure devices	Pressure and massage devices, intermittent positive pressure body suits
	Cutting superficial fibrous septae	RF and optical fiber laser devices	
	Biomodulation	LLLT, LED, and whole body cryotherapy	(Zerona™), efficacy not reproduced consistently

(DC: deoxycholate; EBD: energy-based device; HIFU: high-intensity focused ultrasound; LED: light-emitting diode; LLLT: low-level laser therapy; MNRF: microneedling radiofrequency; PPC: phosphatidylcholine)

stuck to tissue and causing skin burn. Innovation of placing radially emitting optical fiber inside fenestrated tip of cannula allows the energy to reach the tissue but virtually no contact.

The author (Dhepe NV) has an experience of using 1,470 nm LipoLife™ for liposuction in 63 cases with tumescent local anesthesia (Figs. 12.23 and 12.24). All cases have instant recovery that make the patient walk out with a pressure garment within 20–30 minutes of the procedure. Average aspirate was 3–5 liters of supernatant fat. Average pinch thickness measured on caliper was 65%. Addition of 1,470 nm laser added significant skin tightening effect to the procedure. None of the patient develops skin burn or laser-related side effects.

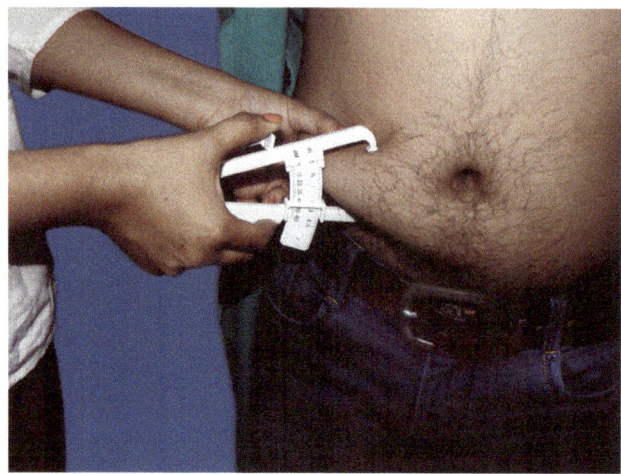

Fig. 12.22A: Measurement of subcutaneous fat. Pinch thickness measured by a caliper before cryolipolysis.

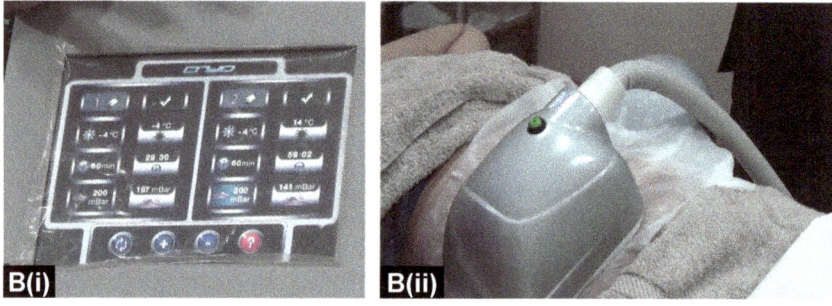

Figs. 12.22B(i) and (ii): Cymedics Cryo™ cryolipolysis using suction probe on 200 mBar negative pressure, reaching tissue temperature −4°C maintained for 60 minutes.

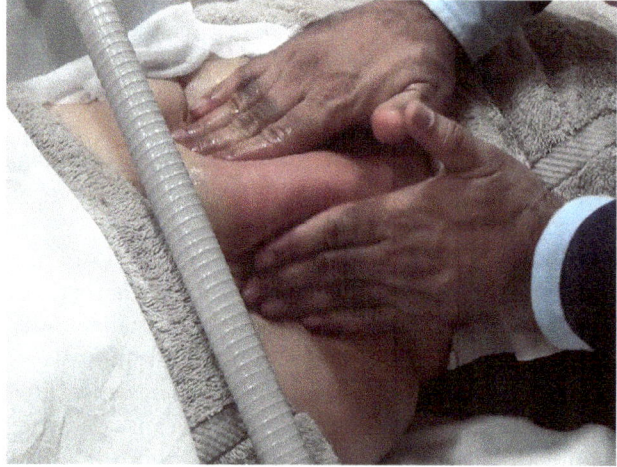

Fig. 12.22C: Manual massage after removal of probe will improve adipolytic activity.

CHAPTER 12: Clinical Indications

Table 12.12: Overview of liposuction procedure.

Parameter	Mechanism	Comment
Anesthesia	General or spinal	Unsafe
	Tumescent local	Safe
Cannula	Large cannula	Unsafe
	Microcannula	Safe
Energy	Manual	
	Power assisted/vibrations	MicroAir™
	High flow water jet	WaterJet™
	Forward emitting bare laser fibers of 980 nm, 1,420 nm, 1,320 nm, etc.	Cynosure and many other devices
	Radially emitting angel fiber in silhouette	1,470 nm Alma LipoLife™

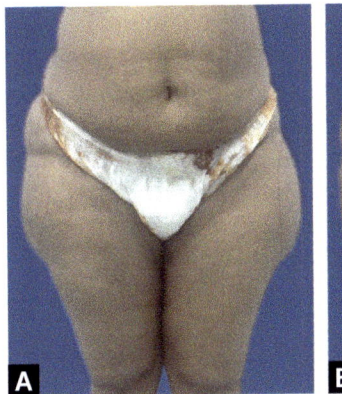
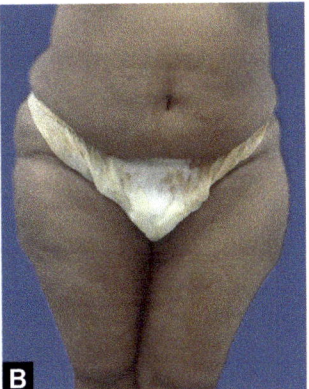

Figs. 12.23A and B: 1,470 nm LipoLife™ laser liposuction under tumescent local anesthesia. Patients walk out within 10 minutes of surgery. Alma LipoLifeTM machine and 1,470 nm radially emitting 600 µ "angel fiber" that sits within fenestrated tip of suction cannula making it "silhouette laser".

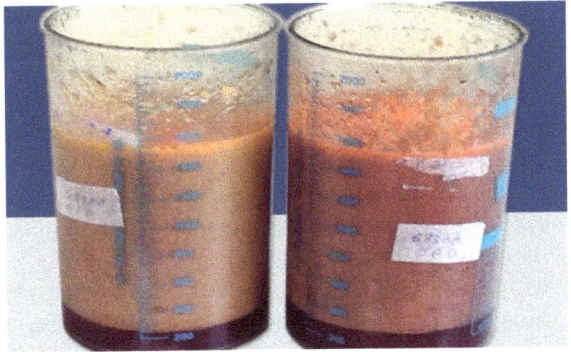

Fig. 12.24: Yellow fat removed with safeLIPO™ using microcanular technique followed by 1,470 LipoLife laser liposuction total blood loss in procedure may not be more than 300 cc.

CONCLUSION

There are a plethora of noninvasive body contouring modalities, including cryolipolysis, RF, low-level laser therapy (LLLT), and high-intensity focused ultrasound (HIFU). Though studies have shown statistical significant effects on body contouring, and removing unwanted fat and cellulite, the clinical effects are mild to moderate, for example, 2–4 cm circumference reduction as a sign of subcutaneous fat reduction after total treatment sessions.

Overall, there is no definitive noninvasive treatment method for cellulite. Additionally, due to the methodological differences in the existing evidence, comparing the technique is difficult (Alizadeh Z). For tissue tightening, cellulite, and fat reduction, the present-time, head-to-head studies comparing the devices are limited, and as a result, it is difficult to definitively compare the efficacy of the devices.

Various EBDs have definitely a role in body shaping but is exaggerated by media and device industries. Almost all the scientific studies on these modalities state their inclusion criteria or the ideal candidate who gets good results; "Young, healthy, not overweight, weight and BMI near normal range, active, and having localized fat deposition not responding to diet and exercise". Such candidates really respond very well. Huge cost incurred in these treatments makes the patient undermine importance of diet, exercise, and healthy lifestyle. Proper counseling of patient to expect realistically, emphasis on lifestyle management, and choosing right technology as per the mechanism suitable that patient will ensure good results in body shaping and happy patients.

BIBLIOGRAPHY

1. Alizadeh Z, Halabchi F, Mazaheri R, et al. Review of the mechanisms and effects of noninvasive body contouring devices on cellulite and subcutaneous fat. Int J Endocrinol Metab. 2016;14(4):e36727.
2. Anderson RR, Farinelli W, Laubach H, et al. Selective photothermolysis of lipid-rich tissues: A free electron laser study. Lasers Surg Med. 2006;38:913-9.
3. DiBernardo BE. Treatment of cellulite using a 1440-nm pulsed laser with one-year follow-up. J Am Soc Aesthetic Plast Surg. 2011;31:328-41.
4. Eldsouky F, Ebrahim HM. Evaluation and efficacy of carbon dioxide therapy (carboxytherapy) versus mesolipolysis in the treatment of cellulite. J Cosmet Laser Ther. 2018;17:1-6.
5. Hexsel DM, Abreu M, Rodrigues TC, et al. Side-by-side comparison of areas with and without cellulite depressions using magnetic resonance imaging. Dermatol Surg. 2009;35:1471-7.
6. Kaminer MS, Coleman WP, Weiss RA, et al. A multicenter pivotal study to evaluate tissue stabilized-guided subcision using the Cellfina device for the treatment of cellulite with 3-year follow-up. Dermatol Surg. 2017;43(10):1240-8.

7. Kapoor R, Shome D, Ranjan A. Use of a novel combined radiofrequency and ultrasound device for lipolysis, skin tightening and cellulite treatment. J Cosmet Laser Ther. 2017;19(5):266-74.
8. Modena DAO, da Silva CN, Grecco C, et al. Extracorporeal shockwave: Mechanisms of action and physiological aspects for cellulite, body shaping, and localized fat-Systematic review. J Cosmet Laser Ther. 2017;19(6):314-9.
9. Neira R, Arroyave J, Ramirez H, et al. Fat liquefaction: Effect of low-level laser energy on adipose tissue. Plast Reconstr Surg. 2002;110:912-25.
10. Nürnberger F, Müller G. So-called cellulite: An invented disease. J Dermatol Surg Oncol. 1978;4:221-9.
11. Sadick NS, Mulholland RS. A prospective clinical study to evaluate the efficacy and safety of cellulite treatment using the combination of optical and RF energies for subcutaneous tissue heating. J Cosmet Laser Ther. 2004;6:187-90.
12. Sasaki GH, Oberg K, Tucker B, et al. The effectiveness and safety of topical PhotoActif phosphatidylcholine-based anti-cellulite gel and LED (red and near-infrared) light on grade II-III thigh cellulite: A randomized, double-blinded study. J Cosmet Laser Ther. 2007;9:87-96.
13. Sylwia M, Krzysztof MR. Efficacy of intradermal mesotherapy in cellulite reduction—Conventional and high-frequency ultrasound monitoring results. J Cosmet Laser Ther. 2017;19(6):320-4.

12E. MISCELLANEOUS LASER RESPONSIVE DISORDERS

Kabir Sardana, Ashraf Badawi, Aastha Gupta, Ananta Khurana, Sidharth Tandon, Khushbu Goel, Red Alinsod, Niteen V Dhepe, Avitus John Raakesh Prasad, Ajay Deshpande, Surabhi Sinha

INTRODUCTION

There are numerous indications for lasers. Most of them are not yet approved, but considering the liberal United States Food and Drug Administration (US FDA) approvals, it is likely that they will be listed soon. We will give a brief overview of them and for the sake of convenience are listing them alphabetically.

Some of the indications like excimer light therapy for psoriasis and vitiligo are approved, but it is the authors' opinion, based on objective evaluation of studies, that in tropical countries with a high ambient ultraviolet (UV) flux, conventional phototherapy is a cost-effective option with good efficacy. Other indications like lasers for onychomycosis and hair growth are also approved, but very few randomized controlled trials (RCTs) have been published. However, as these devices are increasingly being used in practice, an overview will nevertheless be given, hoping that the reader is able to choose the ideal treatment option.

ACNE

Light-based therapies are an attractive alternative therapy because they potentially offer a more rapid onset and better patient compliance with a low incidence of adverse events. However, optimal treatment methods and the relative efficacy of light-based therapies as compared to traditional therapies remain unclear. Light-based acne therapies are generally thought to act via reducing *Propionibacterium acnes* proliferation or by targeting the sebaceous gland to reduce sebum production; however, other mechanisms may exist (Table 12.13).

Mode of Action of Devices

Propionibacterium acnes produce endogenous porphyrins that are photoactivated, thus producing singlet oxygen species and free radicals that may result in bacterial destruction.

Blue light results in the most pronounced photoactivation of endogenous porphyrins. However, its clinical efficacy is limited by a shallow depth of penetration. Combined blue and red light and photopneumatic therapy are potentially the most promising therapies for acne that are believed to work, at least in part, by targeting *Propionibacterium acnes*. The IPL can be used in

Table 12.13: Summary of devices that have a role in acne therapy.

Inhibits Propionibacterium acnes	Inhibits sebaceous gland	Inhibits sebaceous gland and Propionibacterium acnes
Blue and red light	1,320 nm Nd:YAG laser	Photodynamic therapy
IPL	1,450 nm diode laser	
Photopneumatic therapy	1,540 nm erbium:glass laser	
532 nm KTP laser		
585/595 nm PDL		

(IPL: intense pulsed light; KTP: potassium titanyl phosphate; Nd:YAG: neodymium-doped yttrium aluminum garnet; PDL: pulsed dye laser)

appropriate settings with good results (Figs. 12.25A to C). The machine used is crucial and another set of images are depicted (Figs. 12.25D and E) using the Magma by Forma TK (Israel).

Infrared wavelength lasers are often able to treat acne by causing sebaceous gland alterations while preserving epidermal integrity. Variable clinical responses have been observed with the 1,450 nm diode, 1,320 nm neodymium-doped yttrium aluminum garnet (Nd:YAG), and 1,540 nm erbium:glass lasers that target sebaceous glands. Our own experience with the erbium:glass (Lux Palomar) has been that there is a certain degree of improvement of acne, but this cannot justify using it for acne. Most of the studies in literature use the laser devices as adjuncts to conventional therapy in acne.

A recent study used a dual mode Qs and LP Nd:YAG (Bakus AD) in patients *without* any active medical therapy for acne. The logic proposed was that the 1,064-nm Nd:YAG laser can penetrate deeply into the dermis causing diffuse dermal heating while limiting epidermal damage. In this study of moderate to severe inflammatory acne, significant reductions were observed in the acne lesion count immediately after treatment (81% reduction) which persisted even after 2 years. The procedure was done in two steps. The first step entailed the use of a 60 ms LP YAG (10-mm spot size, 60-ms pulse duration, energy fluences of 20 to 23 J/cm^2) which would thermally impact the sebaceous gland, resulting in reduced sebum output. The settings were such that the inflammation from the laser was limited. The second stage used the Q-switched Nd:YAG with low energy (6-mm spot size and energy fluences of 1.1 to 1.3 J/cm^2), that induced power density enough to have a deep and superficial effect with the aim of normalizing the hyperkeratinization of the follicular epithelium. This is a significant study as no concomitant medication was used and moreover this wavelength is safe in patients of skin of color.

A study examined the use of isotretinoin at a low dose of 10 mg followed after 30–45 days by the NAFL using the 1,550-nm Er:glass fractional laser (Sellas, Korea) in a split face study. Three treatments were administered at

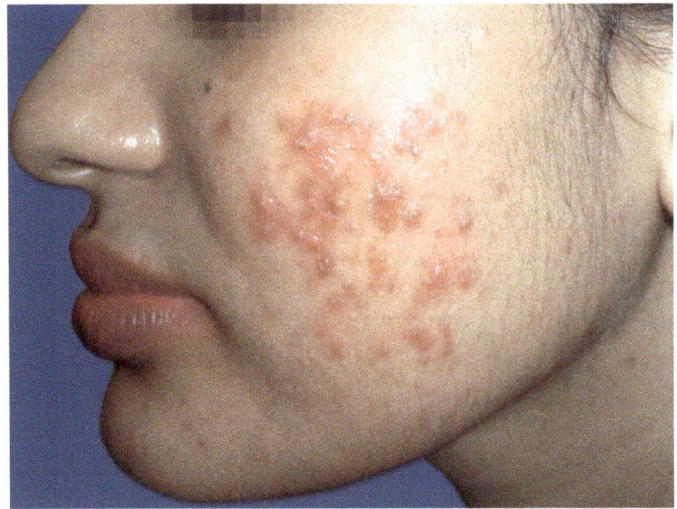

Fig. 12.25A: A case of steroid acne, refused medical management and peels, opted only for IPL. She was treated only with IPL.
Settings: 410 nm filter (Blue) with fluence of 18–20 J/cm², pulse number 3, pulse duration 3, 4, and 5 ms with a pulse delay of 10 ms was done first, followed by 560 nm filter (Yellow) with same parameters and fluence of 23–26 J/cm².

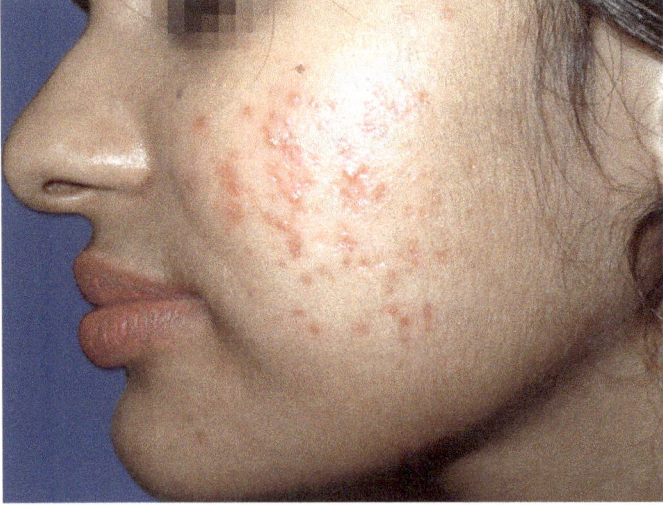

Fig. 12.25B: Two sessions of previous settings 2 weeks apart resulted in reduction of acne with residual macular erythema and scarring. This was followed by the 530 nm filter (Green) with fluence of 21–23 J/cm², pulse number 3, pulse duration 3, 4, and 5 ms with a pulse delay of 10 ms, followed by 590 nm filter (Orange) to improve the scars with same parameters and fluence of 27–29 J/cm².

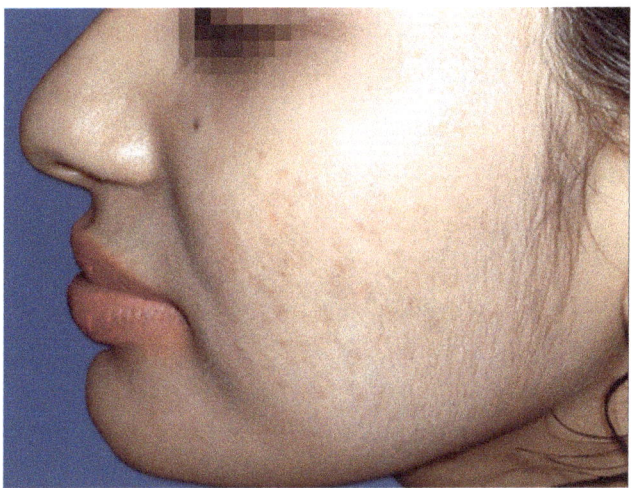

Fig. 12.25C: Three sessions of previous settings 3 weeks apart resulted in reduction of macular erythema and scarring.
The Orange (585–590 nm) filter helps in remodeling the scars once acne treatment is over.

monthly intervals, in a low energy setting (20 mJ/cm^2 and 100–169 points per area). Though both sides improved, comedone formation was less on the laser treated side. Scars, except the ice pick scars, improved. Though this work mirrors previous publications (Sardanak et al.) the highlight is the use of isotretinoin with lasers, here note the sequential use and low dose of isotretinoin used (Xia J et al.).

Photodynamic therapy (PDT) is potentially an effective light-based acne therapy and may cause photodestruction of both *Propionibacterium acnes* and sebaceous glands. The optimal photosensitizer, light source, and therapeutic protocol for PDT as a treatment for acne are unknown.

The PDT using the Indocyanine green-dye is usually done with 805-nm diode lasers because the peak absorption wavelength of ICG is closest to 805 nm. As 830 nm is also close to the peak absorption wavelength of ICG, this can also be used and was shown in a study by Choi SH et al. to have bactericidal effects on *P. acne*. This study showed that ICG-based PDT using an 830-nm LED had a significant clinical effect on reducing acne severity. Also compared with 805-nm diode lasers, 830-nm LED can be used to irradiate lesions all at once and can penetrate deeper into the skin (Choi SH et al.).

Photopneumatic devices that combine gentle negative pressure with broadband pulsed light simultaneously to attack multiple targets in the skin for better treatment outcome have also been used in acne and may represent a extension of the use of IPL in acne (Rajabi-Estarabadi A et al.).

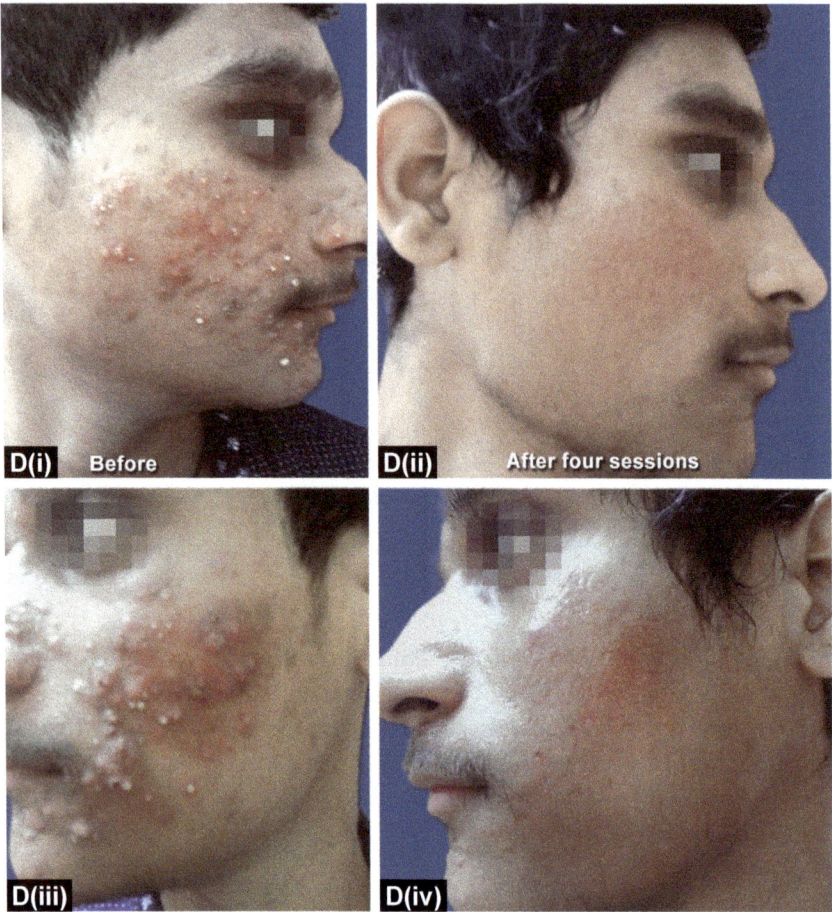

Figs. 12.25D(i) to (iv): Steroid induced acne. 440–1,100 nm filter: 7.1 mJ/cm² continuous mode six passes followed by 14.1 mJ/cm². Single pulse mode over the lesions six passes weekly.
Source: Magma by FormaTK (Israel).

Summary

A recent study has shown that fractional radiofrequency (RF) can also help ameliorate active acne. Though the study designs of the various clinical trials in this area make it impossible to draw firm conclusions at this time, there is considerable evidence that light-based therapies that act via photodestruction of *Propionibacterium acnes*, may be capable of clinically improving acne. As light-based therapies are well tolerated and have a low incidence of adverse events, they may be used as an adjunct to medical therapy.

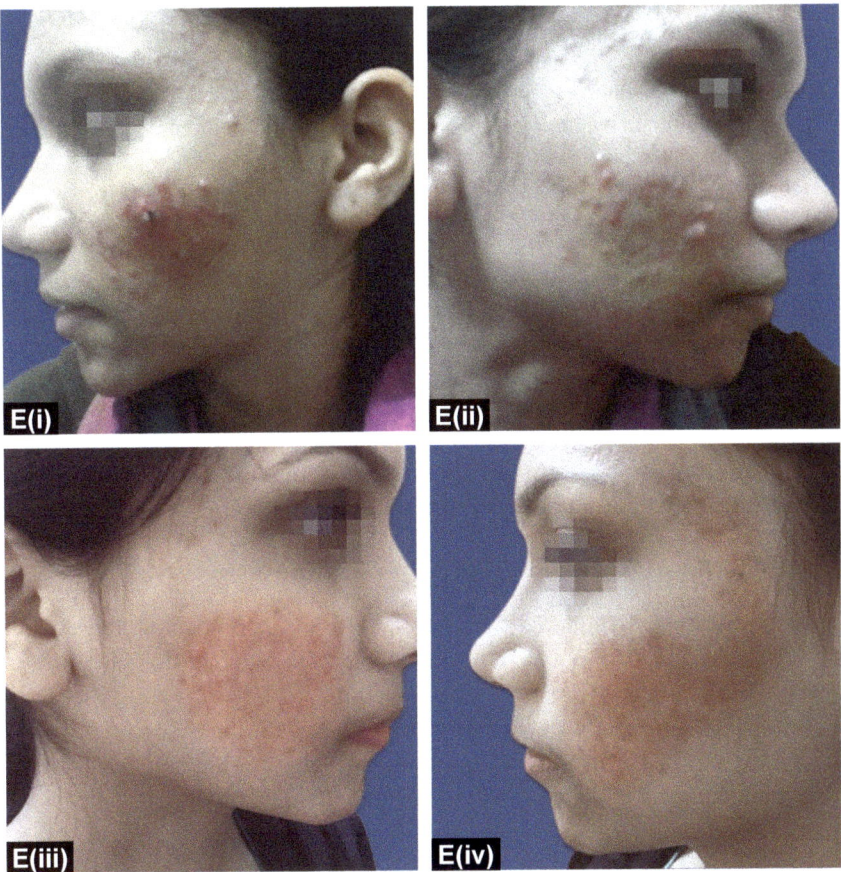

Figs. 12.25E(i) to (iv): Acne vulgaris—papulo-pustular. 440–1,100 nm continuous mode 7.1 mJ/cm² six passes followed by 14.1 mJ/cm².

BIBLIOGRAPHY

1. Bakus AD, Yaghmai D, Massa MC, et al. Sustained benefit after treatment of acne vulgaris using only a novel combination of long-pulsed and Q-switched 1064-nm Nd: YAG lasers. Dermatol Surg. 2018;44(11):1402-10.
2. Bogle MA, Dover JS, Arndt KA, et al. Evaluation of the 1,540-nm erbium:glass laser in the treatment of inflammatory facial acne. Dermatol Surg. 2007;33:810-7.
3. Choi SH, Seo JW, Kim KH. Comparative study of the bactericidal effects of indocyanine green- and methyl aminolevulinate-based photodynamic therapy on Propionibacterium acnes as a new treatment for acne. J Dermatol. 2018;45(7):824-9.
4. Clark C, Bryden A, Dawe R, et al. Topical 5-aminolaevulinic acid photodynamic therapy for cutaneous lesions: outcome and comparison of light sources. Photodermatol Photoimmunol Photomed. 2003;19:134-41.

5. Lee KR, Lee EG, Lee HJ, et al. Assessment of treatment efficacy and sebo-suppressive effect of fractional radiofrequency microneedle on acne vulgaris. Lasers Surg Med. 2013;45:639-47.
6. Rajabi-Estarabadi A, Choragudi S, Camacho I, et al. Effectiveness of photopneumatic technology: a descriptive review of the literature. Lasers Med Sci. 2018;33(8):1631-7.
7. Sardana K, Manjhi M, Garg VK, et al. Which type of atrophic acne scar (ice-pick, boxcar, or rolling) responds to nonablative fractional laser therapy? Dermatol Surg. 2014;40:288-300.
8. Xia J, Hu G, Hu D, et al. Concomitant Use of 1,550-nm nonablative fractional laser with low-dose isotretinoin for the treatment of acne vulgaris in Asian patients: A randomized split-face controlled study. Dermatol Surg. 2018;44(9):1201-8.

BENIGN DISORDERS, TUMORS, AND CYSTS

Though most of these lesions have been discussed in the chapter on Ablative Lasers, a few uncommon indications are discussed here.

Epithelioma Adenoides Cysticum (Trichoepithelioma)

This condition is characterized by small, colorless papules that are located mainly on nasolabial folds. Histologically they are hair follicle tumors (trichoepitheliomas).

There are reports about successful treatment with the argon and carbon dioxide (CO_2) lasers in individual cases. Recurrences depend on ablation depth and are part of the nature of the disease (Sajben FP et al.).

Fibrous Papule of the Nose

These lesions are variously described as a fibroma or a regressive fibrosed nevus. These lesions, which occur mostly isolated on the tip of the nose, are essentially a cosmetic issue. Before laser therapy was introduced, excisions and cauterization were the main treatment options.

Due to the fibrous structure, ablation with the *erbium-doped yttrium aluminum garnet (Er:YAG) or pulsed CO_2* is an excellent choice. The CO_2 laser, used at a setting of *0.1 s, and a total fluence of 1-5 J/cm^2 is ideal* (also see Chapter 2: Ablative Lasers). The pulsed dye laser (PDL) and the argon laser can also be considered as therapeutic options.

Koenen Tumors

Laser vaporization of Koenen tumors with a *CO_2 laser* proved to be similar to conventional surgical techniques in terms of cosmetic satisfaction. There are two advantages though of using this laser, first is the lack of bleeding and second the short operating time with excellent cosmetic and functional outcome.

Neurofibromas

Surgical Excision

This is the simplest option and an elliptical excision is an effective, inexpensive treatment, and is useful when only few lesions are present.

Lasers

- Carbon dioxide laser resurfacing can be utilized for facial lesions but not for nonfacial sites as there is a high risk of hypertrophic scar/keloid formation.
   A cutting technique can be utilized to excise them using a continuous mode, 15–30 W, and the lesion is cut until the desired depth is obtained. To undermine the lesion, the laser probe can be defocused, this also helps to coagulate the vessels.
   For smaller lesions a vaporization technique may be utilized to flatten and remove the lesions using a defocused beam of 3–6 W, ablating to the level of the adjacent normal skin. The use of saline between passes is useful to remove the char.
   Another method used is by opening the epidermis, after which the neurofibroma can be pressed out and ablated. Removal should always be done completely down to the base to prevent quick recurrence (Figs. 12.26A to E).
- *Erbium-doped yttrium aluminum garnet*: Kardorff has published reports about successful therapy of neurofibromas using the Er:YAG laser in combination with surgical excision. This is not usually preferred as the laser does not have an efficient coagulation profile.
   Interstitial photocoagulation can be performed for the treatment of bulkier lesions, including nonfacial lesions.
- *Diode 975 nm*: A prototype, diode laser with a central wavelength 975 nm, that has been used in ENT and penetrates deeply was studied by Szymanczyk J. The results seem impressive but more data would be needed, for establishing commercial viability, though the machine looks like a handy device.

Seborrheic Keratoses

Various treatments options include cryotherapy, electrodesiccation, curettage, and laser therapy. Most often, the traditional methods of treating seborrheic keratoses (SKs) are more appropriate. If there is an acute eruption of widespread lesions, perform a review of systems and consider a full physical examination to rule out any underlying medical condition or carcinoma (sign of Leser-Trélat).

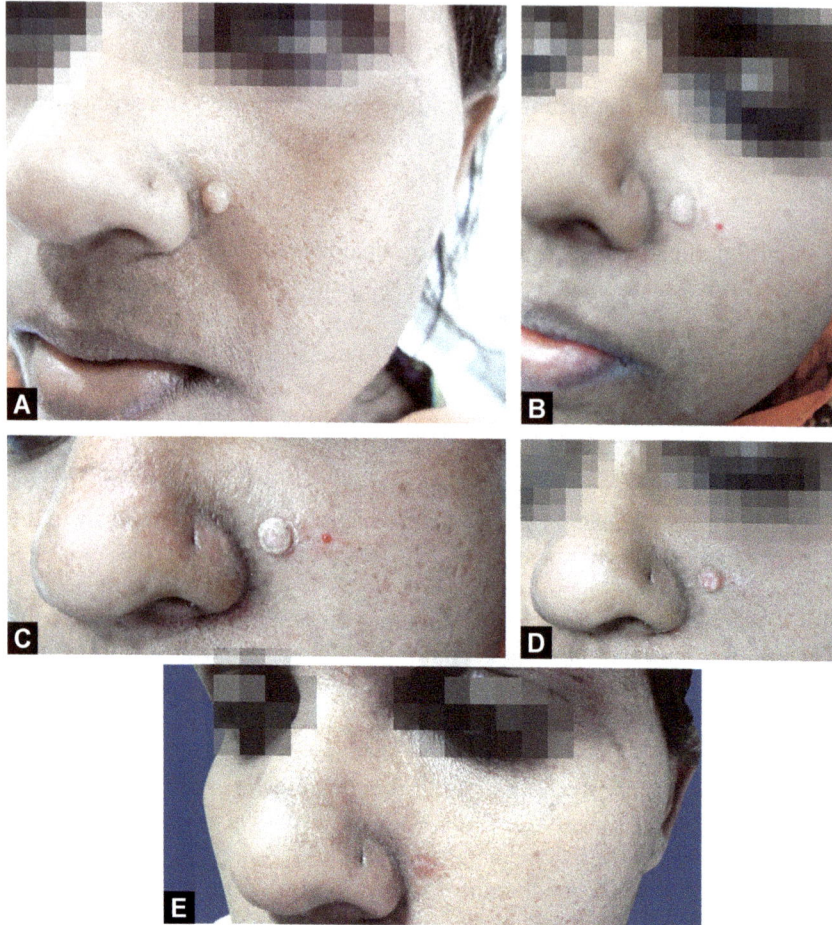

Figs. 12.26A to E: (A) A neurofibroma on the side of the nose; (B) Local anesthesia is given; (C) The Er:YAG (dermablate) is used to first ablate the epidermis (7 J/cm², 2 Hz); (D) The Er:YAG ablation is continued till bleeding occurs signifying lower papillary dermis. After this the pulsed CO_2 is used to destroy the base; and (E) Post-treatment photograph showing complete healing of the lesion. (CO_2: carbon dioxide; Er:YAG: erbium-doped yttrium aluminum garnet).

Treatment

- *Cryotherapy*: Light cryotherapy is a rapid, inexpensive, and effective method for treating SKs.
- *Curettage and light cautery*: Electrodesiccation of SKs is another effective measure and with RF a better surgical cosmesis can be achieved.
- *Shave excision*: Shave excision can effectively remove SKs.
- *Lasers*: Lasers if used should be used at the lowest fluence, with a short pulse duration. If used in a wrong dose it can cause more harm than good. An overview is given here, and our preferred laser is the Er:YAG.

i. *Melanin targeting lasers for thin seborrheic keratoses*: Q-switched ruby (694 nm) and Q-switched alexandrite (755 nm), and the long-pulsed 532 nm lasers can effectively treat thin SKs. The problem is that the results are usually not as good as ablative lasers and may require multiple sessions.
ii. *Ablative lasers*: Seborrheic keratoses are common benign, epidermal neoplasms that are very variable in number, size, and color. There are numerous methods of removal including electrofulguration.

If an ablative laser is used an ultrapulse CO_2 or a superpulsed CO_2 with a pulse duration of 1.2 ms and a long interval of 50 ms is appropriate. If the continuous wave (CW) is used a pulse duration of 0.1 s, and a total fluence of 1–5 J/cm^2 is ideal. The lowest possible fluence should be used. This is to avoid pigmentary sequelae.

Amongst the ablative lasers we favor the use of the Er:YAG as it ensures an accurate depth of penetration and excellent healing. A dose of 3–5 J/cm^2 at 2 Hz gives rapid results (Dmovsek-Olup B). A single laser impulse is adequate for most lesions. Some wipe the area with normal saline, which helps to visualize the dermis, though it is better to leave the residue as it affords a biological healing and sheds off in 3–5 days. A controlled superpulsed CO_2 is another option (Fitzpatrick RE).

A case with the dosimetry is depicted in Figures 12.27A to F. Interestingly this patient kept developing SK rapidly and later on was diagnosed as a case of pancreatic cancer. So, sign of Leser-Trélat can be rarely associated and I (Kabir Sardana) now advise patients for a positron emission tomography-computed tomography (PET-CT), in case of rapidly progressive SK to avoid any medicolegal issues.

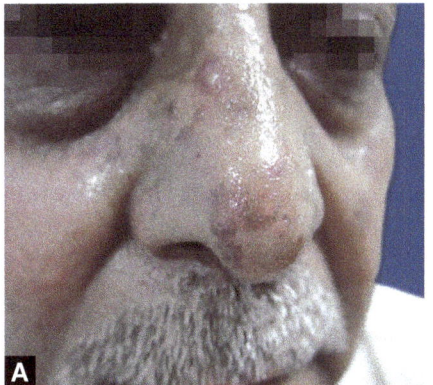 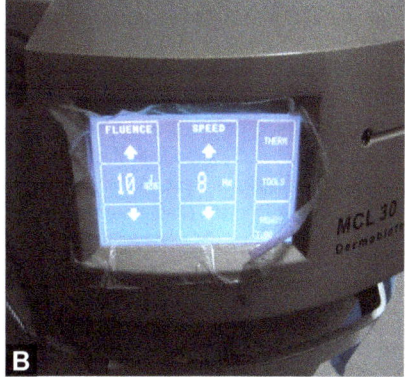

Figs. 12.27A and B: A case with SK. The settings used in the Er:YAG depend on the ease of use, here the settings are of 10 J/cm^2, the speed can vary, if you want fast turnaround time increase the frequency. If the lesion is near the eye one can reduce the Hz. The advantage of the Er:YAG is that the laser removes the skin in layers with predictable end points unlike the CO_2 which tends to coagulate the vessels. (SK: seborrheic keratosis; CO_2: carbon dioxide; Er:YAG: erbium-doped yttrium aluminum garnet)

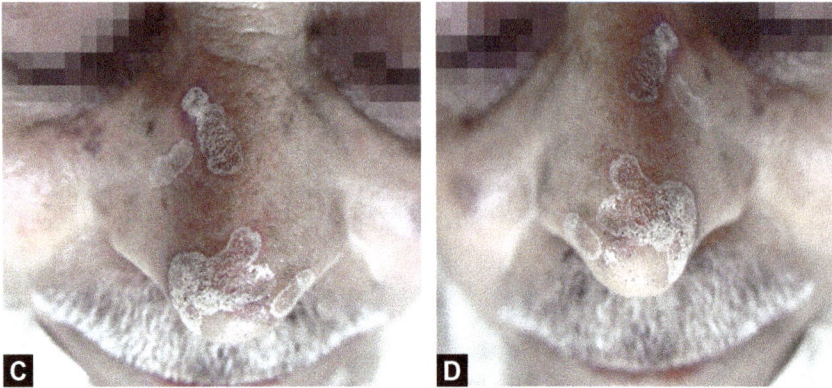

Figs. 12.27C and D: The first pass shows the characteristic whitening of the epidermis. This occurs because the laser has the highest absorption coefficient for water. This also makes it a very safe laser. Another pass (right) removes the lesion and also the epidermis.

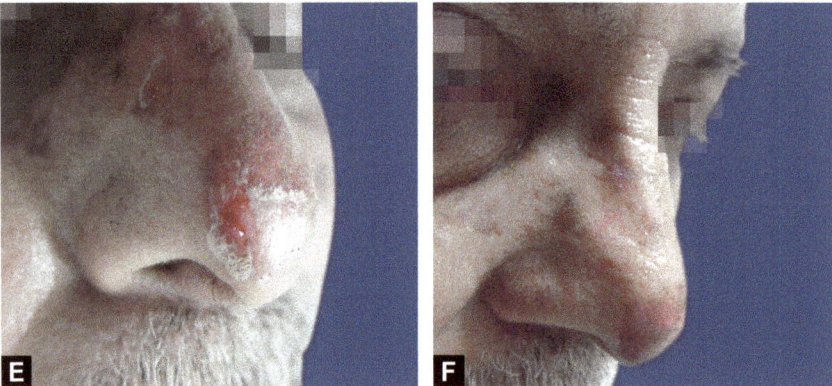

Figs. 12.27E and F: Note the papillary dermis bleed. This is the most accurate indicator of entering the dermis. Most CO_2 lasers are "blind" as clinicians use settings in excess of the optimal pulse duration and interval. The Er:YAG has a pulse duration in microseconds. Most CO_2 used have a setting from 0.1 s to 1 s. This leads to coagulation and thus, there is no clean lasers end point. The ideal settings to replicate such fine end points with an SpCO_2 is to use a pulse duration less than 2 ms and an interval of 50 ms. As most "run of the mill" CO_2 are calibrated in seconds, this (2 ms) corresponds to 0.002 s, and I have rarely seen such a laser with most practitioners. The right image shows the almost perfect ablation with excellent cosmesis. (CO_2: carbon dioxide; Er:YAG: erbium-doped yttrium aluminum garnet)

Sebaceous Hyperplasia

It is a common benign condition of the sebaceous glands of middle-aged adults or older individuals with small yellowish or skin colored papules of size 2-9 mm, normally with a central umbilication, located on the face (particularly the nose, cheek, and forehead) (Fig. 12.27G).

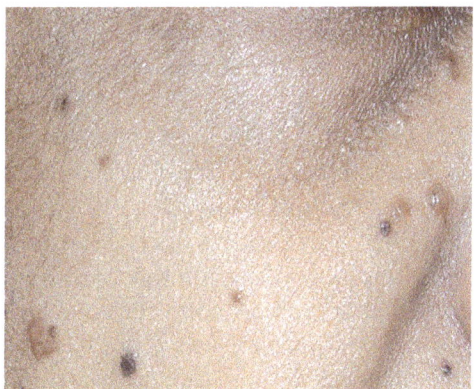

Fig. 12.27G: Note the skin colored, shiny papules with a central depression: Sebaceous hyperplasia.

Treatment

Like most benign sebaceous gland tumors, the patient should be forewarned about the variable response of treatment and the fact that the course and further lesions are not influenced by the laser therapy. Oral isotretinoin has been shown to be effective in removing some lesions after 2-6 weeks of treatment, but the recurrence of the lesions is common after cessation of therapy.

- *Cautery*:
  - "Light" cryotherapy and electrosurgery are fast and cheap options.
- *Laser therapy*:
  i. The 1,450 nm diode laser has been studied in 10 patients.
     Each patient was treated one to five times with fluences of 16-17 J/cm^2 with a cooling interval of 40-50 ms. After two to three treatments with the diode laser, 84% of lesions decreased in size greater than 50%, and 70% decreased greater than 75%.
  ii. Pulsed dye laser (585 nm) has been shown to improve sebaceous hyperplasia.
     The settings were three stacked 5 mm pulses at fluences of 7 J/cm^2 and 7.5 J/cm^2. Most lesions responded after one treatment session with flattening, shrinking, or resolution. However, this does not prevent recurrence.
  iii. Erbium-doped yttrium aluminum garnet or CO_2 can also improve the disorder. The goal is to ablate at a dose less than 5 J/cm^2 and flatten the lesion till the surrounding skin and then give one more pass. With CO_2, use the ultrapulse or superpulse mode. If the latter is used, this is one indication where one can set it to 0.1 s, though the ideal pulse

duration would be less than 50 ms preferably 10 ms (0.01–0.05 s). This achieves rapid ablation with minimum thermal damage.
iv. Laser-assisted PDT.
v. *1720 nm device*: A problem with most of the existing therapies is that they are essentially ablative and as they do not target the chromophore and they do *not* follow the principles of selective photothermolysis and hence either fail or cause scarring. Also most would use conservative settings hence only the superficial component of the lesion is treated, leading to rapid recurrence. A novel report noted almost complete clearance of sebaceous hyperplasia lesions without depressions or scarring that highlights the applicability of the intrinsic selectivity of 1,720 nm laser device (Winstanley D et al.). This was based on the fact it has been shown that human fat has absorption peaks at 1,210 nm and 1,720 nm.

Xanthelasma

This is a benign disorder characterized by yellowish plaques typically located in the periorbital region, especially in the inner corner of the eyes and upper eyelids; it is also the most common form of skin xanthoma. The lesions are permanent and have a tendency to progress and coalesce.

They are due to accumulation of fat within the histiocytes, known as foamy histiocytes, located mainly in the upper reticular dermis. The main component is accumulated cholesterol, which for the most part is esterified.

In 50% of patients, normal serum levels of cholesterol are found. The main association is with hypertriglyceridemia, found in 50% of cases. Reduced high-density lipoprotein (HDL) level can be found in some patients. The diagnosis is clinical, but it should be remembered that about half of patients have abnormal lipid levels; therefore, they should have their values measured frequently. Some drugs, such as nilotinib, used to treat chronic myelogenous leukemia, may cause xanthelasma (Sayin et al. 2016).

Treatment

Xanthelasmas often recur after treatment with any modality.
- *Surgical excision*: Surgical excision is the treatment of choice for xanthelasmas. The lesion is lifted and then excised using a blade or a Gradle scissor. The defect is either left to heal by second intention or sutured using silk or ethilon sutures. This procedure usually results in a very cosmetically acceptable outcome and ophthalmologists are particularly adept at this procedure. In clinical practice though, surgical removal is best indicated for cases of diffuse xanthelasma, deep involvement of the dermis and/or muscle. Recurrence is common, with rate of about 40%.
- *Localized tissue destruction*: Trichloroacetic acid (TCA) (30–90%), depending on the lesion size and thickness is the preferred agent.

- The pingyangmycin family antibiotic bleomycin, can be injected into the lesions with good results (Wang et al. 2016).
- Lasers.
    i. *Why laser therapy for xanthelasma?*
    Laser therapy is well established in the treatment of xanthelasma allowing bloodless removal with minimal scarring, pain, and perilesional inflammation. It is a viable alternative to surgical excision (which is a preferred modality with most ophthalmologists) with fewer side effects and good cosmesis especially in patients who are *not* good candidates for excision (anticoagulated patients or elderly patients with lax periorbital skin who pose greater risk for ectropion as a surgical complication).

    When compared to TCA and cryosurgery, laser therapy requires fewer sessions, has less downtime, better cure rates, and fewer recurrences.
    ii. *Mechanism of action:* The exact mechanism of xanthelasma laser surgery is not understood fully. It is presumed that the caloric energy, which originates from the coagulation of the vessels within the upper corium, leads to a damage of the perivascular foam cells. Also the coagulation of the pathologically hyperpermeable vessels would lead to a blockage of the leakage of lipids into the tissue and thereby prevent recurrent lesions.
    iii. *Lasers available for xanthelasma palpebrarum and literature review (Table 12.14):* Lasers used in the treatment of xanthelasma palpebrarum (XP) include CO_2, YAG, argon, PDL, and 1,450 nm diode. Argon and PDLs use shorter wavelengths of light preferentially absorbed by hemoglobin. In xanthelasma, these lasers may induce coagulation within the vessels of the upper dermis, thereby destroying the perivascular, lipid-laden foam cells, and preventing further leakage of lipid into the surrounding tissue.

    The 1,450 nm diode, Nd:YAG, Er:YAG, and CO_2 lasers all use longer wavelengths of light absorbed best by cellular water. With water as its chromophore, the 1,450 nm diode laser has been shown to induce photothermal destruction of sebaceous glands in the mid-dermis by generating destructive heat at this particular depth. This principle has led to its theoretical use in xanthelasma.

    Carbon dioxide lasers are by far the most commonly reported laser modality for the treatment of XP and is the author's personal choice of treatment. It offers excellent cosmetic results with a range of 1-3 sessions of therapy. The author (Goel K) compared CO_2 laser with 30% TCA in treatment of XP and found that for small lesions, both TCA and ultrapulse CO_2 laser are efficacious and the choice can depend on availability of a particular treatment and choice of the patient or the treating physician. However, for clinically large lesions ultrapulse CO_2 laser is a better option because of better penetration depth leading to clearance of lesions, which are more

Table 12.14: Comparison of different laser modalities in treatment of xanthelasma palpebrarum.

Laser types	Number of studies	Mean number of sessions	Percentage clearance	Percent recurrence (follow-up range, months)	Side effects
CO_2	9	1.9	100	8.5% (1–54)	Palpebral edema, erythema, hypopigmentation, hyperpigmentation, atrophic scars, and upper eyelid retraction
Er: YAG	5	1.1	86.5	0% (1–12)	Dyspigmentation, minor bleeding, erythema, and edema
Nd: YAG	3	1.6	55.5	0% (0.5–2)	Dyspigmentation, hypopigmentation, pinpoint bleeding/crusting, and edema
Argon	2	2.5	100	9.4% (6–16)	Dyspigmentation, hyperpigmentation, hypopigmentation, scar, and erythema
PDL	2	4.5	100	0% (0–1)	Purpura, edema, and hyperpigmentation
1,450 nm diode	1	2.5	47.5	0% (1–1.5)	Hyperpigmentation, edema

(CO_2: carbon dioxide; Er:YAG: erbium-doped yttrium aluminum garnet; Nd:YAG: neodymium-doped yttrium aluminum garnet; PDL: pulsed dye laser)

deep or extensive. Moreover, lesser number of sittings are needed with laser treatment so there is better patient compliance. However, laser would lead to greater chances of pigmentary changes initially (3 months) which would improve with due course of time (6 months in our study), and so the patient should be appropriately counseled. As far as recurrence is concerned, there was no statistical difference between the two modalities.

The Er:YAG laser also appears to be a promising modality, though it is unclear whether the efficacy matches that of CO_2 laser. Notably, the lower number of sessions required may offer an advantage for treatment. In the few studies reporting use of the Nd:YAG laser, outcome was highly variable and appears to be less efficacious than Er:YAG.

Overall, reports on laser therapy for XP suffer from small cohort size, short follow-up, and single-arm design. Further larger-sized randomized trials comparing these laser modalities would be helpful. An algorithmic approach is detailed in **Chapter 2: Ablative Lasers.**

An overview of the procedures and results are given in the Figures 12.28 and 12.29. A commonly used setting with the CO_2 laser using the superpulse mode is depicted in Figures 12.30A and B.

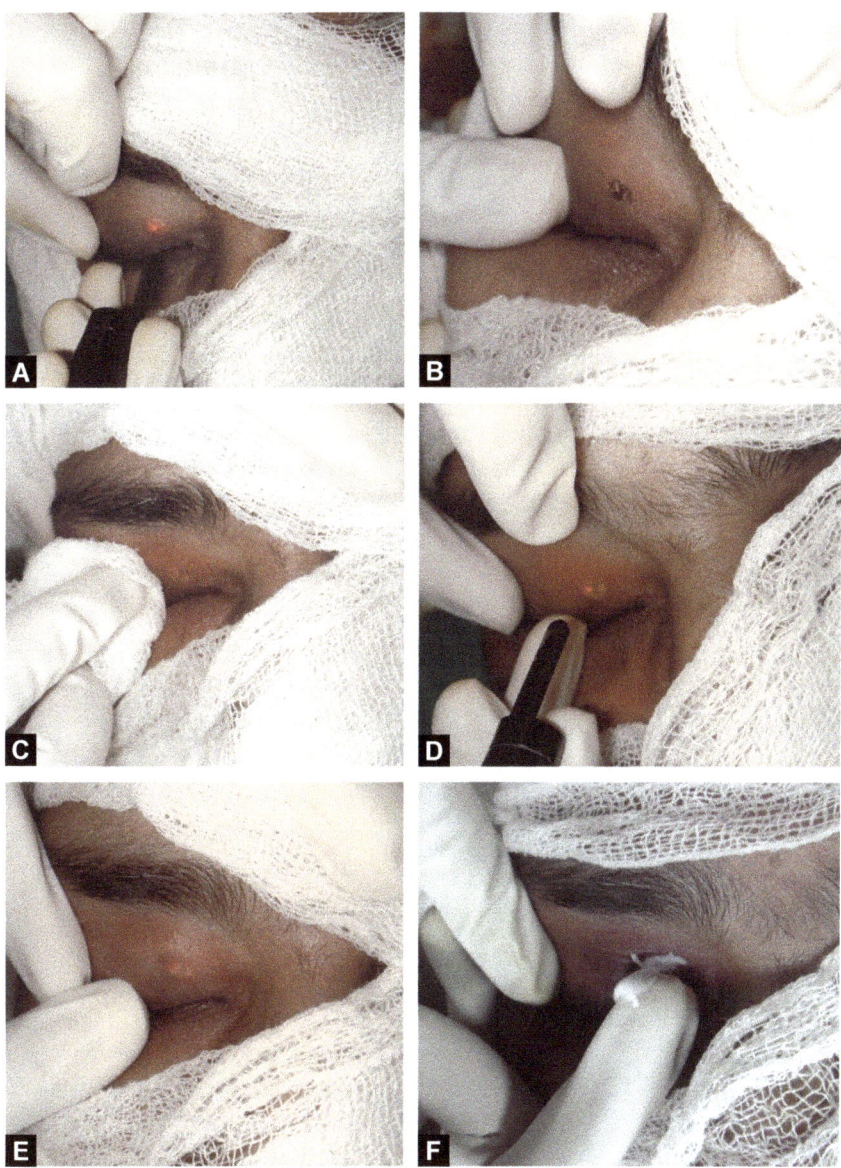

Figs. 12.28A to F: Photographs illustrating procedure of ultrapulse carbon dioxide (CO_2) laser treatment of patient of XP. (A) First pass being given; (B) Formation of coagulated debris; (C) Removal of debris with a wet gauze; (D) Second pass being given; (E) Appearance of bleeding points in laser irradiated area; and (F) Application of antibiotic cream.

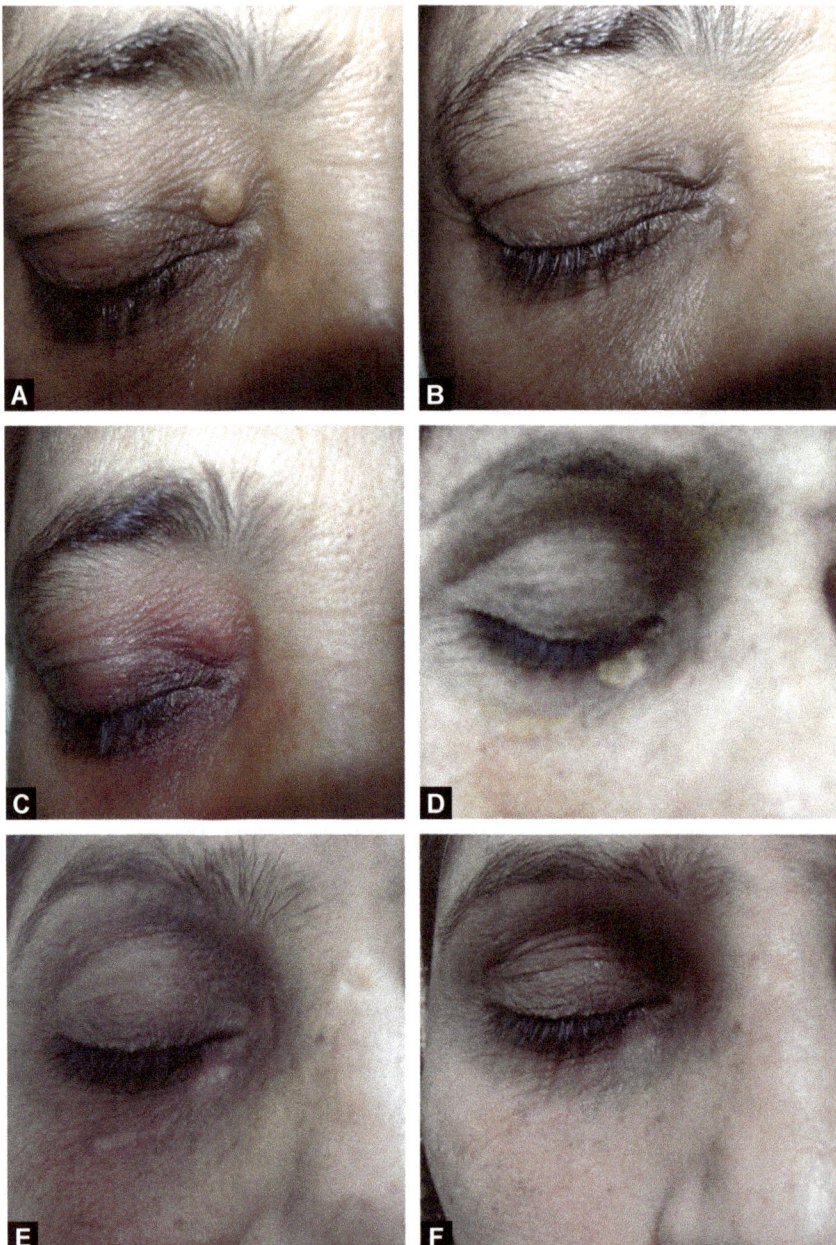

Figs. 12.29A to F: Results with ultrapulse carbon dioxide (CO_2) laser in 2 patients. (A) Initial photograph; (B) Follow-up at 1 month; (C) Follow-up at 6 months; (D) Initial photograph; (E) Follow-up at 1 month; and (F) Follow-up at 6 months.

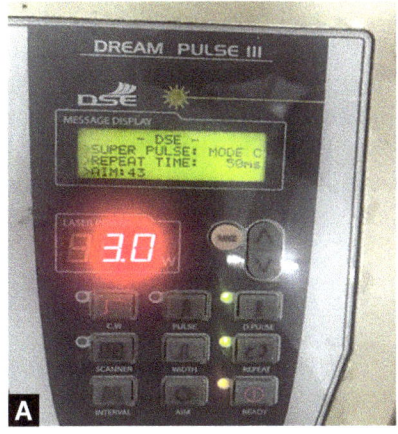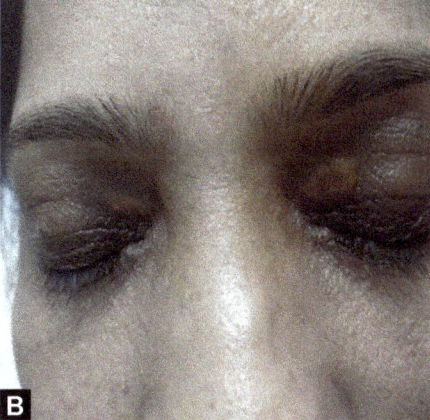

Figs. 12.30A and B: The setting used is 3 W and the mode C is a pulse duration of 1.2 ms. The pulse duration is often very important and to obtain ideal ablation with less thermal damage, a pulse duration of 0.25–10 ms, is ideal with a fluences of 1–10 J/cm^2. The interval we have used is 50 ms. As a thumb rule higher the pulse duration more the coagulation, thermal damage, and carbonization.

BIBLIOGRAPHY

1. Goel K, Sardana K, Garg VK. A prospective study comparing ultrapulse CO_2 laser and trichloroacetic acid in treatment of xanthelasma palpebrarum. J Cosmet Dermatol. 2015;14:130-9.
2. Gungor S, Canat D, Gokdemir G. Erbium:YAG laser ablation versus 70% trichloroacetic acid application in the treatment of xanthelasma palpebrarum. J Dermatolog Treat. 2014;25:290-3.
3. Nguyen AH, Vaudreuil AM, Huerter CJ. Systematic review of laser therapy in xanthelasma palpebrarum. Int J Dermatol. 2017;56:e47-55.
4. Park EJ, Youn SH, Cho EB, et al. Xanthelasma palpebrarum treatment with a 1450-nm-diode laser. Dermatol Surg. 2011;37:791-6.
5. Rohrich RJ, Janis JE, Pownell PH. Xanthelasma palpebrarum: A review and current management principles. Plast Reconstr Surg. 2002;110:1310-4.
6. Sayin I, Ayli M, Oğuz AK, et al. Xanthelasma palpebrarum: A new side effect of nilotinib. BMJ Case Rep. 2016;12:2016.
7. Szymanczyk J, Sawczak M, Cenian W, et al. Application of the laser diode with central wavelength 975 nm for the therapy of neurofibroma and hemangiomas. J Biomed Opt. 2017;22(1):10502.
8. Wang H, Shi Y, Guan H, et al. Treatment of xanthelasma palpebrarum with intralesional pingyangmycin. Dermatol Surg. 2016;42:368-76.
9. Winstanley D, Blalock T, Houghton N, et al. Treatment of sebaceous hyperplasia with a novel 1,720-nm laser. J Drugs Dermatol. 2012;11(11):1323-6.

590 SECTION 2: Therapeutic Indications

Epidermal Nevi

Though this is detailed in **Chapter 2: Ablative Lasers,** we must appreciate that these have a high rate of recurrence and incomplete removal. If a patient presents with a "soft" nevus, the results are good (Figs. 12.31A and B), but with a "hard" nevus, the results are poor (Figs. 12.32A and B).

Since epidermal nevi develop as result of overactivity of pluripotent embryonic epidermal basal keratinocytes and genetic mosaicism, recurrence

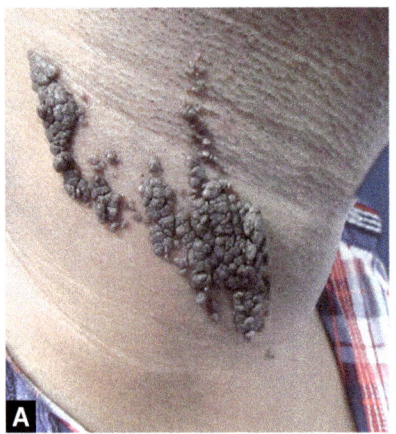
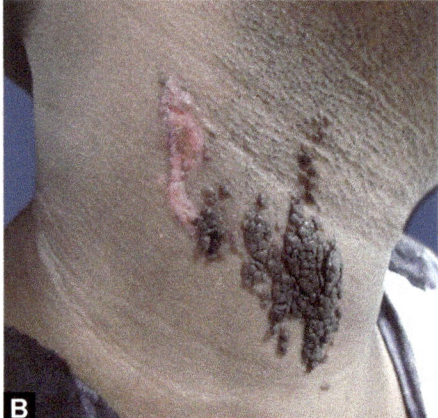

Figs. 12.31A and B: A soft epidermal nevi. Here a test spot with Er:YAG has been done. Note the clean base. We do not like to cross the papillary dermis which is easily recognized with the Er:YAG laser as there is pinpoint bleeding at this point. This is not seen with most CO_2 lasers unless it is set at ultrapulse or superpulse settings. (CO_2: carbon dioxide; Er:YAG: erbium-doped yttrium aluminum garnet)

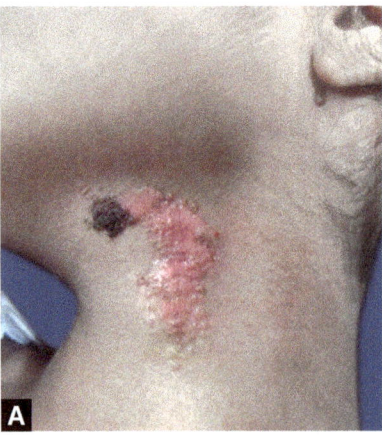
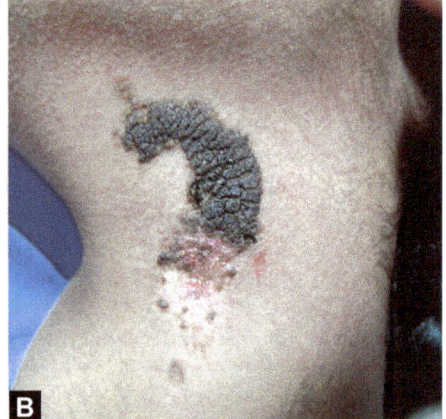

Figs. 12.32A and B: A hard nevi: CO_2 ablation 6 W CW mode. This is universally difficult to treat. Though most books discuss the histological variants, the morphological classification of soft and hard nevi is more useful for laser interventions. (CO_2: carbon dioxide; CW: continuous wave)

is an issue. The pathology shows papillomatosis, acanthosis, epidermal hyperplasia, and hyperkeratosis along with elongated rete ridges. Thus, we need a laser that removes the epidermis effectively and targets the dermis.

Though ablative lasers remain the "work horse" laser, there are some other options that can be used:

- *Picosecond*: This laser is ideal for pigment lesions especially tattoos, but a recent retrospective case series of patients by Levy et al. treated epidermal nevi with a PS 532-nm laser (Picoway, Syneron Candela, CA, USA). The technical features of this laser for the 532-nm wavelength include pulse duration of 375 ps, maximum energy of 200 mJ, and peak power of 0.53 gigawatts. The patients were treated at 8–10 weeks interval for up to 6 sessions, with a spot size of 3 mm and fluence of 1.8 J/cm^2. The remarkable visual results in the patients and the lack of recurrence at 12 months makes this an interesting extension of the pico laser. The rationale that guided the use of the 532-nm wavelength over the 1064-nm wavelength was the greater affinity to melanin and its superficial absorption. The concept was to use the high energy to cause blistering (epidermal-dermal separation) which helped in removing the epidermal nevi (Levi A et al.).
- Some of the other tools used include the excimer light system and a combination of RF and PDT (Zheng X et al. and Grgurich E).

Always use a test spot before treating the whole lesion. Do not cross the papillary dermis to avoid scar formation. And unlike the abstract of publications, the results are usually not as good as it may seem. Thus, it is better not to intervene aggressively. The Er:YAG is better for cosmesis but cannot go deep enough while the CO_2 goes deep enough but can cause scarring so there is not much choice and these ablative lasers still remain the most effective lasers for this indication.

Nevus Lipomatosus Superficialis

Nevus lipomatosus cutaneous superficialis (NLCS) is a localized form of a lipomatous nevus and was first described by Hoffman and Zurhelle in 1921 and is classified into two clinical subtypes.

The classic form usually presents by adolescence and consists of grouped, fleshy, skin-colored to yellow papules and nodules on the lower trunk, buttocks, or thighs in a segmental distribution. The second variant presents in adulthood as a solitary papule or nodule anywhere on the skin, including unusual sites such as the face, scalp, and clitoris.

Treatment

Treatment options for NLCS are minimal and a conservative approach is advised, but lesions tend to increase in size and number and rarely ulcerate. Surgical excision is particularly useful for the solitary variant of NLCS, but it is usually impractical for the classic form of clustered lesions, in which a large area is involved.

Lasers and their Rationale

The use of lasers has largely focused on the use of CO_2 laser ablation. Fatah et al. treated NLCS with one session of *superpulsed CO_2* laser at 10 J/cm² in CW mode, with a 2 mm spot size, which was well tolerated and no recurrence of the lesions were seen at 12-months follow-up.

Kim JY et al. though reported a case of NLCS on the right lower back, which recurred after CO_2 laser treatment and suggested staged excision for large multiple type of NLCS.

Our approach to treatment of this condition was based on the histological depth of nevus lipomatosus superficialis and the use of appropriate settings of the ultrapulse CO_2 based on our earlier use in other conditions.

The basic abnormality is the presence of varying amounts of mature adipose tissue in the dermis, often unrelated to the fat of the underlying subcutis. The fat can constitute from less than 10-70% of the lesion. When there is only a small amount of fat, it is usually localized around the subpapillary blood vessels. There are also abnormalities in the other connective tissue components of the dermis, including some thickening of the collagen bundles, increase in elastic tissue.

Thus, there is a need for a laser that has both ablative and coagulative potential (to seal the blood vessels) with an established dose depth correlation to reach the papillary dermis. The ultrapulse mode of the CO_2 is safer than the CW or superpulse mode, as between 20 µm and 30 µm is ablated with each pass, while leaving an acceptably narrow zone of residual thermal damage: 25-70 µm, in contrast to the 200-600 µm zone produced by the CW CO_2 laser.

Thus, if used cautiously there is minimal dermal damage and consequentially little scarring. Our use of the ultrapulse mode of the CO_2 laser is based on its well-studied tissue effects wherein a dose of 250 mJ effectively removes the epidermis in 1-2 passes with minimum thermal damage (40 µm) thus, minimizing scarring. It has been estimated that at 250 mJ/pulse three passes achieves an ablation up to the papillary dermis. The concomitant coagulation (50-200 µm) would effectively seal the blood vessels encountered.

This principle was applied in our case (Sardana K 2017) where we used a dose of 250 mJ/pulse with which we removed the visible tumor mass in two passes. The third pass was used to coagulate the vessels and also sufficiently ablate the dermal fat, which is a part of the pathology of nevus lipomatosus superficialis (NLS).

If the superpulse mode is used, the settings that would be useful is a dose of 5-9 J/cm² with a pulse duration more than 50 ms. This would achieve sufficient ablation and coagulation (Figs. 12.33A to C).

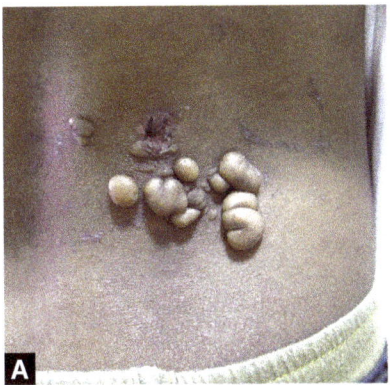
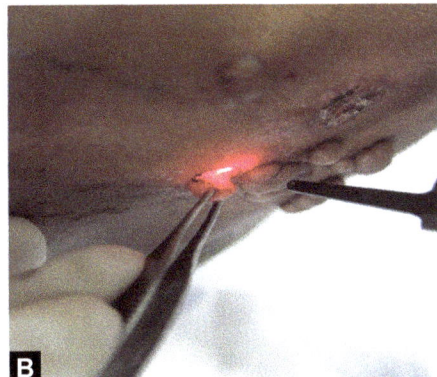
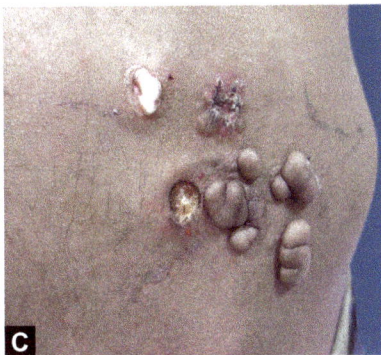

Figs. 12.33A to C: A case of nevus lipomatosus superficialis. The base was removed using CO_2 in CW mode and then the tissue was ablated using Er:YAG. Another option can be ablating the base using the $SpCO_2$ laser. Here keep a high pulse duration more than 50 ms to enable coagulation of the base. (CO_2: carbon dioxide; CW: continuous wave; Er:YAG: erbium-doped yttrium aluminum garnet)

BIBLIOGRAPHY

1. Alster TS. Cutaneous resurfacing with CO_2 and erbium:YAG lasers: Preoperative, intraoperative, and postoperative considerations. Plast Reconstr Surg. 1999;103: 619-32.
2. Fatah S, Ellis R, Seukeran DC, et al. Successful CO_2 laser treatment of naevus lipomatosus cutaneous superficialis. Clin Exp Dermatol. 2010;35:559-60.
3. Fitzpatrick RE, Tope WD, Goldman MP, et al. Pulsed carbon dioxide laser, trichloroacetic acid, Baker-Gordon phenol, and dermabrasion: A comparative clinical and histologic study of cutaneous resurfacing in a porcine model. Arch Dermatol. 1996;132:469-71.
4. Grgurich E, Gupta N, Owen R, et al. Inflammatory linear verrucous epidermal nevus responsive to 308-nm excimer laser treatment. Cutis. 2018;102(2):111-4.
5. Jain S, Sardana K, Garg VK. Ultrapulse carbon dioxide laser treatment of porokeratotic eccrine ostial and dermal duct nevus. Pediatr Dermatol. 2013;30:264-6.
6. Kauvar AB, Waldorf HA, Geronemus RG. A histopathological comparison of "char-free" carbon dioxide lasers. Dermatol Surg. 1996;22:343-8.
7. Kim YJ, Choi JH, Kim H, et al. Recurrence of nevus lipomatosus cutaneous superficialis after CO(2) laser treatment. Arch Plast Surg. 2012;39:671-3.

8. Levi A, Amitai DB, Mimouni D, et al. Picosecond 532-nm neodymium-doped yttrium aluminum garnet laser-a promising modality for the management of verrucous epidermal nevi. Lasers Med Sci. 2018;33(3):597-601.
9. Sardana K, Bansal S, Garg VK, et al. Treatment of nevus lipomatosus cutaneous superficialis with CO(2) laser. J Cosmet Dermatol. 2017;16(3):333-5.
10. Sardana K, Garg VK. Successful treatment of nevus comedonicus with ultrapulse CO_2 laser. Indian J Dermatol Venereol Leprol. 2009;75:534-5.
11. Sardana K, Mendiratta V, Kakar N, et al. Spontaneously improving Michelin tire baby syndrome. Pediatr Dermatol. 2003;20:150-2.
12. Zheng X, He S, Li Q, et al. Successful treatment of verrucous epidermal nevus with fractional micro-plasma radiofrequency technology and photodynamic therapy. J Cosmet Laser Ther. 2018;20(6):357-9. doi: 10.1080/14764172.2018.1511914. Epub 2018 Aug 21.

Keratosis Pilaris

This is a common disorder and the two basic tenets of treatment should revolve around the twin principles of a lack of persistent results and giving a realistic expectation to the patient regarding the results.

The ultimate goal is to target the erythema, follicular keratosis, and textural abnormalities.

- *Topical therapy* is often used and is a good option for maintenance and is a low cost intervention.
    i. Lactic acid and alpha-hydroxy acid lotions (10–12%) applied twice daily may improve the textural roughness. Another option is retinoids where tazarotene is better than tretinoin.
    ii. Corticosteroids applied sparingly may show improvement (use the class 5–7 steroids).
- *Systemic therapy*: Oral retinoids and dapsone have been used for the inflammatory stage of keratosis pilaris atrophicans (KPA) and the former may help the follicular hyperkeratosis.
- *Laser therapy*: Shorter wavelength have been traditionally used to target the erythema and textural alterations. These are more amenable to laser intervention than the follicular lesions.
    i. Pulsed dye laser (595 nm, 7 mm spot, 7–10 J/cm^2, DCD 40/20, and pulse duration of 1.5–3 ms) can be effective in the treatment of the associated erythema.
    ii. *Diode lasers*: Three treatments with the 810 nm diode laser may induce significant improvements in skin texture and roughness/bumpiness in KP patients with Fitzpatrick skin types I through III, but baseline erythema is not improved (Ibrahim O).
    iii. *Hair removal laser*: Laser-assisted hair removal with long-pulsed non-Q-switched ruby laser may be an effective treatment.
    iv. Fractional CO_2 laser has been used to target the follicular lesions.

v. Combination therapy has been used to target multiple aspects of the disorder, using a 595 nm PDL with nonpurpuragenic fluences, a long-pulsed 755 nm alexandrite laser, and microdermabrasion (Lee SJ et al).
- Photopneumatic technology has also been used.

BIBLIOGRAPHY

1. Ibrahim O, Khan M, Bolotin D, et al. Treatment of keratosis pilaris with 810-nm diode laser: A randomized clinical trial. JAMA Dermatol. 2015;151:187-91.
2. Lee SJ, Choi MJ, Zheng Z, et al. Combination of 595-nm pulsed dye laser, long-pulsed 755-nm alexandrite laser, and microdermabrasion treatment for keratosis pilaris: Retrospective analysis of 26 Korean patients. J Cosmet Laser Ther. 2013;15:150-4.
3. Schoch JJ, Tollefson MM, Witman P, et al. Successful treatment of keratosis pilaris rubra with pulsed dye laser. Pediatr Dermatol. 2016;33:443-6.
4. Vachiramon V, Anusaksathien P, Kanokrungsee S, et al. Fractional carbon dioxide laser for keratosis pilaris: A single-blind, randomized, comparative study. Biomed Res Int. 2016;2016:1928540.

VIRAL DISORDERS

Though most viral disorders are self-limiting by nature, with the most consistent results being mediated by immune modulation, destructive methods are often used, where lasers provide the best trade-off between efficacy and side effects.

Lasers Used for Warts and Molluscum Contagiosum

The *CO_2 laser light* (wavelength of 10,600 nm) is mainly absorbed by water and enables vaporization of tissue of any kind. Because a CO_2 laser creates temperatures of 200–300°C, the treatment is painful and requires some type of anesthesia stronger than an eutectic mixture of local anesthetics (2.5% lidocaine and 2.5% prilocaine emulsion in an oil-in-water base). Therefore, most clinicians feel that for the treatment of viral infections, this type of laser may be considered too invasive. But if it is to be used, a CW mode is useful as here ablation with thermal injury is helpful in preventing recurrences. The choice of ablative lasers depends on the site and the facilities, two scenarios are treated with two different ablative lasers (Figs. 12.34 and 12.35).

With the flashlamp-pumped pulsed dye laser (FPDL) (Table 12.15), which emits light in the yellow-orange part of the visible light spectrum at 585 nm or 595 nm (Kauvar AN) can also be used. This light is best absorbed by hemoglobin and oxyhemoglobin and is, therefore, used for the treatment of vascular lesions. With very short pulses (0.45 ms) purpura develops within minutes in the treated areas and needs 10–14 days to resolve as macrophages

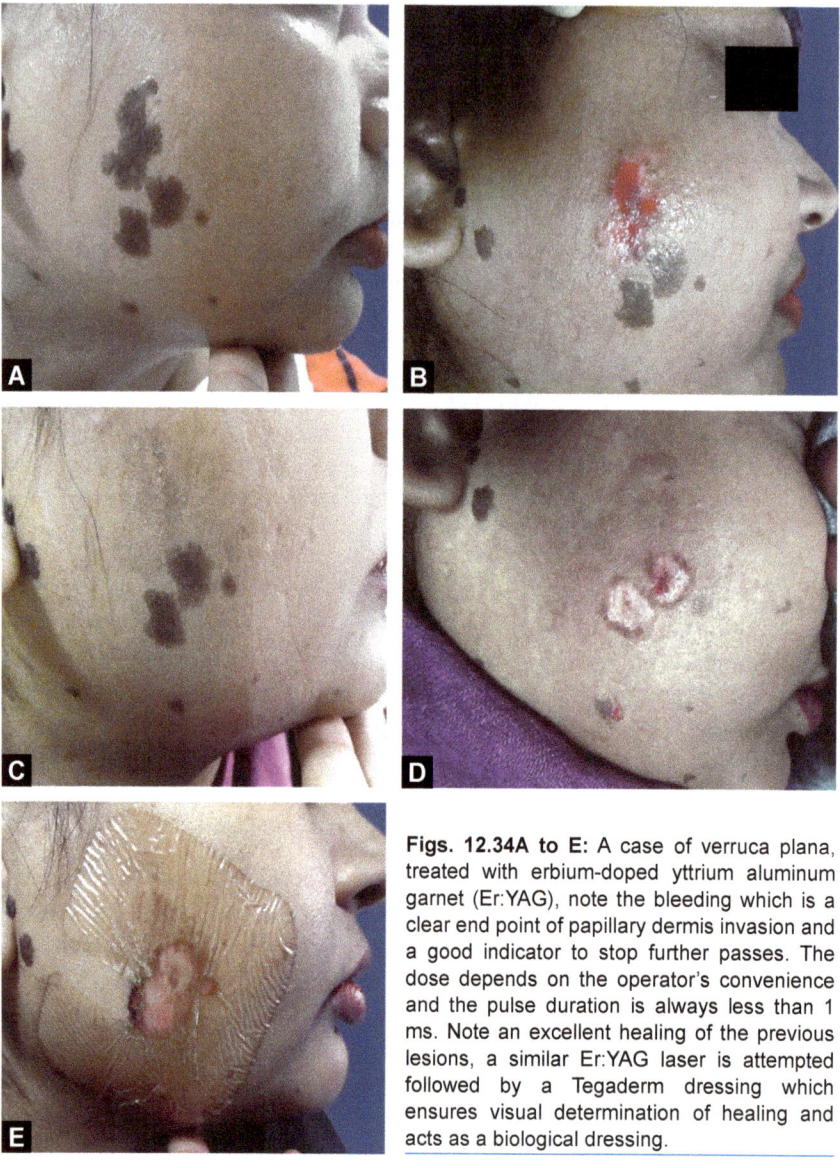

Figs. 12.34A to E: A case of verruca plana, treated with erbium-doped yttrium aluminum garnet (Er:YAG), note the bleeding which is a clear end point of papillary dermis invasion and a good indicator to stop further passes. The dose depends on the operator's convenience and the pulse duration is always less than 1 ms. Note an excellent healing of the previous lesions, a similar Er:YAG laser is attempted followed by a Tegaderm dressing which ensures visual determination of healing and acts as a biological dressing.

digest damaged material and blood residual. The yellow-orange light of this particular laser is designed to destroy superficial blood vessels.

In viral warts, the concept is to destroy the warts' blood supply and supposedly induce their regression, although the studies using the FPDL with the same treatment parameters offer controversial results (Kopera D). Other than transient purpura, side effects from FPDL treatment of viral infections of the skin, when 0.45 ms pulses are used, are rare. They include post-treatment hyperpigmentation, blistering, and sometimes scarring.

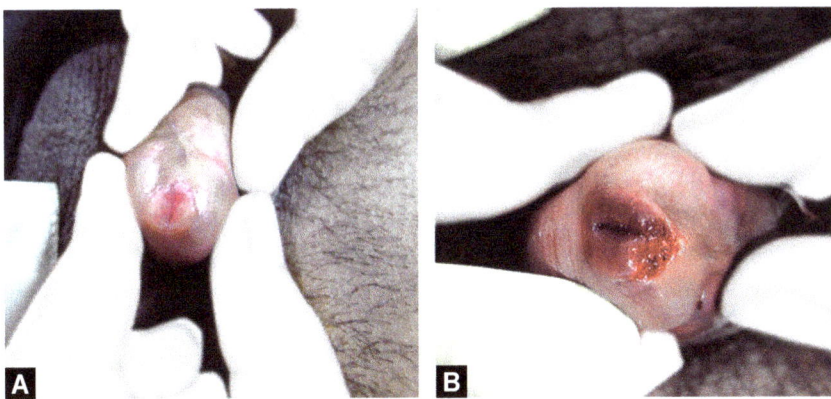

Figs. 12.35A and B: An intraurethral wart treated with $SpCO_2$, here the pulse duration was increased to 0.7 s (700 ms) to enable coagulation. This can be further increased to 1 s to achieve more coagulation.

Table 12.15: Use of pulsed dye laser (PDL) in viral disorders.

Molluscum contagiosum	
• Dose	• 6–7 J/cm^2
• Pulse duration	• 0.45 ms
• Number of sessions	• 1–2
Common warts	
• Dose	8–12 J/cm^2
• Pulse duration	0.45–1.5 ms
• Number of sessions	1–8
Genital warts	
• Dose	6–7 J/cm^2
• Pulse duration	0.45 ms
• Number of sessions	1–5

Treatment for *molluscum contagiosum* must be individualized. Some treatments may be painful and would not be the first choice for children. Other treatments are not painful but require diligence over a long period of time. Sometimes, the best treatment is reassurance that the lesions are self-limited. Most would prefer curettage, cryosurgery, toxic or irritating topical agents [e.g. cantharidin, 5-fluorouracil (5-FU), tretinoin, adapalene, and salicylic acid], and immunomodulating topical imiquimod. Lasers in our view are a rapid therapeutic modality for molluscum. Apart from the CO_2 laser, the FPDL can be used.

This author has treated numerous cases of *molluscum contagiosum* with the CO_2 laser and it provides a rapid, fast method of treatment, and with a mode of action that combines the best of extirpation and TCA/potassium hydroxide (KOH), which is more cumbersome. Also, the high temperature can effectively kill the virus. A single spot mode in a dose of 0.5-2 W, with a pulse duration of 10 ms is sufficient.

INFLAMMATORY DISORDERS

Angiolymphoid Hyperplasia with Eosinophilia

The treatment of angiolymphoid hyperplasia with eosinophilia (ALHE) is known to be difficult. Intralesional corticosteroids, surgical excision, and lasers are the most frequently used therapies, although none of them is effective in all cases. Other options reviewed in the literature are topical or oral corticosteroids, cryotherapy, oral retinoids, imiquimod, tacrolimus, bleomycin, and interferon alpha-2a (INFα-2a).

Laser

Laser therapy can be a useful tool, especially for challenging locations in which surgery cannot be performed. The most frequently used lasers to treat ALHE are those targeting oxyhemoglobin. The use of the argon laser (484–514 nm) was first reported in 1988 but its long pulse duration led to nonselective damage and scarring. There are several reports about the use of PDLs for ALHE; most of them are single case reports in which complete remission has been observed. Longer wavelength PDL (595 nm) seems to be slightly more effective because it enables deeper tissue penetration (around 2.5 mm). The common settings used are 585 nm, 7–10 mm, (5–7.5 J/cm^2), and 0.45 ms (Lertzman BH). But it must be appreciated that the results may require up to seven sessions and are not complete except while using the 595 nm (Angel CA).

Other lasers used include Nd:YAG laser, using a 6 mm round spot size with two pulses of 7 ms duration with a 20 ms interpulse delay and a fluence of 100–150 J/cm^2. A copper vapor laser (CVL) was used for the treatment of ALHE in one patient. CVLs emit yellow light (similar to PDLs) of 578 nm. The pulse duration is 20 ms, with a pulse repetition rate of 15,000 cycles.

Because the CO$_2$ laser is an ablative laser that targets water, it is less selective than vascular lasers. But we prefer this as it has the advantage of ablation with coagulation and is immeasurably cheaper than PDL and millisecond pulsed Nd:YAG lasers (Kaur T). Though there are no reports of the Er:YAG as it has a poor coagulative profile, a dual mode Er:YAG may be used.

Darier's Disease

This genetic condition has been treated by lasers, though chances of recurrence are there unless post-therapy histological confirmation can be done.

Lasers Used

The CO$_2$ laser was successfully used to destroy recalcitrant plaques in two patients with Darier's disease by McElroy et al. with significant improvement and recurrence in only one treatment site. The same laser was used by Minsue Chen et al. to treat a patient with lesions involving 40% of total body area. The authors used a 3 mm spot and energies ranging from 10 W to 40 W in two passes with tumescent local anesthesia, without recurrence at 2 years of follow-up. Nevertheless, the risk of scarring with a CO_2 laser increases with the depth of treatment and the thermal damage.

Beier et al. treated two patients with an Er:YAG laser (2,940 nm) under local anesthesia with the painting technique and with an overlap of 30%. The treatment end point was the exposure of the papillary dermis including a margin of adjacent normal skin, using up to seven stacked pulses, a spot size of 1.6 mm, and fluences of 5–8.5 J/cm^2. No recurrences and/or scarring were observed in the two patients in a follow-up of 20 months. Both patients had remission of the pruritus; post-treatment hypopigmentation was observed in the cubital and popliteal area of one patient and a few spots in the other patient. Post-treatment biopsies showed no signs of Darier's disease in both patients.

It is this author's view that a combination of Er:YAG and CO_2 is a better option as the Er:YAG has a predictable depth and when the end point of ablation is achieved, a pass of CO_2 can enable adequate coagulation.

Dermatomyositis

There have been some reports of poikilodermatous erythema and telangiectasias of dermatomyositis treated with PDLs and argon lasers, with good response (Yanagi T).

Lasers have also been used successfully to treat other connective tissue diseases (Brauer 2014).

Eczema

In 2008, (Syed S) in their pilot study, showed that PDL treatment improves localized areas of chronic eczema. Twelve children with localized chronic eczema were treated with PDL (595 nm). After 2 weeks and 6 weeks, a significant decrease in eczema severity score was seen for the PDL-treated areas compared with the control areas. Treatment was well-tolerated.

This may suggest that dermal vasculature plays an important role in chronic eczema or that PDL treatment may have an effect on cutaneous immunological activation (Woo PN).

Elastosis Perforans Serpiginosa

Treatment with pulsed CO_2 and Er:YAG laser techniques may have been modestly helpful in patients with idiopathic elastosis perforans serpiginosa (EPS) (Vestey JP). The PDL has appeared to be beneficial in one reported case of EPS in a patient with Down syndrome.

Granuloma Annulare

In 1988, CO_2 laser was used with good results to treat granuloma annulare (GA). There are reports of the use of PDL where the lesion was treated three times, initially and at months 5 and 13. After the first session of treatment, significant flattening and reduction of erythema were evident. After the second and third treatments, further improvement was observed and long-term remission was achieved (Sniezek PJ).

In 2008, Karsai et al. (Karsai S) reported a patient with disseminated GA who was treated with fractional photothermolysis using a 1,440 nm Nd:YAG laser. A complete remission was achieved after two treatment sessions.

A recent report describes the use of excimer laser (Bronfenbrener R), though it is the author's opinion that the results of photochemotherapy are better with almost 50% clearance on psoralen plus ultraviolet A (PUVA) with a 79% remission rate (Browne F) (Table 12.16).

Granuloma Faciale

A variety of surgical procedures may be used in the management of granuloma faciale (GF): surgical excision, dermabrasion, electrosurgery, cryotherapy, and different types of lasers.

Laser Therapy

Different lasers have been used in the treatment of GF with promising results, either as an ablative therapy with CO_2 laser or as a selective therapy targeting

Table 12.16: Recent case reports of lasers used for the treatment of granuloma annulare.

Type of laser	Location of treated lesions	Description of treatment	Outcome	Recurrence
585 nm pulsed dye laser	Left wrist	6.75 J/cm², 5 mm spot size, 36–43 pulses per session, 3 sessions over 13 months	Near clearance	None after 3 years
308 nm excimer	Dorsal hands	300 mJ/cm², 5 doses per session × 15 treatments	Clearance of treated area	None after 6 months
1,440 nm Nd:YAG	Arms, neck, chest, abdomen	6 J/cm², 3 ms pulse duration, 2 full passes with 25% overlap every 3 weeks × 2–3 treatment sessions per area	Clearance of treated areas	None after 8 months

(Nd:YAG: neodymium-doped yttrium aluminum garnet)

the prominent vasculature in GF lesions using the Q-switched argon laser, PDL, diode laser, and potassium titanyl phosphate (KTP) 532 nm laser.

Argon laser was first used in 1988, resulting in resolution of the clinical and microscopic abnormalities. The laser most frequently used to treat GF is the PDL.

Hailey–Hailey Disease

While dermabrasion is an option for refractory lesions, with clearance rates as high as 83%, but hypertrophic scarring is commonly observed. The use of the CO_2 laser to vaporize the lesions has been described by several authors (Kartamaa M), with the treatment end point being skin destruction reaching the follicular infundibulum while sparing the adnexal glands to avoid hypertrophic scarring.

Kartamaa et al. used a continuous CO_2 laser to treat six patients with symmetrical lesions, leaving one side as untreated controls. There was improvement on the treatment side in five patients, with hypertrophic scarring occurring in the axillary area of the other patient. Christian et al. reported one patient with refractory axillary lesions treated with three passes of a CO_2 laser using a fluence of 28 J/cm^2; focal recurrences were managed with a short dwell CO_2 laser with a fluence of 15 J/cm^2. Complete resolution was observed in only one side.

Beier et al. treated two patients with an Er:YAG 2,940 nm laser under local anesthesia with the painting technique. These patients had axillary and groin lesions and the treatment parameters were as follows: 0.35 ms pulse duration, up to seven stacked pulses, 5 mm spot size, and 5–8.5 J/cm^2 fluence. Complete remission was observed in one patient at 1 year of follow-up; in the other patient lesion recurrence occurred at the edges and adjacent areas, which were managed with an additional treatment.

Lichen Sclerosus

The first line of therapy is potent topical corticosteroids, such as clobetasol propionate for at least 3 months, combined with emollients.

Recalcitrant lesions can be treated with a CO_2 laser (Peterson et al.). A retrospective study of 50 patients found that 80% of the patients were disease-free at a median follow-up of 14 years (Windahl). The pulsed mode or a repeat mode (3–4 W; 0.20 s) in a defocused beam can be used to vaporize the macroscopically altered area of the glans penis. If there is a phimosis that can be also treated simultaneously.

The PDT has been tried in 12 females with vulvar lichen sclerosus where a dose of 30–70 mW/cm^2 was used with a wavelength of 635 nm. Treatment was well tolerated by eight patients and a marked improvement in pruritus was observed in 10 women, which was maintained for a mean of 6 months.

It must be remembered that surgical treatment by circumcision can be curative, if the disease is treated early when still localized. Once progression to urethral involvement has occurred, treatment is much more difficult and lasers should be reserved for the early stage before meatal stenosis has occurred (Stewart L).

Lupus Erythematosus

Though laser therapy offers novel and often effective treatment for recalcitrant cutaneous conditions in lupus erythematosus (LE), scleroderma, sarcoidosis, and dermatomyositis, the limited number of reports, with outdated technologies and techniques makes it difficult to recommend this as a first-line therapy for CTD (Brauer JA).

The PDL is used in several vascular disorders, such as rosacea telangiectasias or port-wine stains. The wavelengths of 585 nm or 595 nm are selectively absorbed by oxyhemoglobin and allow a selective destruction of the vessel walls. The rationale for the therapeutic success of PDL in LE is the growing evidence that endothelial cells play a major role in the inflammatory process and systemic manifestations in LE. The targeting of endothelial cells in rheumatic diseases is now an important field in the development of new drugs (Szekanecz Z), and even classic drugs used in the treatment of LE, such as chloroquine, have been shown to reduce skin lesions from LE partially through inhibition of angiogenesis.

Published series of patients with LE lesions treated with a PDL (Raulin C) have shown significant improvement of skin lesions, even in those patients with the systemic form of the disease. The older series used a PDL with a wavelength of 585 nm, achieving a clearance rate of 70% in nine patients.

Another application for lasers in the treatment of LE is the atrophic scars, especially in discoid lupus erythematosus (DLE) because this subtype frequently causes disfiguring and cribriform scars. The CO_2 laser in CW mode has been used, though this author favors the use of the Er:YAG laser, due to its measured dose depth response and excellent healing after ablation.

Also, it must be remembered that LE may be aggravated by UV light, though there are no published reports of such an aggravation due to PDL, CO_2, or Er:YAG lasers.

Necrobiosis Lipoidica

In 1999, Currie et al. described a case report of necrobiosis lipoidica (NL) treated with a PDL. At low fluences, minimal therapeutic effect was achieved, and at higher fluences skin breakdown occurred, so they concluded that caution is required when attempting to treat NL with a laser.

Other therapies tried include PDT (De Giorgi V).

Nodular Amyloidosis

A patient with a large scalp lesion of nodular primary localized cutaneous amyloidosis (LCA) was treated with a CO_2 laser with excellent cosmetic results and minimal morbidity (Truhan AP). In 1999, a case report of multiple nodules treated with a PDL was described, with clinical improvement in the color, size, and friability of nodules maintained for 6 months (Alster TS). Histologic examination revealed decreased inflammation and improvement in dermal collagen after laser irradiation.

There are certain important issues to appreciate before using lasers for this condition (Lesiak A). Firstly, the pathology is deep and the amyloid is admixed with a proliferative vasculature with the result that most ablative procedures encounter bleeding that is an issue while treating this condition with lasers (Hamzavi I). Though a report of fractional ablative laser has been published (Anitha B), the concomitant use of a topical steroid salicylic acid ointment means that probably the fractional lasers helped to increase the transcutaneous penetration of the steroid.

Sarcoidosis

Laser therapy has been used mainly for lupus pernio, which is the most characteristic lesion of cutaneous sarcoidosis. It has a predilection for acral sites, most commonly the nose. The lesions are usually violaceous plaques or nodules that can be disfiguring and can cause significant psychological morbidity.

Lasers Used

Pulsed dye laser was first used by Goodman et al. where a 75% improvement after two treatments was seen, but recurrence was observed after 6 months. Cliff et al. confirmed the PDLs effectiveness to clear lupus pernio clinically and histologically, with no recurrence after 2 months.

The CO_2 laser remodeling and healing by secondary intention have also been performed for lupus pernio. Six cases have been reported (O'Donoghue NB) with satisfactory aesthetic results and no recurrence in most cases. Some use intralesional triamcinolone acetonide after laser therapy (Stack BC).

In addition, the 532 nm frequency-doubled Nd:YAG laser has been used to treat lupus pernio with a complete remission after a 3-year follow-up (Ekback M).

Scar sarcoidosis is characterized by erythema, infiltration, and progressive induration of a preexisting scar. It can resemble hypertrophic scars or keloids. Anecdotal use of a Q-switched ruby laser led to a complete clearance of scar sarcoidosis lesions (Grema H).

Successful treatment of this condition was also reported using a 595 nm PDL. No recurrence was observed after 1 year of follow-up. Laser treatment seems to be effective for isolated cases of cutaneous sarcoidosis. Nevertheless, only few cases have been reported so far (Brauer JA).

Conclusion

There are two issues with the use of lasers. Firstly, in most cases the follow-up period has been short for a disease like sarcoidosis where recurrences have been seen even after years of steroid therapy. Secondly, there are cases of aggravation of sarcoidosis with PDL therapy and CO_2 laser. Thus, lasers are not to be used as a preferential treatment in sarcoidosis (Kormeili T).

Psoriasis

The benefits of using the 308 nm excimer laser for psoriasis is well-established and it has been shown that the psoriatic lesions treated with the excimer laser cleared with fewer treatments than narrowband ultraviolet B (NB-UVB) therapy. Though a summary of the indications and advantages are given here, it is this author's opinion that PUVAsol is a reasonably effective option for psoriasis, with a more pronounced immunomodulatory effect than excimer laser.

Indications

- Localized plaques that have not responded to medical therapy
- Mild to moderate psoriasis
- Type II–IV skin with disease limited to the scalp or flexural areas.

Advantages

- It spares the uninvolved skin from UV exposure
- Remissions for up to 2 years have been seen in some patients
- Laser therapy demonstrated efficacy at lower cumulative doses when compared to conventional light therapy
- Used for psoriatic lesions that occurs in the groin and axilla (inverse psoriasis) and scalp
- It can be used in all skin types.

Summary

The ultraviolet B (UVB) phototherapy is an effective treatment modality for psoriasis. For patients with localized plaque-type lesions, 308 nm excimer laser phototherapy offers rapidly delivered, targeted, high UVB doses, while sparing adjacent healthy skin. A study by Mudigonda T compared the advantages and disadvantages of the 308 nm xenon chloride (XeCl) UVB excimer laser with nontargeted broadband ultraviolet B (BB-UVB), NB-UVB, and PUVA phototherapies. Three prospective nonrandomized studies compared NB-UVB with excimer laser phototherapy. No head-to-head studies were found for BB-UVB or PUVA compared to excimer laser. Both the 308 nm excimer laser and nontargeted phototherapies were found to effectively clear localized psoriasis.

Although it is proposed that excimer laser exclusively treats diseased skin with better response rates, split-body trials revealed no differences. Long-term studies are necessary to compare the effects of high-dose excimer laser regimens with nontargeted phototherapies.

Interestingly PUVA has not been compared with excimer laser and it is quite likely that due to the more profound immunomodulatory effect and depth of penetration, PUVA is probably superior in terms of efficacy and relapse rates.

BIBLIOGRAPHY

1. Alster TS, Manaloto RM. Nodular amyloidosis treated with a pulsed dye laser. Dermatol Surg. 1999;25:133-5.
2. Angel CA, Lewis AT, Griffin T, et al. Angiolymphoid hyperplasia successfully treated with an ultralong pulsed dye laser. Dermatol Surg. 2005;31:713-6.
3. Anitha B, Mysore V. Lichen amyloidosis: Novel treatment with fractional ablative 2,940 nm erbium:YAG laser treatment. J Cutan Aesthet Surg. 2012;5:141-3.
4. Beier C, Kaufmann R. Efficacy of erbium:YAG laser ablation in Darier disease and Hailey-Hailey disease. Arch Dermatol. 1999;135:423-7.
5. Brauer JA, Gordon Spratt EA, Geronemus RG. Laser therapy in the treatment of connective tissue diseases: A review. Dermatol Surg. 2014;40:1-13.
6. Bronfenbrener R, Ragi J, Milgraum S. Granuloma annulare treated with excimer laser. J Clin Aesthet Dermatol. 2012;5:43-5.
7. Browne F, Turner D, Goulden V. Psoralen and ultraviolet A in the treatment of granuloma annulare. Photodermatol Photoimmunol Photomed. 2011;27:81-4.
8. Christian MM, Moy RL. Treatment of Hailey-Hailey disease (or benign familial pemphigus) using short pulsed and short dwell time carbon dioxide lasers. Dermatol Surg. 1999;25:661-3.
9. Cliff S, Felix RH, Singh L, et al. The successful treatment of lupus pernio with the flashlamp pulsed dye laser. J Cutan Laser Ther. 1999;1:49-52.
10. Currie CL, Monk BE. Pulsed dye laser treatment of necrobiosis lipoidica: Report of a case. J Cutan Laser Ther. 1999;1:239-41.
11. De Giorgi V, Buggiani G, Rossi R, et al. Successful topical photodynamic treatment of refractory necrobiosis lipoidica. Photodermatol Photoimmunol Photomed. 2008;24:332-3.
12. Dmovsek-Olup B, Vedlin B. Use of the Er:YAG laser for benign skin disorders. Lasers Surg Med. 1997;21:13-9.
13. Ekback M, Molin L. Effective laser treatment in a case of lupus pernio. Acta Derm Venereol. 2005;85:521-2.
14. Fitzpatrick RE, Goldman MP, Ruiz-Esparza J. Clinical advantage of the CO_2 laser superpulsed mode. Treatment of verruca vulgaris, seborrheic keratoses, lentigines, and actinic cheilitis. Dermatol Surg Oncol. 1994;20:449-56.
15. Goodman MM, Alpern K. Treatment of lupus pernio with the flashlamp pulsed dye laser. Lasers Surg Med. 1992;12:549-51.
16. Grema H, Greve B, Raulin C. Scar sarcoidosis—treatment with the Q-switched ruby laser. Lasers Surg Med. 2002;30:398-400.
17. Hamzavi I, Lui H. Excess tissue friability during CO_2 laser vaporization of nodular amyloidosis. Dermatol Surg. 1999;25:726-8.

18. Kardorff B. Neurofibromatose Typ I (Morbus Recklinghausen): Kombinierte Erbium:YAG-Laser- und Exzisionstherapie von kutanen Neurofibromen. Derm. 1998;4:404-6.
19. Karsai S, Hammes S, Rütten A, et al. Fractional photothermolysis for the treatment of granuloma annulare: a case report. Lasers Surg Med. 2008;40:319-22.
20. Kartamaa M, Reitamo S. Familial benign chronic pemphigus (Hailey-Hailey disease). Treatment with carbon dioxide laser vaporization. Arch Dermatol. 1992;128:646-8.
21. Kaur T, Sandhu K, Gupta S, et al. Treatment of angiolymphoid hyperplasia with eosinophilia with the carbon dioxide laser. J Dermatolog Treat. 2004;15:328-30.
22. Kauvar AN, McDaniel DH, Geronemus RG. Pulsed dye laser treatment of warts. Arch Fam Med. 1995;4:1035-40.
23. Kopera D. Verrucae vulgares: Flashlamp-pumped pulsed dye laser treatment in 134 patients. Int J Dermatol. 2003;42:905-8.
24. Kormeili T, Neel V, Moy RL. Cutaneous sarcoidosis at sites of previous laser surgery. Cutis. 2004;73:53-5.
25. Lertzman BH, McMeekin T, Gaspari AA. Pulsed dye laser treatment of angiolymphoid hyperplasia with eosinophilia lesions. Arch Dermatol. 1997;133:920-1.
26. Lesiac A, Rakowski A, Brzezinska A, et al. Effective treatment of nodular amyloidosis with carbon dioxide laser. J Cutan Med Surg. 2012;16:372-4.
27. McElroy JA, Mehregan DA, Roenigk RK. Carbon dioxide laser vaporization of recalcitrant symptomatic plaques of Hailey-Hailey disease and Darier's disease. J Am Acad Dermatol. 1990;23:893-7.
28. Minsue Chen T, Wanitphakdeedecha R, Nguyen TH. Carbon dioxide laser ablation and adjunctive destruction for Darier-White disease (keratosis follicularis). Dermatol Surg. 2008;34:1431-4.
29. Mudigonda T, Dabade TS, West CE, et al. Therapeutic modalities for localized psoriasis: 308-nm UVB excimer laser versus nontargeted phototherapy. Cutis. 2012;90:149-54.
30. O'Donoghue NB, Barlow RJ. Laser remodelling of nodular nasal lupus pernio. Clin Exp Dermatol. 2006;31:27-9.
31. Peterson CM, Lane JE, Ratz JL. Successful carbon dioxide laser therapy for refractory anogenital lichen sclerosus. Dermatol Surg. 2004;30:1148-51.
32. Raulin C, Schmidt C, Hellwig S. Cutaneous lupus erythematosus-treatment with pulsed dye laser. Br J Dermatol. 1999;141:1046-50.
33. Sajben FP, Ross EV. The use of the 1.0 mm handpiece in high energy, pulsed CO_2 laser destruction of facial adnexal tumors. Dermatol Surg. 1999;25:41-4.
34. Sniezek PJ, DeBloom JR, Arpey CJ. Treatment of granuloma annulare with the 585 nm pulsed dye laser. Dermatol Surg. 2005;31:1370-3.
35. Stack BC, Hall PJ, Goodman AL, et al. CO_2 laser excision of lupus pernio of the face. Am J Otolaryngol. 1996;17:260-3.
36. Stewart L, McCammon K, Metro M, et al. SIU/ICUD consultation on urethral strictures: anterior urethra-lichen sclerosus. Urology. 2014;83:S27-30.
37. Syed S, Weibel L, Kennedy H, et al. A pilot study showing pulsed-dye laser treatment improves localized areas of chronic atopic dermatitis. Clin Exp Dermatol. 2008;33:243-8.

38. Sysa-Jedrzejowska A, Narbutt J. Effective treatment of nodular amyloidosis with carbon dioxide laser. J Cutan Med Surg. 2012;16:372-4.
39. Szekanecz Z, Koch AE. Vascular involvement in rheumatic diseases: 'Vascular rheumatology'. Arthritis Res Ther. 2008;10:224.
40. Truhan AP, Garden JM, Roenigk HH. Nodular primary localized cutaneous amyloidosis: Immunohistochemical evaluation and treatment with the carbon dioxide laser. J Am Acad Dermatol. 1986;14:1058-62.
41. Vestey JP, Tidman MJ, Mclaren KM. Primary nodular cutaneous amyloidosis—long-term follow-up and treatment. Clin Exp Dermatol. 1994;19:159-62.
42. Windahl T. Is carbon dioxide laser treatment of lichen sclerosus effective in the long run? Scand J Urol Nephrol. 2006;40:208-11.
43. Woo PN, Finch TM, Hindson C, et al. Nodular prurigo successfully treated with the pulsed dye laser. Br J Dermatol. 2000;143:215-6.
44. Yanagi T, Sawamura D, Shibaki A, et al. Treatment for poikilodermatous erythema of dermatomyositis with the pulsed dye laser. Br J Dermatol. 2005;153:862-4.

PIGMENTARY DISORDERS

A multitude of disorders have been discussed previously in **Chapters 2 to 4**. We will focus on some entities not discussed previously. Though melasma has been detailed in **Chapters 3 and 4**, we will encapsulate the salient facts here again as this is one indication which is fraught with disheartening results and sequelae in pigmented skin and is ill-advised for the discerning clinician.

Melasma

There are three fundamental prerequisites for successful therapy of any dermatosis. *Firstly*, the intervention should target the main cause; *secondly*, it should be superior over the conventional methods, without combining with existing agents and *lastly*, there should be less relapses.

Without even discussing the mechanism of action of lasers in treating melasma, laser interventions fail all the three dictates (Sardana K). Especially in type V and VI skin, they are of little use and this is directly in contrast with the spate of publications on the topic including reviews, when the results remain abysmal in pigmented skin. We will examine the role of lasers, device wise, and suggest a protocol, for the "brave" clinicians who would like to use lasers in an ideal scenario.

There is agreement that melasma, is a chronic disorder with periods of remissions and exacerbations. This means that there is no known way for curing melasma till today. That fact should be shared with any patient of melasma before suggesting any modality of treatment including laser treatment which is certainly not an inexpensive treatment option for a temporary relief of symptoms of this dermatoses.

Laser and Light-based Treatments

Laser and light therapy represent an alternative third-line approach to treat melasma and may be particularly beneficial for patients with melasma that is refractory to topical therapy or chemical peel regimens, or when a patient wishes for an accelerated pace of improvement in light skin types. Analogous to chemical peels, these modalities accelerate the removal of melanin but do not target the melanin production itself. There is a very high risk of rebound flare or postinflammatory hyperpigmentation (PIH) especially in dermal and mixed types of melasma **(see Chapter 3: Pigmented Lesions and Tattoos)**.

Laser Physics and Melasma

The five broad categories of laser and light therapy include: (1) intense pulsed light (IPL), (2) Q-switched lasers, (3) picosecond lasers, (4) nonablative fractionated lasers, and (5) ablative fractionated lasers.

As discussed in **Chapters 1 and 3**, in melasma, the depth and the target size of the organelle varies (melanin, melanocyte, and clumps of melanocyte). The ideal wavelength for Indian skin (1,064 nm) can have a high scatter and reflected energy, which can itself cause initiation of PIH. Hence, there is very little science behind using lasers in melasma. Moreover, the cardinal dictum that lasers are not ideal for "dynamic pigmented lesions" excludes melasma as it is a perpetually dynamic condition (Goldman).

Intense pulsed light: Overall, IPL therapy appears to give modest improvement in patients with epidermal melasma with a high recurrence rate unless an aggressive topical therapy is maintained at least 6–12 months post-treatment. IPL therapy is best suited to treat patients with Fitzpatrick skin types 1–3 because use in patients with darker skin type carries an elevated risk to target endogenous skin pigment.

Q-switched lasers: The results from studies on the use of Q-switched lasers were disappointing and treatments were complicated by significant rebound hyperpigmentation. We published the first article on the lack of response in 2013 (Sardana K et al.) when conferences were replete with "great" results. Sadly, it required more cases of side effects to withhold the use of Q-switched lasers in Indian skin.

A new variant of Q-switched lasers called low fluence or subthermolytic Q-switched treatment (*aka* laser toning) is gaining popularity. The lasers are the same but the fluences are lower than those that are traditionally used to treat pigmented lesions. The low-fluence treatments largely utilize the 1,064 nm wavelength, which penetrates deeper into the dermis and leaves the epidermis relatively spared. The treatment of patients with melasma with subthermolytic low fluences is based on the theory that the pigment disruption takes place through a photoacoustic mechanism that breaks apart the pigment only and spares the keratinocytes and melanocytes from destruction. However, there is often some degree of damage that accompanies subthermolytic Q-switched treatment but this damage is reported to be less than that from traditional photomechanical treatment.

The results belie this "utopian" thought. In a study, three of 22 patients (all with Fitzpatrick skin type V) developed mottled hypopigmentation after five laser treatments and eight patients developed confetti type hypopigmentation. Three months after treatment, four patients had developed rebound hyperpigmentation and there was a 100% recurrence rate although there was some degree of lightening (Wattanakrai et al., 2010).

Various combinations have been tried, including fractionating the laser energy (Yue et al. 2016) or combining low-fluence Q-switched lasers with long-pulsed Nd:YAG [laser toning (Kang et al., 2011) or IPL (Vachiramon et al., 2015; Yun et al., 2014)], but the recurrence rate has been high, making its use unjustified.

***Ablative fractional laser*:** Fractional lasers were supposed to be the ideal intervention. Though in type I and II skin this treatment in general seems to offer a more durable response in comparison with IPL and Q-switched, there is recurrence. Also, the theory of "shuttling out melanin" is tenuous as the minuscule melanin loss cannot help much in melasma. We have used the fractional technology and found it does little on the macroscopic level. The same story applies to the ablative fractionated resurfacing lasers.

***Picosecond lasers*:** These work via the photoacoustic rather than the photothermal effects. Therefore, it may be more efficient at pigment removal without inducing thermal damage to surrounding tissue. This thermal damage seems to be the greatest drawback of conventional Q-switched laser treatment for patients with melasma and is likely the cause of the high PIH rates after treatment.

Though there is evidence of improvement with the pico lasers, the imagery that is shown in the articles do not mirror the "excellent" results in the abstracts. It is our belief that as far as skin of color are concerned if the pico is used, the 1064 nm pico has more use than the 755 nm, as the former is less absorbed by the competing pigment in the skin. Two studies have been recently published using this pico 1064 nm. The first was a combination with topical HQ and the other used the 595 mm pico in addition to the 1064 nm pico.

The first study (Chalermchai T) combined HQ 4% with the 1,064 nm laser (PicoWay®) with the following settings: 1,064 nm laser, resolve fractional mode, 100 dots per 6 × 6 mm diameter, fluence = 1.3–1.5 mJ per microbeam, pulse duration = 450 ps, 4% coverage per pass for 2–3 passes until mild erythema occurred as an end point with a total of 400–1000 shots, rate = 4 Hz. The authors showed that the combination is effective for dermal melasma, though with such a expensive machine, a stand-alone result would have been more convincing.

The second study was an RCT with a split face protocol using the pico laser of Lutronic (Choi YJ), using both the 1064 nm and 595 nm. The highlight was the use of a split faced protocol and dual wavelength picosecond laser. One side of the face was treated with the HQ 2% cream. The logic of using of 595 nm was to target the vasculature which has a minor role in melasma. The settings used were—1064 nm, 7-10 mm spot size, 0.2-1.5 J/cm^2 fluence, 5 or 10 Hz frequency, 2-4 passes followed by 595 nm, 0.1-0.55 J/cm^2, 5 mm, 2 or 5 Hz, and 1-2 passes with 750 picosecond pulse duration until the presence of mild erythema. The results were quantified using a colorimeter with a primary end point to achieve 51% or more improvement of lightness of pigment at 1 week after the final treatment compared with the baseline value. A close look at the data shows that, one the photographic improvement is not as marked as the abstract stated, and most importantly the mMASI, improved at 7 weeks, but the condition recurred at week 10. This study again proves that visible improvement is not profound or sustained in melasma which is a dynamic pigment disorder.

A study using the RCM (Jo DJ) throws up some important observations that can explain the lack of consistent results with lasers. Firstly, most were mixed melasma cases thus the target depth of the pigment would vary and would not be amenable to a fixed dose. Also apart from melanocytes with more stage IV melanosomes in the dendritic processes, there were also dermal melanophages. The two have varying sizes and consequentially the laser would need to be modulated to target both the melanocytes and melanophages. The distribution of melanin aggregates was uneven, so a fixed dose therapeutic strategy of laser treatment would fail. Also aggregated melanosomes may have higher absorbed photothermal energy density than do single melanosomes accounting for the erratic results and mottled hypopigmentation commonly encountered. Most importantly, the lasers were more effective at inducing melanolysis in surrounding normal skin than they are in melasma lesions. Also the laser tends to concentrate more in the follicular epithelium accounting for the mottling seen. These variables add to the already complexities of pigment reduction in melasma thus adding to the, seasoned opinion that lasers might not be the ideal intervention for melasma.

We feel that the results are not markedly superior to the existing modalities, especially when considering the extremely high price of the picosecond lasers which is not justified when treating melasma, which will recur sooner or later. (*see* **Chapter 3: Pigmented Lesions and Tattoos**)

Laser-assisted drug delivery: There is a new wave of facilitating the delivery of topical medications, which is a technique that is known as laser-assisted drug delivery (LADD). Currently, most topical therapeutic treatments have poor bioavailability due to the difficulty to penetrate the skin barrier. With LADD, CO_2 or Er:YAG ablative lasers create a matrix of transepidermal channels that provide direct access to deeper layers of the skin and facilitate cutaneous and transcutaneous drug delivery. By manipulating the density and depth of these channels, it appears possible to manipulate the amount of drug that is absorbed, the delivery rate, and the drug biodistribution, which may lead to improved clinical efficacy. Tranexamic acid has been combined with microneedling in melasma.

Summary

The mechanism of melasma remains to be fully elucidated but current research suggests that it is a multifactorial condition where pathways of pigment homeostasis are disrupted in the epidermis, extracellular matrix, and dermis (Kwon et al., 2016). The sum of these changes is that the pathways for pigment production are greater than the sum of the pathways for pigment elimination (Fig. 12.36). As a result, melanosomes accumulate at the dermal-epidermal junction (DEJ), the papillary dermis, or deeper.

The history of continuous failures of lasers in melasma, should be enough to stop any more discussion. But then how would conference sessions survive? On a more serious note, the dynamic nature of melasma and with a pathology at various levels, needs a dynamic laser to treat this problem. We had published a review on the depth penetration assessment of fractional lasers (Sardana K, 2012) which primarily explained the poor results in ice pick scars (Sardana K, 2014), the same concept can be extended to melasma. Hence if a "safe" device is discovered, which at present is believed to be the

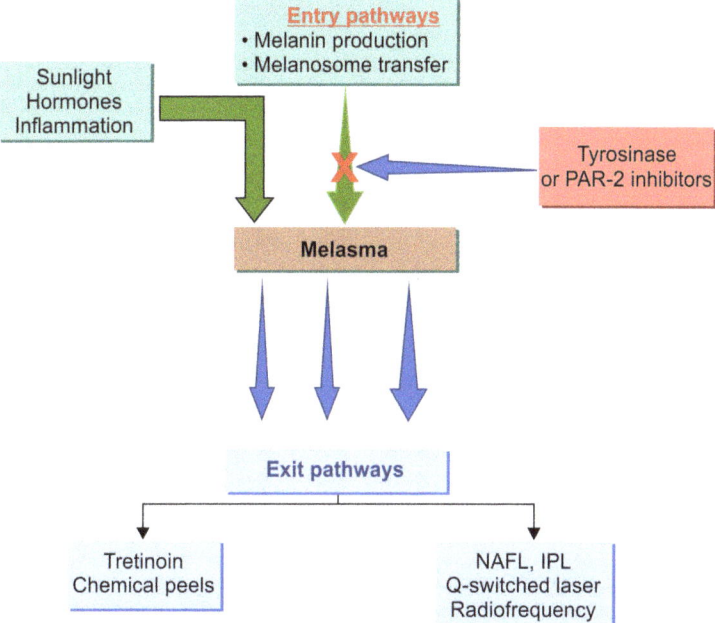

Fig. 12.36: Overview of the various treatment of melasma and their broad site of action. Lasers act at the same step as peels. (IPL: intense pulsed light; NAFL: nonablative fractional laser; PAR-2: protease activated receptor-2)

thulium laser, the depth matters as melasma can be epidermal, dermal, and mixed. Note that most of lasers have been used in combination with other agents, which cannot prove the superiority of lasers (Flowchart 12.2).

As most clinical studies for laser- and light-based treatments are not categorized by the type of melasma (epidermal, mixed, or dermal) and the various ablative fractional laser (AFL) wavelengths have variable penetration, the first step would be to discover a reliable tool to assess level of melasma. Of course we need to go back to the in vitro study to assess depth and in an era where we have moved on to RF, such studies are hard to come by, thus we need to rely on existing data (Fig. 12.37). The data has to be analyzed in respect to in vitro or in vivo models and the device used. As a thumb rule, use of an ablative fractional device, may be counterproductive for melasma, as it would create a large thermal coagulation zone (Fig. 12.37). Also as it is obvious in Figure 12.37, one would need to modulate or interchange lasers to achieve varying depths, which again is only for a static lesion, which is not typified by melasma. Our own work (unpublished) with the fractional Er:YAG, Er:glass, and CO_2 has not found any dramatic results, though all our cases were the mixed type of melasma.

Flowchart 12.2: Overview of lasers in melasma. Note the combination with other agents in most studies.

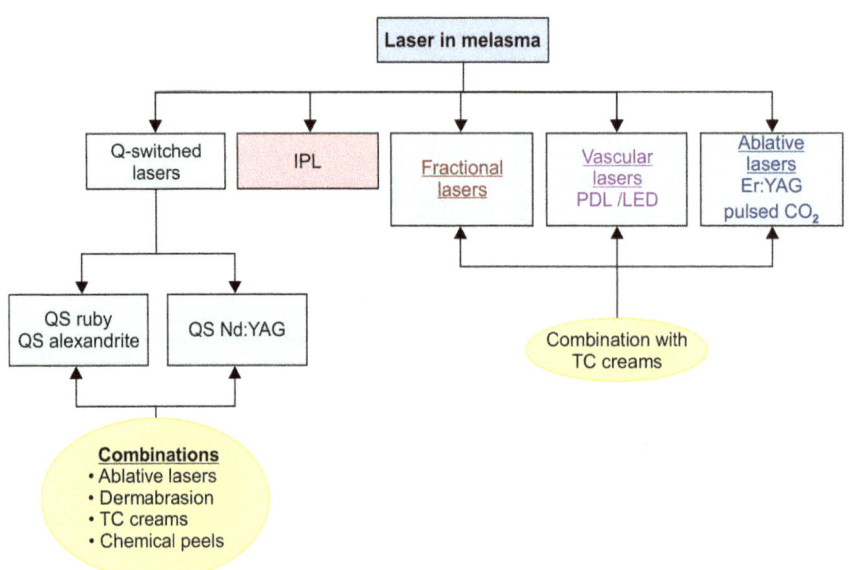

(CO_2: carbon dioxide; Er:YAG: erbium-doped yttrium aluminum garnet; IPL: intense pulsed light; LED: light-emitting diode; Nd:YAG: neodymium-doped yttrium aluminum garnet; PDL: pulsed dye laser)

Source: Sardana K, Chugh S, Garg VK. Which therapy works for melasma in pigmented skin: lasers, peels, or triple combination creams? Indian J Dermatol Venereol Leprol. 2013;79:420-2.

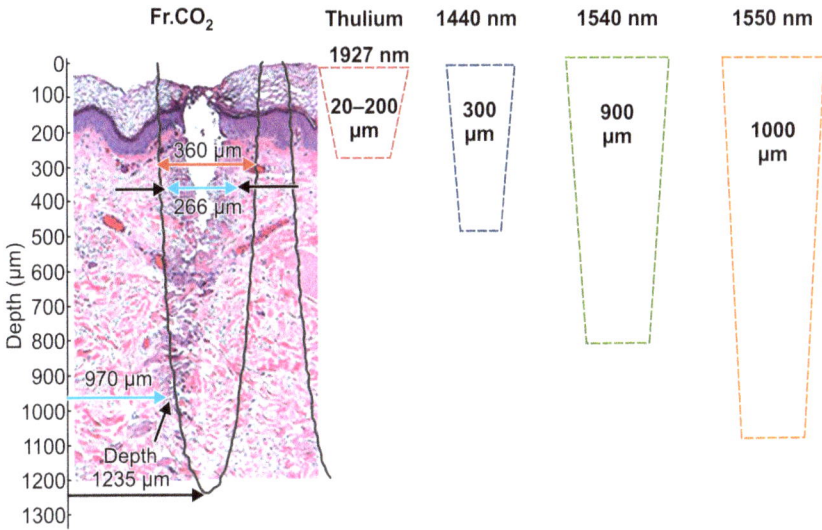

Fig. 12.37: Histological data of depth of various lasers, in comparison to fractional carbon dioxide (CO_2) laser (left to right—thulium 1,927 nm, 1,440 nm, 1,540 nm, and 1,550 nm). Note the coagulation zone and ablation zone with fractional CO_2 laser. The implications are obvious, the ideal laser will have to be tweaked to enable an ideal depth of penetration which will in turn depend on the pathology of melasma which in recalcitrant cases is mixed (epidermal and dermal). Such a device does not exist as yet, making the therapy of melasma a difficult task by lasers.

Table 12.17: Proposed therapeutic ladder for melasma.

First-line therapy	Control of risk factors (sun protection, discontinue hormone treatments or photosensitizing medications) – Topical antityrosinase therapy – Other inhibitors of the melanin synthetic pathway (e.g. protease-activated receptor-2 inhibitor) – Topical exfoliant – Triple combination topical cream, if tolerated
Second-line therapy	Combination of first-line treatment + series chemical peels
Third-line therapy	Combination of first-line treatments with: – NAFL (1927 nm) – NAFL (1550 nm, 1540 nm, or 1440 nm) – Fractional radiofrequency devices
Fourth-line therapy	Combination of first-line treatments with: – Intense pulsed light (test spots) – Q-switch laser

(NAFL: nonablative fractional laser)

Though some authors of recent publications may scoff at this idea, we believe that to some extent, melasma is a "protection mechanism" to the tropical flux of UV light, and it is this natural response that leads to stimulated melanogenesis. Any aggressive tweaking may be grossly counterproductive as it would initiate a repair mechanism with inflammation that would aggravate melasma. A protocol (Table 12.17) is given here to treat melasma which inculcates lasers, which can give a "present day" status to its treatment in melasma. The one caveat that the reader must appreciate as shown in Flowchart 12.2, is that, results tend to be more impressive when energy devices are combined with topical agents and hence this should be understood while analyzing studies that claim superlative results of lasers in melasma.

BIBLIOGRAPHY

1. Badawi AM, Oswan MA. Fractional erbium-doped yttrium aluminum garnet laser-assisted drug delivery of hydroquinone in the treatment of melasma. Clin Cosmet Investig Dermatol. 2018;11:13-20.
2. Chalermchai T, Rummaneethorn P. Effects of a fractional picosecond 1,064 nm laser for the treatment of dermal and mixed type melasma. J Cosmet Laser Ther. 2018;20(3):134-9.
3. Choi YJ, Nam JH, Kim JY, et al. Efficacy and safety of a novel picosecond laser using combination of 1,064 and 595 nm on patients with melasma: A prospective, randomized, multicenter, split-face, 2% hydroquinone cream-controlled clinical trial. Lasers Surg Med. 2017;49(10):899-907.
4. Dunbar S, Posnick D, Bloom B, et al. Energy-based device treatment of melasma: an update and review of the literature. J Cosmet Laser Ther. 2017;19:2-12.
5. Hurliman E, Zelickson B, Kenkel J. In-vivo histological analysis of a fractional CO_2 laser system intended for treatment of soft tissue. J Drugs Dermatol. 2017;16:1085-90.
6. Jo DJ, Kang IH, Baek JH, et al. Using reflectance confocal microscopy to observe in vivo melanolysis after treatment with the picosecond alexandrite laser and Q-switched Nd:YAG laser in melasma. Lasers Surg Med. 2018 Oct 23. doi: 10.1002/lsm.23025. [Epub ahead of print]
7. Kang H, Kim J, Goo B. The dual toning technique for melasma treatment with the 1064 nm Nd:YAG laser: a preliminary study. Laser Ther. 2011;20:189-94.
8. Kist DA, Elm CM, Eleftheriou LI, et al. Histologic analysis of a 2,940 nm fractional device. Lasers Surg Med. 2011;43:79-91.
9. Kwon SH, Hwang YJ, Lee SK, et al. Heterogeneous pathology of melasma and its clinical implications. Int J Mol Sci. 2016;17:E824.
10. Marqa MF, Mordon S. Laser fractional photothermolysis of the skin: Numerical simulation of microthermal zones. J Cosmet Laser Ther. 2014;16:57-65.
11. Sardana K, Chugh S, Garg VK. Which therapy works for melasma in pigmented skin: lasers, peels, or triple combination creams? Indian J Dermatol Venereol Leprol. 2013;79:420-2.
12. Sardana K, Garg VK, Arora P, et al. Histological validity and clinical evidence for use of fractional lasers for acne scars. J Cutan Aesthet Surg. 2012;5:75-90.
13. Sardana K, Garg VK. Lasers are not effective for melasma in darkly pigmented skin. J Cutan Aesthet Surg. 2014;7:57-60.
14. Sardana K, Ghunawat S. Rationale of using hypopigmenting drugs and their clinical application in melasma. Expert Rev Clin Pharmacol. 2015;8:123-34.
15. Sardana K, Manjhi M, Garg VK, et al. Which type of atrophic acne scar (ice-pick, boxcar, or rolling) responds to nonablative fractional laser therapy? Dermatol Surg. 2014;40:288-300.

16. Trivedi MK, Yang FC, Cho BK. A review of laser and light therapy in melasma. Int J Womens Dermatol. 2017;3:11-20.
17. Vachiramon V, Sirithanabadeekul P, Sahawatwong S. Low-fluence Q-switched Nd:YAG 1064-nm laser and intense pulsed light for the treatment of melasma. J Eur Acad Dermatol Venereol. 2015;29:1339-46.
18. Wattanakrai P, Mornchan R, Eimpunth S. Low-fluence Q-switched neodymium-doped yttrium aluminum garnet (1,064 nm) laser for the treatment of facial melasma in Asians. Dermatol Surg. 2010;36:76-87.
19. Yue B, Yang Q, Xu J, et al. Efficacy and safety of fractional Q-switched 1064-nm neodymium-doped yttrium aluminum garnet laser in the treatment of melasma in Chinese patients. Lasers Med Sci. 2016;31:1657-63.
20. Yun WJ, Moon HR, Lee MW, et al. Combination treatment of low-fluence 1,064-nm Q-switched Nd:YAG laser with novel intense pulse light in Korean melasma patients: a prospective, randomized, controlled trial. Dermatol Surg. 2014;40:842-50.

Postinflammatory Hyperpigmentation

Postinflammatory hyperpigmentation is commonly seen after dermatoses or trauma to skin and is a very common issue in Indian skin. The pigment may lie either in the epidermis or dermis. Basal cell layer pigmentation and dermal melanophages are seen.

Treatment

The safest and most effective treatment is time and patience. Overaggressive therapy in our skin type can be counterproductive. Normally, epidermal PIH will resolve on its own over a period of months. Therapeutic options include topical retinoids, bleaching creams, chemical peels, and rarely lasers (Fig. 12.38).

- *Sun protection*: Sun avoidance includes avoiding peak sun hours, wearing a hat out doors to protect the face from sun exposure and an awareness that UVA rays penetrates through windows while driving, while at work, and while at home.
- *Topical treatments*:
    i. Hydroquinone (HQ) formulations, particularly with sunscreens are useful. We do not use more than 2% and abhor the use of triple combination as they contain HQ 4% and steroids that due to overaggressive application by patients make things worse than before. HQ free creams, are a better option. These include deoxyarbutin, ellagic acid, dioic acid, n-butylresorcinol, and azelaic acid, which match the potency of HQ in in vivo trials (Sardana K 2015). A product that is available in India is a non-HQ product with documented results in 3 months (Mazurek K) and contains 20% azelaic acid and mandelic acid, phytic acid, 4-n-butylresorcinol, and ferulic acid (Azelac RU facial serum, Sesderma, Valencia, Spain).

Cause of hyperpigmentation

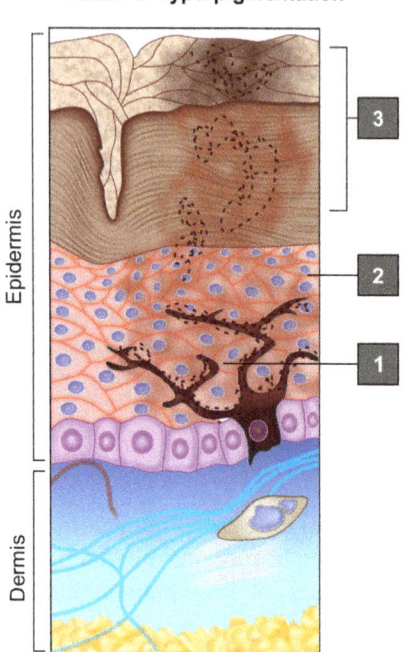

1. Inflammation causes pigment producing cells to become overactive
2. Excess pigment is released into cells, which then work their way upwards through the skin
3. Dead cells carrying extra pigment which collects at the surface, visible as brown spots

Treatment

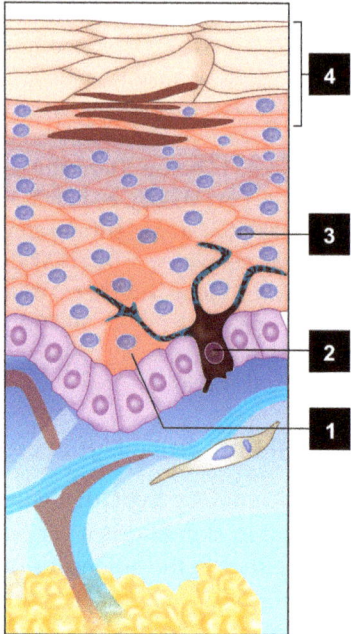

1. **Reduce inflammation**
   Use of mild steroids

2. **Modulation of melanogenesis**
   Lasers?

3. **Increased turnover**
   Use of topical hydroxy acid (GA, salicylic acids, Mandelic acid and retinol)

4. **Exfoliation**
   Removes dead skin cell and reduces amount of visible pigment

Fig. 12.38: Overview of the mechanism and the principle modalities of treating post-inflammatory hyperpigmentation (PIH).

---

  ii. *Retinoids*: Though combinations of 2% mequinol and tretinoin is an option, adapalene somehow works better (personal experience).
  iii. Azelaic acid (20%) cream applied twice daily provides slow lightening of pigmentation so does kojic acid (1–2.5%) cream.
- *Chemical peels*: Chemical peels are an effective treatment option for the reduction of PIH. Though various peels are recommended, salicylic acid peels are the safest for dark skin phototypes. *Never* use the TCA peels

for PIH. In fact, TCA has been used as model to cause PIH (Isedeh P), hence we abhor its use, including the chemical reconstruction of skin scar (CROSS) technique.
- *Lasers*: Several laser types have been studied for the treatment of PIH and other hyperpigmentation, with variable results. The Q-switched ruby and Q-switched alexandrite lasers have been reported to worsen lesions and are *not* recommended for dark-skinned patients. The experience with melasma shows that almost the same problems plague the use of lasers in PIH. We do not recommend its use.

Conclusion

There are two simple caveats that should be understood for PIH. *Firstly*, in pigmented skins PIH is a natural corollary to inflammation, hence any intervention that causes inflammation is to be avoided. Hence, we prefer nothing more than a salicylic acid peel 20% and topical vitamin C which suffices in most cases. *Secondly* the best treatment is "time", which is the best healer. The epidermis would proliferate and the turnover would reduce the PIH without the need for aggressive intervention. In fact, we are surprised at the intricate methods discussed in meetings to treat it as the fundamental caveat is to avoid tissue insult and most of the methods employed do just that. Especially the compounded HQ preparations and TC creams which irritate the skin. If the PIH is due to hemosiderin of course nothing will help. Lasers are minimally useful in this condition. As a thumb rule dermal PIH needs peeling (beta hydroxy peels) while epidermal melasma responds to topical agents in pigmented skin.

BIBLIOGRAPHY

1. Chaowattanapanit S, Silpa-Archa N, Kohli I, et al. Postinflammatory hyperpigmentation: A comprehensive overview: Treatment options and prevention. J Am Acad Dermatol. 2017;77:607-21.
2. Isedeh P, Kohli I, Al-Jamal M, et al. An in vivo model for postinflammatory hyperpigmentation: An analysis of histological, spectroscopic, colorimetric and clinical traits. Br J Dermatol. 2016;174:862-8.
3. Mazurek K, Pierzchała E. Comparison of efficacy of products containing azelaic acid in melasma treatment. J Cosmet Dermatol. 2016;15:269-82.
4. Sardana K, Ghunawat S. Rationale of using hypopigmenting drugs and their clinical application in melasma. Expert Rev Clin Pharmacol. 2015;8:123-34.

Poikiloderma of Civatte

Poikiloderma of Civatte (POC) is a condition that is seen commonly in skin types I and II and is consequent to chronic UV damage on the neck and the chest. The severity of findings is dependent on the duration and intensity of sun exposure, constitutive skin color (Fitzpatrick skin type), and the capacity to tan.

Telangiectases, mild atrophy, reticulated hyperpigmentation and hypopigmentation affecting the lateral and posterior aspect of the neck, anterior chest, and jawline is seen with sparing of the submental area.

Treatment

- *Topical therapy:* Daily sunscreen application with UVB/UVA coverage.
- *Laser therapy*: Though laser therapy is advocated, this has to be done with great caution, as the neck is prone to various sequelae including scar formation, dyspigmentation, "fingerprinting" or treatment skip areas, and textural changes. The neck is prone to scarring as it has less pilosebaceous units. Laser fluences should be lowered by approximately 25-30% of facial parameters to avoid adverse effects. Like most cases of photoaging a multiple laser approach is needed. This is so as there is usually a pigmentary, vascular, and dermal collagen degeneration seen in POC. A single laser will not help. Thankfully, it is uncommon in pigmented skin. If seen the fractional laser may be the only hope as the PDL wavelenghth is absorbed by the melanin with side effects.
    i. *Pulsed dye laser*: Low fluences utilized (e.g. Vbeam 595 nm, 0.45-1.0 ms, 4-6 J/cm^2, 7-10 mm spot, and DCD 30/20). Improvement in telangiectasia and atrophy is seen. There is a possibility of late dyspigmentation hence lower fluences should be used. A recent study by Mejis MM et al. has used a PDL using a 585 nm wavelength and a fixed pulse duration of 450 micros and deduced that the safe dose is 5 J/cm^2, with a 10 mm spot size.
    ii. *Intense pulsed light (e.g. StarLux, 20-30 ms, 28-34 J/cm^2, and 10% pass overlap)*: Improvement of all components may be possible.
    iii. *VersaPulse 532 nm laser*: Low fluences are necessary.
    iv. *Fractionated nonablative and ablative laser*: All components may be targeted. A lower fluence may be needed.

Conclusion

This typifies a difficult disorder to treat as it has multiple components, which would ideally need multiple lasers. In Indian skin, which is type V and VI the fractional RF or nonablative fractional laser (NAFL) may be ideal. The other wavelengths may be absorbed by melanin leading to side effects. The IPL seems to be a option, but as there is very little data on the size of vessels to be treated and the optimal pulse duration will be an issue.

BIBLIOGRAPHY

1. Meijs MM, Blok FA, de Rie MA. Treatment of poikiloderma of Civatte with the pulsed dye laser: A series of patients with severe depigmentation. J Eur Acad Dermatol Venereol. 2006;20:1248-51.

2. Rusciani A, Motta A, Fino P, et al. Treatment of poikiloderma of Civatte using intense pulsed light source: 7 years of experience. Dermatol Surg. 2008;34:314-9.
3. Tierney EP, Hanke CW. Treatment of poikiloderma of Civatte with ablative fractional laser resurfacing: Prospective study and review of the literature. J Drugs Dermatol. 2009;8:527-34.

Vitiligo

Among the various forms of therapy for vitiligo, phototherapy is an important intervention. Excimer laser and light system are basically a form of targeted UVB therapy, which is an option for small areas recalcitrant to conventional therapy.

Excimer System

The 308 nm excimer laser and lamp have been used in dermatology since 1997. These devices emit a wavelength in the UVB spectrum. The monochromatic wavelength at 308 nm provides photobiological effects for those devices that are theoretically superior compared with NB-UVB, especially their immunologic effects. In vitiligo, a more immediate requirement is the migration and the proliferation of melanocytes where there seems to be no advantage of the 308 nm and NB-UVB wavelengths (Casacci M et al.).

An overview of the procedure is given in Table 12.18. The dosing recommendations for each individual laser should be thoroughly studied prior to treating patients, as each machine will differ slightly in its use.

The 308 nm excimer lamp is not strictly monochromatic and the beam of light is not coherent and those systems are much less expensive than lasers. The data concerning the treatment of vitiligo with the 308 nm excimer lamps are much more limited compared with excimer lasers, but they seem to provide a comparable rate of repigmentation (Shi Q et al.).

Advantages: The fluences to be used are low and the immediate side effects are limited to erythema and rarely blisters (especially if sessions are repeated three times a week). Also these devices allow treatment of areas that are usually difficult to reach with UV cabins such as the folds, and they specifically target the affected depigmented patches, preventing hyperpigmentation of the surrounding skin.

Disadvantages: Only relatively small surfaces can be treated and most authors propose the use of these devices for lesions affecting less than 10% of the total surface body area.

Results: The clinical efficacy of the 308 nm excimer laser is well demonstrated. Overall, 20-30% of the treated patches reach a satisfactory aesthetic result, that is, a repigmentation of at least 75%. Those results appear superior to those usually obtained with NB-UVB phototherapy but direct comparison data between NB-UVB and 308 nm emitting devices is still very limited.

Table 12.18: Step-by-step approach of using the excimer laser for vitiligo, psoriasis, and alopecia areata.

Preprocedure	• Skin type of patient and minimal erythema dose (MED) should be determined • MED testing should be performed on non-sun-exposed area of skin such as volar forearm or buttocks at least 1 day prior to treatment
Overview	• Weekly or biweekly treatments are required • Treatments are quick and generally take less than 2–3 minutes for a 10 cm² lesion
Procedure	• Ensure appropriate protective eyewear for the patient and the provider • Apply mineral oil to intended treatment areas to enhance ultraviolet (UV) penetration (for psoriasis) • *Initial dose*: 2–3 × MED for psoriasis; 50 mJ/cm² less than MED for vitiligo or AA • Deliver treatment pulses in nonoverlapping pulses • *End point*: The goal is to produce moderate erythema for psoriasis, and minimal erythema and clinical response for vitiligo and AA • If there is no erythema or response then increase dose by 25% for psoriasis, or 50 mJ/cm² for vitiligo and AA • If minimal erythema is produced, then increase dose by 10–15% at each subsequent visit for psoriasis; maintain this dose for vitiligo or AA • For moderate erythema in treating psoriasis, maintain this dose; for vitiligo or AA, decrease dose by 50 mJ/cm² • If severe erythema, burning, blistering, or pigment alteration occurs then skip one treatment session and decrease dose by 15–25% for the next scheduled visit for psoriasis; for vitiligo or AA, decrease by 100 mJ/cm²
Postprocedure	• To prevent severe erythema or burning of the skin, MED testing is extremely important • Patients should be advised to use sun protection and sunscreen when going outside following treatment • If blistering occurs, the area should be covered with antibiotic ointment or hydrophilic petrolatum until healed • Pruritus may be treated with a low-potency topical steroid twice daily until resolved • Hyperpigmentation may occur at treated sites • Higher fluences of the excimer laser produce faster and longer remissions but are associated with a higher risk of phototoxic reactions and blistering

A study that has been published is an important lesson for clinicians wishing to buy the excimer system in preference over NB-UVB. Verhaeghe E studied the efficacy of 308 nm monochromatic excimer light (MEL) versus localized 311 nm NB-UVB in vitiligo patients. This prospective intrapatient placebo-controlled randomized trial found that while 20% of the lesions treated with NB-UVB achieved repigmentation scores above 50%, none of the lesions treated with MEL achieved a repigmentation higher than 50% after 24 sessions. Thus, localized 311 nm NB-UVB is more effective in the treatment of vitiligo and an unbiased view reinforces the fact that it is better than the 308 nm excimer lasers.

In India, where PUVA is practiced, it is the author's opinion in conjunction with a recent study (Singh S) that probably with the abundant sunlight and low risk of melanoma in our skin, the excimer laser cannot be universally recommended especially for the larger population that cannot afford this therapy.

Other indications of excimer laser: They include postresurfacing leukoderma, leukoderma after laser tattoo removal with a Q-switched Nd:YAG laser, hypopigmented striae, halo nevus, and nevus depigmentosus.

Conclusion: Lasers for vitiligo reinforce certain principles for using lasers. *Firstly*, they should be superior to conventional therapies; *secondly*, the results should be stable and long-term follow-up studies must be published. The safety profile is a recurring theme, that is probably relevant in FST (I-III) but in darker skin types this is not necessarily an issue.

Predictably, some of the advantages with conventional phototherapy and PUVA are also seen with excimer lasers, like, the excellent results on the face, with more than three-fourths of patients reaching at least 75% repigmentation. But the system has not been and probably will not be able to overcome the known issues with conventional phototherapy namely:

- Lack of response on the extremities and the bony prominences.
- Lack of stability of response, which is impossible to predict as long-term results have not been reported. In fact, one study reported no repigmentation after 1 year of follow-up.

A summary of the use of this system is provided in Table 12.19.

The development of the 308 nm excimer lamp is more recent and is much cheaper and the results are comparable to excimer lasers. Le Duff F et al. performed a prospective trial comparing the 308 nm excimer laser and the 308 nm excimer lamp and confirmed that these two devices are equally effective in repigmenting vitiligo patches.

Lasers and Melanocyte Grafting

Surgical approaches are recommended for segmental vitiligo or for localized vitiligo that has been stable for more than 3 years. It is also a useful method for congenital hypomelanosis, such as piebaldism, or for nevus depigmentosus. The preparation of the recipient bed before grafting requires a homogeneous epithelial removal.

Table 12.19: Overview of excimer laser light in vitiligo.

Indications	Limited or localized lesions of vitiligo
Site (most to least responsive)	Face, scalp/neck, genitals, trunk, extremities, hands and feet, including bony prominences
Skin type	Fitzpatrick III or higher skin types respond the best
Size	Small lesions respond more quickly

Both the CO_2 lasers (Kahn) and more recently, the Er:YAG lasers (Pai GS) followed by epidermal skin grafts or epidermal suspension grafts have been used. Such a method has also been used in piebaldism (Guerra L). Recently, dermabrasion with Er:YAG laser followed by fluorouracil applications before NB-UVB therapy was compared to NB-UVB alone in 50 patients with symmetrical patches of vitiligo (Anbar TS). A moderate to marked improvement was observed in 78.1% of the lesions treated with the combination protocol as compared with 23.4% of the lesions that have only received phototherapy. Pain and transient hyperpigmentation was reported in the combination group. These results clearly need to be confirmed, but they suggest an interesting new approach for treating vitiligo.

Our experience with this is restricted to the Er:YAG. This is set at a dose of 5–6 J/cm^2 and multiple passes are made till pinpoint bleeding appears, which is the end point. A study is underway comparing this with conventional surgical grafting, thus this author cannot yet recommend it as a preferential method for recipient site preparation (Figs. 12.39A and B).

Lasers for Inducing Leukoderma

Laser devices were first used for depigmenting the residual pigmented areas in generalized vitiligo. Permanent depigmentation is usually proposed for people older than 40 years and after detailed information is given to the patient. Monobenzylether of hydroquinone (MBEH) causes a permanent depigmentation of the skin that has been used for generalized vitiligo.

Though some lasers have been used, the evidence for their use and their efficacy is limited. A short, retrospective study suggests that a Q-switched ruby laser is as effective as MBEH (depigmentation was observed in 69% of

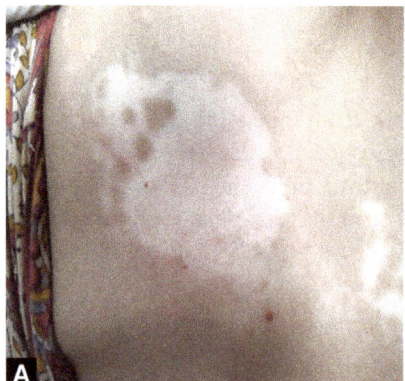 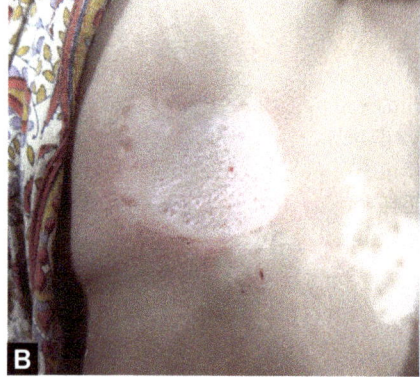

Figs. 12.39A and B: (A) Two passes have been given with the erbium-doped yttrium aluminum garnet (Er:YAG) laser. Note the loss of epidermis and a faint erythema, which signifies the papillary dermis; and (B) Pinpoint bleeding is the end point of the ablation.
Source: Dr Sumit Gupta, New Delhi

the subjects with both treatments) (Njoo MD). Of interest, repigmentation of treated areas was observed in 44% and 36% of the patients treated with lasers and MBEH, respectively. Thus, patients should be informed of the risk of repigmentation after both kinds of treatment.

Isolated success has been reported in a patient with generalized vitiligo who was treated with Q-switched ruby laser, with no repigmentation observed 1 year after the treatment (Kim YJ). More recently, Q-switched alexandrite laser has been shown to be efficacious in depigmentation of one patient. Again, no repigmentation was observed at follow-up after 1 year (Rao J). A study from India (Majid I) used the Q-switched 532 nm, but the concomitant use of MBEH with the laser can potentially influence the results.

Thus, depigmenting lasers seem to be an attractive alternative to MBEH for depigmenting patients with generalized vitiligo but they should be reserved for limited surfaces and they should not be proposed if depigmentation involves less than 50% of the affected area. In all the cases, patients have to be clearly informed of the potential risk of later repigmentation and photoprotection of the treated areas should be systematically prescribed. More importantly if the Q-switched Nd:YAG is used the 532 nm in preference to the 1,064 nm.

BIBLIOGRAPHY

1. Al-Mutairi N. 308-nm excimer laser for the treatment of alopecia areata in children. Ped Dermatol. 2009;26:547-50.
2. Anbar TS, Westerhof W, Abdel-Rahman AT, et al. Effect of one session of Er:YAG laser ablation plus topical 5-Fluorouracil on the outcome of short-term NB-UVB phototherapy in the treatment of non-segmental vitiligo: A left-right comparative study. Photodermatol Photoimmunol Photomed. 2008;24:322-9.
3. Baltas E, Nagy P, Bonis B, et al. Repigmentation of localized vitiligo with the xenon chloride laser. Br J Dermatol. 2001;144:1266-7.
4. Casacci M, Thomas P, Pacifico A, et al. Comparison between 308-nm monochromatic excimer light and narrowband UVB phototherapy (311-313 nm) in the treatment of vitiligo—a multicentre controlled study. J Eur Acad Dermatol Venereol. 2007;21:956-63.
5. Guerra L, Primavera G, Raskovic D, et al. Permanent repigmentation of piebaldism by erbium:YAG laser and autologous cultured epidermis. Br J Dermatol. 2004;150:715-21.
6. Kahn AM, Ostad A, Moy RL. Grafting following short-pulse carbon dioxide laser de-epithelialization. Dermatol Surg. 1996;22:965-7.
7. Kim YJ, Chung BS, Choi KC. Depigmentation therapy with Q-switched ruby laser after tanning in vitiligo universalis. Dermatol Surg. 2001;27:969-70.
8. Le Duff F, Fontas E, Giacchero D, et al. 308-nm excimer lamp vs. 308-nm excimer laser for treating vitiligo: A randomized study. Br J Dermatol. 2010;163:188-92.
9. Majid I, Imran S. Depigmentation therapy with Q-switched Nd:YAG laser in universal vitiligo. J Cutan Aesthet Surg. 2013;6:93-6.

10. Nicolaidou E, Antoniou C, Stratigos A, et al. Narrowband ultraviolet B phototherapy and 308-nm excimer laser in the treatment of vitiligo: A review. J Am Acad Dermatol. 2009;60:470-7.
11. Njoo MD, Vodegel RM, Westerhof W. Depigmentation therapy in vitiligo universalis with topical 4-methoxyphenol and the Q-switched ruby laser. J Am Acad Dermatol. 2000;42:760-9.
12. Novak Z, Bonis B, Baltas E, et al. Xenon chloride ultraviolet B laser is more effective in treating psoriasis and in inducing T-cell apoptosis than narrow-band ultraviolet B. J Photochem Photobiol. 2002;67:32-8.
13. Pai GS, Vinod V, Joshi A. Efficacy of erbium YAG laser-assisted autologous epidermal grafting in vitiligo. J Eur Acad Dermatol Venereol. 2002;16:604-6.
14. Rao J, Fitzpatrick RE. Use of the Q-switched 755-nm alexandrite laser to treat recalcitrant pigment after depigmentation therapy for vitiligo. Dermatol Surg. 2004;30:1043-5.
15. Shi Q, Li K, Fu J, et al. Comparison of the 308-nm excimer laser with the 308-nm excimer lamp in the treatment of vitiligo—a randomized bilateral comparison study. Photodermatol Photoimmunol Photomed. 2013;29:27-33.
16. Singh S, Khandpur S, Sharma VK, et al. Comparison of efficacy and side-effect profile of oral PUVA vs. oral PUVAsol in the treatment of vitiligo: A 36-week prospective study. J Eur Acad Dermatol Venereol. 2013;27:1344-51.
17. Verhaeghe E, Lodewick E, van Geel N, et al. Intrapatient comparison of 308-nm monochromatic excimer light and localized narrow-band UVB phototherapy in the treatment of vitiligo: A randomized controlled trial. Dermatology. 2011;223:343-8.

Becker's Nevus

This topic is discussed in detail in **Chapter 3: Pigmented Lesions and Tattoos** and the one thing we have learnt having used Q-switched Nd:YAG, IPL, Er:YAG, and fractional lasers is that almost nothing works consistently. This can be understood if one looks at the basic of laser–tissue interactions.
- The pathology is both the hair growth and the pigment at various levels
- Hence, one needs to target two different pathologies which usually fails
- The residual pigment helps in repigmentation very fast.

The universal abysmal results of lasers in melasma can be extended here also and here we have a more complicated pathology. One concept is to use laser hair removal to improve the overlying hypertrichosis followed by pigment-specific or ablative lasers. There are marked postinflammatory hypo and hyperpigmentation sequelae and in our skin type lower fluences are needed which reduce the efficacy. We have used the fine ablation potential of Er:YAG but there is frequent recurrence (Flowchart 12.3).

HAIR DISORDERS

Though, lasers have been used for hair transplantation, we will largely focus on the direct effect of lasers on hair growth.

Flowchart 12.3: Therapy of Becker's nevus.

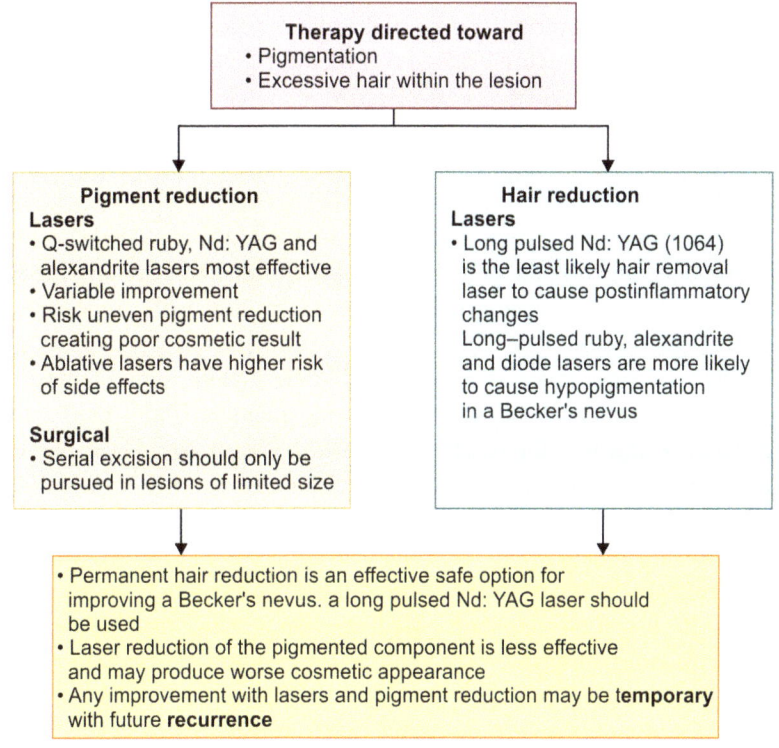

(Nd:YAG: neodymium-doped yttrium aluminum garnet)

Though lasers and light therapies for alopecia include 308 nm excimer laser, fractional photothermolysis, and UV phototherapy, we will largely focus on low-level laser therapy (LLLT).

It has long been known that red or near-infrared laser light promotes tissue repair and regeneration and low-intensity light called LLLT stimulates cellular activity. After the discovery of lasers in the 1960s, there has been tremendous interest in using these laser devices to treat various medical conditions. The most commonly used devices have wavelengths in the range of 500–1,100 nm (the so-called optical window of tissue) and they deliver fluences of 1–10 J/cm^2 with a power density of 3–90 mW/cm^2. LLLT has shown beneficial effects for a variety of medical conditions such as wound healing, nerve regeneration, joint pain relief, stroke recovery, and the prevention and treatment of mucositis. Home-use LLLT devices that emit low-power coherent monochromatic red light have been developed for various skin conditions, including hair growth.

Alopecia

The pathogenesis of alopecia depends on the type of hair loss. The genetic hair loss, androgenetic alopecia (AGA) is consequent to DHT, which binds to the nuclear androgen receptor, which regulates gene expression. Disruption of epithelial progenitor cell activation and cell proliferation due to abnormal androgen signaling forms the essential pathophysiological component of this condition, which in turn leads to continuous miniaturization of sensitive terminal hair follicles, and their conversion to vellus hair follicles. Although the exact genes involved in hair loss are not clearly known, some of the proposed genes responsible for hair growth are desmoglein, activin, epidermal growth factor (EGF), fibroblast growth factor (FGF), lymphoid-enhancer factor-1 (LEF-1), and sonic hedgehog. There are several other forms of hair loss such as alopecia areata (AA), telogen effluvium (TE), and chemotherapy-induced alopecia. AA is an autoimmune inflammatory condition, which presents with nonscarring alopecia.

While the conventional methods of therapy include topical minoxidil, finasteride (males only) and surgical hair transplantation with LLLT having received FDA approval. The HairMax LaserComb was approved by the US FDA and received 510 K clearance as a safe therapy for the treatment of male AGA in 2007 and female AGA in 2011 (Wikramanayake TC). The other FDA approved devices include Sunetics, Laser Hair Brush and Clinical unit, Revage 670 Laser (Chair unit), and Spencer Forrest X5 (Handheld) Hair Laser. Recently, a diode laser, the X5 Hair Laser has been used. Though a sham, device failure and resultant missing data from the control group are a negative aspect, the authors report a positive trend hair growth, due to the chronic use of X5 Hair Laser device. A list of studies on various devices is detailed in Table 12.20.

Basic Science of Low-level Laser Therapy

There are a few mechanisms proposed for its action (Figs. 12.40A and B) and are listed here:
- Stimulates the mitochondrial transport chain
- Enhances adenosine triphosphate (ATP) production
- Stimulates wound healing
- Reduces inflammation, improves neurologic damage, such as with stroke, and improves musculoskeletal and joint pain.

The extension of this form of therapy to alopecia has an interesting history. In the late 1960s, Endre Mester, a Hungarian physician, began a series of experiments on the carcinogenic potential of lasers by using a low-power ruby laser (694 nm) on mice. Mice were shaved as a part of the experimental protocol. To Mester's surprise, the laser did not cause cancer but instead improved hair growth around the shaved region on the animal's back. This was the first demonstration of "photobiostimulation" with LLLT, and it opened a new path in the field of medicine.

This experimental fact was supported by a clinical phenomenon where an increase in hair density, color or coarseness, or a combination of these occurs

Table 12.20: Overview of studies with LLLT devices for hair growth.

Home devices	Power	Treatment regimes	Studies	Subjects	Results	Peer reviewed?
Capillus™ 82 Laser Cap	410 mW	30 min 3–4 ×/week	Double blind RCT	44F	63.7% increase in terminal hair count vs sham	No
Capillus™ 202 Laser Cap	1010 mW	30 min 3–4 ×/week				
Capillus™ 272 Pro Laser Cap	1360 mW	30 min 3–4 ×/week				
HairMax™ Laser Band 41	205 mW	3 min 3×/week	Prospective cohort	28M, 7F	Total hair count and hair tensile strength increased	Yes (Satino)
HairMax™ Laser Band 82	410 mW	90s 3×/week	Double blind RCT	110M	Mean terminal hair density increased by ~20 hairs/cm^2	Yes (Leavitt)
HairMax™ Prima7 Laser Comb	35 mW	15 min 3×/week	Case report	2M	No significant change in hair count or thickness	Yes (Rushton)
HairMax™ Ultima 9 Laser Comb	45 mW	15 min 3×/week	Retrospective cohort	11M, 21F	Global photos – majority w/ moderate improvement	Yes (Munk)
HairMax™ 12 Laser Comb	60 mW	8 min 3×/week	Double blind RCT	128M, 141F	Terminal hair density increased by ~15 hairs/cm^2	Yes (Jimenez)
iGrow™ Hair Growth System	255 mW	25 min every other day	Double blind RCT	41M	35–37% increase in terminal hair count	Yes (Lanzafame)
			Double blind RCT	42F		
iRestore™ Hair Growth System	255 mW	25 min every other day	Double blind RCT	18M, 18F	Pending, study in progress	N/A
Lasercap™ LCPRO	1120 mW	36 min every other day	Case series	7F	Improvement in hair volume and shine	N/A
			Case series	1M, 2F		
NutraStim™ Laser Hair Comb	60 mW	8 min 3×/week	N/A	N/A	N/A	N/A
Theradorme™ LH80 PRO	400 mW	20 min 2×/week	Double blind RCT	80M	Pending, study in progress	N/A

(LLLT: low-level laser therapy; RCT: randomized controlled trial)

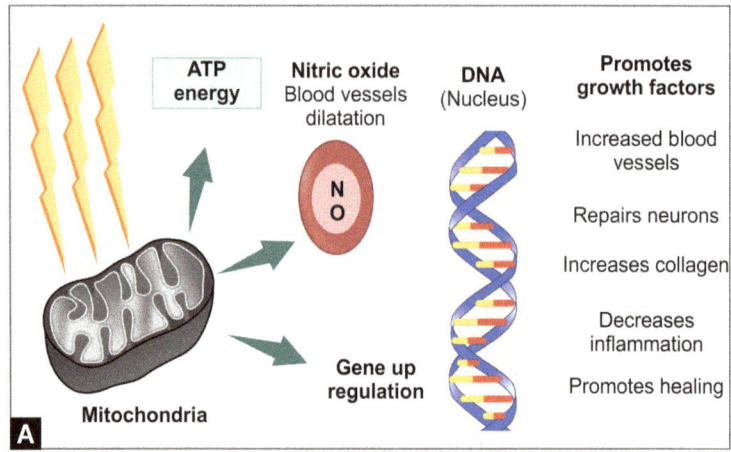
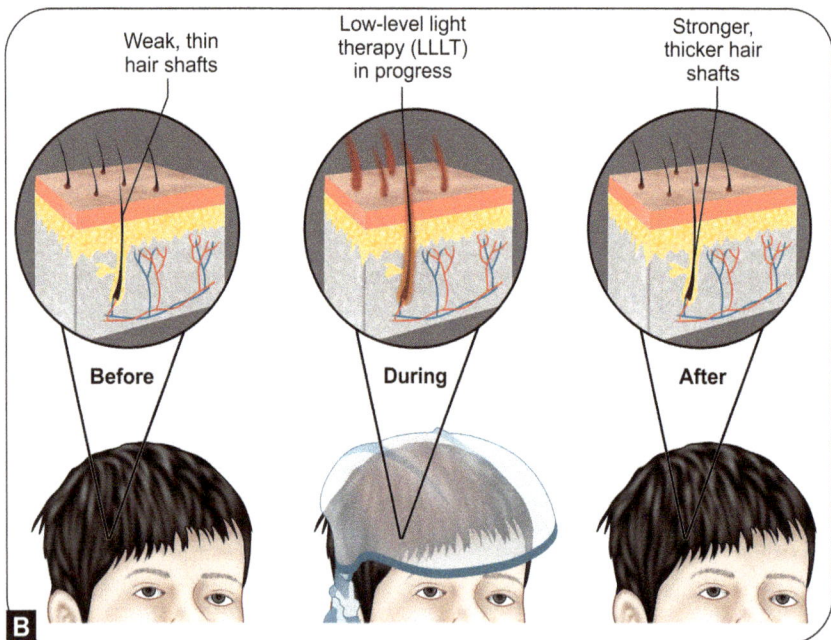

Figs. 12.40A and B: Overview of the mechanism suggested for efficacy of LLLT for alopecia, lower figure shows the mechanism of the iGrow® Laser Hair Growth Helmet. (ATP: adenosine triphosphate; DNA: deoxyribonucleic acid; LLLT: low-level laser therapy)
Source: Adapted from Dr Sajjad Khan, ILHT Hair Transplant Surgery Center, Dubai, 2016.

at or around sites treated for hair removal and is known as "paradoxical hypertrichosis", the incidence of which varies from 0.6% to 10%.

A group of researchers also observed transformation of small vellus hairs into larger terminal hairs upon low fluence diode laser treatment and named this phenomenon as "terminalization" of vellus hair follicles. Why this happens is yet unknown and has been explained by a subtherapeutic heat generation, which induces follicular stem cell proliferation and differentiation by increasing the level of heat shock proteins (HSPs) such as HSP27, which plays a role in regulation of cell growth and differentiation. Thus, subtherapeutic injury caused by the laser could also result in the release of certain factors, which could potentially induce follicular angiogenesis and affect the cell cycling.

Thus, laser phototherapy is assumed to stimulate anagen reentry in telogen hair follicles, prolong duration of anagen phase, increase rates of proliferation in active anagen hair follicles, and to prevent premature catagen development.

Other Lasers

Fractional erbium glass fiber 1,550 nm (Mosaic, Lutronic Co., Ltd, Seoul, South Korea) was used in an experimental study in rats. The radiation was applied over the shaved skin of C3H/HeN rats using various power and density configurations in different radiation intervals. Stimulation effects on hair were observed due to the level of power employed, density, and radiation interval. Histologic findings reveal the conversion of hair in telogen phase into anagen phase. The conversion into anagen hair and the increase of Wnt-5a, β-catenin were regarded as signs of therapeutic response. This was then translated into an in vivo study by Kim et al. 2011 where 20 male volunteers were treated in five sessions and in 2-week intervals with a dose of 5 mJ power with a total density of 300 spots/cm^2. This stimulated growth factors, including vascular endothelial growth factor (VEGF), which induces neoangiogenesis. The heartening results were replicated using the fractional erbium glass fiber 1,550 nm on female pattern alopecia (Lee et al. 2011).

Conclusion

A list of studies using LLLT are detailed in Table 12.21. The results of all the devices depend largely on the parameters used to assess them and long-term follow-up. However, more studies are needed to optimize treatment parameters and determine long-term efficacy as well as safety of emerging LLLT technologies. Most studies investigating effects of LLLT on hair growth have used wavelengths that range from 635 nm to 650 nm, but as of today no study has compared the effect of near-infrared wavelengths such as 810 nm, which have deeper penetrating capacities, to red light. Moreover, further studies are required to compare efficacy of different light sources (continuous vs. pulsed) and methods of light delivery [laser vs. light-emitting diode (LED)].

There are certain overbearing concerns that shroud the use of these devices:
- There is still a paucity of peer-reviewed studies validating LLLT for hair loss. It is unclear why so few studies exist, given the positive anecdotal reports described earlier.

Table 12.21: Clinical studies of LLLT in alopecia.

	Patients	Diagnosis	Device parameters and treatment regimen	
Yamazaki et al. 2003	Six male and nine female patients	Alopecia areata	Super Lizer™ pulsed linear light, 600–1,600 nm, 1.8 W, 3 minutes/week or every other week	The patients received additional supplements and medications and were treated until vellus hair regrowth in at least 50% of the affected area. LLLT only accelerates the process of hair regrowth in AA patients.
Satino et al. 2003	28 male and seven female patients	Androgenetic alopecia	HairMax LaserComb, 655 nm, 5–10 minutes every other day, for 6 months	• Hair tensile strength improved in the vertex area for males and temporal area for females. • Hair count improved (for temporal area: 55% in women, 74% in men; in vertex area: 65% in women, 120% in men) with vertex area in males having the best outcome.
Kim et al. 2007	24 male patients	Androgenetic alopecia	655 nm and 780 nm, once a day for 10 minutes, for 14 weeks	
Leavitt et al. 2009	110 male patients		HairMax LaserComb, 3 times/week for 15 minutes, for 26 weeks	Significantly greater increase in mean terminal hair density compared to subjects in the sham device group
Lanzafame et al. 2013	44 male patients	Androgenetic alopecia	Helmet (Top Hat 655) containing 21, 5 mW lasers and 30 LEDs, 655 nm, 67.3 J/cm^2, 25 minutes every other day, for 16 weeks	35% increase in hair growth among male AGA patients
Kim et al. 2013	40 patients		Helmet type LLLT device, 650 nm laser with 630 nm and 660 nm LEDs, 92.15 mW/cm^2, 47.90 J/cm^2, 18 minutes/day, for 24 weeks	LLLT increased hair count and shaft diameter, however, blinded global images did not support these observations

(AGA: androgenetic alopecia; LEDs: light-emitting diodes; LLLT: low-level laser therapy)

- The treatment of alopecia has moved from the domain of dermatologists to quacks, beauticians, homeopath, and so called "trichologists". While we can appreciate the nuances of the etiology, this is lost on alternative practitioners and patients. Thus, a detailed evaluation and biopsy with its proper interpretation is needed where necessary. If LLLT is made a "home use" device, which it largely is, there will be situations where results will not be commisurate with the diagnosis. Who will protect consumers from

buying expensive items that may not be applicable or aggressive enough for their type of hair loss?
- Fractional lasers have entered this field, with studies on the 1,550 nm nonablative fractional erbium glass laser, the ablative fractional 2,940 nm Er:YAG laser, and the ablative fractional CO_2 fractional laser, though the logic is still fuzzy.

As trained dermatologists, we should be open to the use of such devices where other options have failed, so long as reproducible studies can demonstrate their safety and efficacy. The technology has expanded to include AA and chemotherapy-induced alopecia and more studies will establish its role in these disorders.

BIBLIOGRAPHY

1. Kim H, Choi JW, Kim JY, et al. Low-level light therapy for androgenetic alopecia: A 24-week, randomized, double-blind, sham device-controlled multicenter trial. Dermatol Surg. 2013;39:1177-83.
2. Kim TH, Kim NJ, Youn JI. Evaluation of wavelength dependent hair growth effects on low-level laser therapy: An experimental animal study. Lasers Med Sci. 2015;30:1703-9.
3. Kim WS, Lee HI, Lee JW, et al. Fractional photothermolysis laser treatment of male pattern hair loss. Dermatol Surg. 2011;37:41-51.
4. Leavitt M, Charles G, Heyman E, et al. HairMax LaserComb laser phototherapy device in the treatment of male androgenetic alopecia: A randomized, double-blind, sham device-controlled, multicentre trial. Clin Drug Investig. 2009;29:283-92.
5. Lee GY, Lee SJ, Kim WS. The effect of a 1550 nm fractional erbium-glass laser in female pattern hair loss. J Eur Acad Dermatol Venereol. 2011;25:1450-4.
6. Wikramanayake TC, Rodriguez R, Choudhary S, et al. Effects of the Lexington LaserComb on hair regrowth in the C3H/HeJ mouse model of alopecia areata. Lasers Med Sci. 2012;27:431-6.
7. Yamazaki M, Miura Y, Tsuboi R, et al. Linear polarized infrared irradiation using SuperLizer is an effective treatment for multiple-type alopecia areata. Int J Dermatol. 2003;42:738-40.

Pseudofolliculitis

Pseudofolliculitis is a common, chronic inflammatory disorder that presents with inflammatory papules and pustules in the beard area of males. It is seen commonly in females in the axillary and pubic area.

This disorder is induced by shaving. Shaving sharpens curled hair, which in turn pierce into the skin adjoining the hair follicle and produce an inflammatory reaction. It can also follow hair plucking, especially in females with hirsutism.

Treatment

- The most simple, inexpensive, and effective treatment for pseudofolliculitis is the cessation of shaving. For those who cannot do practice this measure, alteration in shaving habits is required. These include wetting the area prior to applying shaving cream, using a sharp razor, shaving in the direction of the hair growth, and avoiding shaving in more than one direction in the same area. Using a clipper instead of a razor is another option.

- An overview of the shaving advise is given in Table 12.22.
- *Topical treatment*: Topical antibiotics are effective in managing the inflammation. Other agents tried include tretinoin, benzoyl peroxide, and glycolic acids.
- *Lasers*:
  i. The long-pulsed 1,064 nm Nd:YAG laser is the treatment of choice in skin phototypes IV-VI. It is safe and effective. Long pulse durations are necessary for epidermal protection. Pulse durations of 30–100 ms are generally recommended. Optimal fluences range from 20 J/cm^2 to 40 J/cm^2.

Table 12.22: Overview of patient advise for prevention of pseudofolliculitis barbae (PFB).

Shaving should not be resumed until all the inflamed lesions have cleared and all the ingrown hairs have been released	1. Advise patients to discontinue shaving for 1 month for mild cases, 2 to 3 months for moderate cases, and 3 to 6 months for severe cases. During this shaving hiatus, beards can be trimmed with scissors or electric clippers to a minimum length of 1 cm 2. Apply a warm water, saline, or Burow's solution compress for 10 to 15 minutes three times a day to soothe the lesions, remove the crust, stop drainage secondary to inflammation, and soften the epidermis, allowing for the easier and earlier release of ingrown hairs 3. Apply a topical hydrocortisone cream or lotion (for 3 to 4 weeks only) to the shaved area 4. An antibiotic or a short-course of oral steroid for 10 days may be needed
For those who need to shave	1. Ingrown hairs should *not* be plucked 2. Use electric clippers to remove as much preexisting beard hair 3. Apply warm water compresses for approximately 5 minutes 4. Use any brand of shaving cream 5. Choose a sharp razor that cuts best without irritation 6. Shave *with* the grain of the hair, using short strokes while avoiding pulling the skin taut. Twice over one area is usually sufficient. Shave *gently* 7. Use a magnifying mirror to search for any ingrown hairs. To release them gently, insert a toothpick under the loop or brush the beard area with a soft toothbrush 8. In expert hands, a hypodermic needle can be used to release ingrowing hair 9. A steroid application can help in such inflamed areas postrelease of the hair

ii. Newer generation diode lasers with longer pulse durations up to 400 ms can also be utilized with caution in darker skin types.
iii. Typically, 5-10 treatments spaced every 4-8 weeks are needed for 50-75% permanent reduction.

- The addition of topical eflornithine to hair laser treatment decreased hair and inflammatory papules faster when compared with laser therapy alone in the treatment of pseudofolliculitis barbae (PFB).

An algorithm is given here (Flowchart 12.4) of the best available evidence for treating PFB and the crucial aspect, is modifying the ingrained shaving method of patients and learning the art of releasing the embedded hair.

Flowchart 12.4: Algorithm for management of PFB.

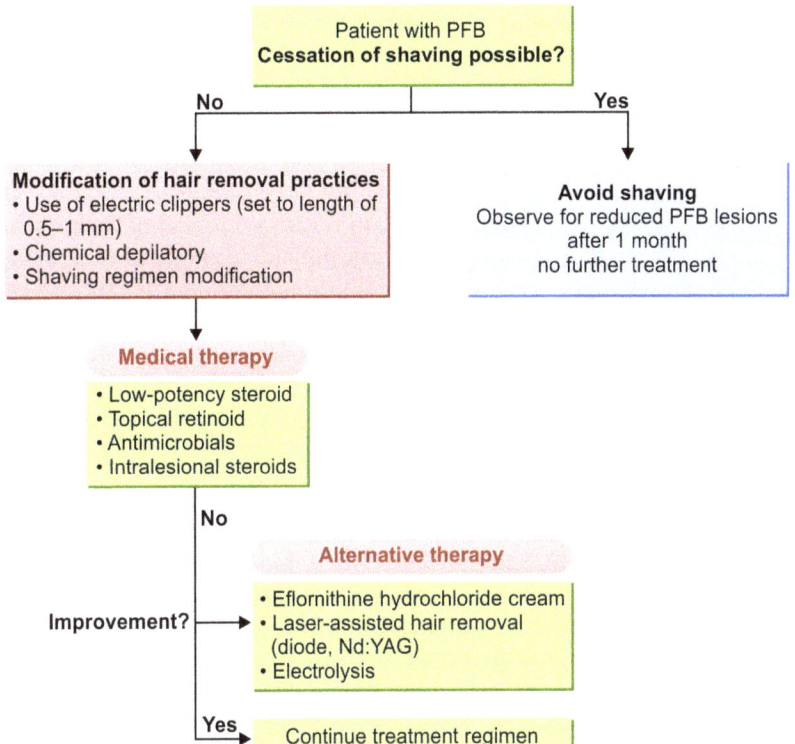

(Nd:YAG: neodymium-doped yttrium aluminum garnet; PFB: pseudofolliculitis barbae)
Source: Adapted from Coley MK, Kelly AP, Alexis AF. Pseudofolliculitis barbae and acne keloidalis nuchae. In: Alexis A, Barbosa VH (Eds). Skin of Color: A Practical Guide to Dermatologic Diagnosis and Treatment, 1st edition. New York: Springer; 2013.

BIBLIOGRAPHY

1. Sardana K. Pseudofolliculitis. In: Sardana K, Khurana A (Eds). Hair Loss Disorders, Restoration, and Management. New Delhi: CBS Publishers and Distributors; 2017. pp. 94-103.

NAIL DISORDERS

The use of lasers for onychomycosis (OM) is the hot new indication though it is fraught with numerous issues. Currently, all of the "approved" lasers for the treatment of OM are Nd:YAG-based lasers (Table 12.23). But as has been discussed in **Chapter 13**, regulatory clearance of medical devices is based on substantial equivalence to a legally marketed preexisting device rather than on the basis of clinical trials data. Therefore, one cannot infer efficacy from FDA clearance.

Mode of Action of Lasers in Onychomycosis

The precise mechanism of action of laser systems in OM is not known, but plausible effects are discussed.

- *Neodymium-doped yttrium aluminum garnet lasers*: These lasers may act by a direct heating effect on the fungi. It has been shown that a temperature of at least 55°C for 5 minutes is required to kill dermatophytes in water suspension (Engelhardt-Zasada C). In vitro studies have shown growth impairment of nail clippings or cell culture media above 50°C when heated with a 1,064 nm or 980 nm laser systems (Paasch U). The problem is that dermatophyte infections are comprised of both hyphae and spores of which spores can be more difficult to eradicate. Also at high temperatures there can be damage to normal collagen (>45°) and skin necrosis can be seen at 50°C. If laser and light-based devices act through nonspecific bulk heating of dermatophytes, there is a high risk of heating and destroying surrounding normal tissue while attempting to eradicate dermatophytes. Thus, selective photothermolysis of dermatophytes, while sparing surrounding skin structures, is preferable. The possible chromophores in this regard include xanthomegnin, chitin, and melanin. Xanthomegnin is abundant in *Trichophyton rubrum* and absorbs 532 nm wavelength. Melanin is abundant in cell walls of all *Trichophyton* spp. and absorbs 1,064 nm wavelength (Figs. 12.41A and B).

  Further, to protect the surrounding tissues, lasers should be delivered in pulses with durations shorter than the thermal relaxation time of the fungus. The thermal relaxation time of hyphae (2-10 mm) is 0.004-0.1 ms, of macroconidia (4-50 mm) is 16-2.5 ms, and of microconidia (2-4 mm) is in the 0.004-0.016 ms range. Thus, selective targeting of dermatophytes likely requires pulse durations in the nanosecond to very low millisecond range.

- *Carbon dioxide lasers*: The effect of CO_2 lasers is possibly photothermal, leading to extreme heating and microexplosions within the fungi. Fractional CO_2 makes microholes improving penetration of topical agents (Bhatta et al.).

- *Diode lasers*: This probably acts by either a direct thermal effect or by decreasing the mitochondrial membrane potential and increasing production of reactive oxygen species (Harris, Landsman).

Table 12.23: Laser systems approved for treatment of onychomycosis.

Laser systems	Type of laser	Wavelength (nm)	Energy fluence (J/cm^2)	Spot size (mm)	Pulse length	Pulse frequencey (Hz)	International approvals for onychomycosis
Dualis SP™, fotona	Long pulse Nd:YAG	1,064	35–40	4	35 ms	1	EU
Q-Clear™ light age, inc.	Qs Nd:YAG	1,064	14	2.5–6	3–10 ns	–	US, EU
Foot-Laser™, Nuvolase	Short pulse Nd:YAG	1,064	25.5	2.5	100–3,000 μs	1	US, Canada, EU, and Australia
Genesis-Plus™, Cutera	Short pulse Nd:YAG	1,064	16	5	300 μs	2	US, Canada, and EU
Varia™, Cool-Touch	Short pulse Nd:YAG	1,064	–	–	600 μs	–	US, EU
Light-Pod® Neo™, Aerolase	Short pulse Nd:YAG	1,064	223	2	650 μs	–	–
Joule Clear-Sense™, Sciton	Short pulse Nd:YAG	1,064	13	–	0.3–200 ms	6	US
Cool-Touch CT3 plus™, Cool-Touch	Short pulse Nd:YAG	1,320	–	2–10	450 μs	–	EU
Mira® 900, Coherent laser group	Mode-locked Ti:sapphire	800	10^{31}–10^{33} m^{2}S^{-1}	0.12–0.45	200 fs	76 MHz	–
Noveon®, Nomir Medical Technologies	Diode	870, 930	212/424	15	–	–	EU
V-Raser®, ConBio/Cynosure	Diode	980	–	–	–	–	–

(Nd: YAG: neodymium-doped yttrium aluminum garnet)

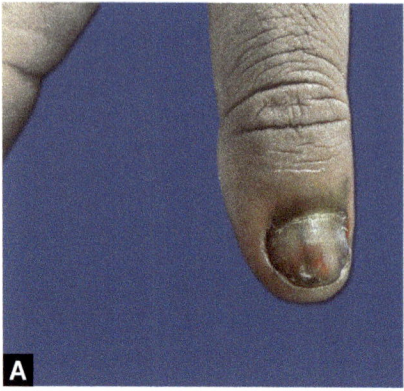 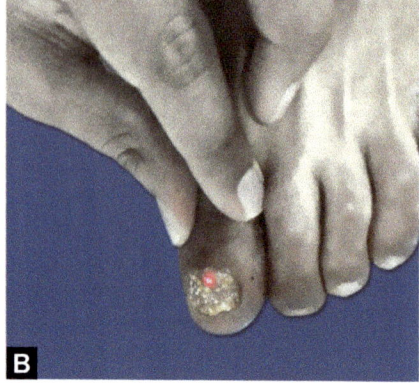

Figs. 12.41A and B: (A) A case of distal lateral onychomycosis; and (B) Use of Q-switched neodymium-doped yttrium aluminum garnet (Nd:YAG) laser for treating onychomycosis (12 J/cm^2, 2 Hz).

Efficacy

Two recent meta-analyses have evaluated the available literature on OM treatment with lasers. Francuzike et al. (2016) reported that 45.45% (10/22) of included laser studies demonstrated an improvement as evident in clinical outcome and/or mycological tests. They found a complete cure rate in 36% (8/22) of their included laser studies with rates exceeding 50% when patients were used as the unit of analysis. Most studies utilized Nd:YAG lasers and were small and uncontrolled. A total of 47.37% of the reviewed studies using a 1,064 nm device reported that all treated patients had a positive response, and 60% of studies reported complete clinical and mycologic cure in at least half of the treated patients. But, given the heterogeneity of data, it was not possible to make comparisons between studies. In a more recent literature review, Gupta et al. concluded that laser studies, to date, provide preliminary evidence of clinical improvemnt and clear nail growth in toenail OM, consistent with the FDA clearance for aesthetic end points. But they do not provide efficacy rates for medical end points that equate or exceed those found with traditional therapies (oral and topical treatments).

Individual systems are discussed here:
- *Short-pulse neodymium-doped yttrium aluminum garnet*: Two RCTs (Hollmig, Karsai) demonstrated no benefit of the laser versus placebo. Results of a company-sponsored phase III efficacy study, registered in 2010, under the title "PinPointe™ FootLaser™ for the Treatment of Onychomycosis" are yet to be published. Small studies have reported benefit with mycological cure rates ranging between 51% and 95% (Hochman, Kimura, Harris).
- *Long-pulsed neodymium-doped yttrium aluminum garnet*: Varying results are reported and the results of two RCTs conducted are not particularly encouraging (Ortiz, El-Tatawy). Some heartening results have been noted

by some users (Avitus John Raakesh Prasad) (Figs. 12.42A to D). In case of black to greenish pigmented onychomycosis, after using of long-pulsed Nd:YAG 1,064 nm, a second pass with Q-switched Nd:YAG 532 nm (fluence around 1–3 J/cm^2, spot size 3–4 mm, and frequency 1 Hz) can be used.

- *Q-switched lasers*: Q-switched lasers might target melanin or chitin in the fungal cell wall leading to photomechanical or photothermal effects. Kalokasidis et al. reported a mycological cure of 95.42% after 3 months

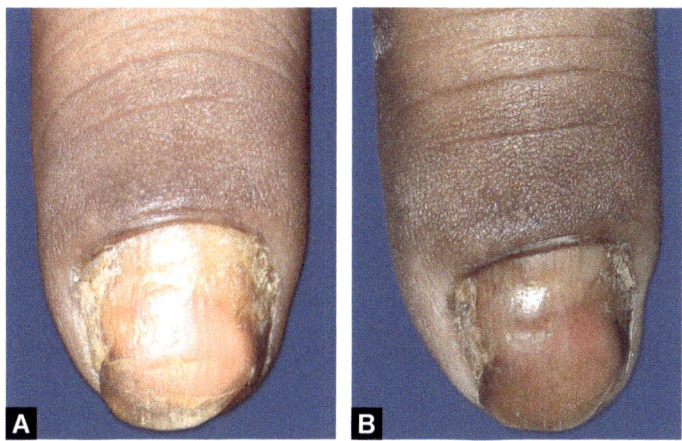

Figs. 12.42A and B: (A) Fluence of 125–150 J/cm^2, spot size 4 mm, pulse duration 20 ms frequency 3 Hz, start from the affected areas with overlap and the remaining normal areas without overlap. Note: Avoid the hyponychium; (B) Second session fluence of 100 J/cm^2, spot size 4 mm, pulse duration 20 ms frequency 3 Hz, firing with overlap over the affected area. After 6 weeks, improvement of the nail plate is seen.

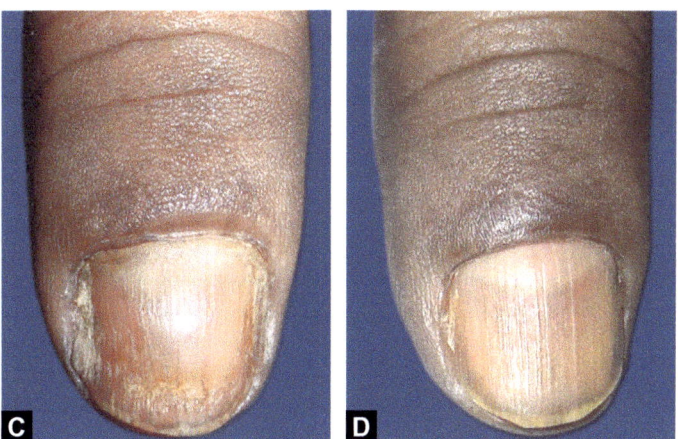

Figs. 12.42C and D: (C) After 8 weeks from second treatment, improvement of the nail plate is seen, third session fluence of 100 J/cm^2, spot size 4 mm, pulse duration 20 ms frequency 3 Hz, firing with overlap over the affected area avoiding hyponychium; (D) After 8 weeks from third treatment, complete resolution is seen. Patient followed up every month for 3 months without re-occurrence.

of treatment with two sessions of Q-switched Nd:YAG. Garcia (2014) reported a clinical response rate of 93%, which increased to 100% after 6 months. In vivo studies with Q-switched Nd:YAG have, however, been conflicting. While Vural et al. demonstrated significant inhibition of growth in irradiated colonies of *Trichophyton rubrum*, Hees et al. did not find any change after using various energy doses of Q-switched Nd:YAG, long-pulsed Nd:YAG, and KTP laser.

We have used a protocol similar to Kalokasidis et al. with successful outcomes in dermatophytic OM (Figs. 12.43A and B) and one case of *Fusarium solani* spp. complex OM (Figs. 12.44A and B).

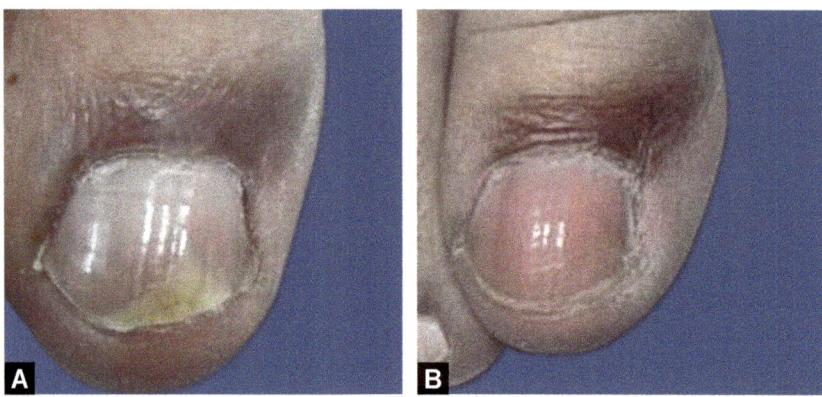

Figs. 12.43A and B: KOH positive case of dermatophytic OM, failed 3 months of terbinafine 250 mg OD, completed 1 year before. The patient was treated with a single session of Qs 1,064 nm (9.3 J/cm^2, 4 mm SS, and 1 Hz), combined in the same session with Qs 532 nm (5 J/cm^2, 2 mm SS, and 1 Hz). Complete clearing with negative microscopy after 1 year. (KOH: potassium hydroxide; OM: onychomycosis; Qs: Q-switched).

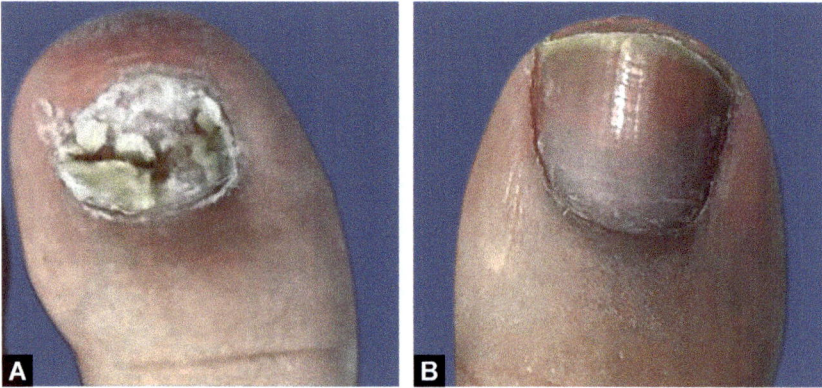

Figs. 12.44A and B: A culture positive case of *Fusarium solani* spp. OM, previously failed multiple adequate oral antifungal treatments. The patient was given two sessions with combined Qs Nd:YAG 532 nm and 1,064 nm (as mentioned in Figs. 12.43A and B). Complete clinical and mycological cure at 1 year. (Nd:YAG: neodymium-doped yttrium aluminum garnet; OM: onychomycosis; Qs: Q-switched).

- *Diode lasers*: Benefit has been demonstrated by one group, with 30% mycological cure rate at 180 days and 38% at 270 days (Landsman). The status of the phase II and phase II/III trials for the Noveon laser in OM (NCT00771732 and NCT00776464), however, remains unknown till date.
- *Fractional carbon dioxide lasers*: Combination with topical antifungal agents has shown higher cure rates than topicals used alone (Lim et al., Zhou et al.).

Conclusion

To summarize, as per the scientific evidence available so far, evidence of unequivocal benefit with lasers as monotherapy/combination therapy is laching. Although, it may be possible to target fungus with selective photothermolysis, the effects of the nail plate on laser optics are unknown and need to be investigated. However, a few trials are encouraging.

While in the short-pulsed Nd:YAG group, both RCTs done so far are negative, there is one positive RCT to the credit of long-pulsed Nd:YAG. Q-switched Nd:YAG has all positive results to its credit, though the available literature is scant so far. A single trial on diode laser shows beneficial response. Fractional CO_2 has demonstrated benefit in combination with topicals compared to topicals alone.

Going by the proposed mechanisms and available data, Q-switched lasers seem to hold promise. The likely chromophores are abundantly present within the common causative dermatophytic species and the laser is thus capable of producing a selective action damaging fungal cells. However, confirmation from in vitro studies is not absolute and the best parameters are yet to be defined.

BIBLIOGRAPHY

1. Bhatta AK, Keyal U, Wang X, et al. A review of the mechanism of action of lasers and photodynamic therapy for onychomycosis. Lasers Med Sci. 2017;32:469-74.
2. Bornstein E, Hermans W, Gridley S. Near-infrared photoinactivation of bacteria and fungi at physiologic temperatures. Photochem Photobiol. 2009;85:1364-74.
3. Carney C, Cantrell W, Warner J, et al. Treatment of onychomycosis using a submillisecond 1064-nm neodymium:yttrium-aluminum-garnet laser. J Am Acad Dermatol. 2013;69:578-82.
4. Engelhardt-Zasada C, Prochacki H. Influence of temperature on dermatophytes. Mycopathol Mycol Appl. 1972;48:297-301.
5. Food and Drug Administration (FDA) (2011). 510(k) Summary K110370. Q-Clear, Light Age, Inc. [online] Available from: www.accessdata.fda.gov/cdrh_docs/pdf11/K110370.pdf. [Accessed April, 2018].
6. Galvan-Garcia HR. Onychomycosis: 1064-nm Nd:YAG Q-switch laser treatment. J Cosmet Dermatol. 2014;13:232-5.
7. Gomez BL, Nosanchuk JD. Melanin and fungi. Curr Opin Infect Dis. 2003;16:91-6.

8. Gupta A, Simpson F. Device-based therapies for onychomycosis treatment. Skin Therapy Lett. 2012;17:4-9.
9. Gupta AK, Simpson FC. Medical devices for the treatment of onychomycosis. Dermatol Ther. 2012;25:574-81.
10. Harris D, McDowell B, Strisower J. Laser treatment for toenail fungus. Proc SPIE. 2009;7161:1-7.
11. Hees H, Raulin C, Baumler W. Laser treatment of onychomycosis: An in vitro pilot study. J Dtsch Dermatol Ges. 2012;10:913-8.
12. Hochman LG. Laser treatment of onychomycosis using a novel 0.65-millisecond pulsed Nd:YAG 1064-nm laser. J Cosmet Laser Ther. 2011;13:2-5.
13. Hollmig ST, Rahman Z, Henderson MT, et al. Lack of efficacy with 1064-nm neodymium:yttrium-aluminum-garnet laser for the treatment of onychomycosis: A randomized, controlled trial. J Am Acad Dermatol. 2014;70:911-7.
14. Kalokasidis K, Onder M, Trakatelli MG, et al. The effect of Q-switched Nd:YAG 1064 nm/532 nm laser in the treatment of onychomycosis in vivo. Dermatol Res Pract. 2013;2013:379725.
15. Khurana A, Chowdhary A, Sardana K, et al. Complete cure of *Fusarium solani* sp. complex onychomycosis with Qs NdYAG treatment. Dermatol Ther. 2018;31:e12580.
16. Kimura U, Takeuchi K, Kinoshita A, et al. Treating onychomycoses of the toenail: Clinical efficacy of the sub-millisecond 1,064 nm Nd:YAG laser using a 5 mm spot diameter. J Drugs Dermatol. 2012;11:496-504.
17. Landsman AS, Robbins AH, Angelini PF, et al. Treatment of mild, moderate, and severe onychomycosis using 870- and 930-nm light exposure. J Am Podiatr Med Assoc. 2010;100:166-77.
18. Landsman AS, Robbins AH, Angelini PF, et al. Treatment of mild, moderate, and severe onychomycosis using 870- and 930-nm light exposure. J Am Podiatr Med Assoc. 2010;100:166-77.
19. Landsman AS, Robbins AH. Treatment of mild, moderate, and severe onychomycosis using 870- and 930-nm light exposure: Some follow-up observations at 270 days. J Am Podiatr Med Assoc. 2012;102:169-71.
20. Lim EH, Kim HR, Park YO, et al. Toenail onychomycosis treated with a fractional carbon-dioxide laser and topical antifungal cream. J Am Acad Dermatol. 2014;70:918-23.
21. Moon SH, Hur H, Oh YJ, et al. Treatment of onychomycosis with a 1,064-nm long-pulsed Nd:YAG laser. J Cosmet Laser Ther. 2014;16:165-70.
22. Nomir Medical Technologies. Treating onychomycosis. In: ClinicalTrials.gov (Ed). Medical Devices for the Treatment of Onychomycosis. United States: National Institutes of Health; 2008.
23. Nomir Medical Technologies. Using light therapy to treat toenail fungus. In: ClinicalTrials.gov (Ed). Study of the Use of Low-level Light Therapy to Treat Toenail Fungus. United States: National Institutes of Health; 2008.
24. Paasch U, Mock A, Grunewald S, et al. Antifungal efficacy of lasers against dermatophytes and yeasts in vitro. Int J Hyperthermia. 2013;29:544-50.
25. Vural E, Winfield HL, Shingleton AW, et al. The effects of laser irradiation on trichophyton rubrum growth. Lasers Med Sci. 2008;23:349-53.

26. Weiss D. 3 Month Clinical Results Using Sub-Millisecond 1064 nm Nd:YAG Laser for the Treatment of Onychomycosis. Hammonton: Weiss Foot and Ankle Center; 2011.
27. Wiznia LE, Quatrano NA, Mu EW, et al. A clinical review of laser and light therapy for nail psoriasis and onychomycosis. Dermatol Surg. 2017;43:161-72.
28. Zhang J, Lu S, Huang H, et al. Combination therapy for onychomycosis using a fractional 2940 nm Er:YAG laser and 5% amorolfin lacquer. Lasers Med Sci. 2016;31:1391-6.
29. Zhang RN, Wang DK, Zhuo FL, et al. Long-pulse Nd:YAG 1064-nm laser treatment for onychomycosis. Chin Med J (Engl). 2012;125:3288-91.
30. Zhou BR, Lu Y, Permatasari F, et al. The efficacy of fractional carbon dioxide (CO_2) laser combined with luliconazole 1% cream for the treatment of onychomycosis: a randomized, controlled trial. Medicine (Baltimore). 2016;95:e5141.

VASCULAR DISORDERS

Though this topic has been discussed previously in **Chapter 5: Lasers for Vascular Indications**, a few other indications and principles are detailed below.

While using the vascular lasers, some generic principles are to be followed [Figs. 12.45A(i) to (iv)]. There are three different techniques that can be employed for treating vascular conditions (as detailed here):

1. Single spot technique [Fig. 12.45B(i)]:
   - The treatment is performed by shooting spot-by-spot on the lesion
   - It is recommended to use a suitable spot size according to the lesion size and location.

   Obviously a device with a variable spot size would be a useful adjunct.
   Clinical use: Coagulation of isolated vascular, pigmented, or solid lesions (e.g. cherry or senile angiomas).

2. Single vessel technique [Fig. 12.45B(ii)]:
   - The treatment is performed by following the course of the vessel continuously without any overlaps
   - Continue the treatment until the required results are met
   - Do not treat the interstices between the vessels
   - If necessary, treat the main vessels first, before continuing with the peripheral smaller vessels (e.g. with spider nevi).

   Clinical use: Where single vessels are clearly visible (e.g. telangiectasia, rosacea where single vessels are recognized, and spider nevi).

3. Spot-by-spot technique [Fig. 12.45B(iii)]:
   - The treatment is performed by shooting several spots one close to the other one
   - Make sure that no overlaps occur.

   Clinical use: For coagulation of isolated vascular, pigmented, or solid lesions (e.g. cherry or senile angiomas).

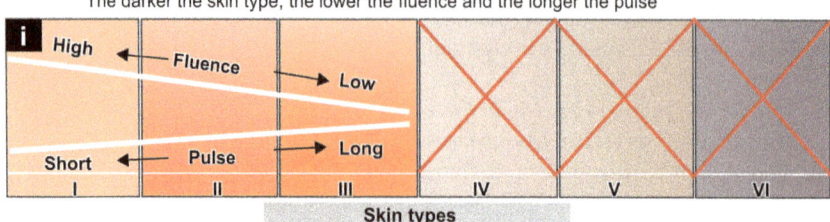
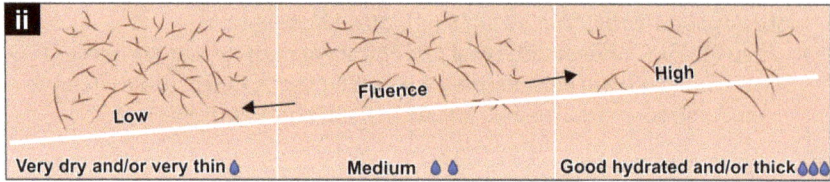
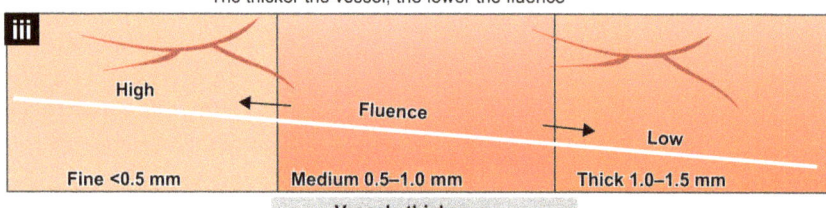
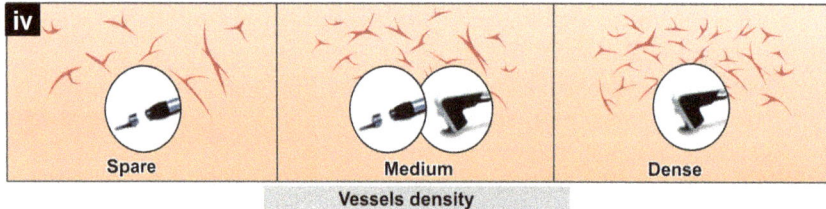

Figs. 12.45A(i) to (iv): General principles to be followed while treating vascular lesions with lasers.

Though conventionally vascular-specific lasers are used in many indications, the CO_2 laser works equally well. The basic principles that are enshrined in the use of the CO_2 laser are:

- Increasing the *pulse duration* to help in hemostasis (0.5–1 s)
- Increasing the pulse interval
- Avoid exceeding a fluence of 5 J/cm^2.

An ideal scenario would be to balance the residual thermal damage (RTD) and the coagulation, which are mutually antagonistic. It has been seen that there is selective epidermal damage for fluences of less than 10 J/cm^2. But the more important parameter is the pulse duration and for pulse durations of 10 ms, fluence (and not power density or achievement of ablation) is a more

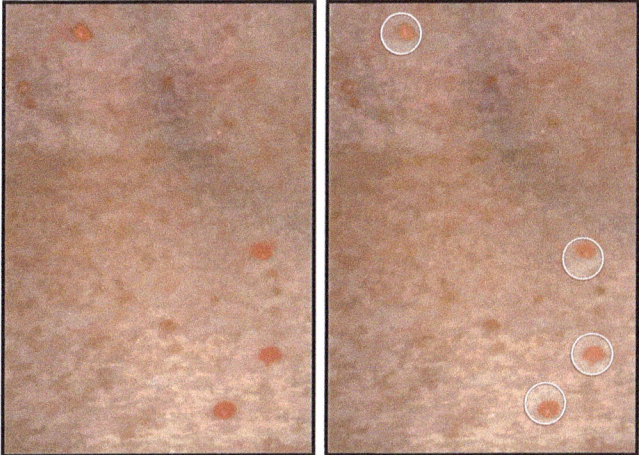

Fig. 12.45B(i): Single spot technique.

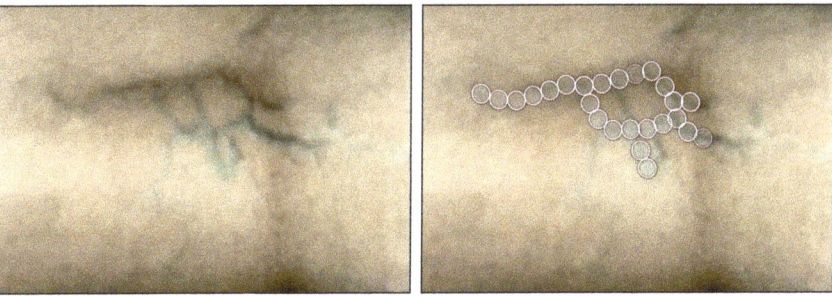

Fig. 12.45B(ii): Single vessel technique.

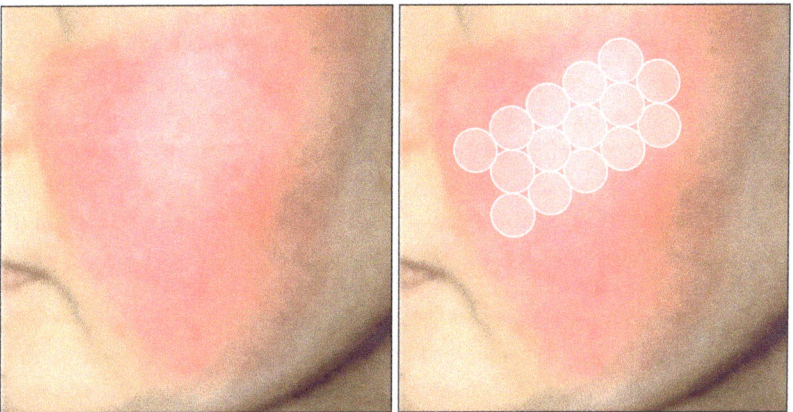

Fig. 12.45B(iii): Spot-by-spot technique.

important parameter in determining the extent of RTD; that is, lower fluences usually result in less RTD.

But remember that high-flow vessels larger than 500 µm are likely to bleed after CO_2 transection. In contrast, without blood flow, vessels up to 2 mm would be coagulated. Ideally, one should choose the laser parameters with the least RTD that still achieves adequate control of bleeding. As a thumb rule the *vaporization mode* with a pulse duration of 0.5-1 s can work well for coagulation vessels, though it would as a corollary increase tissue damage.

Cherry Angiomas/Spider Angiomas

Cherry angioma presents as a 1-3 mm bright red to violaceous, smooth, and dome-shaped papule. Spider angioma displays a network of dilated capillaries radiating from a central vessel. Both may bleed when traumatized.

Cherry angiomas show loss of rete ridges as well as congested and ectatic capillaries and postcapillary venules in the papillary dermis. Spider angiomas reveal a central ascending arteriole that branches and communicates with multiple dilated capillaries.

Treatment

- *Electrosurgery*: Electrodessication with coagulation (monopolar setting, 1-2 W, followed by gentle curettage with end point as lesional flattening and hemostasis) has been the traditional treatment modality for these lesions. It is cheap and effective. There is a chance of scarring and for multiple lesions it may be cumbersome.
- *Lasers*:
  i. *Pulsed dye laser* is the treatment of choice. A spot size should be selected that matches diameter of the angioma. With spider angiomas, the central feeding vessel as well as the surrounding vessels should be treated. It is best to compress the lesion with a microscope slide to blanch all but the central feeding vessel. A purpuric laser pulse should be delivered. The microscope slide should be removed to allow for cooling of the area. Subsequently, a purpuric laser pulse can be employed to target the telangiectasias radiating from the feeding vessel. The purpuric treatment end point represents coagulation of the targeted vessels.
  ii. *Potassium titanyl phosphate lasers*: The KTP 532 nm laser produces a favorable response. Spot size should match the lesion diameter. The vessels should be traced out completely for most effective treatment. Treatment end point is lesional clearance or superficial whitening. Erythema can be expected post-treatment, lasting for 24-48 hours.
  iii. *Carbon dioxide laser* (ultrapulse 3 mm collimated handpiece, 300-400 mJ/pulse, nonoverlapping pulses; Sharplan FeatherTouch 1.25 mm handpiece, 14-40 W, 3 mm scan size, nonoverlapping

pulses) has been employed as second-line therapy with success. Treatment end point is lesional flattening. Potential scar formation must be considered.

iv. *Long-pulsed Nd:YAG (1,064 nm) laser* has been shown to be effective in treatment of angiomas.

Procedure: Depending on the size and morphology of the lesions, the spot size can be adjusted between 3 mm and 6 mm, energy between 15 J and 20 J (fluence varying from 50 J/cm^2 to 250 J/cm^2 depending on lesion—see Box 12.3 here), pulse width 10-30 ms depending on lesion (pulse duration of 5 ms can be used if lesion is small and energy is lower), and frequency 1 Hz is preferred to treat smaller lesions.

When higher fluence is required, lower spot size or higher energy should be used. Though the fluence earlier might seem very high, the author (Dr Avitus) has tried various doses and arrived at this by trial and error (of course this is machine specific and a lower fluence, 30-60 J/cm^2 can be used initially).

- Local anesthesia is given perilesional if required as lesional will dilute or dissipate the pigment. Use of adrenalin will can vasoconstriction, so it should be avoided.
- Always fire from a distance of two fingers (2-3 cm), this is to prevent the lens of the probe from getting damaged. In this case, keeping the spot size higher to compensate for the lift, for example, if spot size of 7 mm or 8 mm is used and if you lift by 3-4 cm from lesion, it will be around 6 mm spot size when it hits the lesion.
- Fire in the center of the lesion first and look for shrinkage of lesion. In case of persistent lesion in surrounding, you can fire few shots around it with reduced fluence.
- Post-treatment will form scab in next 24-48 hours with complete healing and resolution in 2 weeks.

A depictive case is shown in Figures 12.45C(i) to (iii).

- *Light therapy*: Intense pulsed light has also been employed with some success. As coagulation is needed for lesional resolution, higher fluences may be required for treatment efficacy. The author (Dr Avitus) uses a

Box 12.3: Calculating fluence for long-pulsed neodymium-doped yttrium aluminum garnet (Nd:YAG).

- If you want to calculate fluence for a given energy and spot size, the following can be done.
Fluence is dependent on the spot size and energy. For example, if spot size is 6 mm, with an energy of 25 J, fluence generated will be 127 J/cm^2
- *Calculation:* Fluence = Energy/spot size area
  = J/πr^2 (r = half of spot size); π = 3.14
If J = 25, r^2 = (diameter 5 mm = 5 cm/2 = 0.25 mm) so it will be (0.25 × 0.25 = 0.0625 mm^2)
Thus, 25/3.14 × 0.0625 = 25/0.19625 = 127.388 J/cm^2
  = 127 J/cm^2

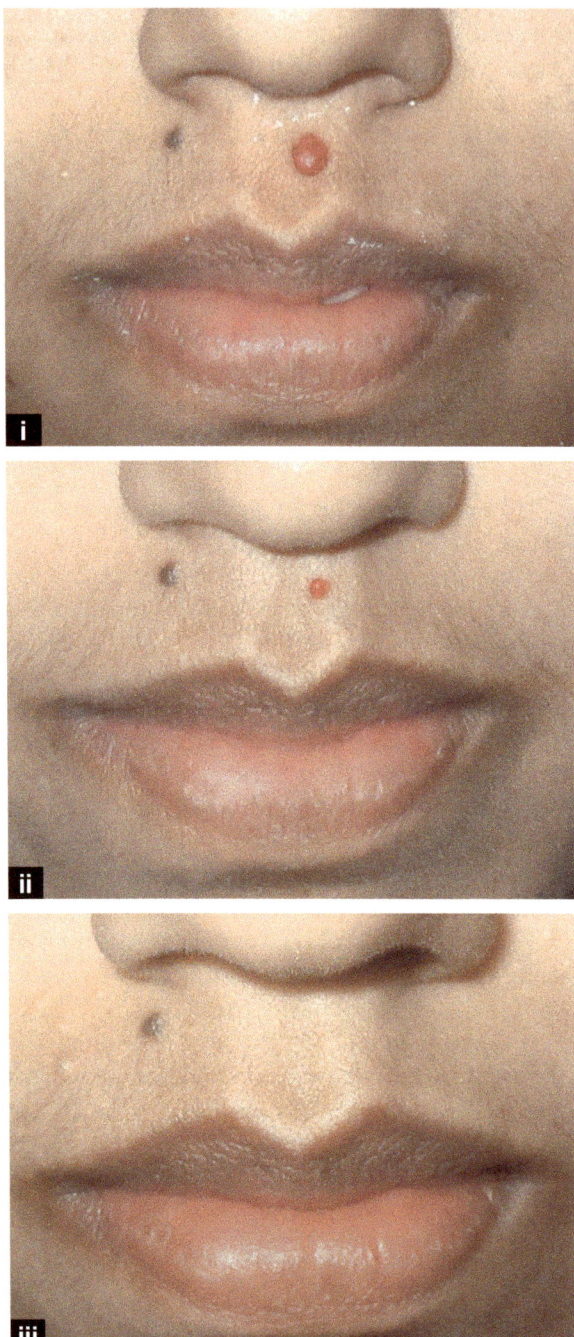

Figs. 12.45C(i) to (iii): Treatment of angioma using LP Nd:YAG. (i) Fluence of 100 J/cm^2, spot size 6 mm, pulse duration 10 ms, frequency 1 Hz, two shots; (ii) After 1 month, fluence of 50 J/cm^2, spot size 3 mm, pulse duration 10 ms, frequency 1 Hz, single shot; (iii) 1 month after second session healed without scarring.

510–530 nm (green filter) and 560–570 nm (yellow filter) with a pulse number of 3–5 and pulse duration (on time) of 3 ms, 5 ms, and 7 ms with pulse delay of 10–20 ms in between pulses. Energy varies depending on the skin type, in our skin, for green filter 15–25 J/cm^2 and for yellow filter 18–28 J/cm^2 is used. Higher than this range can be employed if skin type is type 1 or 2.

- *Surgical excision*: Excision should be reserved for lesions that are resistant to other treatments. A postoperative scar is expected which may be less cosmetically pleasing than the angioma.

The advantage of lasers over conventional methods is the speed of response and cosmetic acceptability. An illustrative seminal study of Dawn G et al. showed that both the KTP vascular laser and the hyfrecator were able to clear vascular spiders and angiomas, but the KTP laser was superior as fewer treatments were required and patients preferred this treatment modality because of the lack of side effects.

BIBLIOGRAPHY

1. Dawn G, Gupta G. Comparison of potassium titanyl phosphate vascular laser and hyfrecator in the treatment of vascular spiders and cherry angiomas. Clin Exp Dermatol. 2003;28:581-3.
2. Fodor L, Ramon Y, Fodor A, et al. A side-by-side prospective study of intense pulsed light and Nd:YAG laser treatment for vascular lesions. Ann Plast Surg. 2006;56:164-70.
3. Solak B, Sevimli-Dikicier B, Oztas-Kara R, et al. Single-center experience with potassium titanyl phosphate (KTP) laser for superficial cutaneous vascular lesions in face. J Cosmet Laser Ther. 2016;18:428-31.

Angiokeratomas

Angiokeratomas (AKs) are telangiectasias with keratotic elements. They present in different clinical scenarios including:
- Solitary or multiple angiokeratomas occurring predominantly on lower extremities
- Angiokeratoma of Fordyce affecting the scrotum and the vulva
- Angiokeratoma of Mibelli, an autosomal dominant disorder affecting dorsum of hands and feet, elbows, and knees
- Angiokeratoma corporis diffusum associated with Fabry's disease, an X-linked recessive disorder, and
- Angiokeratoma circumscriptum usually grouped on one extremity.

Histology shows marked dilated, thin-walled blood vessels in the papillary dermis, associated with an overlying acanthotic hyperkeratotic epidermis. Apart from lasers, other surgical treatments include excision, electrocautery, electrofulguration, or cryosurgery.

Treatment

Lasers: Angiokeratomas are ideally treated by lasers, as surgical methods carry high risks of scarring and hemorrhage. Argon, PDL, Nd:YAG, copper vapor, KTP, CO_2, and Er:YAG lasers have emerged as alternative options. Vascular lasers like PDL, Nd:YAG, and argon are the most studied and of these, PDL offers the safest side effect profile. Nd:YAG may be more effective for hyperkeratotic angiokeratomas. Combination treatment with multiple laser modalities has also demonstrated some success.

The basic principle is to target the vascular component, but in our experience using such lasers do not circumvent the variable thickness of skin overlying the AK. Hence, though various lasers have been tried, we have relied on the workhorse, CO_2 laser. We may be biased, but in our experience CO_2 is a vastly superior option, 1-2 sessions are enough to enable predictably "happy" results. Of course, recurrence is a possibility.

- *Pulsed dye laser*: The PDL is an effective device for the improvement of the vascular component of AKs, but frequently some keratosis remains. The target chromophore is hemoglobin. The settings reported to help are at 595 nm, 5-7 mm spot, and 9-11 J/cm^2. Covering the angiokeratoma with a glass slide, that is, diascopy, is helpful. The end point is lesional purpura. It requires multiple sessions.
- Resurfacing lasers such as CO_2 and Er:YAG lasers can be utilized for lesional vaporization. Patients generally require local infiltration with 1% lidocaine with or without epinephrine prior to treatment. The ultrapulse CO_2 3 mm collimated handpiece, with an energy of 300-500 mJ with non-overlapping pulses is used. Another option is to use the CW CO_2 laser.
    - **Procedure:** First two laser passes can be performed on each lesion with a CW focused mode at a power density of 6-10 W/cm^2, to eliminate the hyperkeratotic and hypertrophic epidermis. After this pass, the partially desiccated tissue can be removed with a saline-soaked gauze, which reveals the superficial dermis with several hemorrhagic points. The second pass can be performed with a defocused mode at the same power density to achieve a slight contraction of tissue and coagulation of the dermal vessels. If the superpulsed CO_2 is used, prolonging the pulse duration and the pulse interval can help achieve the same results (Figs. 12.46 to 12.48).

        Treatment sites should be cleansed with saline-soaked gauze between laser passes.
    - **Postoperative care:** It requires twice daily washing with soap and water and application of an antibiotic ointment. Healing occurs in 2-6 weeks. As with all ablative procedures, scarring may be observed.
- Other lasers that have been used in the past with variable success include KTP laser, argon laser, and copper vapor laser. Long-pulsed Nd:YAG (1,064 nm) laser has been shown to be effective due to its selectivity and its deeper penetration into the skin.

CHAPTER 12: Clinical Indications

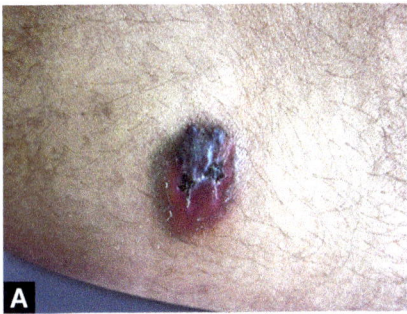
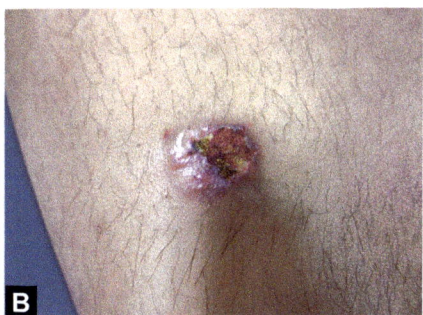
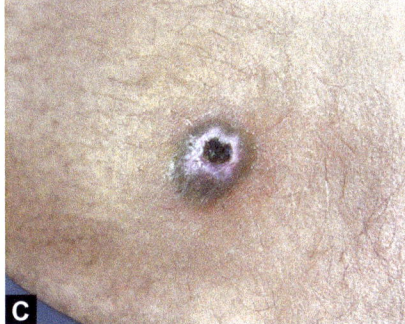

Figs. 12.46A to C: A case of angiokeratoma, ideal laser is CO_2 as it has a coagulation profile better than Er:YAG and helps to seal the vessels. Note the marked healing with a central crusting corresponding to the intense thermal damage consequent to the CO_2 laser. The settings were 6 W, pulse duration was 0.20 s. (CO_2: carbon dioxide; Er:YAG: erbium-doped yttrium aluminum garnet).

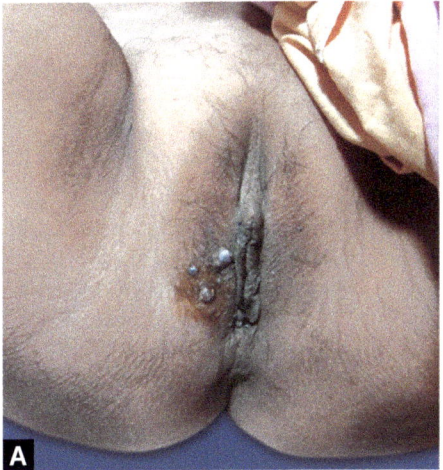
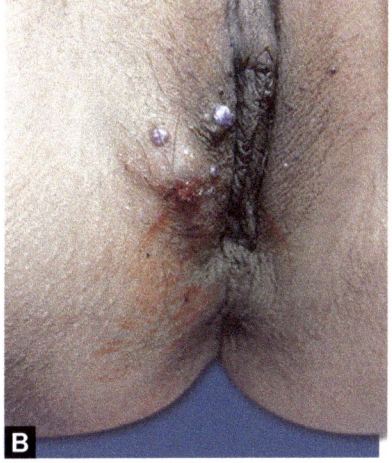

Figs. 12.47A and B: A case of vulval AK treated by pulsed CO_2. Note the coagulation of the base that prevents bleeding which is seen classically with such tumors. Here, the CO_2 has to be defocused in the CW mode or the pulse duration has to be increased in the superpulse mode (0.5–1 s). (AK: angiokeratoma; CO_2: carbon dioxide; CW: continuous wave).

With the long-pulsed Nd:YAG, a preferred setting (Dr Avitus) is a fluence of 100–150 J/cm^2, spot size 4–6 mm with a frequency of 1 Hz.

Successful treatment with a *dual-wavelength laser system* (595 nm and 1,064 nm) has been recently reported (Cynergy with Multiplex™, Cyno-

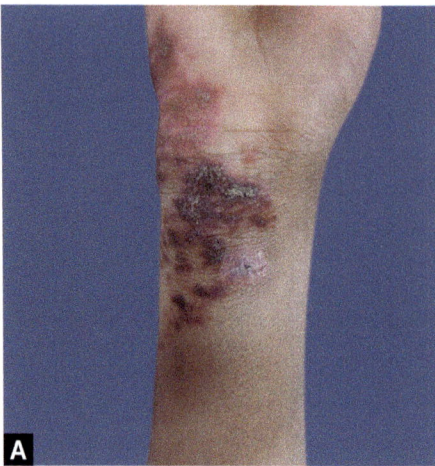 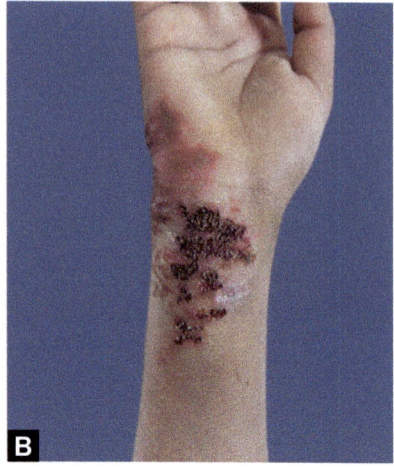

Figs. 12.48A and B: Another case of AK treated with pulsed CO_2. Use settings that can coagulate the vessels. Either defocus a CW CO_2 or increase the pulse width of a pulsed CO_2 (ideal pulse width/duration between 0.5 s and 1 s). (AK: angiokeratoma; CO_2: carbon dioxide; CW: continuous wave).

sure, Westford, MA, USA). The idea is to target superficial and deep vessels. A recent study combined PDL and long-pulsed Nd:YAG laser. Combined dual PDL-long pulsed Nd:YAG (PDL: 595 nm, 5 mm/7 mm, 0.5 ms, 8–10 J/cm^2; long-pulsed Nd:YAG: 3 mm/5 mm, 15 ms, 90–120 J/cm^2) treatment was used to treat lesions with moderate to severe hyperkeratosis and hyperplasia.

BIBLIOGRAPHY

1. Gorse SJ, James W, Murison MS. Successful treatment of angiokeratoma with potassium titanyl phosphate laser. Br J Dermatol. 2004;150:620-2.
2. Nguyen J, Chapman LW, Korta DZ, et al. Laser treatment of cutaneous angiokeratomas: A systematic review. Dermatol Ther. 2017;30.
3. Oni G, Mahaffey P. Treatment of angiokeratoma of the vulva with pulsed dye laser therapy. J Cosmet Laser Ther. 2010;12:51-2.
4. Zeng Y, Li XQ, Lin QZ, et al. Treatment of angiokeratoma of Mibelli alone or in combination with pulsed dye laser and long-pulsed Nd:YAG laser. Dermatol Ther. 2014;27:348-51.

Glomus Tumor

Hereditary multiple glomus tumors constitute an autosomal dominant skin disease that is known to demonstrate cutaneous mosaicism typified by type 1 and 2 segmental arrangements. These lesions can be spontaneously painful. PDL treatment can be used to relieve pain but may not be curative.

Telangiectasias

These represent dilated capillaries and postcapillary venules with thickened walls. They are superficial (200–250 µm deep) and have small cross-sections (200–500 µm in diameter).

Treatment

Facial telangiectasias are frequently treated for cosmetic purposes. Multiple effective treatment options exist. As in most conditions, lasers cannot prevent the likelihood of patients to develop more telangiectasias.

Lasers

- *Pulsed dye laser*: The ideal laser is PDL though the associated purpura is a concern.

    The traditional PDL with a short pulse duration of 0.45 ms or 1.5 ms provides the most effective treatment for facial telangiectasias. However, post-treatment purpura occurs which generally lasts for 7–14 days.

    Newer generation 595 nm PDL (i.e. V-beam or V-beam Perfecta lasers, Candela) with variable pulse durations (0.45 ms, 1.5 ms, 3 ms, 6 ms, 10 ms, 20 ms, 30 ms, 40 ms) can provide a reduced purpura treatment of facial telangiectasias when longer pulse durations are utilized, but is somewhat less effective and usually requires multiple treatments.

    Dose: Commonly, subpurpuric fluences of less than 10 J/cm^2 at pulse duration of 10 ms, with a 7 mm spot size are utilized.

    An ideal setting with the variable pulse PDL is by using purpuric fluences or by pulse stacking with subpurpuric pulses (stacked 2–4 subpurpuric pulses at a 1.5 Hz repetition rate, 7.5 J/cm^2, 10 ms pulse duration, and 10 mm spot size), or by performing multiple passes during the same session.

    Larger thicker linear vessels can be treated with the newest generation 595 nm long PDL (V-beam Perfecta, Candela Corp) using a 3 × 10 mm elliptical spot size, 40 ms pulse duration, and 15–17 J/cm^2.

    End point: Immediate coagulation/graying that quickly clears is the desired end point.

- *Intense pulsed light*: The IPLs have also been shown to be effective against telangiectasias and have a lower risk of inducing purpura and generally induce a mild erythema.

    Using the yellow filter (560–570 nm) the effective fluences range from 32 J/cm^2 to 40 J/cm^2 with pulse width of around 20 ms. While using IPL for vascular lesions, do not give pressure on the lesion and avoid cooling for more than 1 or 2 seconds. This results in vasoconstriction, making the target devoid of chromophore.

    These are useful for larger matted telangiectasias and the diffuse erythema associated with rosacea. The treatment end point is immediate vessel clearance or selective vessel darkening. Multiple treatments may be required for the greatest treatment benefit. As has been repeatedly emphasized the results of IPL are highly dependent on the machine, we are detailing results with an IPL [Magma by Forma TK (Israel)] in various conditions with erythema, telangiectasias and rosacea using very conservative settings (Figs. 12.49A to F).

- *Variable pulse 1,064 nm*: The variable pulse width 1,064 nm Nd:YAG laser has proven to be effective in the treatment of facial telangiectasias. Shorter pulse widths with higher fluences might be necessary for effective treatment of smaller vessels but have an increased risk of blister and scar formation. The sequential delivery of 595 nm and 1,064 nm wavelength has been reported to be more effective than a single wavelength treatment.

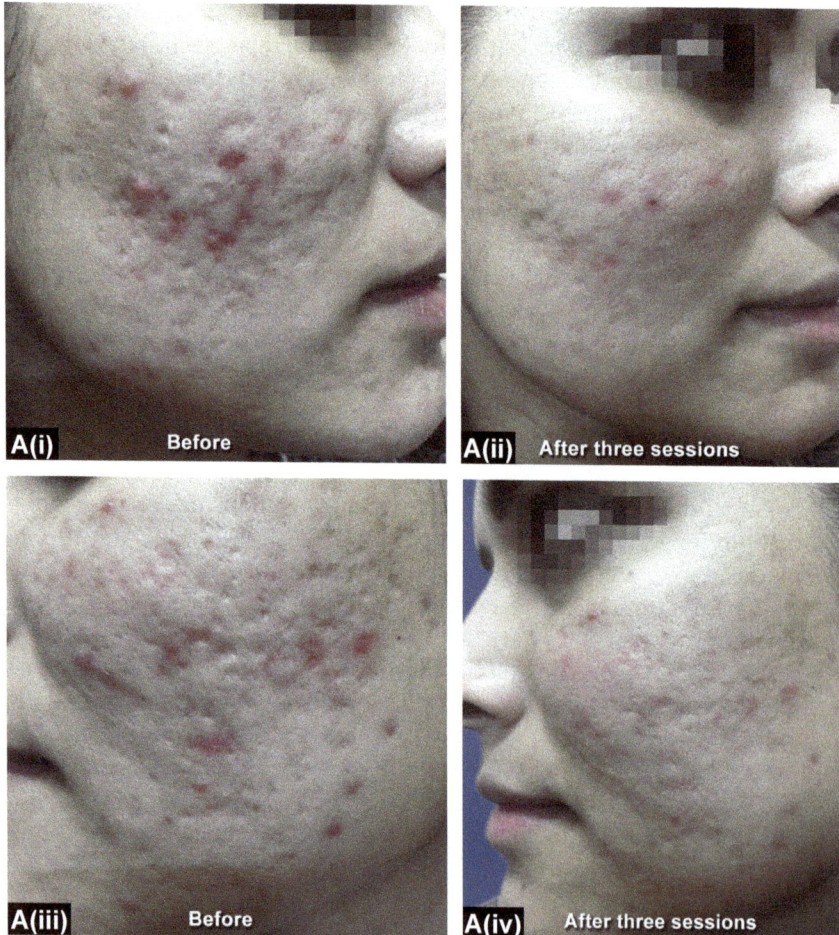

Figs. 12.49A(i) to (iv): Persistent erythema post-retinoid therapy (550–1,100 nm filter 7.1 mJ/cm² continuous mode followed by 14.1 j/cm² single pass mode six passes each).

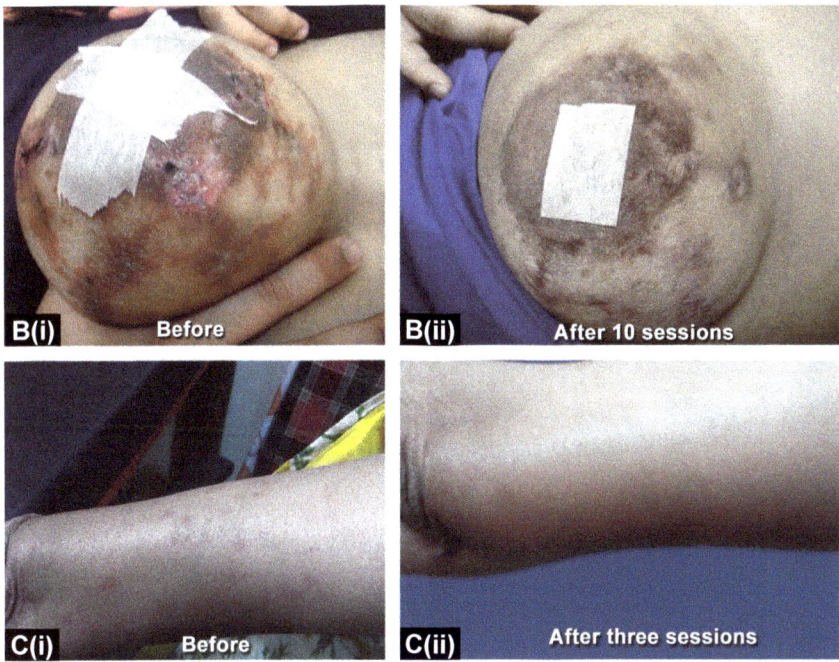

Figs. 12.49B and C: B(i) and (ii) Cutis marmorata telangiectasia congenital (550–1,100 nm 14.1 mJ/cm² single pulse mode six passes weekly); C(i) and C(ii) Telangiectasia macularis eruptiva perstans. 550–1,100 nm single pulse mode 14.1 mJ/cm² three passes weekly.

- *Potassium titanyl phosphate*: Frequency-doubled 532 nm Nd:YAG laser also called KTP laser provides effective absorption of hemoglobin with a pulse duration of 1–50 ms making it ideally suited to treat superficial vessels without purpura formation. Tracing of individual vessels is a useful technique for patients.

  A study from Turkey (Solak B) found that the rate of clearance plus marked improvement (favorable outcome) was 66.1% for telangiectasia group. This compares well with the use of traser, where 44% maintained "complete vessel clearance", at 1 year.

  The QuadroStarPRO is a KTP lasers used for the treatment of vascular and pigmented lesions and is available in two different versions: (1) the QuadroStarPRO yellow, features the 577 nm wavelength while (2) the QuadroStarPRO green, features the 532 nm wavelength. The former can be used for treating telangiectasia in an ideal skin type patient (Figs. 12.49E and F).

Conclusion

The problem is that the wavelengths that are often used will be an issue in our skin type as the melanin will compete with these lasers and there is a high chance of dyspigmentation. The long-pulsed Nd:YAG is probably the best bet.

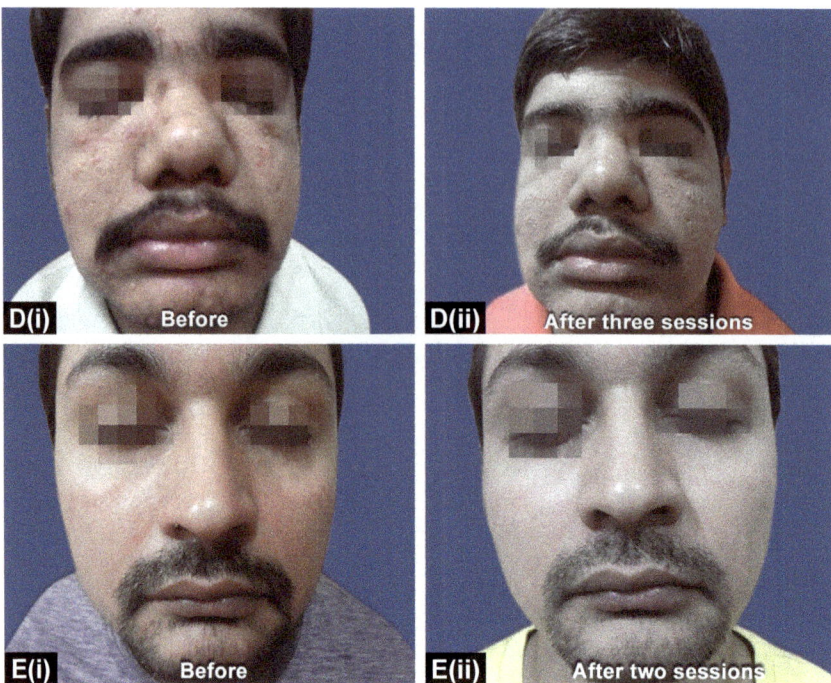

Figs. 12.49D and E: D(i) and (ii) Rosacea. 550–1,100 nm filter 14.1 mJ/cm² in single pulse followed by 7.1 mJ/cm² in continuous mode six passes each weekly. E(i) and (ii) Rosacea—erythematotelangiectatic (ET) type. 550–1,100 nm filter 14.1 mJ/cm² in single pulse followed by 7.1 mJ/cm² in continuous mode six passes each weekly.

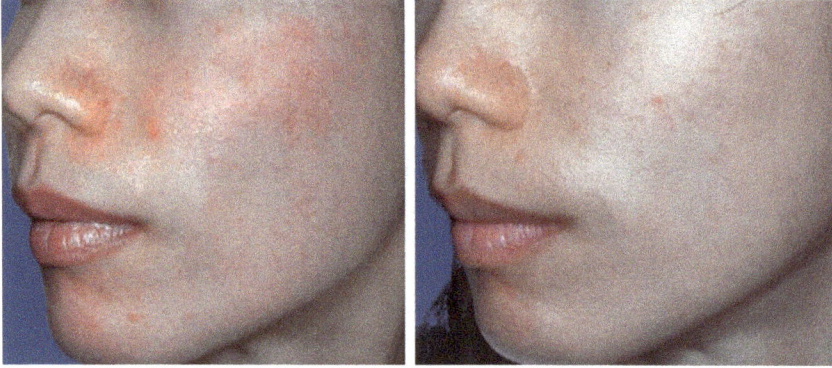

Fig. 12.49F: Treatment of telangiectasias with KTP 577 nm (14–16 J/cm², 1 mm spot size).

Though the PDL is the preferred device, there is post-treatment purpura for 7-14 days with purpuric settings while with nonpurpuric settings, the efficacy will be lower, with facial edema, erythema, and discomfort.

BIBLIOGRAPHY

1. Geddes-Bruce E, Hamill SS, Zachary CB, et al. One-year follow-up of a TRASER clinical trial for the treatment of nasal telangiectasias. Lasers Surg Med. 2018;50:61-3.
2. Karsai S, Roos S, Raulin C. Treatment of facial telangiectasia using a dual-wavelength laser system (595 and 1,064 nm): A randomized controlled trial with blinded response evaluation. Dermatol Surg. 2008;34:702-8.
3. Rohrer TE, Chatrath V, Iyengar V. Does pulse stacking improve the results of treatment with variable-pulsed-dye lasers? Dermatol Surg. 2004;30:163-7.
4. Ross EV, Uebelhoer NS, Doman-Kevitz Y. Use of a novel pulse dye laser for rapid single-pass purpura-free treatment of telangiectases. Dermatol Surg. 2007;33:1466-9.
5. Sarradet DM, Hussain M, Goldberg DJ. Millisecond 1064-nm neodymium:YAG laser treatment of facial telangiectases. Dermatol Surg. 2003;29:56-8.
6. Solak B, Sevimli-Dikicier B, Oztas-Kara R, et al. Single-center experience with potassium titanyl phosphate (KTP) laser for superficial cutaneous vascular lesions in face. J Cosmet Laser Ther. 2016;18:428-31.

Venous Lakes

The venous lakes are very common about the lips and other mucosal areas. They are large vascular channels, which are often deeply situated and respond to most high-powered, long-pulse devices with pulse durations of 20–60 ms. The histology is characterized by dilated thin-walled venules in the superficial dermis. Thrombosis may be observed.

Treatment

- *Lasers*: Laser therapy is often effective and needs to be tailored to the depth of the target vessels. The lasers used include PDLs, 755 nm alexandrite lasers, long-pulse Nd:YAG lasers, and the combined 595 nm/1,064 nm multiplex device.
    i. *Pulsed dye laser* is often effective for *superficial* venous lakes, but the *longer wavelengths* of diode (800–900 nm), alexandrite (755 nm), or Nd:YAG (1,064 nm) lasers are necessary for thicker or deeper lesions. The aim with a PDL is to produce mild purpura and edema. With diode and Nd:YAG lasers, the goal is reduction in lesion thickness and clearance of the ectatic vessels. For the larger and deeper lesions an Nd:YAG laser with a spot size of 3 mm, pulse widths of 30–100 ms, and fluences of up to 150 J/cm^2 may be needed.
    ii. *Diode laser*: 800–810 nm, 30 ms, and 30–50 J/cm^2 can be a very useful treatment (Figs. 12.50A and B). It is preceded by a 3 s compression of the lesion with the chill tip prior to the laser pulse. A physical "kick-back" is often felt by the laser surgeon at the time of the laser pulse impact. The clinical end point is immediate purpura.

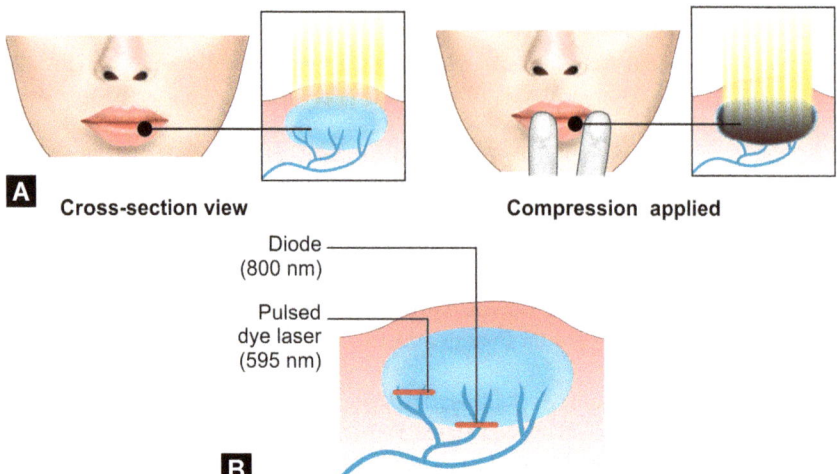

Figs. 12.50A and B: Compression helps in treating venous lakes by vascular lasers as the laser penetrates deeper. Diode is superior to PDL.

    iii. *Carbon dioxide*: Most of the vascular lasers are not effective as there is an issue of the depth of penetration and occasionally multiple sessions are required. We prefer the CO_2. In case of a pulsed laser the superpulse mode is useful. A conventional CW can also be used. If a superpulse mode is used, increase the pulse duration to 2–3 ms and the interval to 100 ms to ensure coagulation of the vessels. A study of 23 cases by del Pozo J et al. used two passes with a continuous and defocused mode, with a power density of 5 W/cm², in the first pass, and a continuous focused mode with the same power density in the second pass.

    iv. *Neodymium-doped yttrium aluminum garnet*: 1,064 nm, pulse duration: 30 ms, fluence: 110 J/cm2, and spot size: 4 mm. With this laser, the treatment area is precooled with an ice cube for 5 s without applying pressure. A single laser pulse is delivered and the ice cube applied immediately for 5–10 s to alleviate the pain and prevent excessive thermal damage. The first laser pulse would result in moderate shrinkage with graying/dulling of the lesion, which is considered the appropriate reaction.

    Practice points:
- As compared to telangiectases, which are the most frequent vascular lesions to be treated on the face, venous lakes are much bigger targets. The bigger the target, the *longer the pulse* and the *lower the fluence* should be used to avoid overtreatment and scarring.
- Spot size should be matched to the diameter of the lesion. Usually, the 4 mm or 6 mm spot size can be used for venous lakes.
- Generally, smaller venous lakes can be safely treated with the earlier parameters, and the larger ones with 6 mm spot, 90–100 J/cm²,

and 40–50 ms.
- Before treatment, the depth of the lesion should be assessed. If the lesion is very thick and protruding, it should be compressed with a glass slide during treatment to press some of the blood out (the laser should be fired through the glass slide). With this simple measure, overtreatment and scarring can be prevented.
- Treatment will be successful if the end point is reached, i.e. moderate shrinkage and color change of the lesion. This effect is seen immediately. If the end point is not reached, first a second pulse should be applied. If there is still no response, the fluence should be increased by 10 J/cm^2 or the pulse length decreased by 10 ms, but never both in one step.
- If necessary, a follow-up treatment should be done in 4–6 weeks.
- In the treatment of venous lakes, contact cooling with an ice cube is more effective than cold air, and also more comfortable for the patients.
- Usually only one treatment session is required, with only one or two pulses delivered.

Sclerotherapy

Intralesional injections with 1% polidocanol have been shown to be effective in clearing two venous lakes after two sessions of sclerotherapy.

Other Options

Electrosurgery, surgical-excision, and cryotherapy are other alternate treatment options. However, these modalities can result in scarring.

BIBLIOGRAPHY

1. Del Pozo J, Peña C, García Silva J, et al. Venous lakes: A report of 32 cases treated by carbon dioxide laser vaporization. Dermatol Surg. 2003;29:308-10.
2. Kuo HW, Yang CH. Venous lake of the lip treated with a sclerosing agent: Report of two cases. Dermatol Surg. 2003;29:425-8.
3. Mlacker S, Shah VV, Aldahan AS, et al. Laser and light-based treatments of venous lakes: A literature review. Lasers Med Sci. 2016;31:1511-9.
4. Wall TL, Grassi AM, Avram MM. Clearance of multiple venous lakes with an 800 nm diode laser: A novel approach. Dermatol Surg. 2007;33:100-3.

Pyogenic Granuloma

This condition is a common disorder that is known to be caused due to a reactive vascular process arising at sites of previous trauma or irritation. It is also known as lobular capillary hemangioma. Amelanotic melanoma as well as squamous cell carcinoma (SCC) and other skin cancers can mimic pyogenic granuloma (PG). A biopsy should be performed for any suspicious lesions in the appropriate clinical setting.

Treatment

Though most of us employ surgical procedures, recently some very simple methods for treatment have been tried and may predate procedures. An overview of treatment options is depicted in Box 12.4.

- *Laser treatment*: Pulsed dye laser (585–600 nm, 0.45–1.5 ms, 7–10 mm, and 6–15 J/cm^2, with or without diascopy) is a safe and effective device for the treatment of small lesions and for pediatric patients. Serial treatments are usually required. Treatment is well-tolerated without anesthesia. Shave excision followed by immediate PDL for larger lesions is a useful adjunct.

    Carbon dioxide is also effective with an appropriate setting, where the pulse width is more than 0.5 seconds to ensure coagulation. Lesional flattening is the clinical end point (*see* **Chapter 2: Ablative Lasers**).

    Long-pulsed Nd:YAG can be employed with fluence of 150–250 J/cm^2 depending on the size of lesion (spot size 4–6 mm, frequency 1 Hz). Always fire in the center of the lesion with higher fluence and then reduce the fluence or increase spot size with same energy and work on the surrounding lesion (Figs. 12.51A to C).

- *Surgical treatment*: Shave excision followed by electrodessication of the base is the procedure most commonly employed. Recurrence is common. Elliptical excision can be performed with low recurrence but will leave a scar. Another time-tested method is ligation of the base with nylon or silk (Holbe HC).

- *Topical agents* tried include:
    i. *Sclerotherapy*: Sclerotherapy with injection of sodium tetradecyl sulfate, or polidocanol has been described in a small series of patients, with complete resolution and inconspicuous scarring. It is a simple, cheap, and effective measure.
    ii. *Chemical cauterization*: Silver nitrate has been used in a small series of patients with PG on the hand. The mass was removed bluntly and the base of the lesion cauterized with silver nitrate. It requires 1–3 sessions.

Box 12.4: Summary of treatment options for pyogenic granuloma (PG).

- *Pedunculated pyogenic granuloma*: Shave excision or curettage followed by cautery of the base
- *Nonpedunculated (sessile) pyogenic granuloma*: Surgical excision of a narrow, deep, ellipse of skin beneath the lesion followed by wound closure with sutures to minimize the risk of recurrence. It is easier to control bleeding with full thickness surgical excision than with shave excision or curettage. Punch excision may be used for small PGs
- *Recurrent pyogenic granulomas*: Offer treatment with shaving or nonsurgical modalities. Surgical excision is a last option
- Topical and intralesional therapies
- *Lasers*: The benefits of decreased scarring with laser therapy must be weighed against the lack of histopathologic confirmation.

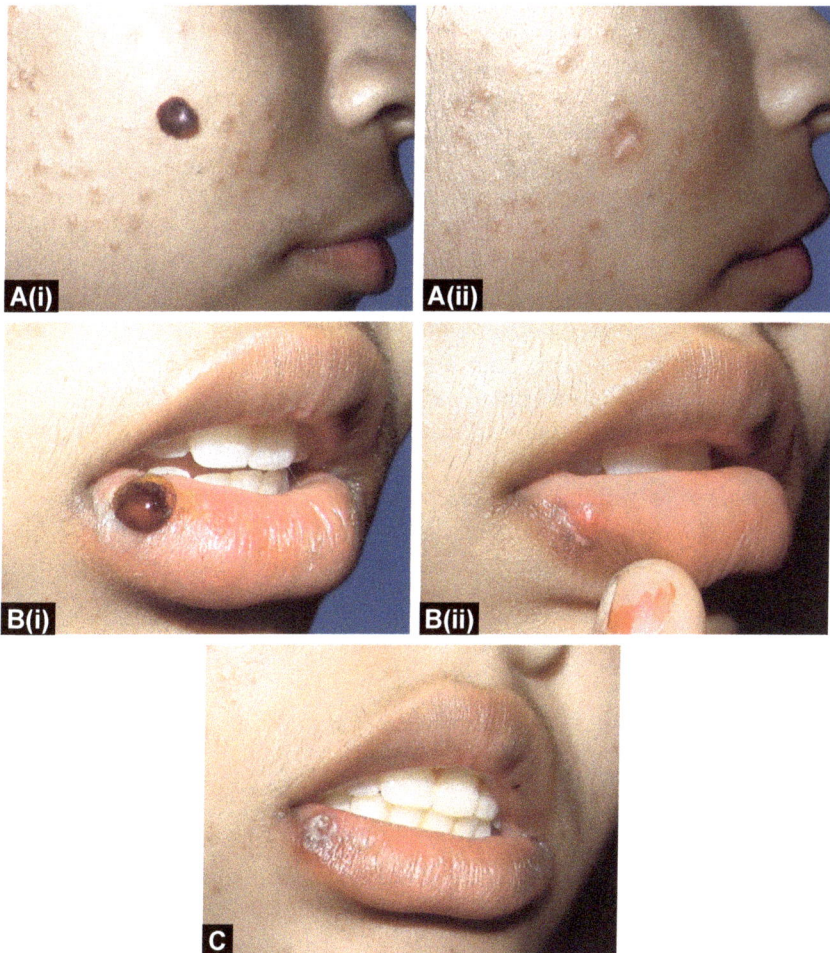

Figs. 12.51A to C: A treatment protocol for pyogenic granuloma using LP Nd:YAG. A lower fluence can be used in clinical practice (30–60 J/cm^2). A(i) Fluence of 200 J/cm^2, spot size 4 mm, frequency 1 Hz, single shot in center. This is followed by and 4–5 shots in the remaining part of lesion using a fluence of 50–100 J/cm^2, spot size 6 mm, pulse duration 20 ms, frequency 1 Hz; A(ii) After 10 days complete resolution of the lesion with minimal scarring. (A lower fluence can be sued initially); B(i) Fluence of 200 J/cm^2, spot size 4 mm, pulse duration 15 ms, frequency 1 Hz, single shot in center followed by 4–5 shots in the remaining part of lesion (Fluence of 50–100 J/cm^2, spot size 6 mm, frequency 1 Hz); B(ii) After 2 weeks, residual lesion was treated with fluence 50–90 J/cm^2, pulse duration 15 ms, spot size 4 mm, frequency 1 Hz; (C) Postoperative morphology after 2 days.

iii. *Topical phenol*: Topical phenol has been used for treatment of periungual PG. A piece of cotton dipped in phenol 98% solution is placed over the PG for 1-3 minutes applications, repeated weekly until resolution. Recurrence is a issue but is useful for patients who refuse surgery or for smaller periungual PG.

iv. *Topical imiquimod*: Topical imiquimod has been used to treat PG in children and adults. Application is from three times per week up to two times per day, as tolerated. It is an expensive option.
v. *Topical beta blockers*: Topical timolol, a nonselective beta-adrenergic antagonist, has been used to treat PG. It may help in children but in adults it is not very effective.

- *Suture ligation*: Ligation of the lesion base using soft (absorbable) suture material has been used in children with facial PG. Following ligation, the tumor becomes necrotic and falls off in days to weeks.

   An elegant procedure is a combination of timolol with ligation. The method by DR Yoo Sang Baek, from Korea uses ligation of the base with 4-0 Black Silk followed by application of timolol maleate ophthalmic 0.5% solution (four times daily with two drops per dose). This is a combination of physical (ligation) and pharmacological (timolol) strangulation. It helps in preventing the PG from enlarging and frequently reduces the tumor size before the planned surgery. It might also resolve PG.

- *Intralesional injection*: Intralesional injection of bleomycin, corticosteroids, or absolute ethanol is described in a small number of case reports.

BIBLIOGRAPHY

1. Baek YS, Kwon SH, Jeon J. Combination of ligation and timolol before surgical excision of pyogenic granuloma. J Am Acad Dermatol. 2018;78:e141-e142.
2. Holbe HC, Frosch PJ, Herbst RA. Surgical pearl: Ligation of the base of pyogenic 57 granuloma—an atraumatic, simple, and cost-effective procedure. J Am Acad Dermatol. 2003;49:509-10.
3. Khandpur S, Sharma VK. Successful treatment of multiple gingival pyogenic granulomas with pulsed-dye laser. Indian J Dermatol Venereol Leprol. 2008;74:275-7.
4. Maloney DM, Schmidt JD, Duvic M. Alitretinoin gel to treat pyogenic granuloma. J Am Acad Dermatol. 2002;47:969-70.
5. Matsumoto K, Nakanishi H, Seike T, et al. Treatment of pyogenic granuloma with a sclerosing agent. Dermatol Surg. 2001;27:521-3.
6. Neri I, Baraldi C, Balestri R, et al. Topical 1% propranolol ointment with occlusion in treatment of pyogenic granulomas: an open-label study in 22 children. Pediatr Dermatol. 2018;35:117-20.
7. Raulin C, Greve B, Hammes S. The combined continuous-wave/pulsed carbon dioxide laser for treatment of pyogenic granuloma. Arch Dermatol. 2002;138:33-7.

WOUND HEALING

Wound healing is a complex process and numerous treatment principles guide its successful implementation (Box 12.5).

Box 12.5: Basic principles: Vascularized bed, free of devitalized tissue, clear of infection, and moist.

- Sharp surgical debridement more than nonsurgical methods for the initial debridement of devitalized tissue
- Topical agents such as antiseptics and antimicrobial agents can be used to control locally heavy contamination. But significant improvements in rates of wound healing have not been found
- For deep wounds, negative pressure wound therapy may protect the wound and reduce the complexity and depth of the defect
- Acute wounds can often be closed primarily. Chronic wounds that demonstrate progressive healing as evidenced by granulation tissue and epithelialization along the wound edges can undergo delayed closure or coverage with skin grafts or bioengineered tissues
- *Adjunctive* Hyperbaric oxygen therapy, ultrasound, electrical, and electromagnetic energy.

The use of lasers for wound healing can be divided into two types:
1. Lasers to augment the healing of acute wounds (e.g. tissue welding, tissue soldering).
2. Lasers for chronic wounds (e.g. low-intensity laser devices).

Lasers for Acute Wounds

The main techniques of laser-assisted wound closure of acute wounds are: simple tissue welding, tissue soldering, dye-enhanced tissue welding, and addition of growth factors. The potential advantages of laser-assisted tissue bonding over conventional methods include increased immediate wound strength, fluid-tight closure, decreased operative repair time, reduced probability of infection and bleeding, and improved cosmetic results. However, lasers have disadvantages such as their high cost, risk of dehiscence, risk of thermal damage, and inconsistency of results.

The exact mechanism involved in laser-assisted wound closure is not completely understood. The heat produced by laser energy in the tissue causes collagen fibers to lose their triple helix structure and become fused, intertwined, swollen, and dissolved and thus, lead to better wound healing.

Lasers for Chronic Wounds

Different lasers for treating chronic wounds include helium-neon, gallium-arsenide (GaAs), gallium-aluminum-arsenide (GaAlAs), Nd:YAG, CO_2, ruby, krypton, and argon dye lasers.

The exact mechanism of action of low-intensity laser therapy is not known. Current hypotheses are: stimulation of calcium influx and mitosis rate, increased expression of HSPs (e.g. HSP70), increased expression of growth factors such as transforming growth factor-α (TGF-α), alteration of mitochondrial activity and increased ATP synthesis, augmented formation of messenger ribonucleic acid (mRNA) and protein secretion, enhancement of fibroblast and keratinocyte proliferation and migration, angiogenesis, improvement of phagocytosis, and increased rate of transformation of fibroblasts into myofibroblasts.

Conclusion

Several in vitro and in vivo studies have demonstrated that LLLT has a significant influence on a variety of cellular functions and clinical conditions. Photobiomodulation influences a variety of biological processes, including the acceleration of wound healing and enhances collagen synthesis in the wound area, thereby increasing wound tensile strength. Stimulation of cell proliferation results from an increase in mitochondrial respiration and ATP synthesis.

To better understand the role of low-intensity lasers in healing of chronic wounds, well-controlled studies that correlate cellular effects and biologic processes are needed. In the absence of such studies, the literature does not appear to support widespread use of lasers in wound healing at this time.

BIBLIOGRAPHY

1. Hawkins D, Houreld N, Abrahamse H. Low-level laser therapy (LLLT) as an effective therapeutic modality for delayed wound healing. Ann N Y Acad Sci. 2005;1056:486-93.
2. Hopkins JT, McLodat TA, Seegmiller JG, et al. Low-level laser therapy facilitates superficial wound healing in humans: A triple-blind, sham-controlled study. J Athl Train. 2004;39:223-9.
3. Karu TI. The Science of Low Power Laser Therapy. London: Gordon and Breach Science Publisher; 1998. pp. 14-33.

MALIGNANT AND PREMALIGNANT DISORDERS

Though an overview of some conditions is given here, the use of lasers cannot replace the role of oncological referral, which should follow histological confirmation and precede any surgical intervention. Though Mohs surgery is the ideal intervention in certain scenarios, lasers can be used. Updated guidelines can be accessed at www.nccn.org/. These guidelines suggest that for precancerous disorders skin-directed therapies may be tried, including lasers, though they cannot match the results of Mohs surgery.

Zoon's Balanitis

The first goal of therapy is the promotion of good hygiene; circumcision is the most consistently effective treatment. Topical steroids, antimicrobials, and hormonal therapy have all showed inconsistent results.

The CO_2 laser is an effective treatment for Zoon's balanitis, especially if circumcision is not a feasible option, and, more recently, good results with an Er:YAG laser were reported (Albertini JG). The patient was treated with an Er:YAG by Albertini et al. and showed no clinical or histological evidence of relapse with complete reepithelialization occurring 1 week after treatment, similar to the patient treated with a CO_2 laser by Baldwin and Geronimus. Nevertheless, in a series of five patients treated with a CO_2 laser (Retamar RA) two patients relapsed after 1 year or 3 years, with the third patient later developing lichen sclerosus.

Basal Cell Carcinoma/Squamous Cell Carcinoma

For low-risk nonmelanoma skin cancer (NMSC), skin-directed therapies can be used, including imiquimod 5%, RT, PDT, and cryotherapy (NCCN guidelines).

Thus, before laser therapy, one or more biopsies must always be taken to confirm the diagnoses histologically. The following laser procedures have been tried:

- *Ablative lasers (carbon dioxide and erbium-doped yttrium aluminum garnet)*: The limits of laser procedures are inherent in the depth of penetration of the lasers vis-à-vis the disorder that requires treatment.

  According to Horlock et al. treatment with the CO_2 laser is advantageous especially for patients with histologically superficial basal cell carcinoma (BCC). In addition, the extent of the ablation increases with the practitioner's clinical experience. In a study with 30 lesions [17 BCCs, 13 squamous cell carcinomas (SCCs) in situ], Humphreys et al. also found that superficial lesions responded very well to treatment with the CO_2 laser. In this study, an energy density of 500 mJ/cm^2 in two to three passes was used. However, with increasing thickness of the lesions, there was histologically minimal thermal damage to the underlying tissue, so that after completion of the laser treatment, residual tumor cells were still present.

- *Neodymium-doped yttrium aluminum garnet*: Because of its limited penetration of 4-7 mm, the Nd:YAG laser is particularly suitable for the treatment of smaller and flatter tumors.

- *Photodynamic therapy and similar approaches*: Photodynamic therapy is becoming more widely used, especially in the treatment of superficial basaliomas and SCCs of up to 2 mm in depth. Although, this is an interesting and promising therapeutic approach, the lack of long-term data means that it should not yet be regarded as a routine procedure for nodular lesions.

Erythroplasia of Queyrat/Bowen's Disease

The standard treatment is micrographically monitored excision, preceded in all cases without exception by a biopsy to confirm the diagnosis and determine the depth of penetration. Alternatives available are curettage, electrodesiccation, cryotherapy, topical application of fluorouracil and imiquimod, PDT, and laser therapy.

The pulsed CO_2 laser is now generally used for the treatment of Bowen's syndrome and erythroplasia of Queyrat. Numerous case reports of successful treatment are available (Del Losada JP, Greenbaum SS). Martinez-Gonzalez et al. described a lasting success achieved in 85% of their cases after only one treatment session with the CO_2 laser. In 8% of cases, there was a later recurrence. A total of 2% of patients did not respond to laser therapy. Vaïsse et al. also report similar results in Bowen's syndrome in one study (eight patients, ten lesions). In a period of almost 3 years, there was a single recurrence of one lesion.

A case report published by Wang et al. also describes a combined treatment with the Er:YAG laser followed by topical application of 5-fluorouracil in one patient. It is not certain whether this procedure will eventually be accepted as standard, because no long-term observations of patient populations are yet available that would allow extrapolation of the results to other patients.

To keep the recurrence rate as low as possible, an adequate safety margin must also be created in the healthy tissue when a laser surgical technique is used. As seen in Figures 12.52A to C, bleeding makes the use of lasers difficult. Very close follow-up is necessary, as with all techniques, especially because complete removal of tumor complexes cannot be absolutely guaranteed and there are still no adequate long-term observations on recurrence rates available.

Paget's Disease

Extramammary Paget's disease is, by definition, an intraepithelial adenocarcinoma that occurs with particularly high frequency in the genitoanal region. There have been several reports of its treatment with the pulsed CO_2 laser and the pulsed Nd:YAG laser.

Louis-Sylvestre et al. described recurrence rates of up to 67% after a year after treatment with the pulsed CO_2 laser; these rates can be reduced to 23% minimum by combining the laser therapy with extensive surgical excision. In a few cases, it proved possible to achieve a disease-free state lasting up to 4.5 years with the combined treatment (Ewing TL).

For some time, PDT has been used with increasing frequency as an alternative to the laser for treatment of Paget's disease (Shieh S). As of this writing, however, there still have not been any studies about this disease

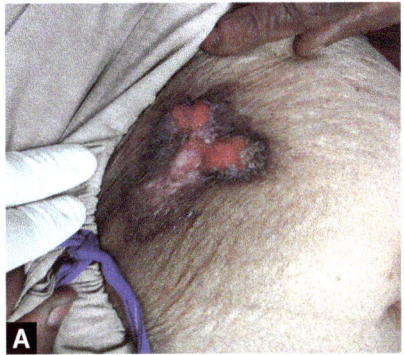
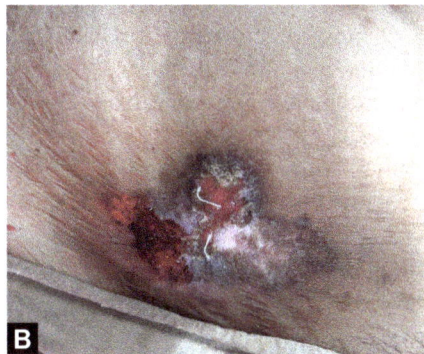
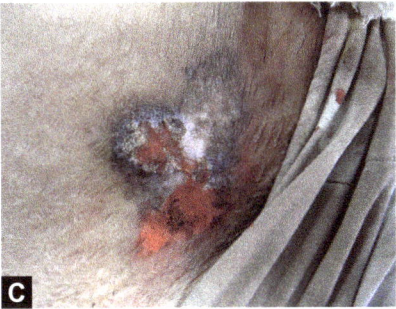

Figs. 12.52A to C: (A) A case of erythroplasia of Queyrat; (B) A spot is treated with pulsed carbon dioxide (CO_2) laser (repeat mode, 4 W, 0.20 s). Note the bleeding as the epidermis is ablated; and (C) A few more passes are given till the elevated surface is ablated. A staged approach should be used for laser therapy of malignant tumor.

in large patient populations. The application of laser systems to date has been based mostly on case reports. Because there also have been reports of ineffectual treatments with the CO_2 laser, careful consideration must be given to whether laser treatment is indicated, and very close follow-up is essential (Puppala S).

Parapsoriasis/Mycosis Fungoides

Mycosis fungoides (MF) is a T-cell, non-Hodgkin lymphoma. Only in the early stages where systemic involvement is not marked, skin-directed therapies are used. These include steroids, topical chemotherapy, RT, phototherapy, imiquimod, and retinoids (NCCN guidelines).

Goldberg et al. had reported a successful treatment of palmoplantar lesion with the pulsed CO_2 laser in 1997. During a follow-up period of 5 years, the patient remained free of recurrence.

Excimer laser has been used both in MF and parapsoriasis but in the early stages of the disease. This type of laser is used because it is thought that, compared with total body irradiation with UV light, the selective application of lasers makes it possible to protect healthy skin at the same time. Passeron et al. showed that complete healing of circumscribed plaques can be attained with a mean of 7–15 sessions and an average of 7 J energy applied per cm^2. These results remained stable for a total of 3 months. Mori et al. also used the excimer laser in seven stage 1A lesions with complete lack of recurrence after 3–28 months. This was improved by Nicticó et al. who achieved a recurrence free interval of more than a year after treating ten lesions in the same stage; a cumulative energy dose of 6–12 J/cm^2 was applied. Upjohn et al. in a study with eight stage 1A or 1B patients, showed that after 20 treatment sessions with the excimer laser, there was complete clinical and histological remission in 37% of cases, which persisted for at least 30 months. In a further 37%, there was an initial clinical and histological remission. However, during follow-up there was a recurrence.

The PDT has also already been successfully applied in these conditions, although as of now there are no long-term data about recurrence rates.

In summary, laser therapy can be a helpful complement to the treatment of MF, especially in its early stages. Long-term results and studies of large patient populations are not yet available.

BIBLIOGRAPHY

1. Albertini JG, Holck DE, Farley MF. Zoon's balanitis treated with Erbium:YAG laser ablation. Lasers Surg Med. 2002;30:123-6.
2. Baldwin HE, Geronemus RG. The treatment of Zoon's balanitis with the carbon dioxide laser. J Dermatol Surg Oncol. 1989;15:491-4.
3. Del Losada JP, Ferré A, San Román B, et al. Erythroplasia of Queyrat with urethral involvement: Treatment with carbon dioxide laser vaporization. Dermatol Surg. 2005;31:1454-7.
4. Ewing TL. Paget's disease of the vulva treated by combined surgery and laser. Gynecol Oncol. 1991;43:137-40.
5. Greenbaum SS, Glogau R, Stegman SJ, et al. Carbon dioxide laser treatment of erythroplasia of Queyrat. J Dermatol Surg Oncol. 1989;15:747-50.
6. Horlock N, Grobbelaar AO, Gault DT. Can the carbon dioxide laser completely ablate basal cell carcinomas? A histological study. Br J Plast Surg. 2000;53:286-93.
7. Humphreys TR, Malhotra R, Scharf MJ, et al. Treatment of superficial basal cell carcinoma and squamous cell carcinoma in situ with a high-energy pulsed carbon dioxide laser. Arch Dermatol. 1998;134:1247-52.
8. Louis-Sylvestre C, Haddad B, Paniel BJ. Paget's disease of the vulva: Results of different conservative treatments. Eur J Obstet Gynecol Reprod Biol. 2001;99: 253-5.
9. Martinez-Gonzalez MC, Pozo JD, Paradela S, et al. Bowen's disease treated by carbon dioxide laser. A series of 44 patients. J Dermatolog Treat. 2008;11:1-4.
10. Mori M, Campolmi P, Mavilia L, et al. Monochromatic excimer light (308 nm) in patch-stage IA mycosis fungoides. J Am Acad Dermatol. 2004;50:943-5.
11. Nicticó S, Costanzo A, Saraceno R, et al. Efficacy of monochromatic excimer laser radiation (308 nm) in the treatment of early stage mycosis fungoides. Br J Dermatol. 2004;151:877-9.
12. Passeron T, Angeli K, Cardot-Leccia N, et al. Treatment of mycosis fungoides by 308 nm excimer laser: A clinical and histological study in 10 patients. Ann Dermatol Venereol. 2007;134:225-31.

13. Puppala S. Failure of carbon dioxide laser treatment in three patients with penoscrotal extramammary Paget's disease. BJU Int. 2001;88:986-7.
14. Retamar RA, Kien MC, Chouela EN. Zoon's balanitis: Presentation of 15 patients, five treated with a carbon dioxide laser. Int J Dermatol. 2003;42:305-7.
15. Shieh S, Dee AS, Cheney RT, et al. Photodynamic therapy for the treatment of extramammary Paget's disease. Br J Dermatol. 2003;146:100-5.
16. Upjohn E, Foley P, Lane P, et al. Long-term clearance of patch-stage mycosis fungoides with the 308-nm laser. Clin Exp Dermatol. 2007;32:168-71.
17. Vaïsse V, Clerici T, Fusade T. Bowen disease treated with scanned pulsed high energy CO_2 laser. Follow-up of 6 cases. Ann Dermatol Venereol. 2001;128:1220-4.
18. Wang KH, Fang JY, Hu CH, et al. Erbium:YAG laser pretreatment accelerates the response of Bowen's disease treated by topical 5-fluorouracil. Dermatol Surg. 2004;30:441-5.

HYPERHIDROSIS

Hyperhidrosis (HH) is a chronic autonomic disorder that is marked by excessive sweating that lasts at least 6 months without any distinguishable cause. Diagnosis includes at least two of the following that is mentioned in Box 12.6.

Though sweating is physiological, excessive sweating is troublesome. It is classified as primary focal HH versus secondary generalized HH. One can find a cause like systemic disease, medication side effect, hormones, etc. for secondary variety whereas primary focal is essentially idiopathic. Primary focal HH is a chronic autonomic disorder that is marked by excessive sweating that lasts at least 6 months without any distinguishable cause.

Unless specified, the word HH mentioned anywhere here in this chapter refers to primary focal variety.

Though there are multiple treatments, the idea is to administer them keeping the financial needs of the patients in mind (Fig. 12.53). Each modality has its advantages, and topical and oral medications are less effective, while Botox achieves long lasting results. Surgical therapy is a more invasive procedure and compensatory hyperhidrosis secondary to sympathectomy limits its use.

Box 12.6: Diagnostic criteria for primary focal hyperhidrosis: any two of six is diagnostic.

- Impairs daily activities
- Bilateral and relatively symmetric
- Occurring at least once per week
- Age of onset younger than 25 years
- Family history
- Cessation of focal sweating during sleep.

Source: Hornberger J, Grimes K, Naumann M, et al. Recognition, diagnosis, and treatment of primary focal hyperhidrosis. J Am Acad Dermatol. 2004;51:274-86.

Hyperhidrosis

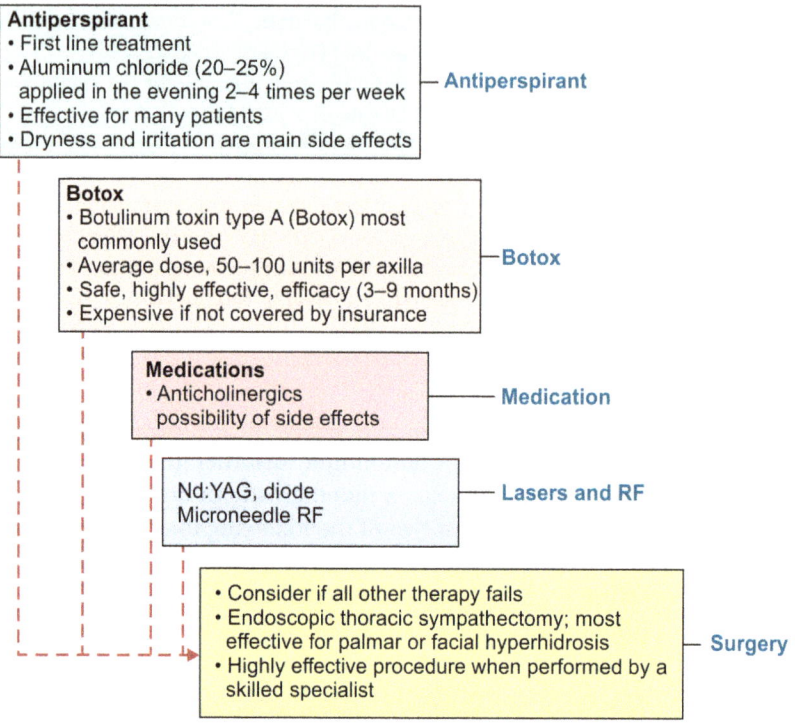

Fig. 12.53: Hyperhidrosis: Overview of treatment modalities for hyperhidrosis. (Nd:YAG: neodymium-doped yttrium aluminum garnet; RF: radiofrequency).

Treatment

Autosuggestion, meditation, and biofeedback mechanisms are useful in reducing frequency of HH attacks. It is worth noting that primary focal HH typically stops during sleep and is worse with stress. An overview of region wise treatment options are detailed in Table 12.24 and the individual therapies are discussed here.

Medical Therapy

- *Topical agents*:
    i. *Aluminum chloride hexahydrate*: Application of 10–30% aluminum chloride hexahydrate solution to unshaven skin for 6–8 hours nightly for 3–4 days can be beneficial. After about 3 weeks, a weekend therapy suffices in most cases.
    ii. **Tap water iontophoresis** can be effective.
       These devices pass a small voltage of direct current (DC) into tap water. This current disrupts polarization of cell walls of sweat glands

Table 12.24: Region wise treatment options for hyperhidrosis (HH).

Treatments/Areas	Axilla	Palms	Soles	Forehead/face
Autosuggestion and meditation	Yes	Yes	Yes	Yes
Medication	Yes	Yes	Yes	Yes
Antiperspirants	Yes	Yes	Yes	Yes
Iontophoresis	–	Yes	Yes	–
Botulinum toxin A	Yes	Yes	Yes	Yes
MiraDry™	Yes	–	–	–
Lasers LSA	Yes	–	–	–
Surgeries	Yes	–	–	–
ETS	Caution	Caution	–	–

and temporarily blocks sweat production. OTC devices are low voltage and battery operated and prescription devices are of plug in type. Alternate daily treatment session of 30–45 minutes can be effective in 60–80% of cases, but patient compliance is an issue due to its temporary results.

- *Systemic agents*: Oral anticholinergics including glycopyrrolate, propantheline, and oxybutynin are useful adjuncts.
  i. *Oral glycopyrrolate*: Typical doses for adults range from 1 mg to 2 mg once or twice daily (i.e. 1–4 mg per day).
  ii. *Oral oxybutynin*: Typical adult doses of oxybutynin are 5–10 mg per day; however, doses up to 20 mg per day have been utilized.

  Responses to systemic anticholinergics usually take about 1 week for the maximum effect. Dose adjustments may be needed to achieve sufficient improvement for individual patients. Continued treatment is necessary to maintain the response to treatment.

- *Botox*: Although other formulations of botulinum toxin may improve hyperhidrosis, most studies have used **ona**botulinum toxin A or **abo**botulinum toxin A. Dosing of these agents is not equivalent; 1 unit of **ona**botulinum toxin A is equal to approximately 3 units of **abo**botulinum toxin A. **USFDA** approval for botulinum toxin for hyperhidrosis is limited to **onabotulinum toxin** A for axillary hyperhidrosis.

  In the biggest trial of 145 patients with primary axillary hyperhidrosis responsive to topical therapy with aluminum chloride, patients were injected with 200 units of abobotulinum toxin A in one axilla and placebo in the other; after 2 weeks, the treatments were revealed, and the axilla that had been treated with placebo was injected with 100 units of abobotulinum toxin A. Two weeks after the initial injection, the rate of sweat production was significantly less on the side treated with abobotulinum toxin A (24 mg/min vs. 144 mg/min). Two weeks after the injection with

100 U, the rate of sweat production decreased from 144 mg/min to 32 mg/min. The mean reduction in sweating was greater with the 200 units injection (81.4% vs. 76.5%).

- *Response*: A response to treatment is usually evident within 2-4 days and improvement in sweating typically persists for 3-9 months.
- *Procedure*:
  - *Anesthesia*: Topical anesthetic cream and/or ice gives sufficient anesthesia but in expert hands nerve blocks should be considered prior to plantar and palmar treatments.
  - A starch-iodine test performed prior to treatment can help delineate the areas to be injected. Iodine is placed on the affected area, followed by the application of corn starch, this should be washed off prior to Botox injections.
  - Botox A (100 U/vial) dilution of 2.0 U/0.1 cc is effective. They are given at 1-2 cm intervals intradermally throughout the affected area. 2 U should be injected per site. A total of 50-100 U/axilla, palm, or sole can be injected, for a total dose of 100-200 U for both treatment sites (Figs. 12.54 to 12.56). A decreased dose can be used for localized hyperhidrosis. Temporary hand and finger muscle weakness may be seen and usually recovers in 4 weeks. Decreased sweating is observed within 1-2 weeks.

Surgical Therapy

Surgery is more invasive and risky approach to HH and is falling out of favor due to the advent of less invasive procedures. Dermal curettage was found to be effective in axillary HH with variable results and reasonable safety in various studies but now subdermal ablation of sweat glands with EBDs like laser and RF (Table 12.25) are favored.

Endoscopic thoracic sympathectomy (ETS) is the last resort for intractable palmar HH with efficacy of 95-100% and 73% satisfaction rate. T1, T2, T3,

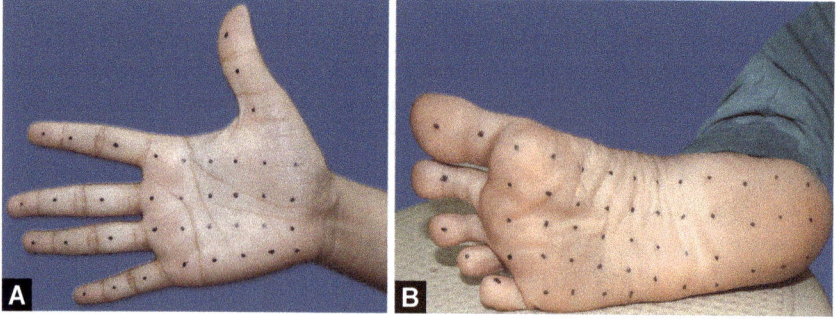

Figs. 12.54A and B: Botulin toxin injection markings for palmoplantar hyperhidrosis: botulinum neurotoxin A (Xeomin® or BOTOX®) 100 units of lyophilized powder are diluted in 4 mL normal saline.

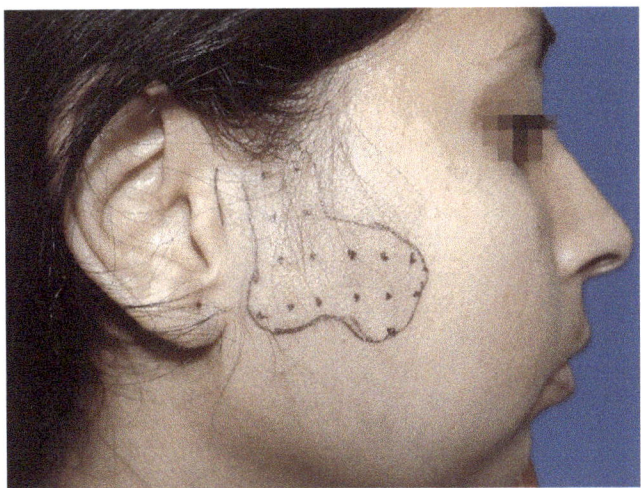

Fig. 12.55: Marking for botulinum toxin (Xeomin® or BOTOX) for gustatory hyperhidrosis. Dilution of 100 units in 4 mL and injecting 0.05 mL to 0.1 mL each site 1 cm apart.

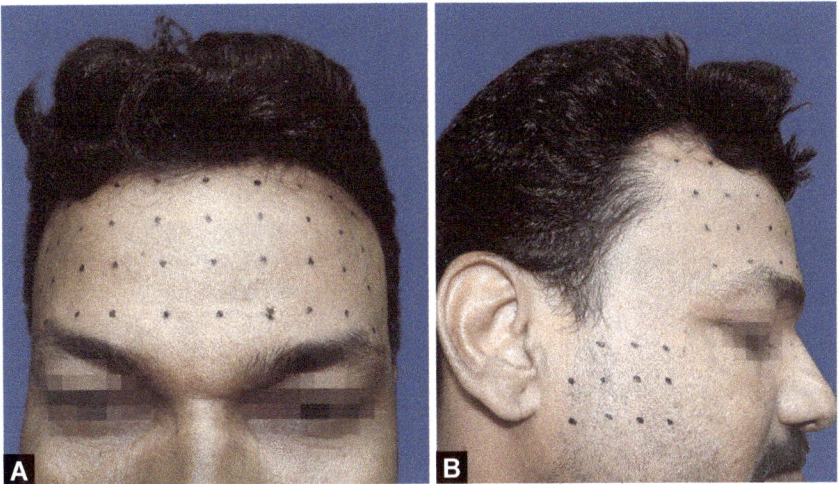

Figs. 12.56A and B: Marking for botulinum toxin (Xeomin® or BOTOX) for gustatory hyperhidrosis. Dilution of 100 units in 4 mL and injecting 0.05 mL to 0.1 mL each site 1 cm apart.

and T4 ganglion are ablated for palmar cases. Multiple ganglion ablation has better efficacy but has higher morbidity. In axillary, only 52% patients had more than 50% improvement. Its effect is negated by compensatory HH in other areas. Side effects of ETS include compensatory HH on abdomen, chest, back, thighs, and face, gustatory phantom sweat, Horner's syndrome—unilateral upper eyelid ptosis, pupil constriction, and facial anhidrosis (0.8%), neuralgia, cardiac effects, and pneumothorax.

Table 12.25: Surgical options for hyperhidrosis.

	Axilla	Palms	Soles	Face
Radical excision with grafting	Not used now	No	No	No
Subdermal curettage	Caution, effective	No	No	No
Superficial liposuction/ laser liposuction	Somewhat effective	No	No	No
Endoscopic thoracic sympathectomy (ETS)	Caution, not used now, compensatory hyperhidrosis	Yes, last option	No	No
1470 laser sweat ablation (LSA)	Most preferred, effective	No	No	No

Lasers and Energy Devices

An overview of the various energy devices are given here in Table 12.26. We will focus on the major approved devices and rationale therein.

A. *Laser and their Logic*: The lasers that have been used include the Nd:YAG and diode lasers, but the literature supports the superiority of the former (1,064 nm Nd:YAG laser) at least in axillary hyperhidrosis (Cervantes J).

   i. *Neodymium-doped yttrium aluminum garnet*: In a study by Goldman and Wollina, alterations and necrosis/collapse of eccrine glands were noted on histologic examination suggesting that direct thermal damage to eccrine glands was responsible for the reduction in sweat. But a study by Letada et al. did not appreciate any histologic changes before and after laser treatment.

   Thus, it is believed that the **mode of action** could be due to cellular or subcellular alterations through heating of melanin or water chromophores, indirectly impacting the sympathetic cholinergic transmissions in the axilla.

   Other wavelengths used include the 1,320 nm Nd:YAG laser and the 1,440 nm laser. Like the 1,064 nm Nd:YAG, eccrine gland necrosis was evident on histology after one treatment with 1,440 nm Nd:YAG.

   ii. *Diode*: With the diode laser (800 nm) though a reduction in sweat was noted by Bechara et al. histologic examination of treated specimens was normal. No endogenous chromophores in apocrine and eccrine glands have been found that absorb the 800 nm pulsed light.

   The 924/975 nm diode laser in combination with curettage provided better results than the 975 nm diode laser (Leclere FM et al.). The 924/975 nm diode laser treatment was equally effective as curettage. The logic of using this is that while the 975 nm is only able to reach the superficial dermis due to its affinity for water, the 924 nm wavelength is preferentially absorbed by fat, which is abundant in the deep subcutaneous tissue. Thus, this would also target the

Table 12.26: Lasers EBDs for HH.

	Energy	Specification	Prototype	Area	Status
Noninvasive/ fractional	Microwave		MiraDry™	Axilla	
	Noninvasive RF	Unipolar, bipolar, and monopolar	Accent™, SweatX™	Axilla, face	
	MNRF	2.5–4 mm, insulated or noninsulated tip	Scarlet™	Axilla	
	RF	Subdermal RF with infrared temperature sensor in situ and infra red camera for skin temperature	ThermiDry™ Monopolar RF by Thermi USA	Axilla, may be face, body	Very safe due to temperature control
	Laser hair reduction	800 nm diode, 1,064 nm Nd:YAG, 755 nm alexandrite, and triple wavelength	Lightsheer™, Gentle YAG™, Soprano ICE™, Sprite Super Diode™ by Active	Axilla	
	HIFU	Microfocused ultrasound with visualization. 4.5 mm depth	Ulthera™	Axilla, may be face	
Ablative/invasive/ optical fiber lasers	Laser	Skin directed		Axilla, may be face	Very safe due to skin-directed tip
	Laser	Radial emission and silhouette	Alma 1,470 nm fiber diode laser	Axilla	
	Laser	Forward emitting bare laser fibers	Alma 1,470 nm fiber diode laser LipoLife™	Axilla	
			800 nm, 890 nm, 924 nm, and 975 nm diodes 1,064 nm, 1,440 nm, and 1,370 nm Nd:YAG lasers	Axilla	
		LSA with endoscopic visualization	ELSA with various fiber lasers mainly 890 nm, 924 nm, and 975 nm	Axilla	

(EBDs: energy-based devices; HH: hyperhidrosis; HIFU: high-intensity focused ultrasound; LSA: laser sweat ablation; MNRF: microneedling radiofrequency; Nd:YAG: neodymium-doped yttrium aluminum garnet)

sweat gland that lie abutting the subcutaneous tissue. The logic of a simultaneous emission of 924 nm and 974 nm is that these wavelengths could damage both the superficial dermis and the deep cutaneous tissue. The problem being that a more prolonged energy delivery is necessary for the 975 nm wavelength to target the sweat glands and at higher temperatures, thus a greater risk of superficial burns is well documented.

iii. *Laser sweat ablation with bare optical fibers*: Various optical fiber lasers used in liposuction are tried in axillary HH. Diode fibers of various wavelengths like 800 nm, 890 nm, 924 nm, and 975 nm are used with same technique like liposuction with tumescent local anesthesia and laser fiber is used to scrap undersurface of dermis to target sweat glands. Most of the fibers are forward emitting hence, lack of focus on dermis, can get stuck in tissue and have chances of lateral thermal damage, nerve paresis, skin necrosis, and scarring.

LipoLife™ by Alma lasers is radially emitting optical fiber emits 1,470 nm wavelength in all direction and also called angel fiber. It is mounted inside the tip of a metal cannula hence is also referred to as a silhouette fiber. It is used with same technique as liposuction except using in very superficial plane.

Another modification of optical fiber is tissue directed tip in 1,470 diode 600 µ optical fiber by Alma, HydroLife™. The tip of optical fiber bends at 90° to direct to skin. It is tough enough to scrap the undersurface of dermis.

- *Authors' experience of laser sweat ablation with 1,470 nm diode laser fiber*: Author (Dhepe NV) has experience of using Alma 1,470 nm tissue-directed optical fiber laser HydroLife™ on 26 patients with technique and parameters described here. Average age of patients was 24 years, predominantly males with average duration of HH more than 8 years.
- *Technique of laser sweat ablation*:
  - Starch-iodine test is done to map the exact area of HH.
  - Each axilla is infiltrated with 100 mL of tumescent fluid.
  - Two or three entry points are made up with 18 G needle.
  - HydroLife™ by Alma with 1,470 nm laser energy emitted from a diode source (Fig. 12.57). The probe with optical fiber inside is inserted. Tip of the fiber should be facing skin. While power settings are kept on 3–4 W, and on pulsed mode with on time 100 ms and off time 50–100 ms, the probe scraps the undersurface of skin giving popcorn-like sound of water boiling indicating ablation in dermis. Total energy used in each underarm is 500 J.
  - As it is freehand technique, the movement of probe should be fast but continuous. Slow movement at any point may cause

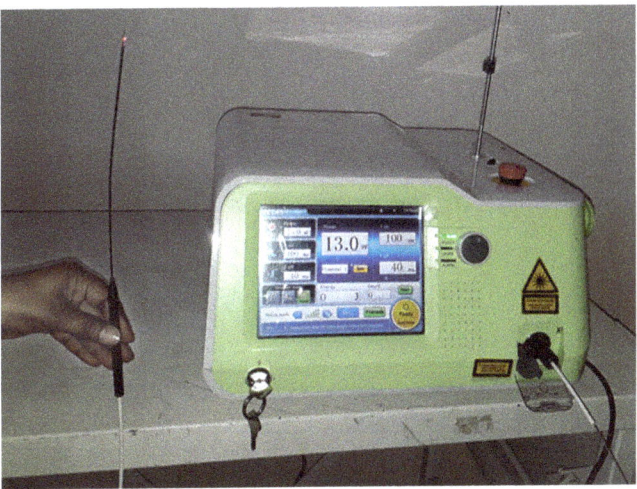

Fig. 12.57: 1,470 nm tissue directed 600 μ optical fiber with cannula on Alma HydroLifeTM.

skin burn. Entire area is covered from different directions through various entry points. Treated areas are cooled with ice packs and patient is sent home with oral and topical antibiotics and pain killers.

Results: All 26 patients experienced immediate relief from HH and maintained at 90 days follow-up. At second follow-up at 6 months, 21 patients still maintained significant result (>75% area of sweat reduction on starch-iodine test) [Figs. 12.58A and B]. 16 patients had complete sweat reduction while remaining eight patients have small discrete areas of HH, probably skipped areas during last treatment. Half of them (four of eight) preferred to wait for another 3 months before deciding for second session. Subsequent treatment was focused on "hot areas" or skipped areas topographically marked on starch-iodine test though entire area was uniformaly covered.

Six patients recruited in study were drop out from MiraDry study for various reasons. All of them got significant reduction in their sweating. Only one of them needed a second session for skipped "hot spots". At 9 months follow-up, all patients maintained significant sweat reduction.

Side effects included erosions and minor scars (<5 mm) at points of prolonged contact of probe with skin and assumed to be technique dependent. Thus, laser sweat ablation (LSA) with tissue-directed anchor fiber emitting 1,470 nm laser is effective and safe out-patient procedure producing long-lasting results. As it is freehand manual, surgical skill is involved results and safety may vary with physician to physician and his learning curve.

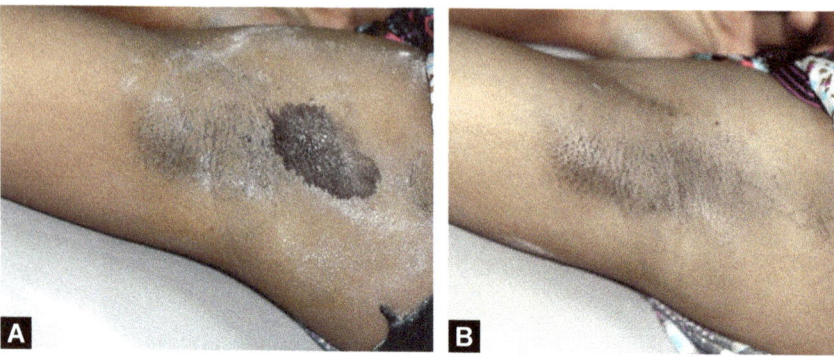

Figs. 12.58A and B: Starch iodine test result before and after 1,470 laser sweat ablation (1,470 nm tissue directed 600 μ optical fiber with cannula on Alma HydroLifeTM) Day 90.

B. *Radiofrequency*: Radiofrequency is largely based on the heat energy that is released by the placement of needles within the skin. Using the logic that there is no laser that ideally targets eccrine glands, RF is ideal in such situations as it is believed to be a "chromophore blind" energy device.

Glaser et al. in a landmark study conducted a randomized trial of 120 adults with primary axillary hyperhidrosis who were given one to three treatments with a microwave energy device (n = 81) or a sham device (n = 39). Patients treated with the microwave device were more likely to notice a subjective reduction in the severity of axillary hyperhidrosis 30 days after treatment than patients in the sham treatment group (89% vs. 54%). The difference in favor of active treatment remained statistically significant for up to 6 months.

In 2012, Hong et al. found that microwaves can be used to treat axillary hyperhidrosis with long lasting effects. Kim et al. conducted one of the first pilot studies in 2013 looking at fractional microneedle radiofrequency (FMR) for primary axillary hyperhidrosis. In 20 cases with two sessions at 1-month intervals, there was a significant decrease in the amount of sweating and 70% of subjects said they experienced greater than a 50% improvement in sweating after 2 months of the last session. Histology confirmed damage of glands at a depth between 2 mm and 4 mm, with a decrease in the density and size of the apocrine and eccrine glands. The side effects noted were transient tingling, swelling, and erythema, though two patients experienced compensatory hyperhidrosis.

A series of articles by Abtahi-Naeini and Fatemi-Naeini et al. in 2014 found that in the 25 cases studied, three sessions of FMR at 3-week intervals were administered and one side was treated, 3 months after the last session, 80% reported more than 50% satisfaction. Histological samples also showed a decrease in the number of sweat glands on the treated side. In 2016, they followed these cases and 1 year later, they found 10 patients who did not experience any relapse of their hyperhidrosis. Importantly they found that there was a significant correlation between hyperhidrosis relapse and change in body mass index. These results were replicated by Schick et al. (2016) in a trial for axillary hyperhidrosis.

Microwave thermolysis is typically administered in two, 20–30 min treatment sessions separated by 3 months. The most common side effects of treatment are altered skin sensation (median duration 25 days, range 4–225 days), discomfort, and other local reactions. Transient median and ulnar neuropathy after microwave thermolysis also has been reported in a patient treated for axillary hyperhidrosis.

A recent study has used surgical ablation of T2, T3, and T4 levels for palmar HH using RF while another used stimulation to achieve heartening results. Thus, RF may soon replace lasers for treating HH.

- *Subdermal radiofrequency sweat ablation ThermiDry^{TM}:* ThermiDry^{TM} is a monopolar RF at 460 kHz reaching temperature at tip 65°C. Subdermal electrode is used to scrap undersurface of dermis in aim to destroy sweat glands. Its safety lies in real-time temperature monitoring and control. Real-time temperature sensors at tip measures subdermal temperature while external infrared camera measures skin surface temperature. RF emission is coupled with safe temperature limit hence safety is ensured. This claims to be single session treatment for axillary HH, though consumable cost is an inhibiting factor.

- *MiraDry^{TM} microwave sweat ablation:* This is the first and the only EBD approved by US FDA for axillary HH. It has 90 W RF generator and used disposable biotips. Vacuum sucks skin in while hydroceramic cooling tip protect epidermis. It fires microwave in a grid sequentially. Easily delegable to assistant. Glaser et al. in a landmark study conducted a randomized trial of 120 adults with primary axillary HH, who were given one to three treatments with a microwave energy device (n = 81) or a sham device (n = 39), 70% of MiraDry^{TM} recipients said that their sweating no longer bothered them after 1.5 years. At energy level 3–70% reduction in one go, 90% in two. In level four or above, it may be a single session treatment. Thus, MiraDry^{TM} may be the safest and lasting option for axillary sweat. In 2012, Hong et al. found that microwaves can be used to treat axillary HH with long-lasting effects.

The author (Dhepe NV et al.) is the first user in India and has used the device in 43 Indian cases. All of them have immediate reduction of sweating within an hour of treatment. All patients tolerated the treatment very well. The parameters used were at power setting of three (3–4 mm) depth. Treatment time was 90 minutes. Two patients developed a swelling in treated area that lasted for 10 days. Most of the patients received a course of prednisolone 40 mg per day for 5–10 days. Only limitation was the entire area that requires infiltration with local anesthesia.

Follow-up at 6 months: Only 14 patients felt they will need one more treatment. Rest are happy with follow-up period of 4-6 months. All the patients felt it improved their social life. 32 out of 43 patients felt that the treatment is costly, but it was worth spending. All of them said they will recommend this to their friends.

Follow-up at 1 year: 18 out of 43 patients needed second session. Six patients needed third session. Six patients opted out of the study after one session and were recruited for LSA treatment. None of the patients developed any adverse reaction. Most of them received energy level 3 and 4. Results would have been better if energy level 5 would have used though at cost of higher incidence of adverse effects.

C. *High-intensity focused ultrasound and ultherapy^{TM}:* Microfocused ultrasound with visualization called Ultherapy^{TM} by Ulthera USA is the first extensively tried device for axillary HH. Protocols of using various energy levels and their combinations are currently under investigations. Many other devices with HIFU without visualizations are also tried in HH with inconsistent results.

Nestor MS, Park H in their two randomized double-blind, sham-controlled pilot studies treated two sessions of MHUV at months interval, male and female patients of 18-75 years of age with moderate-to-severe bilateral axillary HH refractory to prior topical therapies keeping a control treated with sham device. At day 60 (30 days after the second treatment), a positive hyperhidrosis disease severity score (HDSS) response rate of 67% was achieved by the MFUV group versus 0% in the sham group ($p = 0.005$). HDSS response rate was more than or equal to 50% in the MFUV group at all-time points except day 7 versus zero in sham group. At day 60, the areas of greatest improvement were sweat production (92%) and social embarrassment (83%).

Conclusion

The use of minimally invasive surgery and devices for controlling axillary hyperhidrosis is not new. Various techniques, especially the high energy microwave with tumescent anesthesia, or multidirectional firing lasers, or even combining liposuction curettage with diode and near-infrared lasers, makes a one-treatment protocol a very real possibility. But as has been seen but sadly not reported in melasma, the ability of the devices to produce focal injury, is counteracted by the body's ability to repair it, and some rebound back toward baseline and like in melasma, sweating inevitably reoccurs with time. It is this because of repopulation of glands over time or a dermal reenervation after procedure, as some investigators have reported.

Palmoplantar HH is debilitating condition, affecting quality more than severe in patient skin diseases. Though botulinum toxin A is the only effective intervention available till date, it has not been very popular due to its huge cost and temporary nature of the results. EBDs are not evolved for this indication due to its potential risk to its delicate neurovascular and vascular structures. EBDs used for axillary HH may be in future safely adopted for palms and soles.

The use of minimally invasive surgery and devices for controlling axillary HH is not new. MiraDry™ microwave is the only FDA approved noninvasive device available for axillary HH though it may require two to three sessions at safe parameters and cost being prohibitive. Various energies are used to destroy sweat glands directly reaching undersurface of skin in tumescent local anesthesia. 1,470 nm tissue-directed anchor fiber is very safe more promising with possibility of making it single session daycare procedure. But being a freehand surgical technique, its results and safety may vary from surgeon to surgeon. Subdermal RF ablation with temperature control has similar potential at experienced hands.

It must be appreciated that there are instances where a contrarian result has been reported with energy devices. Aydin et al. for instance, found that during epilation, deep penetration with the 1,064 nm Nd:YAG laser may actually stimulate rather than destroy eccrine sweat glands when applied through the skin surface, ultimately causing or exacerbating the issue of hyperhidrosis. Additionally, a case series has shown that the depilatory laser may actually trigger the onset of hyperhidrosis.

The main limitation of the data on HH is that there are a lack of well-defined studies to assess the efficacy and safety of laser treatment. Only some of the studies used the contralateral axilla as a control to rule out spontaneous remission. Lastly, there is a large variation in laser parameters and treatment regimens. For now, though the Nd:YAG seems to be superior than other lasers, RF might be another option. Any future work should demonstrate histological ablation of eccrine glands coupled with prolonged results to enable replication.

ENLARGED PORES

Enlarged facial pores is a lay term that is poorly defined in the medical literature and often is categorized in terms of arbitrary circular diameters determined through cosmetic skin analyzers. The term refers to pilosebaceous follicular enlargements (with or without open comedonal horny impactions) that can be visualized by the naked eye, most commonly occurring on the face and scalp. An article defined a pore as any circular shape with a size wider than 0.02 mm. Facial pores are not fixed but are dynamic structures.

The epidermal architecture around facial pores, as viewed through confocal laser microscopic imaging, consists of epidermal elongations hanging down into the dermis-like stalactites, and dermal papillae rising into the epidermis-like stalagmites. Interestingly, the undulating, so-called stalagmite-like (SL) structure of the epidermodermal junction structure has commonly been associated with larger hollows and an uneven skin tone, and this is the only characteristic structure observed in enlarged pores.

Causative Factors

It is now thought that seborrhea, loss of skin elasticity and tension, and hair follicle size are most clinically relevant to the pathogenesis of enlarged pores.

Other potential associated and causative factors include genetic predisposition, acne, comedogenic xenobiotics, chronic photodamage, chronic radiodermatitis, and vitamin A deficiency.

- The direct relationship between *sebum* output and pore size has been well established particularly in men, who generally have higher sebum output levels than women, which likely is testosterone driven. But this is confounded by females who exhibit enlarged pores without raised androgens. However, a cyclical variation is well established in females, due to increased progesterone affecting sebaceous gland activity. Admittedly, acne and facial pores are interlinked, given the frequent occurrence of open comedones within the pores (Figs. 12.59A and B).

  The direct relationship between sebum output and pores is evident from the fact that the sites of predilection, on the nose and medial aspects of the cheeks, is explained by the increased sebum excretion (Fig. 12.60).

- *Skin elasticity and tensile strength* when defined visually and mechanically has shown a negative correlation with facial pore size and density. It is logically surmised that in some cases, enlarged pores could be a consequence of aging, that effects the collagen and elastin framework that allows the skin to maintain its resilient properties.

  Pore density and size appears to vary diversely across ethnicities, though Chinese women exhibit notably lower pore size and density across all ages as compared to other ethnicities. Black individuals have

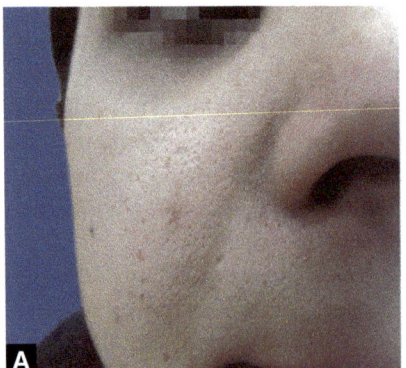 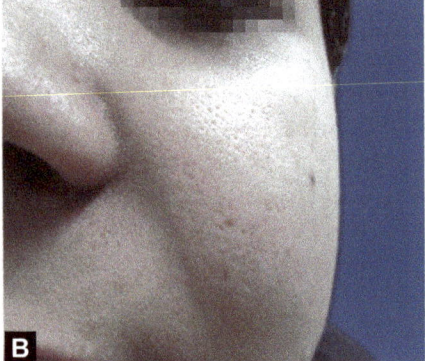

Figs. 12.59A and B: Enlarged pores in a girl who had been treated for acne.

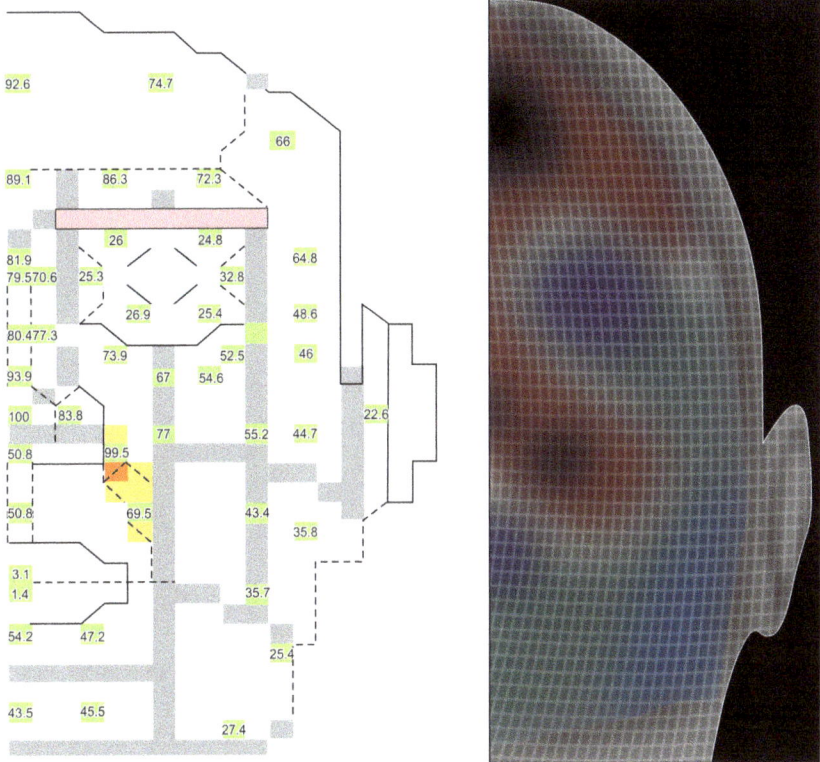

Fig. 12.60: A depiction of the variable skin sebum levels. The highest levels were in the medial aspects of the nose and cheek which correspond to the enlarged pores.

aberrant epidermal architecture, defined as the presence of SL structures at the dermoepidermal junction, correlating with enlarged pore size compared to other ethnicities.
- Increased *hair follicle* volume including thick hair is another cause.

Treatment

The therapy revolves around targeting the mechanisms earlier and most therapies are targeted at the sebum excretion and skin remodeling.

Topical Agents

- Various agents have been tried including retinoids, though their ability to normalize keratinization would logically cause enlarged pores. Thus, it is erroneous to conclude that retinoids reduce facial pore size and density irrespective of concomitant acne vulgaris.

    Both tazarotene 0.1% and tretinoin 0.025% have been tried and as an extension peels, this includes both glycolic acid (30% solution) every 2 weeks for a total of five treatments and salicylic acid.

- Novel agents tried include botanicals, like, natural plant-derived chlorophyllin-copper complex sodium salt (CHLcu) and tetrahydrojasmonic acid (LR2412). Chlorophyllin-copper complex sodium salt is derived from chlorophyll, a green pigment found in plants, and has been investigated as a topical gel in liposomal dispersions for application in photodamaged and aged skin. Chlorophyllin-copper complex sodium salt exerts in vitro hyaluronidase inhibitory activity to maintain hyaluronic acid in the extracellular matrix and counteracts the structural breakdown of cutaneous aging.

Systemic Agents

The most commonly used oral therapies for enlarged pores are antiandrogens, such as, combined oral contraceptives, spironolactone, and cyproterone acetate, which modulate sebum production due to the presence of androgen receptors within sebaceous glands.

Lasers and Energy Devices

The various devices tried include the gold particle 800 nm diode laser, 1,450 nm diode laser, microneedle apparatuses, fractional RF devices, 2,790 nm Er:YAG laser, nonablative 1,410 nm fractionated erbium-doped fiber laser, and nonablative 1,440 nm fractional laser.

Their effect is in reducing the aging process, and help in collagen remodeling that indirectly may help in pores. The results are variable and not consistently persistent or complete. A summary of the devices used are given in Table 12.27.

Diet

Diet may be an important source of substrate for sebum synthesis. Diets rich in carbohydrates with a high glycemic index are associated with hyperglycemia, reactive hyperinsulinemia, and increased formation of insulin-like growth factor-1 (IGF-1). Except cheese, milk, and all other dairy products also have potent insulinotropic properties, far exceeding those expected from their low glycemic indexes.

Botulinum Toxin

Recent reports have suggested that intradermal botulinum toxin may play a role in decreasing sebum production and pore size.

Conclusion

The problem with published data is that they focus on how a reduction in the number or diameter of facial pores accompanied treatments, which caused

Table 12.27: Overview of lasers and energy devices for facial pores.

Interventions	Number of patients	Results
Three times, one side of the nose, 1,450 nm *diode laser* (SmoothBeam; Candela Corporation, Wayland, MA)	n = 8, age range 25–42 years	Sebum-producing follicles reduced by 8.5% and 16.7% at week 4 and week 6 ($P < 0.05$)
One time, full face, fractional *RF microneedle* device (Infini; Lutronic Co., Goyang-si, Korea)	n = 20, age range 22–34 years	Casual sebum level and sebum excretion rate: 30–60% and 70–80% reduction, at week 2 ($P < 0.01$)
Four times, forehead and cheeks, *radiofrequency microneedle* (IME-HR 5000, IME Co. Ltd., Tokyo, Japan)	n = 15, age range 23–36 years	• Fewer sebaceous glands and the development of fibrosis • The mean rate of skin surface lipids reduced by 31.5% ($P < 0.01$)
Three times, full face, gold particles (Nanospectra, Houston, TX), 800 nm diode laser (LightSheer, Lumenis, Yokneam, Israel)	• RCT 1: n = 48, age range 16–35 years • RCT 2: n = 51, age range 16–26 years	• Thermal injury to sebaceous follicles and glands RCT 1: The mean percent inflammatory lesion count reduced by 61% at 28 weeks ($P = 0.009$) • RCT 2: Inflammatory lesion count reduced in 12 weeks ($p = 0.015$) and 16 weeks ($P = 0.04$), respectively
Three consecutive sessions of low-energy level treatments with a fractional CO_2 laser at 4-week intervals	32 patients	The mean number of enlarged pores was decreased by 28.8% after the second session and by 54.5% at posttreatment evaluation
Three times, full face, non-ablative 1,410 nm fractionated erbium-doped fiber laser (Fraxel re:fine; Solta Medical, Hayward, CA)	n = 15, age range 26–46 years	51% improvement in dilated pores (14/15). Decreased sebaceous glands in the dermis
Six times, full face, low-energy nonablative 1,440 nm fractional laser (Clear 1 Brilliant laser system; Solta Medical Inc., Hayward, CA)	n = 20, age range 29–50 years	*Pore score:* 17% average reduction ($P < 0.002$)
Four times, full face, fractional bipolar RF (Matrix RF; Syneron Medical Ltd., Yokneam, Israel)	n = 31, age range 19–38 years	• Improvement of smoothness of the scars (2.61), pore sizes (2.32), brightness (1.97), and overall appearance (2.9) • Improvement of melanin index ($P = 0.001$), erythema index ($P = 0.049$), gross elasticity ($P = 0.004$), net elasticity ($P = 0.001$), and biological elasticity ($P = 0.002$). Thicker collagen fibers and prominent dark blue fine elastic fibers

(CO_2: carbon dioxide; RCT: randomized controlled trial; RF: radiofrequency)

the improvement of other symptoms, instead of focusing on the improvement of facial pores themselves. Thus, a combination of therapies are advisable, which may not always satisfy the patient's visual need for a perfect face.

BIBLIOGRAPHY

1. Alexiades M. Clinical assessment of a novel jasmonate cosmeceutical, LR2412-Cx, for the treatment of skin aging. J Drugs Dermatol. 2016;15:209-15.
2. Lee SJ, Seok J, Jeong SY, et al. Facial pores: definition, causes, and treatment options. Dermatol Surg. 2016;42:277-85.
3. Tran C, Michelet JF, Simonetti L, et al. In vitro and in vivo studies with tetra-hydro-jasmonic acid (LR2412) reveal its potential to correct signs of skin ageing. J Eur Acad Dermatol Venereol. 2014;28:415-23.
4. Uhoda E, Pierard-Franchimont C, Petit L, et al. The conundrum of skin pores in dermocosmetology. Dermatology. 2005;210:3-7.

FACIAL REJUVENATION

Introduction

As noted in **Chapter 10: Combination Laser Therapy: Rationale and Indications**, facial rejuvenation, targeting multiple aspects of aging, is one of the few classic indications where combination of lasers is a useful concept. The concept of multimodal combination treatments for facial rejuvenation was proposed in a paper on tatoo removal (Ruiz-Esparza J). This approach was also proposed for treating reticular and telangiectatic leg veins (Goldman MP, Fitzpatrick RE).

A recent paper by Douglas C Wu, and Richard E Fitzpatrick, has published an aggressive **sequential multimodal laser protocol** that safely and selectively targets specific components of the photoaging process while simultaneously producing significant global facial rejuvenation in a single treatment session.

Protocol

As has been discussed previously in **Chapter 10: Combination Laser Therapy: Rationale and Indications**, there are multiple aspects that result in aged skin and they need to be addressed separately.
- *Telangiectasia and erythema*: This is treated with the 595 nm long PDL (10 mm spot, 3-6 ms, and 6-8 J/cm^2).
- *Pigmented lesions*: These are treated next with the Q-switched 755 nm alexandrite laser with focused spot and spot size varying by distance from the skin (10 J/cm^2, 5 Hz).
- *Fine lines*: The superficial fractionated CO_2 laser (Active FX) is used for fine lines in the perioral region, the cheeks, and the eyelids (100 mJ, 600 Hz, and 1,300 mm spots distributed utilizing a computer-generated

square pattern measuring between 2 mm^2 and 11 mm^2). The density used to the perioral region was 100% coverage, and one or more passes were applied with wiping away of epidermal debris between passes. The density used to the cheeks was 91%/72%/55% coverage sequentially, and the eyelids 72% coverage. This might be high for pigmented skin and may be reduced. Further sculpting of perioral lines and any scars is then achieved with the pulsed Er:YAG laser using a focused spot size and varying distances to control the amount of ablation to an approximate depth of 25–50 µm per pulse.

- *Last pass*: A full face and neck treatment with deep fractioned CO_2 laser (Fraxel re:pair) is performed. The periorbital region and eyelids were treated with 20–30 J/cm^2 and 30–35% density; the face was treated with 30–50 mJ and 50–55% density; and 20–30 mJ was used to treat the neck in tapering fashion with 30% density at the submental region, and then 25%, 20%, and 15% proceeding inferiorly.

All these procedures were performed in a single session with good results, minimal side effects (such as transient burning, stinging, erythema, and edema), and no major adverse events. Previous studies for facial rejuvenation that use of non-AFLs, and RF devices—all of which are considered minimally invasive strategies focused mainly on minimizing downtime hence, the results were not as dramatic.

Conclusion

This protocol is an aggressive method, but can achieve marked results in a single session. Other protocols do exist, but the basic principle is to first treat the vascular and pigmented lesions followed by the fine and deep lines. We would still prefer a sequential approach than a simultaneous approach as our skin type is prone to PIH. But the basic idea remains that such a approach can help to maximize results in minimum time in an ideal skin type for aged skin.

BIBLIOGRAPHY

1. Fitzpatrick RE, Goldman MP, Dierickx C. Laser ablation of facial cosmetic tattoos. Aesthetic Plast Surg. 1994;18:91-8.
2. Gold MH, Biron JA, Sensing W. Facial skin rejuvenation by combination treatment of IPL followed by continuous and fractional radiofrequency. J Cosmet Laser Ther. 2016;18:2-6.
3. Goldman MP, Fitzpatrick RE. Pulsed-dye laser treatment of leg telangiectasia: with, without simultaneous sclerotherapy. J Dermatol Surg Oncol. 1990;16: 338-44.
4. Kearney C, Brew D. Single-session combination treatment with intense pulsed light and nonablative fractional photothermolysis: A split-face study. Dermatol Surg. 2012;38:1002-9.

5. Kim JE, Chang S, Won CH, et al. Combination treatment using bipolar radiofrequency-based intense pulsed light, infrared light, and diode laser enhanced clinical effectiveness and histological dermal remodeling in Asian photoaged skin. Dermatol Surg. 2012;38:68-76.
6. Ruiz-Esparza J, Goldman MP, Fitzpatrick RE. Tattoo removal with minimal scarring: the chemo-laser technique. J Dermatol Surg Oncol. 1988;14:1372-6.
7. Wu DC, Fitzpatrick RE. Facial rejuvenation via the sequential combined use of multiple laser modalities: Safety and efficacy. Lasers Surg Med. 2016;48:577-83.

NONINVASIVE VAGINOVULVAL TIGHTENING AND ORGASMIC DYSFUNCTION: REJUVENATION WITH LASERS AND RADIOFREQUENCY

Introduction

Vaginal rejuvenation is commonly defined as a combination of minimally invasive procedures that stimulate regeneration of female lower genital tract, aiming to regain aesthetic and functional features lost with the aging process in menopausal women. It is also indicated to treat vagina relaxation in young women.

Vaginal atrophy (also referred to as vulvovaginal atrophy, urogenital atrophy, or atrophic vaginitis) caused by estrogen loss often results in vaginal complaints (e.g. dryness, burning, and dyspareunia) that cause distress in menopausal women. Urinary frequency and recurrent bladder infections may also occur.

Vaginal relaxation is one of the major causes of sexual dissatisfaction and is defined as the loss of the optimum structural architecture of the vagina, generally associated with natural aging and specially affected by childbirth, whether vaginal or not. Multiple pregnancies increase the alteration of these structures, making vaginal muscles relaxed with poor tone, strength, control, and support. The vaginal canal becomes wider and stretched, and sexual gratification consequently diminishes, since it has been attributed to frictional forces generated during intercourses. This is one of the components of the constellation of symptoms grouped as genitourinary syndrome of menopause (GSM).

Treatment

Vaginal laxity remains usually underreported, although the majority of women patient's consider this condition as bothersome with significant impact to their relationship. The visual aspect and functionality of introitus is marked most often as being responsible for sexual disorder and reduced quality of life (QoL) (Pauls RN).

There are several treatment options to minimize GSM symptoms, including nonhormonal products for mild cases, local vaginal hormone therapy for persistent symptoms, and systemic hormonal replacement therapy (HRT) as a broader approach for severe symptoms.

The nonhormonal therapy are mostly, vaginal lubricants and moisturizers, which admittedly provide only a temporary relief prior to intercourse. Lubricants have been demonstrated to decrease vaginal irritation during sexual activity but do not provide a long-term solution. A summary of the holistic management is given here in the Box 12.7 but we will focus on lasers and energy devices.

Following the recent recommendations "cosmetic vaginal/vulvar surgery" includes labiaplasty, labia minora reduction, excess or redundant clitoral prepuce reduction, labia majora reduction or augmentation, labia majora divergence repair, perineal skin reduction, and mons pubis reduction (McDaniel D). Of all the devices, lasers and RF-based devices have a potential use in this indication.

Devices Used

The CO_2 and the Er:YAG lasers are among the most studied technologies aiming vaginal rejuvenation. More recently, RF has also gained some strength in treating this area, with prominent findings, specially using a transcutaneous temperature-controlled RF for vulvovaginal rejuvenation (see here).

Some laser devices used are the CO_2 laser (Femilift™ from Alma Lasers) for vaginal rejuvenation, which has a special sterile, disposable, and individual cover for each patient. This facility makes the procedure more hygienic and allows the operator to perform multiple laser sessions subsequently, without the long wait for sterilization. The Er:YAG laser used is of Fotona (IntimaLase™ and IncontiLase™) or from LMG (Solon Femina™), and both of them have a laser speculum (Fig. 12.61) that avoids the contact between the laser device and the vagina, but needs to be sterilized before the next patient. RF devices have also been used (Fig. 12.62).

Box 12.7: Overview of genitourinary syndrome of menopause.

- *First-line R_x*: Vaginal moisturizing agents supplemented by water-based lubricants during vaginal intercourse
- *Second-line R_x*: Low-dose vaginal estrogen therapy, twice-weekly dosing
- *Delivery*: Insert, ring, cream depends on patient preference. The ring and the 10 μg estradiol insert provide the lowest-dose options. For low-dose vaginal estrogen ring (7.5 μg/day) or insert (10 μg two to four times weekly) or a minidose of conjugated estrogens cream (0.25 g twice weekly), opposing progestin to prevent endometrial neoplasia is not need
- *Third-line R_x*: Ospemifene
- *Fourth-line R_x*: Laser.

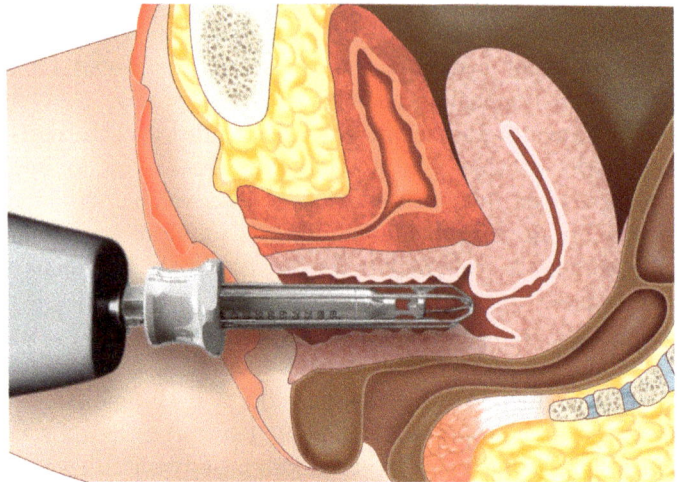

Fig. 12.61: A depiction of the erbium-doped yttrium aluminum garnet (Er:YAG) probe used for vulval and vaginal rejuvenation.

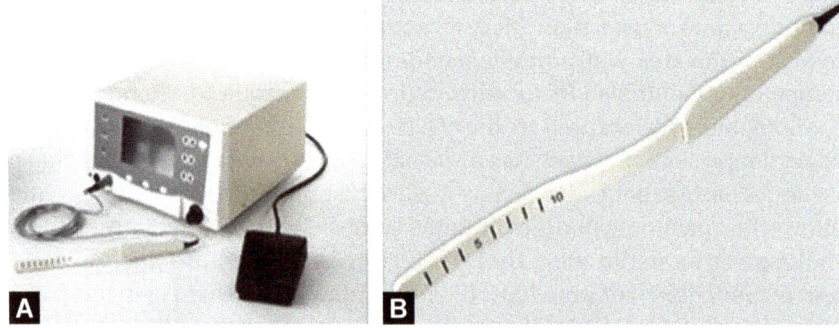

Figs. 12.62A and B: The transcutaneous temperature controlled radiofrequency (TTCRF) device (ThermiVa, ThermiAesthetics, Southlake, TX) with probe and foot switch (A) as well as a close-up of the treatment probe (B).

Indications

The vaginal laser is indicated for women between 20 years and 80 years old with one of the following symptoms:
- Hypotrophy and/or vaginal atrophy.
- Mild to moderate urinary incontinence.
- Sexual dysfunction such as dyspareunia, dryness, low vaginal sensitivity, and vagina wall bleeding during intercourse.
- Postpartum and lactation (temporary estrogen-reduced levels).
- Vagina relaxation/laxity.
- Post-treatment for gynecological cancers (breast and endometrial), to improve vaginal symptoms of the lack of estrogen.

Contraindications

- Pregnancy.
- *Bacterial or fungal vaginal infection*: Laser treatment can be performed only 30 days after vaginal infection treatment.
- Human papillomavirus (HPV) infection.
- *Active herpes viral infection*: Laser treatment can be performed without active infection and during prophylaxis treatment.
- Gynecological oncology pathologies.
- Previous surgical orthesis implant for urinary incontinence, like transvaginal mesh/sling.
- Impaired immune system or chronic corticoid therapies.
- Scleroderma, lichen sclerosus, vitiligo, or psoriasis.
- Uncontrolled diabetes.
- Anticoagulant therapy.
- Patients who have used isotretinoin in the last 12 months.

Procedure (Laser)

- The patient should be in lithotomy position.
- Insert a disposable or sterile vaginal speculum to look for active lesions, signs of infection, or alterations of either the vaginal fluid or the mucosa. If the normal aspect is observed, dry the pathway with sterile gauze to avoid burning from water absorption.
- After taking out the speculum, carefully introduce the laser device completely, until you feel touching the cervix or the patient complains of pain. Some lubricant oil, like mineral oil, might be used in the introit if it is too dry, avoiding the laser window. Usually, the laser probes are marked circumferentially and have a sign that represents the vaginal depth, between 7 cm and 13 cm. They also have a security distance from the tip to the laser window, which prevents the patient from cervix irradiation.
- Some devices have a 360° laser beam delivery system, enabling 360° irradiation of the vaginal canal, whereas others carry a limited laser window, which needs to be clockwise rotated systematically to reach the totality of vaginal wall circumference. These last devices are also assigned to make rotation easy and patterned, so the doctor is sure to perform the 360° irradiation.
- After the first circumferential deep shot, pull back the device as marked (1 cm), making subsequent shots until the whole marked area is outside the vagina. Patient's usually report some heating sensation when the laser window is coming closer to vaginal introit. This is when you shall fully insert it again and perform a new pass, starting from the deep to the introit.

- The number of subsequent passes and laser sessions are also described by the manufacturer's protocol, depending on the patient's complaints and the results achieved by each session.

Treatment Protocols

- The higher the power, the bigger is the depth and thus, a proportionately higher effect of the thermal injury provoked.
- If the main objective is tightening, higher energies are required. The doctor must perform three consecutive passes, throughout the whole vagina wall, circumferentially, in each laser session, with a total of three sessions with an interval of 30 days for the best outcomes.
- The same protocol with high energy is also applied to urinary incontinence treatment. Here, at least two passes should be applied focusing on the anterior wall of the vagina (using a clock as a reference, the laser window must be focused between 10:00 clock and 02:00 clock), and one circumferential pass.
- When vaginal dryness and atrophy are the main complaints of the patient, lower energy is indicated. One or two circumferential passes are enough for each session. Three sessions are necessary for better results.

Post-treatment Advise

- No sexual intercourse for 3–7 days.
- No tampons for 3 days.
- No antibiotic cream is needed.
- Some translucent or blood discharge might occur within the following 3–7 days after the procedure.

Radiofrequency for Vulval Rejuvenation

Radiofrequency has been employed widely in many protocols for skin laxity treatment. A 2010 study by Millheiser et al. (Millheiser LS) of introital/transvaginal monopolar RF (with cryogen cooling) for vaginal laxity after vaginal childbirth reported statistically significant improvement in vaginal laxity in 87% of subjects. Perceived improvement of sexual function (a secondary study end point) was noted in all patients originally reporting reduced sexual function. An investigation by Sekiguchi et al. applied low-energy RF for vaginal introital laxity in premenopausal women, revealing significant improvements in vaginal laxity and sexual function maintained through 12-month follow-up with no reported adverse events.

In Dr Ivan Fistonić's paper a monopolar RF is used. The procedure was performed with a device that delivers 3.25 MHz focused monopolar RF energy by a noninvasive contact electrode with power range from 1 W to 90 W, with a therapy circle time of 30 s and encompassing a treatment area of 3.2 cm^2 (Exilis Protege Intima, BTL Industries Inc., Boston, MA). A disposable adhesive return pad was used for the grounding. Starting parameters were the initial power of 90 W with continuous energy emission (100% duty factor). Generous amount of the ultrasound gel was applied to the treated area for close contact between the handpiece and the skin. During the treatment, surface temperature of treated skin was between 40°C and 43°C. Each patient received four consecutive treatments at 1-week intervals for labia tissue tightening.

The studies on this topic, have shown that the RF device helps not only to improve tightening (Fistonic̀ I) but also improves orgasmic function (Alinsod RM). The results can last up to 12 months (Clark Z). Here, we detail the findings of Dr Alinson who has shared his personal observations on his results, which would help those attempting to replicate his findings (Figs. 12.63 to 12.67).

Protocol (Dr Alinsod RM)

- No anesthesia is required.
- Each patient received three sessions at intervals of about 1 month.
- Treatment was performed using a slim S-shaped probe with a stamp-sized metal RF emitter on one surface of the tip (25 minutes total time on average) (Fig. 12.62).
- External treatments covered the labia majora and minora, lower mons pubis, perineal body, clitoral hood, and clitoris.
- Full length treatment of the vagina with concentration on the anterior wall can be performed. Tissue temperature during therapy was elevated to and maintained between 40°C and 45°C.
- After treatment, patient's immediately resumed normal activities, including sex.

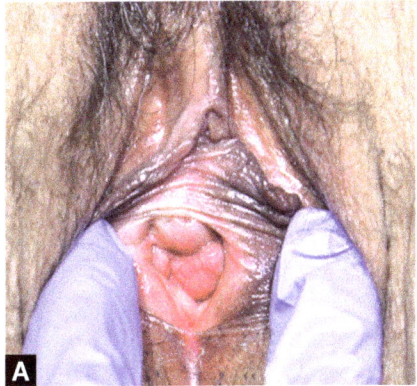 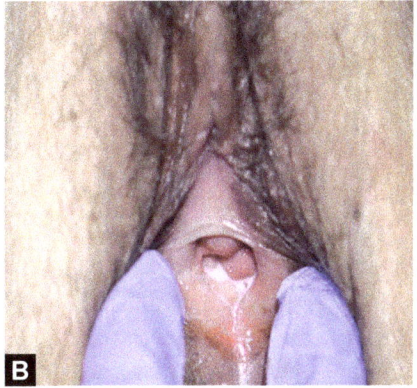

Figs. 12.63A and B: (A) Symptomatic postmenopausal patient with genitourinary syndrome of menopause (GSM) and dyspareunia underwent three ThermiVa treatments of the labia majora and full depth of the vagina; and (B) After three ThermiVa treatments the patient was able to produce a normal transudate resulting in elimination of dyspareunia and symptoms of GSM. Shrinkage of her cystocele also relieved the moderate pelvic pressure experienced. *Courtesy:* Red Alinsond, MD

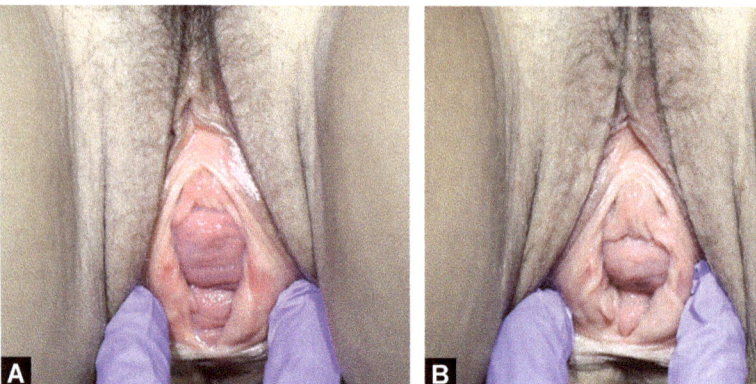

Figs. 12.64A and B: (A) Multiparous woman complained of pelvic pressure and visible bulging vaginal structures. She did not want a surgical solution. A moderate cystocele and rectocele was diagnosed and she underwent full vaginal depth ThermiVa x3. Photos are taken at maximal Valsalva; and (B) After monthly ThermiVa x3, her bladder and rectal prolapse were reduced by one-half to one stage with resultant elimination of her symptoms of pelvic heaviness and pressure as well as visible bulge. Photos are taken at maximal Valsalva.
Courtesy: Red Alinsond, MD

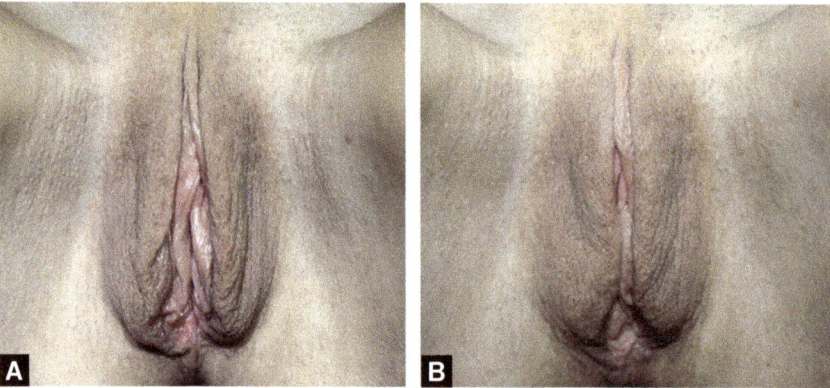

Figs. 12.65A and B: (A) Perimenopausal woman complaining of vulvar laxity of the labia majora underwent one ThermiVa treatment; and (B) Significant majora laxity reduced with resulting increased confidence.
Courtesy: Red Alinsond, MD

The results of Dr Alinsond cannot be generalized as something other devices can do. **Viveve** cannot achieve any of these results as they only do introital tightening and do not do labia majora or deep vaginal treatments. **Pelleve** only does external treatments and cannot go internal. **UltraFemme** 360 cannot specifically target the mid urethra. *ThermiVa* is the only RF device to use low wavelengths (460 kHz) while other devices use 1 MHz and higher. Only the low wavelengths have been shown histologically to increase the small nerve fiber density and improve sensitivity. Only low wavelength RF

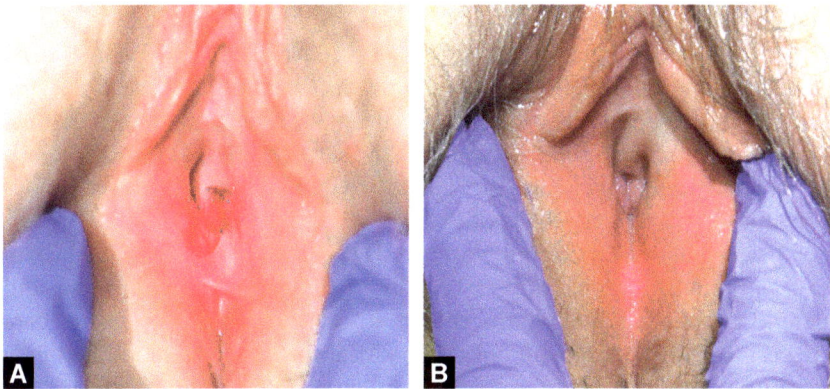

Figs. 12.66A and B: (A) Menopausal woman with severe genitourinary syndrome of menopause (GSM), dyspareunia, rigid vaginal tissue, and vaginal bleeding underwent full treatment of labia majora and perineum and full depth of the vagina with ThermiVa monthly x3; and (B) After three treatments with ThermiVa there was soft and pliable vulvovaginal tissue allowing for normal pain free intercourse and daily comfort. Healthy skin with excellent blood flow was seen in vulva and vagina with normal production of vaginal transudate.
Courtesy: Red Alinsond, MD

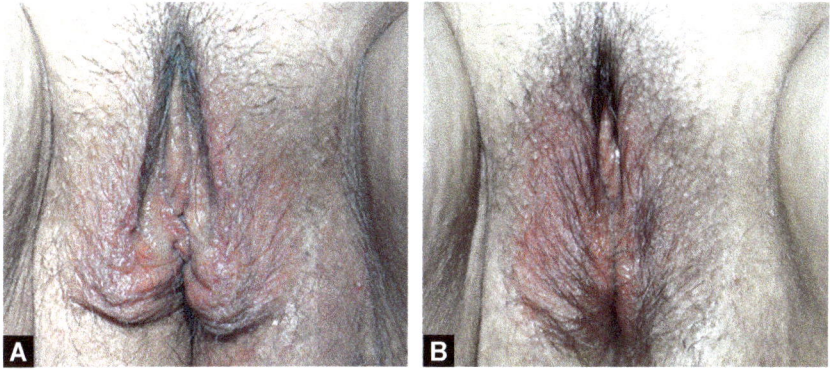

Figs. 12.67A and B: (A) Menopausal woman with severe genitourinary syndrome of menopause (GSM) and dyspareunia underwent ThermiVa treatments x3; and (B) Normal premenopausal appearing tissues with resolution of GSM symptoms.
Courtesy: Red Alinsond, MD

has been shown histologically to increase both collagen and elastin and angiogenesis and neurogenesis. CO_2 and erbium lasers have not been shown to increase elastin content like RF does. This explains why RF treated tissues have better stretch and softness compared to laser treated tissues. Hence, to mirror results, the same device would be needed to avoid inordinate results and/or complications (Figs. 12.63 to 12.67).

Conclusion

There is no doubt that lasers and energy devices are useful for vulval rejuvenation. The issue as always is what device to use. As there are very few comparative trials, it seems any device that produces localized thermal energy can produce results. Considering the safety profile of Er:YAG, it seems to the ideal device, but RF has proved itself to be a very versatile device and is probably a very cost-effective option.

A systematic review and meta-analysis reported that despite the lack of well-designed controlled studies, laser intervention appears to be a safe and potentially effective nonpharmacologic intervention for GSM. Some data suggest that laser therapy in postmenopausal women reduces vulvovaginal symptom severity and restores vaginal mucosa, resulting in improved QoL. According to another review, this technology is promising for treatment vulvovaginal atrophy, but cost issues need to be addressed.

Laser devices have not been approved by the US FDA for the treatment of vulvovaginal atrophy. The American College of Obstetricians and Gynecologists has advised that: (1) Although initial observational data indicate potential utility, additional data from randomized trials are needed to further assess the efficacy and safety of this procedure in treating vulvovaginal atrophy, particularly for long-term benefit; and (2) Obstetrician-gynecologists should be cognizant of the evidence regarding innovative practices and should be wary of adopting new or innovative approaches on the basis of promotions or marketing. Additional large clinical trials are actively recruiting subjects.

In conclusion, the spin off between lasers and RF is akin to skin tightening and acne scars, wherein technology comes in waves and time will tell which "wave" has a long-lasting impact.

BIBLIOGRAPHY

1. Arunkalaivanan A, Kaur H, Onuma O. Laser therapy as a treatment modality for genitourinary syndrome of menopause: A critical appraisal of evidence. Int Urogynecol J. 2017;28:681-5.
2. Clark Z. Labial tissue rejuvenation and sexual function improvement using a novel noninvasive focused monopolar radiofrequency device. J Cosmet Laser Ther. 2017;30:1-5.
3. Fistonić I, Sorta Bilajac Turina I, Fistonić N, et al. Short time efficacy and safety of focused monopolar radiofrequency device for labial laxity improvement-noninvasive labia tissue tightening. A prospective cohort study. Lasers Surg Med. 2016;48:254-9.
4. Florentino AV, Bretas TL, Issa MC. Lasers for aesthetic and functional vaginal rejuvenation. In: Issa MC, Tamura B (Eds). Lasers, Lights and Other Technologies: Clinical Approaches and Procedures in Cosmetic Dermatology, 1st edition. New York: Springer; 2018. pp. 1-13.

5. McDaniel D, Weiss R, Weiss M, et al. Two-treatment protocol for skin laxity using 90-Watt dynamic monopolar radiofrequency device with real-time impedance intelligence monitoring. J Drugs Dermatol. 2014;13:1112-7.
6. Millheiser LS, Pauls RN, Herbst SJ, et al. Radiofrequency treatment of vaginal laxity after vaginal delivery: Nonsurgical vaginal tightening. J Sex Med. 2010;7: 3088-95.
7. Pauls RN, Fellner AN, Davila GW. Vaginal laxity: A poorly understood quality of life problem; a survey of physician members of the International Urogynecological Association (IUGA). Int Urogynecol J. 2012;23:1435-48.
8. Pitsouni E, Grigoriadis T, Falagas ME, et al. Laser therapy for the genitourinary syndrome of menopause. A systematic review and meta-analysis. Maturitas. 2017;103:78-88.
9. The American College of Obstetricians and Gynecologists (ACOG). (2016). Fractional Laser Treatment of Vulvovaginal Atrophy and U.S. Food and Drug Administration Clearance: Position Statement. [online] Available from: www.acog.org/Resources-And-Publications/Position-Statements/Fractional-Laser-Treatment-of-Vulvovaginal-Atrophy-and-US-Food-and-Drug-Administration-Clearance. [Accessed April, 2018].

CONCLUSION

The data and experience given here is a "birds-eye" view of the plethora of indications and lasers that can be used. But it is the experience of this author that for most of the common indications, consistent and visible response is by using the conventional ablative lasers. For pigmented lasers, epidermal and static disorders respond the best. Fractional lasers are primarily of use in acne scars. The use of excimer lasers in pigmentary disorder may be justifiable, but in pigmented skin, the result may not be different from conventional treatments (e.g. PUVA in vitiligo). As far as malignant cases are concerned, lasers do not find any mention in the NCCN guidelines (http://www.nccn.org/default.aspx) and should be used only in the premalignant conditions. The use of lasers in hair growth and nail disorders has received FDA approvals, but there is still a need for multiple, RCT, on these conditions with long-term follow-up with preferably comparison with conventional modes of therapy.

The laser practitioner must in the end remember that apart from the "science and fiction" of sponsored talks, there is an important consideration of return of income, wherein the cost of procedures and visible patient satisfaction play the most important role in the indications for laser and energy devices.

Section 3
Practical Aspects and Complications

CHAPTER 13

How to Setup a Laser Center in a Private Setup?

Apratim Goel, Masuma Molvi

KEY POINTS

- Introduction
- Why set up a laser center?
- Essentials of setup:
    - Capital investment
    - Facility
    - Rooms
    - Power supply
    - Air conditioning
    - Device maintenance
    - Safety protocols
    - Emergency protocols
    - Staff training.
- Equipment for a startup:
    - Laser device
    - Mobile laser unit
    - Additional tools
    - Qualified physicians and technicians
    - Patient records
    - Drugs.
- How to design a laser center?
    - Space utilization
    - Designing rooms
    - Noise reduction
    - Branding and marketing
    - Website and social media
    - Designing the staff appearance.
- *Requirements:* Legal, statutory, and insurance
    - Insurance
    - Legal issues
    - Statutory.

INTRODUCTION

Aesthetic medicine has now become a fundamental and renowned branch of dermatology, pioneered by the emergence of laser and light based procedures for cosmetic and therapeutic purposes. An amalgam of clinical dermatology, dermatosurgery and cosmetology constitutes an integrated dermato-aesthetic practice, all of which require the use of various lasers as combined or monotherapy to treat an array of conditions optimally. For this reason, lasers are now becoming an integral part of dermatological practice in India, with more and more dermatologists starting laser dermatology practice all over the country. An appropriate laser setup based on guidelines formulated to take care of every aspect associated with it such as device maintenance, lighting, rooms, placement, and ventilation and so on is utmost essential in this scenario. This chapter aims to guide aspiring as well as established clinical dermatologists to setup a professional, legal and secure laser center which will make practice simple, safe and fruitful. The International Survey on Aesthetic/Cosmetic Procedures was performed in 2014 and 2015 by the International Society of Aesthetic Plastic Surgeons (ISAPS), including data compiled from a total of 1,391 plastic surgeons worldwide. It concurred laser hair removal and laser skin resurfacing as the two most common laser procedures performed by plastic surgeons practicing aesthetic medicine worldwide, constituting 12.1% and 4.5% of the all the nonsurgical procedures performed that year, respectively. Laser hair removal (9.1%), photo rejuvenation (4.7%) nonsurgical fat reduction (3.5%), and skin tightening (2.8%) emerged as the commonest ones carried out in the 2015 survey.

WHY SETUP A LASER CENTER?

Even in the midst of economic recession, cost cutting and the most recent demonetization in India, cosmetic practice is and always will remain one of the fastest growing segments of medicine. A decade earlier, this field was mainly dominated by dermatologists and few plastic surgeons, but today general practitioners, dentists as well as specialists from all fields including alternate medicine are impinging into it. The reason being, there is an ever increasing demand for enhancing and maintaining one's physical appearance which never goes out of fashion. So, as dermatologists who have the most knowledge and experience in this stream, it would be their short-sightedness not to make way into laser and aesthetic practice. Further, with the cosmetic boom that the society is experiencing; we also expect more and more research and technology emergence. It will prove interesting as well as lucrative for professionals to opt for a laser and cosmetic setup (Box 13.1).

Box 13.1: Advantages of laser and aesthetic practice.

- Cosmetic surgeries like liposuction and tummy tucks are not everyone's favorite option. Nonsurgical treatment for any aesthetic issue is generally the first choice as it eliminates the pains of admission, risk of anesthesia, suture related complications, possibility of scarring and prolonged downtime.
- Laser and aesthetic treatments are popular with immense scope for expansion. It is the need of the hour!
- As dermatologist we must practice ethically and look beyond financial concerns.
- Aesthetic procedures can have life altering effects on a person. An aesthetic patient is not typically a patient but a client as he may medically be completely fit yet wishes to undergo treatment to alter an unwanted but normal facet of him/her.
- In case you are looking for a multi-clinic practice model, it is easy to setup processes and duplicate an aesthetic setup as compared to surgical skills.
- It is an excellent corporate health wellness business model.

ESSENTIALS OF LASER CENTER

Capital Investments

The amount of capital required to start a laser center depends on the target population, opening inventory, rent and utility deposits, fixtures, leasehold improvements and required equipment. Before you take the plunge, scrupulously assess target population, locality, competitors and their services and carefully formulate what you intend to offer. Ponder why your facility should be chosen over any other. Be open to calculated risks. However, expect the best and prepare for the worst!

Facility (Figs. 13.1A and B)

- Choose the right location, strategically situated, posh yet sublime and adequate. Close proximity to a prominent landmark such as temple, bank, famous building, etc. will make it easy for clients to locate and refer to others as well.
- In the facility, the area allotted for laser treatments should ideally be safe and convenient to use and navigate through for patients and operators in order to facilitate suitable and optimal handling of costly equipments.
- The facility should be designed to handle procedures under local anesthesia and sedation. An emergency trolley and staff trained to handle medical emergencies should be available at all times.
- Laser procedures can be surgical or nonsurgical in nature. Surgical laser procedures requiring extensive nerve block, general anesthesia like hair transplantation surgery, with risk of extensive bleeding or involving large raw areas may demand the need to have a minor operation theater for dermatosurgical interventions.

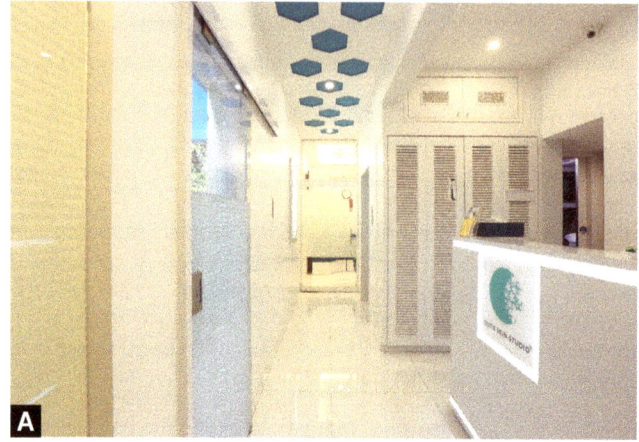

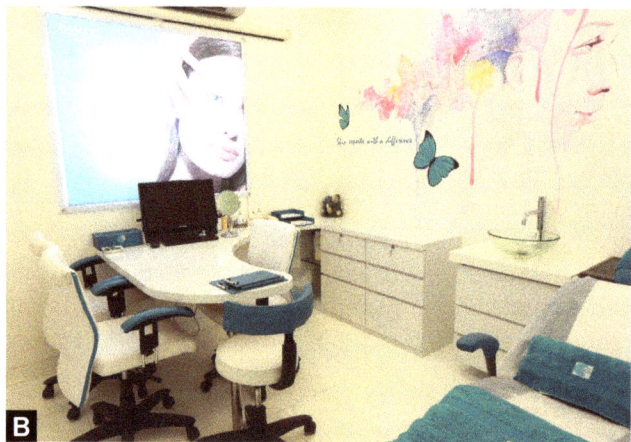

Figs. 13.1A and B: A depiction of an ideal laser facility.

Rooms

The laser room, formally called the *controlled area laser*, should ideally incorporate the following features:
- *Location*: Should be wisely chosen in accordance to local fire, safety, sanitation and building regulations to avoid issues later. The room should be marked with a sign board or red bulb. Preferably, a single patient to be treated at a given time in a laser room.
- *Dimensions*: In order to accommodate the laser machine, patient chair, operator chair, trolley for tools and place for three personnel to move around, i.e. patient, operator and assistant, preferably a 12 × 12 feet room should be designed.
- *Door*: It should be at least 3 feet in width to allow easy transfer of laser machines and made of opaque material to prevent accidental laser light transmission.

- Nonreflective and laser opaque surfaces to be provided. All walls and floors to be kept clean. Laser devices to be methodically cleaned by trained personnel only.
- Wash basin can be present, however assure the laser device never comes in contact with water.
- Area should be well-lit with mobile and adjustable overhead lamps.
- The following notice must be fixed to the laser machine itself: "Device to be operated by Authorized Personnel only".
- Shelves or wall cabinets to store consumables and instruments of approximately 1 foot depth may be provided to ease use.

Power Supply

- A three-phase electric connection is preferably recommended.
- High capacity meter with thick cables to prevent meltdowns and short circuits.
- Imported machine cables may not be supplied with a grounding pin and this may need to be provided separately. Earthing of the equipment is essential to avoid damage to the equipment and electrical shocks to the operator.
- Individually circuit each plug point to protect other machines in case of a short circuit in one plug.
- Custom made extension cords with grounding should be opted for in case the same patients need to be treated with more than 1 machine at a time.
- A laser machine should always be plugged in with a stabilizer and/or uninterruptible power supply (UPS).
- A back-up lighting system must be installed to allow completion of any ongoing procedure and periodically checked.
- UPS and batteries should be installed in cool and ventilated spaces. In the laser room, points fed by UPS, stabilizer, or directly from mains should be labeled separately. Plugging high voltage devices to UPS points may trip UPS affecting function of machine already on UPS.

Air Conditioning

- Temperatures of 18–22°C for normal functioning of the laser device are advisable.
- Air conditioner requires a three-phase electric meter connection which should be incorporated in the initial planning and designing of the center itself.

Device Maintenance

- Dust-free environment, low surrounding temperatures and uninterrupted power supply without voltage fluctuation are utmost essential for long-term optimal functioning of the laser machine.

- Keeping the laser rooms clean and covering the machines when not in use can help minimize dust collection.
- Keep laser room cool at all times and place machine away from direct sunlight to maintain device temperature and prevent over-heating when in use.
- Only authorized personnel should clean the device following every use. Outer surface and laser tips to be cleaned with alcohol or acetone.
- In case of intense pulsed light (IPL) device, gel over filters should be wiped off using acetone wipes. Unclean IPL glass filters can catch fungus and turn opaque, blocking output.
- Based on manufacturer service guidelines, service engineer maintenance visits should be scheduled for the laser device during warranty period.
- Post expiry of warranty period, annual maintenance contract (AMC) from supplier should be essentially opted for. AMC will also be required for insurance purpose.

Safety Protocols

- Local area fire protocols should be enlisted and put up based on guidelines. Fire safety equipments like extinguishers should be installed, the staff trained on its use and its maintenance done on regular basis.
- External eye shield for patient and operator is a must at all times. Goggles of sufficient optical density (OD) for specific laser wavelength are to be used. For procedures around eyes or on eyelids, internal eye shield made of laser opaque material are to be used.
- *Cooling devices*: Cooling is mainstay in patient safety. External cooling devices like Zimmer contains compressor and therefore requires a separate electric circuit.
- Ice packs or cooling gel packs should be kept handy and used during laser procedures to improve patient comfort and safety.
- *Safe laser use*: It will help to avoid burns or eye damage to patients or operator. Reflective surfaces like mirrors, reflective jewelry, and mobile phones are not allowed in laser room. Machine should always be on standby mode when not in direct use. It should be used by authorized operator only. Avoid using spirit immediately before laser use.
- In case of therapeutic procedures like warts removal, etc. facial masks and gloves should be employed.
- In case of seropositive patients, universal precautions to be employed.
- Obtain proper drug history for xylocaine hypersensitivity, sulfa-drug allergy, β-blockers, aspirin or any other antiplatelet drug.
- If any instruments like comedone extractor, forceps, etc. used, sterilization should be looked upon meticulously.

Emergency Protocols

- Vasovagal attack, anaphylaxis, uncontrolled bleeding, fire, accidental eye exposure, etc. are unwanted possibilities, which you should be prepared to manage.
- An electrocautery machine to control bleeding, equipment for airway maintenance, instruments for emergency resuscitation and an emergency drug tray are essential.
- The patient chair should have the option to tilt head down or "syncope position" to allow resuscitation.

Staff Training

Regular training of staff on fire protocol, power failure protocol, sterilization, device use, internal clinic protocols, etc. should be arranged and overlooked personally.

EQUIPMENTS AND MAN POWER

Laser Device

- Device for laser hair removal like diode, etc. is always the first one you should buy followed by laser for acne scars or pigmentation.
- An IPL with multiple handpieces specific for conditions like hair reduction, acne, photo-rejuvenation, etc. can be opted for during the initial period. It may also serve as a useful tool to be offered as a secondary option to patients resistant or inadequately responsive to other devices in future.
- Survey the market and choose machines, which are already deemed effective. Do not experiment in the beginning.
- Pick companies which offer favorable maintenance, service and payment policies. Cooperative and efficient company personnel will be an added benefit.

Mobile Laser Unit

In the Indian scenario, these are highly useful. A laser with fiberoptic delivery system can be made mobile after consultation with supplier. However, a laser with an articulated arm delivery cannot be made mobile. Proper packing using shock absorbing material is necessary for transportation.

Additional Tools

- *Patient chair*: (Approximately 6 × 2.5 feet) A dental chair serves the purpose well.

- Operator's chair.
- *Treatment trolley*: All procedural material and consumables should be arranged systematically and easy to access.
- Materials for a laser procedure should be in a labeled draw in the trolley and may contain the following:
  - Razor, marking pen, patient external eye shield, facial wipes, sterile gauze, gloves, antiseptic ointment, laser consent form, post-treatment instruction sheet, EMLA cream, etc.

Drugs

Drugs and anesthesia: Basic drugs like paracetamol, diclofenac, ondansetron, omeprazole, hydrocortisone, hyaluronidase, etc. should be readily available. Topical and injectable anesthesia is mostly required for laser procedures and should be at your disposal.

Qualified Physicians and Technicians (Table 13.1)

- *Physician's qualification*: A dermatologist, plastic surgeon or general practitioner trained and certified to perform laser procedures needs to be employed as an assistant doctor to run the center or do treatments along with you. Such training may be obtained during postgraduation or later in specified workshops or at center, which routinely performs such procedures.
- *Personnel/Team*: The personnel needed to hire depends on the services offered and caliber of the clinic. Typically, a team comprising of clinic manager, receptionist, technicians (at least one male), helpers, accountant and marketing and sales in-charge should be taken up. Technicians should be qualified and trained to assure high quality treatment and avoid mishaps.
- Primary legal responsibility of result and complications of treatment lies with the treating physician only, irrespective of the operator. So chose your team wisely!

Table 13.1: Basic staff requirement for a laser/aesthetic medical center.

Personnel	Qualification required
One Clinic Manager	Management degree/diploma
One Clinic Assistant Manager	Management degree/diploma
Two Doctors	MD, DNB, MBBS, BAMS, BHMS
Two Front Office Executives	Good Communication Skills
Two Skin Therapists	CIBTAC, CIDESCO
One Clinic Assistants/Nurses	Undergraduate Science degree

Patient Records

- Patient's health declaration questionnaires.
- Software based summary of patient treatment and other details requiring mention at every visit.
- Detailed informed consent in the language understood by patient for each procedure explaining its nature, anesthesia used, machine used, postoperative down time, etc. and duly signed by patient is the most essential record to avoid medicolegal complications.
- *Digital photography*: Patient pictures taken before and at regular intervals after each procedure is an essential record and a savior at multiple occasions. It should be stored in a hard disk and should be backed up as well.

DESIGNING A LASER CENTER

Designing a laser and aesthetic center is an art and needs to be carried out meticulously and passionately with fair amount of far-sightedness to allow scope of future expansion. Architects and interior designers may be employed for technical assistance but cannot be allowed to take the lead as very often it turns out either functionally inconvenient or results in improper space utilization. Have the final layout in mind and work toward it to meet your goals. Few start-up pointers are listed in Box 13.2.

Space Utilization

Make the most of what you have!
- Depending on the type and variety of services you wish to render to patients, an area of 500–2,500 square feet may encompass all. Considering the high rental cost in metro cities, a space of 800–1000 carpet would be sufficient for a start up.
- The center should have the following essential sections for easy management and flow of events, designed in a way which is convenient for staff, patients and daily management errands (Fig. 13.2).

Box 13.2: Laser center startup mini checklist.

Where to start?
1. Know your investments
2. Plan the clinic area/site
3. List your priorities
4. Enlist the technology
5. Scope for expansion
6. Invest in marketing
7. Employ trained staff
8. Plan for 1 year advance
9. Know your competitors
10. Be ready to face failure

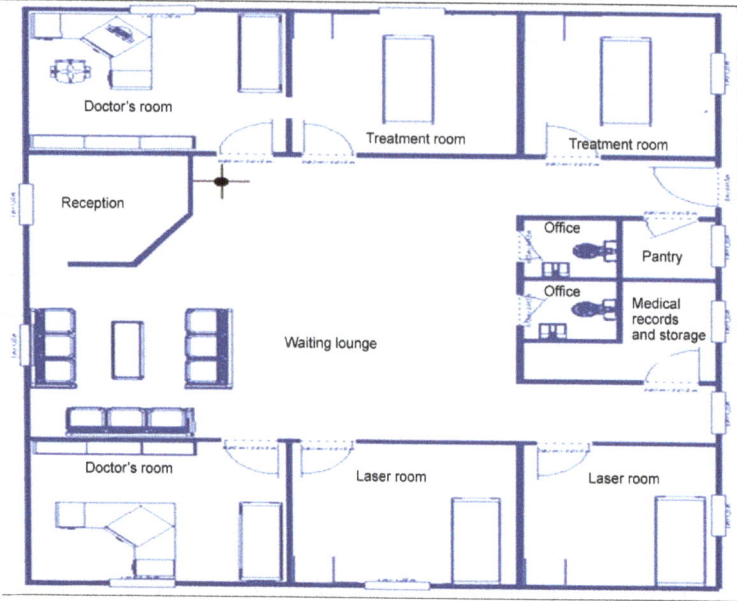

Fig. 13.2: A layout plan of a laser clinic.

- Consultation rooms.
- *Treatment rooms*: Labeled according to specific procedures or facilities.
- *Laser rooms*: Equipped with specific utilities and marked with a sign or red bulb.
- Reception, enquiry and billing counter.
- Administrative room for clinic manager, marketing and sales in-charge, accountant, etc. It may also accommodate patient records.
- Pantry and storage area.
- Waiting lounge.
- Counter to dispense products.
- Have smaller but more rooms/cubicles to accommodate several patients at a time and to maintain their due privacy.
- Foldable doors can provide room for expansion when required.
- Smooth floors for wheel transport of machines.

Designing Rooms

- *Consult room*: Attractive and elaborate
- *Laser and procedure room*: Solid colors with treatment posters
- *Examination room/medical procedures*: Preferably white interiors to indicate sterility
- *Lounge or waiting area*: Warm, welcoming, soothing, and creative.

Noise Reduction

- Choose a suitable location keeping visibility as well as serenity in mind. Aesthetic patients are always looking for a wholesome rejuvenating experience.
- In case of glass cubicles, use double or soundproof glass.
- Use silicon wool or thermocol in partitions.
- Keep the treatment rooms at a distance from the main door and reception.
- Play soft instrumental music at all times.

Branding and Marketing (Box 13.3)

- Use a representative color code and logo to establish recognition. For example, print logo on visiting cards, stationery, clocks, main door, sign boards, etc. using standard color schemes.
- Most areas of the clinic can be used to showcase available technologies and procedures done such as lift, staircase, lighted boards with clinical artwork in treatment and consultation rooms; all of which should be changed periodically.
- Detailed treatment brochures with brief answers to frequently asked questions.
- Television in the lounge area playing information on available treatments or patient reviews on use of lasers present at the center.
- *Personalize your practice*: Show in-house procedural videos to lay at rest any patient apprehension or confusion. Do not use borrowed ones from companies but your own; this will indirectly help you boast your experience and caliber.
- Any offers/discounts should be displayed in the waiting area.

Box 13.3: The 14 Ps of aesthetic practice.

1. **Place:** Choose based on geographic location and demographics of patients
2. **Purpose**
3. **Practice and personnel**
4. **Patients**: Be an aggressive listener and communicate effectively
5. **Procedures:** Before doing any procedure, explain adequately to the patient. During start-up, opt for basic procedures and then gradually improvise and expand
6. **Photography** with scientific communities during presentations and publications
7. **Professional skills:** Fellowship programs, workshops, etc.
8. **Performing evaluation trials:** For new machines
9. **Products and equipment**
10. **Patient records**
11. **Publicity**
12. **Promote**
13. **Problems**
14. **Protection:** Property damage insurance, fire insurance, etc.

- The sign board outside the clinic should be attractive and specific. Avoid cluttering and make it interesting.
- Remember, out of sight means out of mind! Make your presence felt through newspapers, inserts, write ups, radio and television talks, pamphlets, signage at prominent visible places in town, delivering talks at clubs, schools and corporate offices, etc.

Website and Social Media

- Website should have the same feel as the clinic in terms of logo, color coordination, etc.
- Website should be simple and user friendly, easy to navigate through and interactive.
- Make your presence felt on social media, post regularly on Facebook, Twitter, Integra, etc.
- Patient reviews should be encouraged through both: website and social media; that is the only way you will improve your shortcomings.

Designing the Staff Appearance

- Uniform and color-coded from top to bottom
- Match look to the brand color scheme with uniforms bearing logo and name badges for a personal touch
- No ornaments and crisply dressed at all times.

REQUIREMENTS: INSURANCE, LEGAL AND STATUTORY

Insurance

- Fire insurance is quintessential for all expensive equipment and overall facility.
- Breakdown insurance, though beneficial, has a very high premium. Fragile or heavily used machines may be covered under this.
- In mobile laser units, insurance for mobility from between centers should be obtained.

Legal Issues

- Though extensive for a start-up, an associated lawyer will prove beneficial in the long run. Medicolegal issues as a result of accidents and botched procedures (from rashes resulting from cosmetic treatments to the first or second degree burns from lasers) can make you anxious without proper legal assistance. Check with your insurance company on policies that can protect you and your business from liability and lawsuits that may arise from customer complaints.

- A full time accountant will ensure fund management, help you to assess future expansion scope and even help to decide revision of strategies and policies.

Statutory Approvals

Statutory requirements are the requirements or standards identified and defined by the various state regulatory authorities which must be complied with before starting a cosmetology clinic (Fig. 13.3).

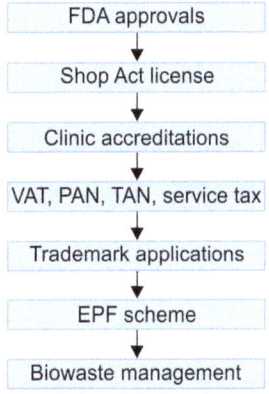

Fig. 13.3: Statutory requirements.

BIBLIOGRAPHY

1. [Internet]. 2016 [cited 22 November 2016]. Available from: http://www.isaps.org/Media/Default/global-statistics/2016%20ISAPS%20Results.pdf
2. [Internet]. 2016 [cited 22 November 2016]. Available from: https://www.isaps.org/Media/Default/global-statistics/2015%20ISAPS%20Results.pdf
3. American Medical Association. Standards and guidelines for cardiopulmonary resuscitation (CPR) and emergency cardiac care (ECC). J Am Med Assn. 1986;255:2905-84.
4. Dhepe N. Minimum standard guidelines of care on requirements for setting up a laser room. Indian J Dermatol Venereol Leprol. 2009;75(Suppl S2):101-10.
5. Hayman MR. Accreditation of the office-based surgical facility. Am Coll Surg Bull. 1995;80:8-11.
6. Olson R. Continuous power to the OR and other critical care areas. Dimensions Health Serv. 1975;52:29-30.
7. Sachdev M, Britto GR. Essential requirements to setting up an aesthetic practice. J Cutan Aesthet Surg. 2014;7(3):167-9.
8. Smalley PJ. Laser safety: Risks, hazards, and control measures. Laser Therapy. 2011;20(2):95-106.

CHAPTER 14

How to Setup a Laser Clinic in a Public Funded Institution

V Dhir, Kabir Sardana, Ananta Khurana

INTRODUCTION

Though a previous chapter covers the topic in a private setup, as some readers may be in Government-aided colleges, a perspective of how to setup a laser center is being given below.

WHY BUY LASERS?

A trivial question with far reaching implications. Laser has become a part of dermatological practice, but it is not justified to expend money on all sorts of lasers. It is the authors' opinion, that *three basic* principles must be met before ordering a laser, presuming of course that trained personnel are there to run it:

1. Lasers with a purely cosmetic need (like hair removal) should not be bought in a medical college government setup. Firstly they are time-consuming procedures and secondly are so well researched that there is little need for further studies on it. Moreover, the numbers of hair removal procedures in private setup are so many that nothing new can emanate out of a medical college experience. Another issue is that the laser clinic tends to be overrun by such patients leaving little time or energy for anything else! Finding approvals to spend public money on them of course is another matter.
2. Lasers where a research into new therapies or aspects of laser physics is needed should be bought. This includes fractional lasers and possibly novel pigment specific lasers.
3. Lasers should be bought for conditions that have organic and cutaneous needs, like scars, benign tumors, tattoos, nevus of Ota and vascular conditions where the costing in private centers is prohibitively high. Conversely where the cost of machine is not so high, like a good pulsed CO_2 laser, is a sensible buy as this can tackle most tumors, though having used the erbium-doped yttrium aluminum garnet (Er:YAG) for a long time an ideal situation would be to have both the ablative lasers.

CHAPTER 14: How to Setup a Laser Clinic in a Public Funded Institution

As in Delhi most centers have lasers, it is better to avoid lasers which are already available in other institutes. We should avoid duplication of same laser to save money. This will also help in smooth purchase of lasers and will save time. As per MCI norms, a hair removal laser, Qsw neodymium-doped yttrium aluminum garnet (ND:YAG) and a CO_2 lasers are necessity for PG courses, so this is a good justification for buying a laser.

WHICH LASERS TO BUY?

We are detailing a list of lasers that could be bought. This is based on almost 10 years of running, buying and maintaining lasers at our institutions. Every center tends to justify its purchases and it is possible that there may be differences of opinion, but as tendering (see below) goes through multiple committees, justifying laser buys is difficult, if the needs of the government and the patients are not matched. It is difficult to justify and say laser lipolysis or a radiofrequency (RF) machine in most medical colleges! The latter as the microneedling RF has disposable tips.

Ablative Lasers

Though most centers buy the CO_2, we would recommend that if possible this should be specified as a *ultrapulse CO_2* and possibly an *Er:YAG*, the latter of which is one of the safest lasers with a predictable depth dose equation. The newer modulated Er:YAG lasers are even safer and better. Remember most ultrapulse CO_2 lasers have superpulse and continuous waves (Cw) modes, but the so-called superpulsed lasers usually are *trumped up* Cw lasers!

As a thumb rule for epidermal and most dermal disorders, the Er:YAG is ideal and for certain vascular and lymphatic tumors, the CO_2 laser is ideal.

Pigment Specific

The large number of pigmented disorders in Indian skin calls for special techniques and apparatus to treat them. For most epidermal disorders, any Q-switched (QS) laser will suffice, though in our skin type the Nd:YAG is preferred. This comes in two forms, *1,064 and 532 nm* which cover most disorders.

For dermal disorders like nevus of Ota and tattoos, ideally a laser with variable spot size is useful. As not all tattoos will respond to the Nd:YAG, so if finances allow a ruby laser would be a useful addition! Though we can forewarn the reader that justifying it will be difficult in Indian skin types!

The pico is a lot of hype *(see Chapter 3)* and it is not in any way superior to the switched laser except in treating some colored tattos.

Vascular Laser

Though the pulsed dye laser (PDL) is the ideal laser, it has three issues. Firstly, the wavelength and pulse duration has to be optimized; secondly, the results in port-wine stain (PWS) are good only if treated early and lastly, the specifications have been set largely for western skin types. The added problem of the consumable (dye) makes it a costly endeavor. But as the cost of therapy, say for PWS is so high in practice, we feel that a government setup should have one, if finances allow! Maintenance is an issue (see case scenarios further).

Fractional Laser

The laser system is used largely for acne scars and rejuvenation, though a multitude of other uses exist. The advantage of buying this is that usually two or more probes can be bought with a system that can cover a range of indications. If a platform is bought, an ablative and a pigment selective probe can also be bought subsequently, which would be easy to justify.

But there is little in vivo difference between buying a fractional (Fr) Er:YAG, Fr Er:Glass and Fr :CO_2 though there may be in vitro differences, thus it is better to buy any one fractional laser and optimize the settings!

It is a *must* to insist on *US Food and Drug Administration (FDA) or European Conformity (CE)* approved laser (see below) *with histological dose depth studies*. The latter is useful to use the proper dosage to target the pathology. We find it amusing to hear speakers extolling the virtues of one over the other without knowledge of how deep the laser goes. In fact that is crucial. We have always believed and said and published data on the variability of response and maintain that any fractional technology cannot eliminate the deep scars.

Hair Removal Lasers

We do not find sufficient reason to justify its use in government medical colleges as it has little use apart from hair removal. Though the intense pulsed light (IPL) was touted as a multiple use laser, in our experience, it is a *jack of all trades, master of one*, the *one* being hair removal!

Moreover, purely on a research point of view, the numbers of hair removal procedures done in private center are so many that little can be added to the existing data. Except for certain procedures like hair removal for scalp grafts, there is little use of this system in a public funded setup.

But there is another view that poor and middle class have every right to get this benefit of hair removal from lasers as the cost of hair removal is very high in private. Plus the MCI recommendations for MD course interestingly have a requirement for a hair removal laser too as mentioned before.

Excimer Laser

The cost of the system, the abundant sunlight in India, cheaper phototherapy units and focused area of impact make it of little use in disorders like psoriasis and vitiligo. Even if a local area is resolved, these being generalized systemic disorders; we cannot justify this equipment in a government setup. We have detailed on this aspect in the Chapter 12D.

Subsurface Lasers, Radiofrequency, Laser Lipolysis, and Low-level Laser Therapy

These systems, no doubt useful, achieve subsurface tightening, marginal growth of hair and minor reductions in fat. None of these can be justified, especially as they are prohibitively costly! Interestingly though they are all FDA approved, not all FDA-approved systems should necessarily be bought in a public funded institution.

TO DELEGATE OR NOT TO DELEGATE?

Energy-based devices have rapidly become *delegated* procedures. It is advisable not to do this as they are costly equipment and most *passing* residents tend to *hone* their skills, sometimes based on little formal knowledge. Each laser has nuances and it is our experience that the life of the laser is directly proportional to the use and the latter is related a lot to the *misuse* of lasers. Also a dedicated day should be allotted to laser clinic to avoid misuse. A compulsory meticulous record keeping and proformas for individual disorders are ideal. This should be handled partly by a nursing staff and by the treating doctor, and the distribution of duties must be crystal clear to avoid snags.

At the end of the day, it is the department head on whom the problems will *lie on* if things go wrong. It is better that the control be with one or more interested faculty members. The indications must be prioritized and decided by consensus to avoid use for conditions unlikely to benefit. At that time, placing a blame on the concerned person will be an issue if all and sundry have had a *free* hand with lasers. We recommend a dedicated day, place, and trained personnel to operate lasers (See case scenarios).

LASER PROCUREMENT IN GOVERNMENT INSTITUTIONS

How to buy the right laser with public funds?
Laser treatment is the new buzz word for dermatology, is growing day-by-day while the side effect profile is going down.

Though a detailed discussion of procurement is beyond the scope of this book as laser purchases are expensive. An overview is given below:
1. **Need Assessment:**
    a. *Scope of services of the hospital:* A primary or even a secondary level hospital does not need lasers and such a request is rarely entertained.
    We should call meeting of all head of departments (HODs) of all the institutes which are within 10 to even 20 km distance (like in Delhi

we have Lady Hardinge Medical College, Maulana Azad Medical College, All India Institutes of Medical Sciences, Safdarjung Hospital, Ram Manohar Lohia, Employees' State Insurance, Army College of Medical Sciences). This is useful to know where lasers are installed and share experiences. Government of India may be asked to form a technical committee from these institutes to:
- Formulate guidelines for indications, specifications and research in this field because a lot of fancy statements are claimed with little science
- Government should ensure that these are followed by other private and government aided institutes
- This committee may work as an Indian FDA or Indian approval agency
- They may also be involved in the purchase of lasers for government medical colleges
- Training program may be formulated and conducted.

b. *Free or paid services:* Though not always the norm some institutions charge a fee that helps to justify a purchase of what is largely believed to be a cosmetic need. Here there are medicolegal issues. (*see* **Chapter 16**).

c. *Cosmetic or therapeutic machine:* This is probably the most important indicator. Thus, it is impossible to justify a hair removal laser, though an IPL which has, at least in theory, multiple uses can be requisitioned. Taking it further, a hospital with a narrow band: ultraviolet B (Nb:UVB) unit should not ideally ask for an excimer laser as again it is difficult to justify it for largely the same indications as phototherapy.

d. *Manpower/space requirements:* The former is probably more important and thus it is better for a medical college where there are residents to assist the primary care providers, to have a laser unit, as then usually routine cases can be handled even if there is a paucity of staff. As for the space, certain basic specifications must be aimed for preferably at the time of starting the process of procurement, as in a government setup things may often be slow to move.

Avoidance of reflective surfaces, planning electrical points carefully (as extension cords must be avoided), doors wide enough for easy passage of the unit and trolley, and air conditioning and ventilation are some of the things which must be kept in mind.

e. *Budget considerations.*

2. **Framing the Specifications:** This is probably one of the few things that can decide the future of the machine. We have detailed the steps for US FDA approval and verification which can help the buyer to decide *worthiness* of the laser company: remember that in private practice, it may not matter as volumes are less, but in a public funded setup a laser with a US or CE certification with studies on the machine make sense (Box 14.1).

> **Box 14.1:** Precise specifications for lasers.
>
> - It should **not be specific** for one company otherwise will be rejected or only one company will apply which will result in rejection
> - At least **2–3 tenders** are required to make the specifications broad based
> - Always go for renowned and reliable companies [preferably US Food and Drug Administration (FDA) or European Conformity (CE) approved]
> - The machines should have **variable spot sizes**
> - Warranty and annual maintenance contracts (AMC): Another important point for which you have to do lot of bargain. Ask for warranty at least for **2–3 years** with parts and AMC for **10 years**. Add penalty clause if they failed
> - All electrical connections and stabilizers should be provided by the company itself because if anything goes wrong the company might blame it on these systems
> - Training requirement should be met by the company
> - A field visit of the company office is advisable. Some have no office or engineers and are just importers
> - Seeing the working parameters and functionality of the machine by asking for demonstration of the machines is a good idea. This should ideally be done in the setting where the machine is supposed to be installed, else in another government/medical college setup with a similar work load

    a. *Discussion in the departmental scientific committee:* A good discussion should be held with other faculty members especially the younger one because you may be going to retire after sometime the others must continue working with laser. The total life of laser in government set-up is around 10 years if a good US FDA approved laser is bought!
    b. Formulation of generic specifications
    c. Discussion on minimum standards acceptable
    d. Consensus
    e. Optional accessories required
    f. Patient load on the laser and the cost effectiveness
    g. Space requirement.
3. **Forwarding the Proposal:**
    a. Sample standard demand performance
    b. Signature of at least three consultants
    c. Adequate justification for the procurement.
4. **Discussion with the Hospital Purchase Committee/Third Party Co-ordinator:** To add a level of fairness (occasionally delays) an external expert is asked to vet the proposal. This helps to take care of any legal or financial issues that may arise:
    a. Scrutiny of proposal
    b. Comments on justification
    c. Is the purchase commensurate with the treatment services scope of the hospital?
5. **Procurement Process:** This step is crucial to purchase and requires a deep understanding of procurement policies of the government. The listed points might seem bureaucratic but happen to serve the dual

process of verification and validation. It is the authors' opinion that these steps have to be accepted and negotiated to properly purchase a machine
   a. Understanding the general financial rules (GFR)—Fundamentals of e-procurement
   b. The tender document
   c. Vetting the proposal—HOD, accounts, competent authority
   d. Terms and conditions including after sales service, annual maintenance contracts (AMC)
   e. Notice inviting tender (NIT)
   f. Tender schedule
   g. Formation of committees
   h. Tender-opening prequalification bid
   i. Technical bid and demonstration
   j. Financial/price bid
   k. Negotiations (if any)
   l. Agreement to purchase
   m. Letter of credit
   n. Dispatch of machine
   o. Freight and delivery
   p. Installation
   q. Trials
   r. Commissioning of machine—standard operating procedure (SOP)
   s. Installation certificate
   t. Release of balance payment
   u. Annual maintenance contracts.
6. **Regulatory Approvals:** This means appropriate FDA 510(k) approvals in the USA, premarket approval (PMA), Health Canada in Canada, Therapeutic Goods Administration (TGA) in Australia, Ministry of Health, Labor and Welfare (Kohseishou) in Japan, appropriate CE marking for medical devices in Europe, and so on.

   Beware of claims like *Approved by the FDA*, the letter of which usually simply means a letter from FDA recognizing that the system is a nonsignificant risk device (NSR) or minimal risk device (MSR). This is *not an approval* to market, but is simply a guide based on which the institutional review board (IRB) of a research center can classify the system when it does take part in a properly structured study.

   FDA 510(k) Clearances: Section 510(k) of the Food, Drug and Cosmetic Act requires device manufacturers who must register, to notify FDA of their intent to market a medical device at least 90 days in advance. This is known as premarket notification—also called PMN or 510(k). This allows FDA to determine whether the device is *equivalent* to a device already placed into one of the three classification categories.

   Thus, *new* devices (not in commercial distribution prior to May 28, 1976) that have not been classified can be properly identified. Specifically, medical device manufacturers are required to submit a premarket notification if they intend to introduce a device into commercial distribution for the first time or reintroduce a device that will be significantly changed or modified to the extent that its safety or effectiveness could be affected. Such change or modification could relate to the design, material, chemical composition, energy source, manufacturing process, or intended use.

A simple way of confirming this is by, one, asking the company for a letter from FDA (see Figs. 13.1A to C sample letter). A second method, which is a *backup* method is depicted in Figures 13.2 to 13.4.

For any individual spending money on a laser, it makes a lot of sense *checking the clearance on the FDA site*. Another sample is given in Figures 13.5A to C.

Of course, once you settle for a non-US FDA machine then this approval does not matter. But it should be made clear that inappropriate use of an unapproved laser is a common litigation claim and at least a CE approval must be obtained.

7. **Looking Beyond the Price:** Ask the following questions before just haggling the price, which though is important may not matter if the device does not deliver results.
   - Internal **trials** if any?
   - Published **data** if any? (see below)
   - **Histological** depth penetration studies for fractional lasers.
   - **Dose intensity parameters** for your skin type.
   - **Follow-up** studies if any?
   - Postmarketing and service team site and offices. Verify the numbers and address.
   - Import license and dealership registration.
   - Proof of a *firsthand device*. Some lasers have been reused and sold!
   - Any legal issues, merger, acquisitions of the company.
   - Any complications reported.

8. **What has been Published on the System/Technology?** There are various types of publication and though most believe or are made to believe that not all lasers can have publications, but it is our opinion that investing in a machine with published studies has a lot more value, even though we admit that occasionally authors may have conflict of interests.

   What you are looking for here are papers by reputable authors published in the indexed and peer-reviewed literature, or at least in well-established and peer-reviewed journals (15 or more volumes). An alternative source is appropriate chapters in books from reputable publishers. What you should not fall for are so-called *white papers* which any manufacturer can produce to look like a genuine publication or articles from the commercially-oriented medical press unless they are also in turn backed up by *real* papers. In India, like in many parts of the world, such scientifically sounding *journals* abound and are not listed for obvious reasons in the bibliography!

Figs. 14.1A and B: Sample letter of approval by US FDA

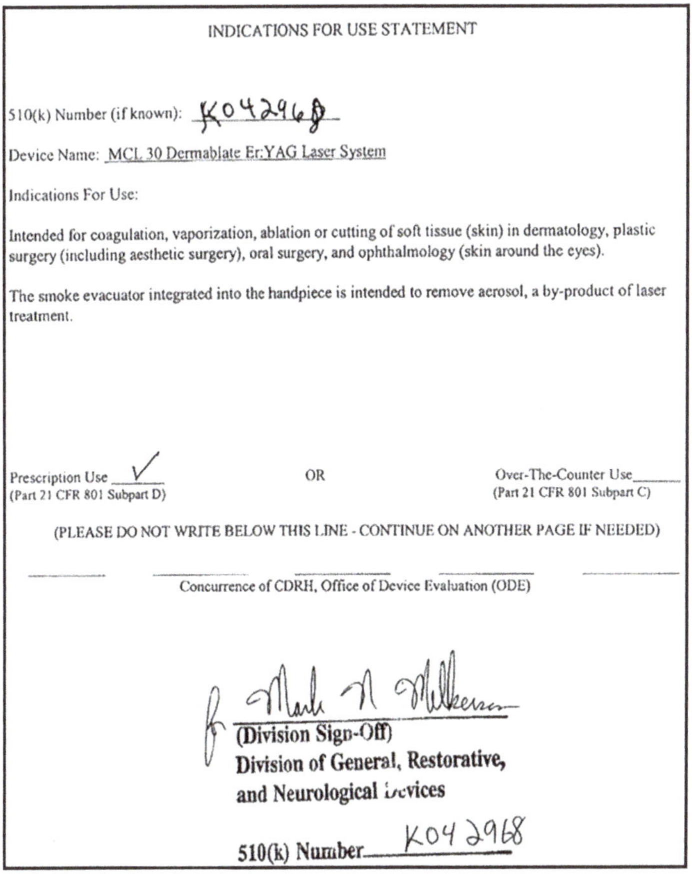

CHAPTER 14: How to Setup a Laser Clinic in a Public Funded Institution

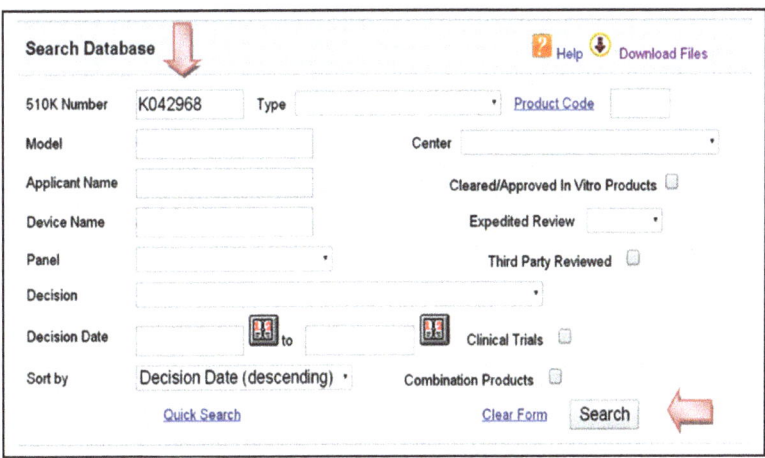

Figs. 14.1C: Sample letters of US Food and Drug Administration (FDA) approval for a medical device (note the 510 k number).

Fig. 14.2: Site of the US Food and Drug Administration (FDA) 510(k) approval. *Enter* the approval number and click on *search*.

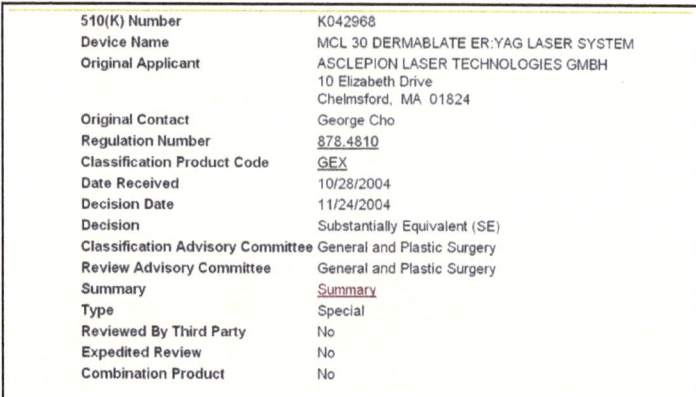

Fig. 14.3: Site of the US Food and Drug Administration (FDA) 510(k) approval. The exact approval date and device is verified.

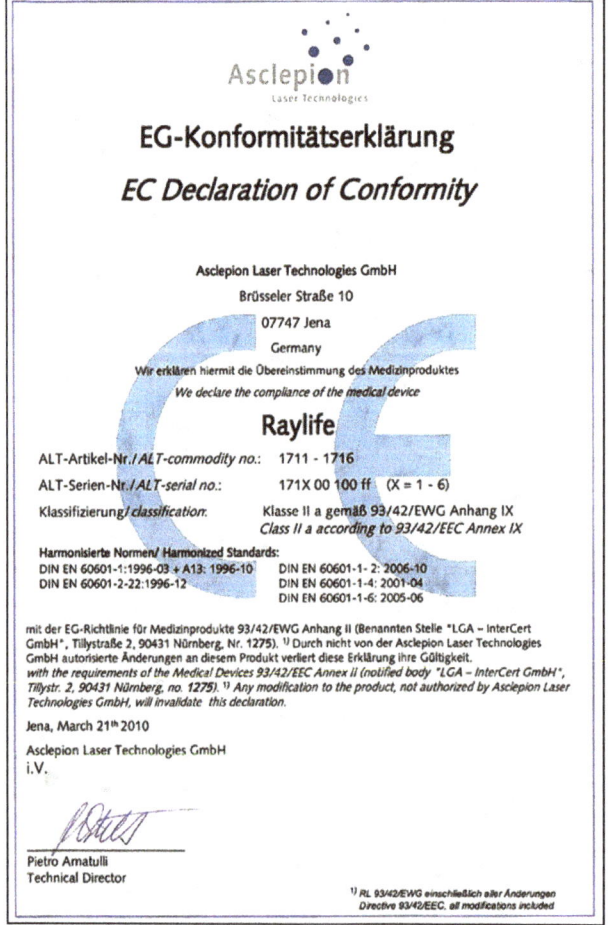

Fig. 14.4: European Conformity (CE) approval letter for medical device.

CHAPTER 14: How to Setup a Laser Clinic in a Public Funded Institution

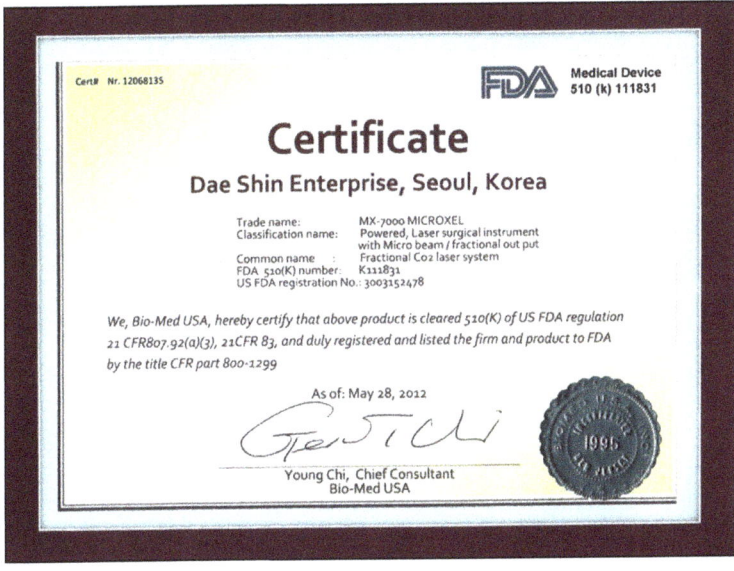

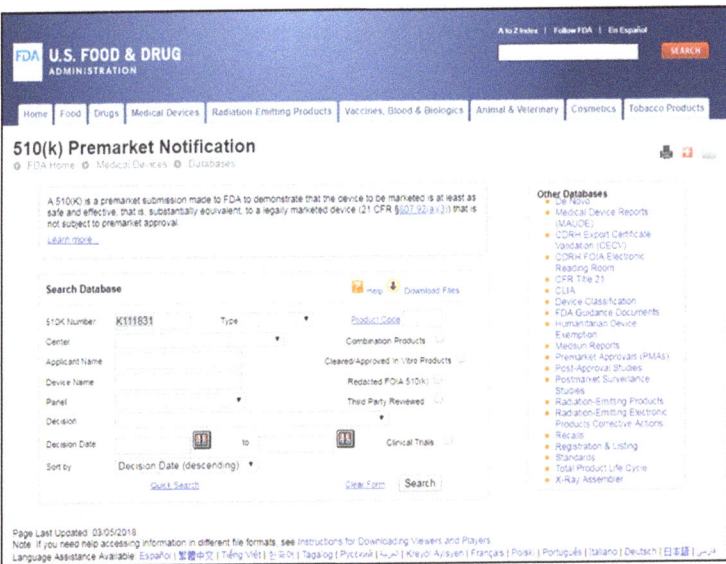

Figs. 14.5A and B: (A) A sample of an FDA approval letter. Note the approval number K111831; (B) As some suppliers are adept at *faking* such data it is good to check on the FDA site (https://www.accessdata.fda.gov/scripts/cdrh/cfdocs/cfpmn/pmn.cfm). Click on search.

The most deceptive *ploy* is where the sales person gives a study on the technology, but of a different company! Make very sure that the articles offered by the manufacturer/salesperson are on their specific system and wavelength(s). There is a lot of differences between approved systems and an unapproved system and often the intensity, dose or even wavelength is not the same as in the published articles.

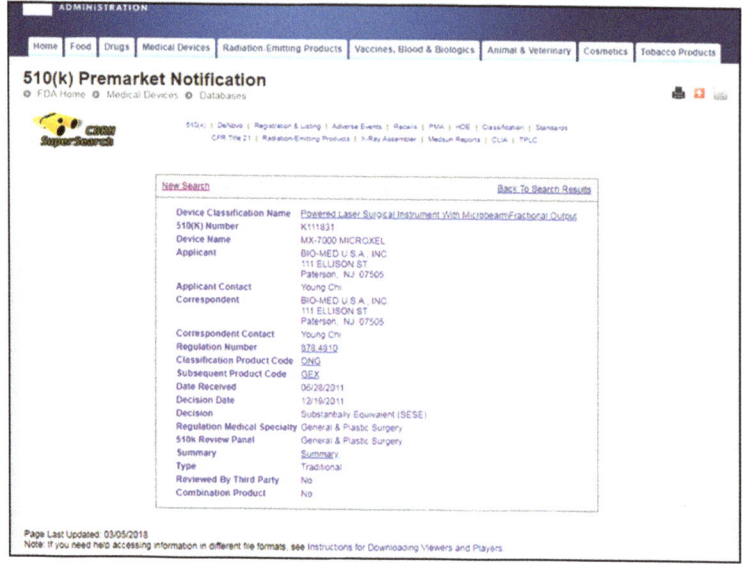

Fig. 14.5C: Food and Drug Administration approval letter. The details are verified. You have a good buy!

CASE SCENARIOS

1. Buying a Laser without Background Knowledge of Spare Parts/Maintenance Issues

A premier institution while setting up a laser system, invested in a vascular laser. The basics of laser physics show that even in ideal cases, the results are abysmal. In Indian skin, the pigment complicates the whole equation as this is never accounted for in the original machines which are researched in Western skin. As there is just one vendor, the machine was bought. The laser AMC was signed. After a few months, it suddenly transpired that the dye is a consumable and not accounted for, and the cost of dye is stupendous. The vendor refuses to supply the same without payment.

Moral: This scenario shows a lack of knowledge of the machine and also the ability of suppliers to cheat buyers. In PDL lasers, the dye has a shelf-life and is a consumable.

2. Lack of Control over Laser Usage

Lasers are not cautery machines. Hence, there should be a designated person who is made responsible and handles the machines and signs in the stock register.

A premier college invested in QS ND:YAG lasers. It was decided to keep one laser on backup and restrict both use and indications. Some indications with a known poor result like nevus of Ota were restricted. Due to a change in the person(s) handling the clinic, new charges were anointed. In the new spirit of apparent freedom, all the lasers were made functional. All residents were given a free hand. The new charges did not consider the life of the lasers or maintenance. In 2 years, both the lasers were defunct.

Moral: If a back-up machine is bought it should be preserved. There should be restricted use of lasers and person responsible should be handed over charge after signing the stock register.

3. Record Keeping under General Financial Rules and Stock Register Verifications

In an annual inspection, which is mandatory under rules in March, the inspecting officer signed on the stock register, without physical verification of the lasers. When the next inspection was done the next inspecting officer asked for a list of the costly items and asked for a stock count. It was noted that one laser machine did not match the make of the machine on record. On inspection of records it was noticed that the machine were handed over in the stock register. It also transpired that three different officers were using the machines with only one of them officially handling the lasers. The supplier was asked and he stated that the machines were supplied as per file record.

Moral: The only proof is the stock register and in case of a discrepancy the officer who has taken charge, the inspecting officer and the HOD are all responsible for the errors.

4. Legal Ramifications of Maintenance of Lasers

A plea by a 23-year-old engineering student who has been unable to get treatment since May 2015 for his skin ailment - PWS, as the machine PDL has not been working was taken up by the High Court (HC). The center had been charging nominally for the procedure. The honorable HC opined *If you have bought a machine, you should maintain it. If the institute does not have funds, which I don't think is the case, then the government should pay for its repairs.* A new machine had to be bought worth 60 lakh, even though it was obvious that the results in PWS were not good.

Moral: Once a machine is bought maintenance is the headache of the institution. The most hardy machines remain the ablative lasers! But if that is used like a cautery machine, it will also get defunct. Also the repairs can be costlier than a new machine!

5. Buying Lasers without Verifying Food and Drug Administration Records

An institution bought an Er:YAG laser after tendering. Three suppliers quoted and all were US FDA certified. The committee that vetted technical specifications asked for certifications and all had certificates of US FDA. After the lowest bidder was approved and bought the machine was installed. After 3 months, a complaint was made by another vendor to the Central Vigilance Commission (CVC) of corruption and buying a non-FDA approved machine. The US FDA site was logged in and it was found that the laser had no US FDA certification. On closer inspection when the machine back panel was opened it was found to have Korean FDA approvals. The vendor had meantime sold his company to another business. The committee is under investigation for corruption and incompetence.

Moral: Here it was the mistake of the supplier but the committee was placed under scrutiny. Hence, a verification of the FDA site is always advisable and background knowledge is a must.

6. Lack of Space for Buying a New Laser

An institution had bought two lasers, both US FDA approved. As they had outlived their life, it was decided to purchase new machines. As per rule, the old lasers were condemned. While preparing the specifications the committee put up the file for approval. The HOD decided to take advice from another department that had bought an MRI machine. The advice given was to include in the tender *buy back policy so that the vendor reduces the cost of the old machine* and takes it away. This was as there was a space crunch. The administration objected, but GFR rules stated that this can be done. Ultimately the headache of disposing of the old machine lay with the new vendor.

Moral: Always take advice of other department that buy expensive equipment's as they have decades of experience in these matters. Remember in government institutions a laser is an expensive buy and errors can be costly.

CONCLUSION

Though the regulatory approvals and procedural systems involved are daunting, the take home message is simple, ask for **validation**, proof of **effectiveness**, **regulatory** approvals and published **studies**. Buying a machine on hearsay and exhortations of speakers in conferences is probably the most foolish method of buying lasers. A classic example is buying lasers to treat pigmentary disorders like melasma.

More importantly, as all such procedures are open to medicolegal scrutiny, it is better to have the right device as the approvals are a useful method of buttressing claims of *good practices* in the court. The cost of litigations and damages can often negate the temporary gains that may ensue by buying an unapproved and cheaper device.

Lastly restrict use, lasers are not radiofrequency machines or cautery, and public funded institutions are responsible for teaching Dermatology and exposing students to cosmetology, not to hone their skills on the A-Z of indications. On a cheeky note, the section II of the book can be referred to know where they work. As the old saying goes *wise men learn from others mistakes, while fools learn from their own.*

CHAPTER 15

Why, When, and How to Buy a Laser?

Anil Ganjoo, Kabir Sardana

INTRODUCTION

Use of lasers, in dermatology, has been rapidly increasing. Over the last 4–5 decades, that lasers have been around, there have been rapid advances in the technology and therapeutic efficacy of lasers. Extensive research has given a better understanding of the laser tissue interaction and this has allowed us to expand the therapeutic options with lasers and has improved the clinical outcome. Lasers have now become the treatment of choice for a number of conditions that were thought to be virtually untreatable about 5 decades ago. Since their inception about 50 years ago, lasers have come a long way. From the initial use of ruby laser for almost every condition to highly precise laser for each condition we have progressed a lot.

Advances in technology have brought with it the availability of large number of different types of systems and large numbers of dealers dealing in similar systems, which has made the laser scene very complex and confusing. Selecting the right system and the right dealer is of utmost importance for a good laser practice.

We have been using lasers in India for the last about 15 years and this decade and a half experience has taught a lot of lessons. While working on our patients we have found that our kind of skins behaves differently than the Western skins. Therefore, we have developed our own parameters that suit our patients' skins. We now know that if used judiciously lasers are wonderful but they have their shortcomings.

PLANNING A LASER CLINIC

When planning a laser setup, one should be well aware of the laser physics, which will help in selecting the system with the right parameters. This is discussed in **Chapter 1** in detail and here we will focus on other aspects that are important to the dermatologists including:
- His/her budget
- His/her patient profile

- His/her patient volume
- His/her patients' paying capacity.

The budget situation decides what kind of investment can be put in and therefore what kind of machines can be bought. Depending upon the type of patients one sees in practice, he can decide as to which system should be his first priority. One should be able to foresee what procedure would be in greatest demand in one's practice. For example, if the physician has a lot of young and old hirsute women walking in then the first system that is bought should obviously be a hair reduction system, while if you get a lot of scars then a fractional resurfacing system should be your choice. Only those with a good volume of patients should plan to setup a laser practice as *high turnover* of patients is *necessary* for recovering the high cost of the machines. Last of all, the *area* that you are practicing in is very important as that determines whether the patients will be able to pay the high costs involved.

A *break-even analysis* (BEA) is often used in the business world to determine exactly when the business will be able to cover all of its expenses and generate profit. *Break-even point (BEP)* is the point in time in which total costs and total revenue are equal and one is able to generate profit thereafter.

A *formula* that can be used is $R = P \times X$

Here laser revenue (R) is equivalent to the procedure fee (P) for each laser treatment multiplied by unit sales (X) (number of procedures performed for that particular laser treatment).

Total *costs* = Include fixed costs (FCs) and variable costs (VCs).

Fixed costs do not change with the volume of patients treated (laser purchase price, warranty, cost of operation such as overhead and cost of staff time, leasing, and maintenance of certification). VCs fluctuate with the number of patients treated and laser activity (cost of consumables/disposables (tips), and occasionally marketing expenses).

Ideally, the BEP should occur within 2 years of a laser purchase. Beyond this time frame, there is a risk that technology changes might make the equipment obsolete, with more attractive and competitive products in the community (Figs. 15.1A and B).

AESTHETICS OF A LASER CENTER

Remember that you are entering the world of aesthetics, which is the world of beauty. Your setup needs to be aesthetically pleasing and welcoming. It is very important that your center is well placed, easily approachable with good parking space. The center should be done up well and should be comforting to the eye at the first look. The staff has to be very courteous and smiling with a ready to help attitude. The reception, treatment rooms, washrooms, etc. should always be clean. The patients should feel that they are well taken care of and their queries are being answered properly (Figs. 15.2 to 15.5).

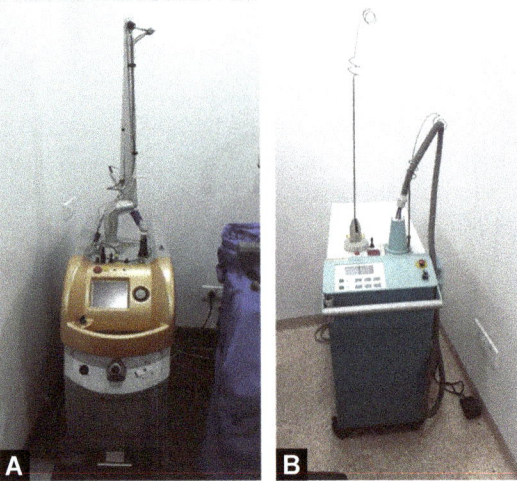

Figs. 15.1A and B: A depiction of some older laser systems which need to be replaced as newer technologies are acquired.

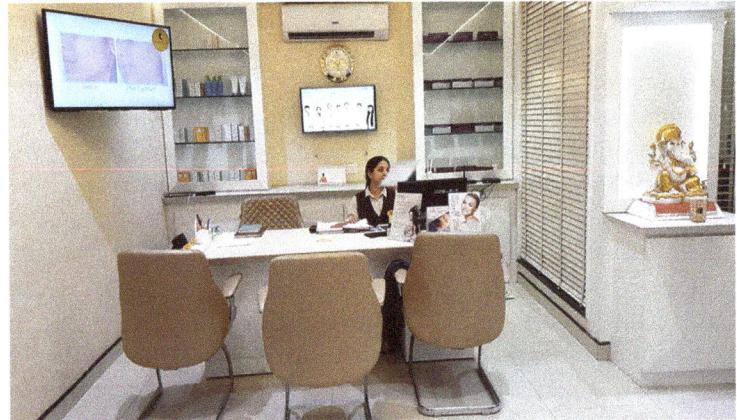

Fig. 15.2: An aesthetically reception.

RISK FACTORS

There are some risk factors which should be assesses before attempting any procedure. Some common caution points include:
- Patients with a history of post-traumatic or postinflammatory hyperpigmentation or melasma are at increased risk of hyperpigmentation.
- Isotretinoin treatment within the past 6 months is a contraindication to ablative lasers.
- A history of hypertrophic scarring and keloid formation increases scarring risk with deeper laser treatments.

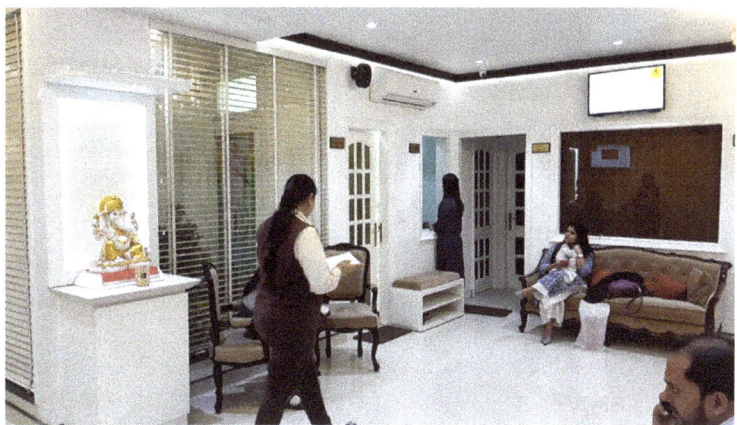

Fig. 15.3: Soothing environment.

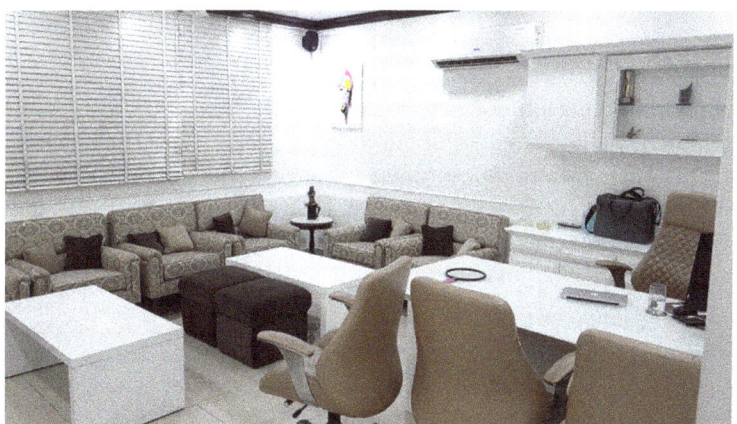

Fig. 15.4: Dermatologists chamber.

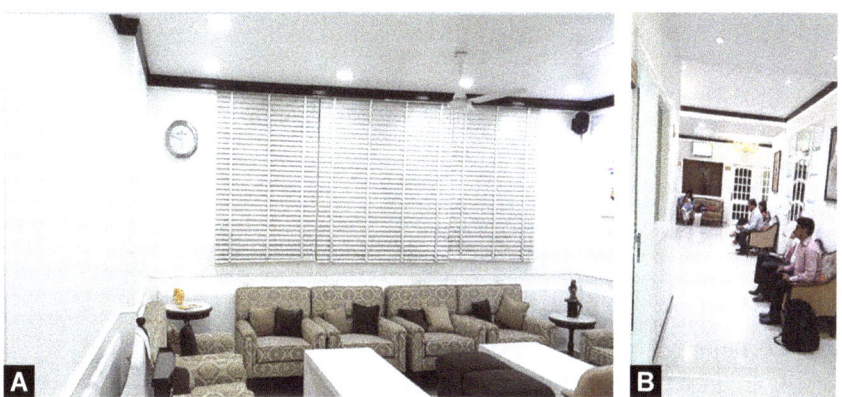

Figs. 15.5A and B: Waiting area for patients.

- In India, steroid abuse is an issue and thus prolonged topical or systemic corticosteroids can delay wound healing and result in areas of atrophic skin healing.
- Immunocompromised patients or those who have collagen vascular disease, can also experience delayed wound healing.
- A history of perioral or facial herpetic lesions creates a higher risk of recurrence after treatment.
- As a general rule, patients who are currently pregnant or breastfeeding should also avoid laser resurfacing because no studies regarding safety exist.
- As a thumb rule laser therapy is ideal for patients with the lightest skin tones, specifically those with Fitzpatrick skin types I through III. Darker skin types carry a risk of postprocedure dyschromia. Additionally, patients with previous postinflammatory hyperpigmentation or melasma, regardless of skin type, are at increased risk of dyschromia.

SPECIFICATIONS OF ENERGY DEVICES

One of the most common questions asked by the starters is whether to start with a *platform* with multiple functions or to go for a *stand-alone machine*. In practice, buying stand-alone systems is always more beneficial as they are more effective than the combinations and also if a platform breaks down all your lasers will breakdown while if a stand-alone machine breaks down only that particular wavelength is gone.

While buying a *new system* one should look for:
- The best specifications.
- Whether that particular system is being used by other colleagues.
- The reliability of the dealer.
- The after sales record of the dealer.

Hair Reduction Lasers

Specifications of the machine are the most important deciding factor to pick up a system.

For *hair reduction* following systems are available in India:
- *Long-pulsed neodymium-doped yttrium aluminum garnet (LP Nd:YAG)*—1,064 nm
- *Diode*—810 nm
- *Alexandrite*—755 nm
- *Intense pulsed light (IPL)*—400–1,200 nm.
- *In motion technologies:*
  - Diode
  - Intense pulsed light.

Long-pulsed neodymium-doped yttrium aluminum garnet is the *safest* due to the longest wavelength. Diode is slightly more efficacious but can produce side effects like burns and pigmentary disturbances, particularly in our kind of dark skins. However, with the *modern diode systems* with the state of the art of cooling tips the side effects have been reduced to a large extent. That makes diode a better alternative to LP Nd:YAG. Even *alexandrite laser* at 755 nm with the modern sapphire cooling tips has become safe with good efficacy particularly for the thin and less pigmented hair. We now also have systems that deliver all three wavelengths: (1) The 1,064 nm Nd:YAG, (2) The 810 nm diode, and (3) The 755 nm alexandrite with the same handpiece in a single shot. This makes the machine more efficacious targeting hair roots at different depths and of different thickness and color at the same time more effectively. IPL systems are the classic "jack of all trades, masters of none". They can do multiple jobs but their efficacy is not comparable to the stand-alone wavelengths. In general, the machine you buy should have a *large spot size* available as larger the spot size, lesser is the scattering and deeper is the penetration. The system should *have variable pulse width*—10–100 ms, which ensures targeting hairs of various thicknesses. Earlier all the machine should have good power and should be sturdy (Figs. 15.6A to C).

Pigment-specific Lasers

The lasers used for *pigmented* lesions are the Q-switched lasers. These include:

- *Q-switched frequency doubled neodymium-doped yttrium aluminum garnet laser*—532 nm
- *Q-switched ruby laser*—694 nm
- *Q-switched alexandrite laser*—755 nm
- *Q-switched neodymium-doped yttrium aluminum garnet laser*—1,064 nm
- *Intense pulsed light*—590–1,200 nm.

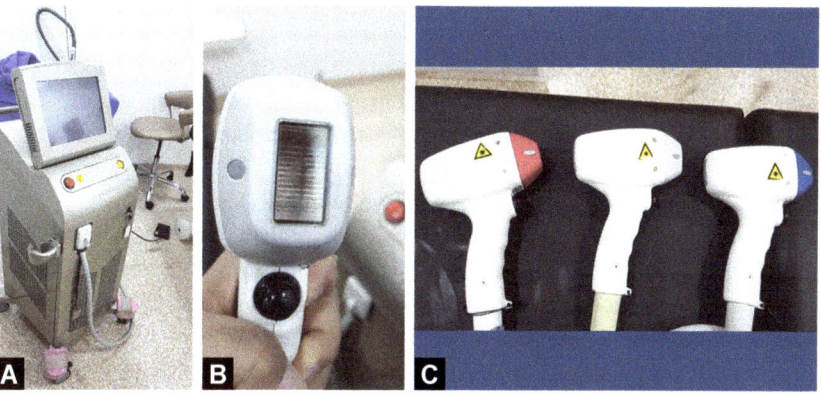

Figs. 15.6A to C: The new age diode lasers with multiple wavelengths improve the efficacy and safety of the procedures.

In India, the most commonly used is the Qs Nd:YAG system:
- 1,064 nm
- 532 nm.

The Nd:YAG laser produces laser energy at a wavelength of 1,064 nm. It will penetrate up to 2–3 mm into the dermis, making it useful in the removal of deeper natural and artificial dermal pigmentations.

When the laser beam is passed through a potassium titanyl phosphate (KTP) crystal, the laser energy frequency is doubled and the resultant light wavelength is halved to 532 nm. This wavelength is absorbed more superficially in the skin, making it useful for the removal of benign superficial epidermal pigmentations.

All Q-switched machines have pulse widths of less than 10 ns. High-end machines with variable spot sizes of 2/4/6/8 mm *and above* are desirable. The machine should have a good power, with maximum fluence of at least 12 J/cm^2, using the smallest spot size. *The large spot size* helps you do the laser toning a very useful new technique that treats a wide range of pigmented conditions including melasma. A peak power output of *1,200–2,000 mJ/cm^2* at 1,064 nm and half of that at 532 nm is the least that one should look for in a Q-switched machine. The newer machines also provide a *quasi-long wavelength of 300* µs that can be used to stimulate collagen buildup to improve the texture and superficial scars. Also the newer machines provide handpieces with wavelengths of *595 nm* and *630 nm* used for gold toning, erythema, and rosacea. Some systems also provide fractionated handpieces and the PTP or the twin pulsing mode both improving tolerability and safety. So, try and look for all these features in your machine. Considering the cost constraints, people often prefer to buy the cheaper machines. However, cheaper machines with a single spot size of 2 mm and maximum energy output of 500–600 mJ/cm^2 are not recommended. IPL is not a very good option for pigmented lesions (Figs. 15.7A to D).

Fractional Lasers

Fractional lasers are the new wonder machines that are now used for an increasing number of indications, major one being resurfacing for scars and aging skin. These are available as ablative and nonablative versions and both are quite effective. The ablative carbon dioxide (CO_2) fractional laser gives the fastest and the best results but has a long downtime (Fig. 15.8).

Superficial scars can be taken care of with erbium-doped yttrium aluminum garnet (Er:YAG) 2,940 nm fractional. It is thus the author's opinion that the results of *nonablative fractional lasers*, like Er:Glass 1,540 nm, are *not comparable* to that of *ablative lasers*. While buying a CO_2 fractional machine one should make sure that the power of the machine should be at least *30–40 W*, the pulse width should be *500–600 ms*, and the machine should have variable density of spots so that less density with high power can be used for

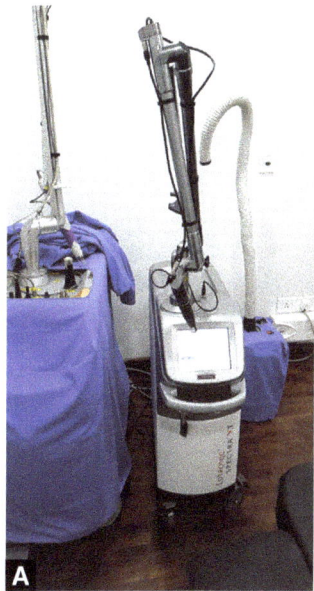
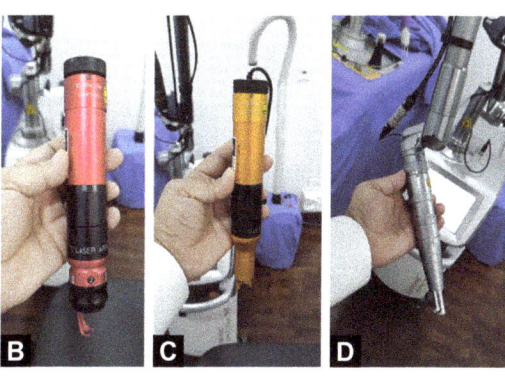

Figs. 15.7A to D: (A) Latest Q-switched machines with different handpieces makes them very versatile; (B) 595 nm handpiece for *gold toning*; (C) 660 nm handpiece for safer treatment of *epidermal lesions*; (D) 532/1,064 nm collimated handpiece with top hat beam for better and safer treatment. Spot sizes from 2 mm to 10 mm increase versatility.

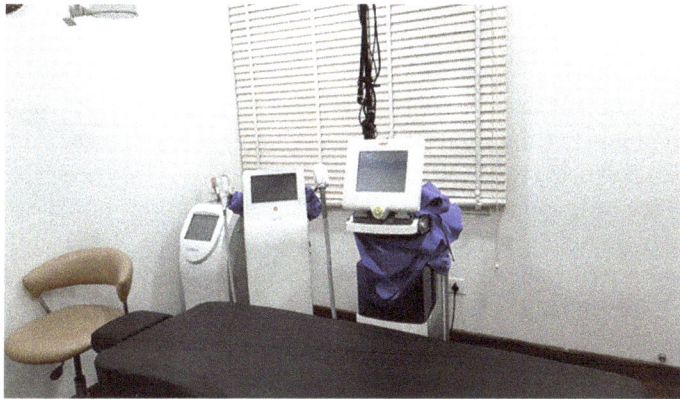

Fig. 15.8: The clinic needs to be equipped devices with the latest high-end systems like the CO_2 laser, the HIFU, RF resurfacing, and tightening among others. (CO_2: carbon dioxide; HIFU: high-intensity focused ultrasound; RF: radiofrequency)

deep scars, while more density with low power can be used for *rejuvenation and textural improvement*.

The highly successful 1,550 nm fractionated erbium laser expanded the use of erbium lasering for both cosmetic and reconstructive indications. This is a milder fractional laser with a "modest but significant improvement" in texture, rhytides, and superficial lentigines with markedly reduced downtime. However, because the results can be insufficient for a number of clinical conditions, the popularity of the fractionated CO_2 platforms continue.

Other superficial ablative and nonablative technologies are available and include 2,790 nm, 1,440 nm, 1,540 nm, 1,550 nm, and 1,064 nm, but the results are not as dramatic as with the ablative and fractionated technologies described earlier.

Vascular Lasers

Vascular lesions are targeted by a variety of wavelength lasers including the pulsed dye (585–595 nm), the KTP frequency-doubled Nd:YAG (532 nm), and the Nd:YAG (1,064 nm) laser systems. Current available pulsed dye lasers (PDLs) emit a wavelength of 585 nm or 595 nm with longer pulse durations. The 585 nm wavelength gives it excellent specificity to hemoglobin with a minimal risk of hyperpigmentation, hypopigmentation, or skin breakdown.

The PDL has been used in fair skin types for port-wine stains, telangiectasias, and hemangiomas. The KTP frequency-doubled Nd:YAG (532 nm) laser is usually used for smaller lesions such as spider veins and telangiectasias, and the Nd:YAG (1,064 nm) laser has utility in treating reticular veins.

WHAT LASERS DO PRACTITIONERS BUY?

In a unique study, a survey was conducted with members of the American Academy of Facial Plastic and Reconstructive Surgery. Members were polled using an online five question survey to evaluate preferences regarding laser purchases and uses (Fig. 15.9).

The 100 respondents reported that the lasers they purchased most commonly included fractionated CO_2 (46%), ablative CO_2 (31%), Nd:YAG (27%), and Er:YAG (25%). Many members owned more than one laser.

The lasers most frequently used via lease agreement were fractionated CO_2 and ablative CO_2 (25% and 21%, respectively).

When queried regarding the laser they would like to have access to, 47% responded that they would like access to a fractionated CO_2 laser, with 29% citing a PDL.

The laser used most commonly was the fractionated CO_2 (31%), followed by the ablative CO_2 (13%). Members advised that physicians starting a new practice acquire a fractionated CO_2 laser (63%), a PDL (17%), and an Er:YAG laser (15%).

In India, the results of vascular lasers are not as good as in the West with the cost of the dye being an added factor. Most buy the CO_2 but not the Er:YAG which in the author's view (Dr Kabir Sardana) is a remarkably safe, predictable laser with almost perfect dose of depth dynamics. Of course, a hair removal and pigment laser is a good investment. We do not feel that the picosecond laser is such a great investment as it is touted, but this is discussed elsewhere.

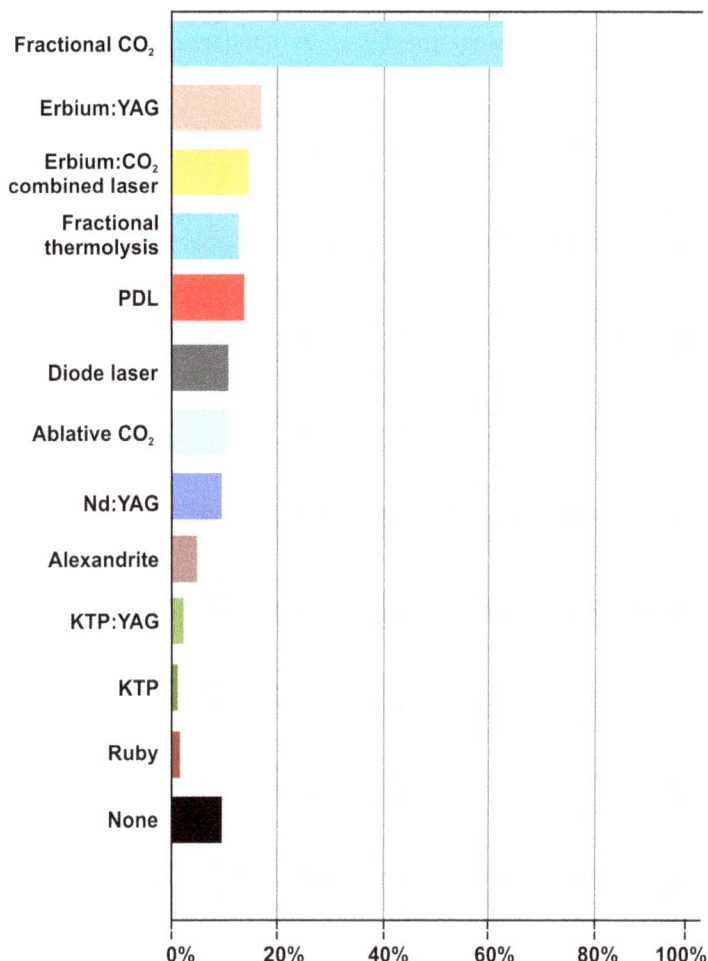

Fig. 15.9: A depiction of the common lasers systems bought by practitioners.
Source: Data from Park SS, Khalid AN, Graber NJ, et al. Current trends in facial resurfacing: a survey of American Academy of Facial Plastic and Reconstructive Surgery members. Arch Facial Plast Surg. 2010;12(1):65-67.

DEALER RELIABILITY

Before buying a system try to integrate the evidence-based literature and experience of your peers who have been using that particular system or who know about it. Literature-based evidence is hard to find since most of the machines have different specifications. But if available, can be a big help and confidence building measure. Peer advice is easy to get. Try to get in touch with colleagues who have been using the same system for some time. They are the best people to guide you about the working of the machine and also about the reliability of the dealer. It is better to believe what the peers say than to listen to what the manufacturers or the dealers say.

Reliability of the dealer is a huge concern. Checking the credentials of the supplier is as important as the specifications of the machine itself.

- One should do a thorough market survey with inputs from colleagues and market experts before putting faith in a particular dealer.
- The dealer should be of good repute, should have an expert team of engineers who can provide a good postsale service.
- The office of the dealer should preferably be in your city so that he can be easily approached.
- Execute a proper contract of purchase, which should include all aspects of warranty.

    Make sure that the warranty clearly mentions the time of warranty and the parts covered under it. Sometimes, the parts that really need to be covered are not covered under warranty. These include parts that are more likely to wear out soon like the flash lamp, the optic cable, the lenses, and the mirrors.
- Keep your eyes open to the possibility of getting a refurbished machine instead of a new one. So, ask for import details of the machine including the papers of point and date of entry into the country and check whether the serial number mentioned on the papers is the same as that of your machine.
- Be in touch with the parent company through emails to make sure that a new machine has been imported directly from the parent company.

Once the machine has been procured, have a written agreement with the company mentioning:

- Likely breakdowns.
- *Warranty*—parts covered.
- Cost of components that usually breakdown.
- Annual maintenance contract (AMC) after the warranty is over.
- Most AMCs do not cover the commonly required components like fiber, flash lamps, power supply, etc. Service contract may also serve the purpose. At times, you need to send your machine to the parent company in Europe/US to get it repaired. So, do a proper homework and assess the postsales performance of the company whose machine you intend to buy.
- Insuring your machine is a good idea.
- Installing a uninterruptible power supply (UPS) is very useful as it ensures:
    - Uninterrupted power supply
    - Prevents damage due to voltage fluctuations.

Also remember that maintenance is an expensive affair as spares are quite costly. Considering the high initial cost and the expensive maintenance, it is always better for a few colleagues to get together to setup laser practice. This shares the cost of buying and maintenance and also increases the patient pool and more the number of patients treated better the cost effectiveness.

AVOIDING COMMON MISTAKES

The single most common mistake is to obtain every single device in the market, buy every single handpiece on the platform, and to get the latest and the greatest. While it is always tempting to do so it can be a big mistake also. Patients are looking for results and good outcomes. Bad results can spoil the reputation of the physician very easily. So, try to get time-tested and result-oriented machines rather than the latest and the most expensive.

The second common mistake is not accounting for all costs (direct and indirect). True costing should include all the overheads like electricity, time, staff, breakdowns, etc.

A business plan with real return on investment (ROI) should be chalked out for each machine. Do not rely on the manufacturer's ROI plan. Instead, ROI should be based on maturity of practice, size, and type of practice and competition in the market.

CONCLUSION

The field of lasers and light devices is undergoing a huge revolution. There are a large number of machines available in the market that makes decision making a very difficult exercise. It is imperative for the physician to approach the issue in a stepwise manner. This includes:
- Evidence-based review and discussion with peers on the specifications of a particular system.
- Assessment of the reliability of the dealer/manufacturer.
- Working out a proper contract on sale and postsale service including the warranty.
- Working out the real "ROI" on the product considering ones practice in volume and demography as also the market competition.

Remember if procured carefully and used judiciously, lasers can be a big boon to the dermatology practice.

BIBLIOGRAPHY

Books
1. Goldman MP. Carbon dioxide and erbium YAG lasers. In: Goldman MP (Ed). Cutaneous and Cosmetic Laser Surgery, 1st edition. USA: CRC Press; 2006.
2. Goldman MP. Skin resurfacing with ablative lasers. In: Goldman MP (Ed). Cutaneous and Cosmetic Laser Surgery, 1st edition. USA: CRC Press; 2006.

Journals

1. Alster TS. Clinical and histologic evaluation of six erbium: YAG lasers for cutaneous resurfacing. Lasers Surg Med. 1999;24:87-92.
2. Alster TS. Cutaneous resurfacing with CO_2 and erbium: YAG lasers: preoperative, intraoperative, and postoperative considerations. Plast Reconstr Surg. 1999;103: 619-32.
3. Jasin ME. Achieving superior resurfacing results with the erbium: YAG laser. Arch Facial Plast Surg. 2002;4:262-6.
4. Tse Y, Manuskiatti W, Detwiler SP, et al. Tissue effects of the erbium: YAG laser with varying passes, energy, and pulse overlap. Lasers Surg Med. 1998;22:70.

CHAPTER 16

Medicolegal Aspects of Lasers in Dermatological Practice

Anil Aggrawal, Kabir Sardana

INTRODUCTION

The use of high energy light sources [laser, intense pulsed light (IPL)] is booming in dermatological and aesthetic surgery. Lasers were introduced in the specialty of dermatology in the *mid-1960s*. Since then, their wide acceptance and use provide striking evidence of their extraordinary ability to treat, precisely and effectively, several skin diseases that were previously incapable of being managed by other medical or surgical methods. Continued evolutionary changes in both the laser IPL technology as well as the understanding of the mechanisms involved in the laser-tissue interaction have improved the precision with which cutaneous laser surgery can be performed and have also increased the indications for it.

LASER COMPLICATIONS AND MEDICOLEGAL LIABILITY

Laser and intense pulsed light (IPL) treatments are however not without their hazards, especially at the hands of a non-specialist, as has become the trend lately. Typical complications arising from laser and IPL treatments are allergic reactions (due to unknown tattoo inks), blistering, burning, color changes (with removal of permanent make-up), contact dermatitis (after hematogenous dissemination of the allergens), crusts, folliculitis, hypertrophic scarring/keloids, localized herpes virus infections, loss of pigmentation/hyperpigmentation (depending on laser/IPL setting, skin type, and pre-interventional or post-interventional sun exposure), paradoxical hair growth (especially with IPL technology) and pruritus. The biggest problems are the treatment of pigmented lesions of uncertain benign/malignant nature without prior diagnosis or histological controls, which often leads to the appearance of an atypical postoperative recurrent nevus or pseudomelanoma. Sometimes amelanotic melanomas may be allowed to progress without detection and may even metastasize.

Laser burns is another injury, which may occur during hair removal. Although usually safe and well tolerated, with the widespread use unexpected side effects can be seen. In recent years, a new laser technology has been introduced to aid in pain and other side effects in laser applications. Diode laser systems are produced for this technology. The major disadvantage with this laser is the gel application during procedure. Epidermal burn reactions can occur due to accumulated debris on the guide.

A number of laser-specific complications is detailed in a separate chapter and needless to say, the patient should be told about the complications and the course of the sequelae in advance (Box 16.1). A list of conditions for which litigation was initiated in a study (Jalian HR) is listed in Box 16.2.

It is not surprising that as laser hair removal is the most common *outsourced* procedure, it is the most common cause of litigation. Apart from that, note that in some cases using the laser for indications that are better treated by *other means* can be a *valid cause for litigation*. The classic examples are psoriasis and vitiligo. For both these, the excimers laser/light are used which are in no way superior to other forms of therapy, including

Box 16.1: Injuries sustained because of laser surgery (Jalian HR, et al.; Svider PF, et al.).

- Burns
- Scars
- Pigmentation
- Disfigurement
- Emotional distress
- Physical suffering
- Erythema
- Diminished quality of life
- Ulceration
- Embarrassment
- Eye injury
- Death
- Disability
- Infection

Box 16.2: Laser procedures performed resulting in litigation (Jalian HR, et al.; Svider PF, et al.).

- Hair removal
- Rejuvenation
- Vascular
- Leg veins
- Tattoo
- Neoplasm
- Scar
- Pigmentary disorder
- Pigmented lesion
- Others*

*These cases included 6 cases in which the specifics of the procedure were not disclosed, 2 cases related to fat removal, 1 case of skin tightening, and 1 case of psoriasis treatment.

phototherapy. If not charged (as in certain institutions), it may not be an issue, but if charged, can be a *recipe* for trouble. Nonsurgical sculpting and tightening are classic examples of indications where there is a mismatch of expectations and results, unless patients are counseled well in advance. Melasma treated in Indian skin is a cardinal mistake as the pigmentary sequelae can lead to major cosmetic concerns and will be difficult to defend in a court of law.

Here it is pertinent to examine medical malpractice suits in USA, which would largely mirror what happens in India, as most of our cosmetic procedures follows their practice and there is a burgeoning environment of malpractice suits in India. As Figure 16.1 shows dermatologists face the maximum litigations (Peter F Svider et al.). Figure 16.2 gives an outlook of the disorders treated.

Dermatologists were the most frequently named physician defendants followed by otolaryngologists and plastic surgeons. The most frequent procedures included laser treatment for age-related changes, followed by revision of acne marks and hair removal (Fig. 16.2). Vascular indications are another cause of litigation including PWS and telangiectasia. Here please note that pigmentary changes were a common cause, the reason why we abhor the use of lasers for conditions like melasma (Fig. 16.3). Also please note that undergoing unnecessary or inappropriate procedures (Fig. 16.3) are a cause for litigation, hence trying to resolve lichen planus pigmentosus, poikiloderma, ice pick scar, laser *tightening* of an aged face without proper counseling and written consent about the quantum of improvement can become an expensive litigious affair.

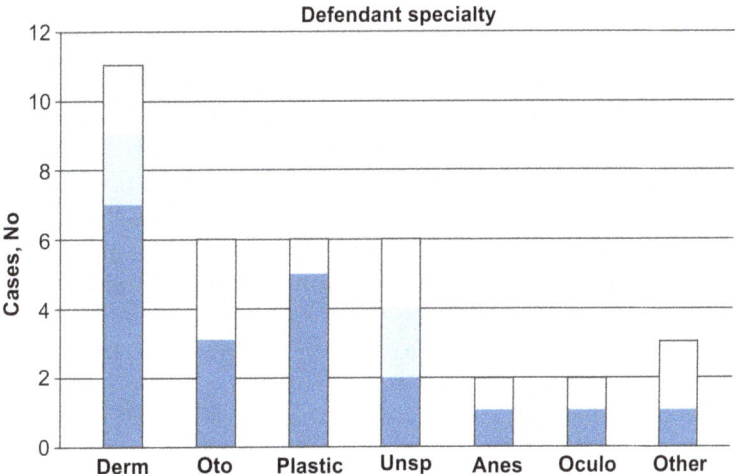

Fig. 16.1: A list of specialty of physician defendants. **Anes** indicates anesthesiology; **Derm**: Dermatology; **Oculo**: Oculoplastic surgery (fellowship-trained surgeons); **Oto**: Otolaryngology; **Plastic**: Plastic surgery; and **Unsp**: Unspecified.
Source: JAMA Facial Plast Surg. 2014;16(4):277-83.

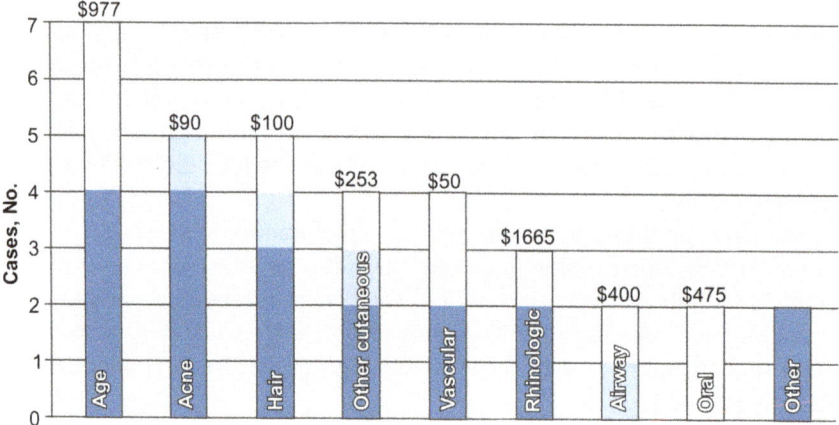

Fig. 16.2: Indications for procedures/types of procedures included in current analysis. **Acne** indicates resurfacing for acne marks; **Age**, cutaneous laser resurfacing for age-related changes; **Hair**, hair removal; **Oral**, oral/oropharyngeal; and **Vascular**, removal of vascular lesions.

Median payments (in thousands of dollars) for each type of procedure are noted above bars. Top portions of bars represent plaintiff decisions; middle portions, settlements; and bottom portions, defendant decisions.
Source: JAMA Facial Plast Surg. 2014;16(4):277-83.

WHO IS QUALIFIED TO DO LASER SURGERY?

This question is often asked, especially as the cosmetic laser trend continues to grow, a number of unqualified practitioners have started doing laser cosmetic procedures. Physicians are also increasingly using physician extenders (PE) to assist them with such procedures.

A physician extender (most commonly a nurse practitioner or physician assistant) is a healthcare provider who is *not a physician* but who performs medical activities typically performed by a physician. Without appropriate supervision and training, one can expect a higher incidence of complications for these non-physicians. At many places, most notably wellness facilities, cosmetology institutes, and hair and tattoo studios, PEs are employed solely, without any supervision by a trained dermatologist. The underlying legal premise supporting this situation is that these practitioners are not treating disease. Thus, there is no need for a diagnosis by a physician, and procedures may be performed by trained laypersons.

A study by Hammes S et al. found that the following complications occurred, with laser procedures performed by medical laypersons: 81.4% pigmentation changes, 25.6% scars, 14% textural changes, and 4.6% incorrect information. The sources of error were the following: 62.8% excessively high energy, 39.5% wrong device for the indication, 20.9% treatment of patients with darker skin or marked tanning, 7% no cooling, and 4.6% incorrect information.

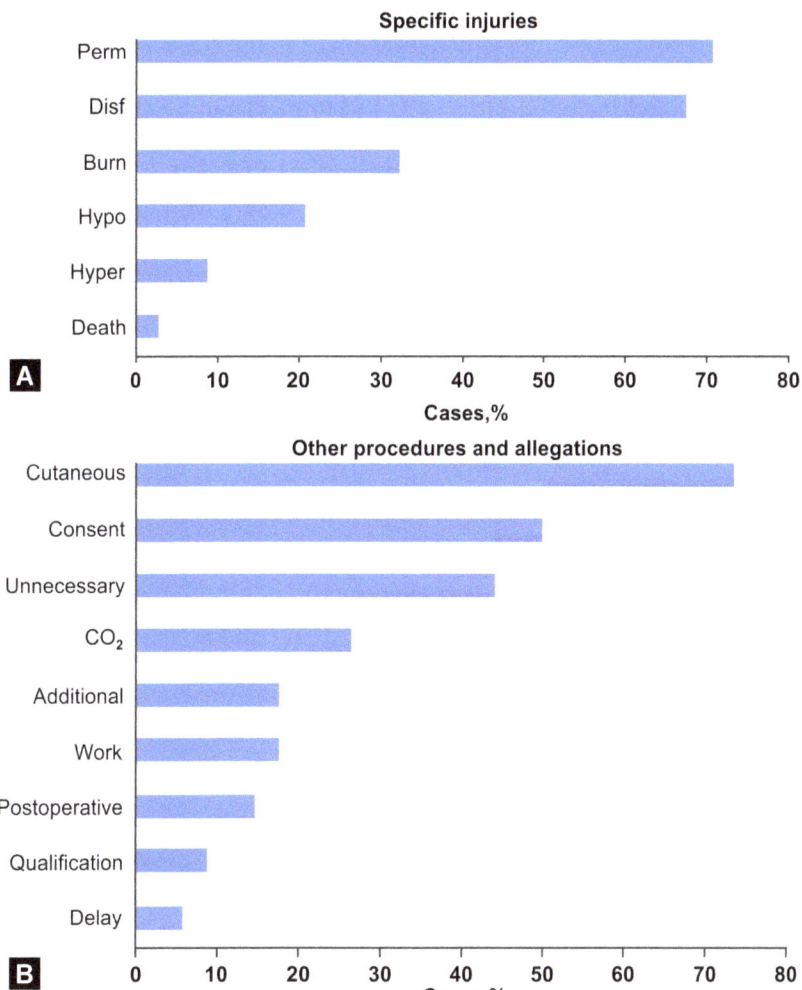

Figs. 16.3A and B: (A) Depicts specific alleged injuries; (B) Types of procedures and allegations not regarding specific injuries.

Additional indicates additional procedures required because of adverse event; CO_2, cases in which use of a carbon dioxide laser was explicitly mentioned (most others did not specify laser type); *consent*, alleged deficits in informed consent; *cutaneous*, cutaneous procedure; *delay*, delay in diagnosis of complication; *Disf*, poor cosmesis, disfigurement, or scarring; *Hyper*, hyperpigmentation; *Hypo*, hypopigmentation; *Perm*, permanent injury; *postoperative*, postoperative negligence; qualification, defendant allegedly not qualified to perform procedure; *unnecessary*, unnecessary or inappropriate procedure; and *work*, employment or income affected by injury.
Source: JAMA Facial Plast Surg. 2014;16(4):277-83.

While *The American Society for Lasers in Medicine and Surgery, American Academy of Dermatology*, and the *American Society for Dermatologic Surgery* have all developed guidelines for PE using lasers in the dermatologic and cosmetic laser setting, corresponding Indian societies have failed to formulate similar guidelines **with** a legal angle. In the US, according to most guidelines a PE, where allowed by state law to do laser treatments is required to have a supervising physician on site and immediately available while the laser procedure is being performed.

Since lasers may have untoward effects on the body if incorrectly used, only those persons are legally allowed to use lasers who are qualified in medicine and surgery, i.e. who hold a proper MBBS degree from an MCI recognized medical college. Here it must be noted that section 27 of *the Delhi Medical Council Act, 1997* deals with *false assumption of Medical Practitioner or Practitioner under this Act to be an offence* and states. *Any person who falsely assumes that he is a medical practitioner and practices the modern scientific system of medicine, shall be punishable with rigorous imprisonment which may extend up to three years or with fine which may extend up to ₹20,000 or with both.*

Shared Decision Making

Shared decision making (SDM) is often required in LASER applications. It is broadly defined as a collaborative effort between the dermatologist and patient to make an informed clinical decision that enhances the chance of LASER treatment success as defined by each patient's preferences and values, when no *best* treatment options are available.

MEDICOLEGAL LIABILITY

Most of the issues arise from the Consumer Protection Act and the intricate details are a must read. For now, an overview is given in **Annexure 1**. Other issues are discussed here.

Differences between Civil and Criminal Negligence

Many dermatologists have asked me the difference between civil and criminal negligence. There is *no absolute or watertight differentiation* between cases of civil negligence and criminal negligence. If a patient decides to go to a civil court or consumer forum to ask for compensation, it is called *civil negligence*. However, if the harm caused to the patient is so great (e.g. death) that he decides to report the matter to police instead, it becomes a case of *criminal negligence*. A *patient can simultaneously sue the doctor in a civil court and can lodge a complaint with the police also*. Thus, the same case would be fought in both civil and criminal courts. In such a case, the same negligent action of the doctor would be civil as well as criminal in nature. *The differentiation between the two thus depends on patient's action* (Fig. 16.4, Table 16.1).

CHAPTER 16: Medicolegal Aspects of Lasers in Dermatological Practice

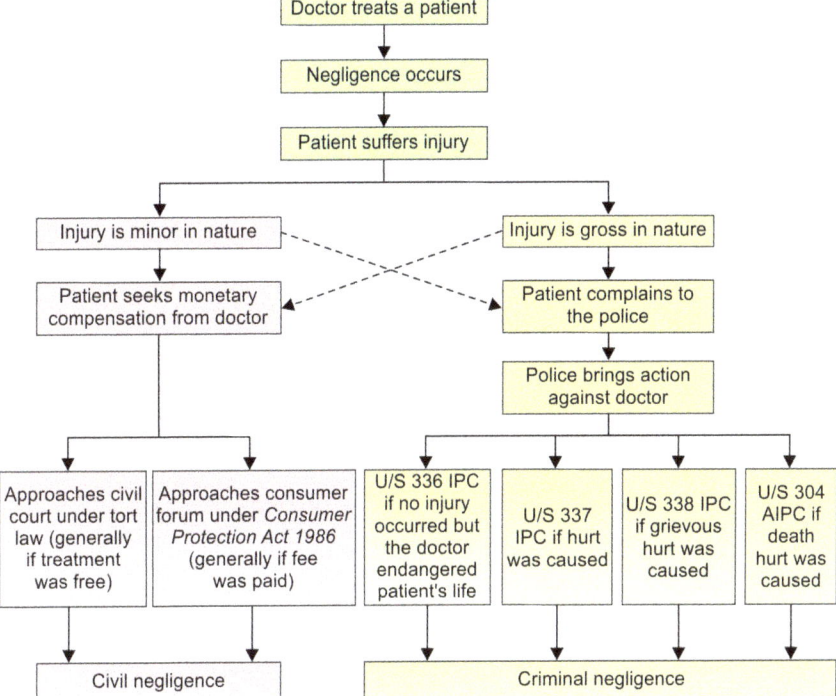

Fig. 16.4: Civil and criminal negligence. Action along the dotted line generally does not occur, but is possible.

Defenses against Negligence

In this section, I am going to tell you about a very little known defense, which is rarely taken by dermatologists, but which can be very effective in selected cases. This is *Novus actus interveniens (NAI)*. It *refers to a situation, where the doctor has been negligent, but a completely unexpected and unforeseen act happened which further worsened the patient's condition.*

Salient Features

1. The new act intervening should be completely unexpected and unforeseen. Sometimes referred to as an *Act of God*.
2. Breaks the chain of causation between the act of negligence and the resulting damage (Figs. 16.5A and B).
   Thus, injury no more remains a proximate cause of doctor's negligence. The concept can also be understood by falling dominoes (Fig. 16.6).
3. This defense is *not available in criminal negligence* or *criminal activity*.
4. *Analogy:* Student does not prepare for exams thinking that he can cram up on the last night → On the last night there is suddenly a failure of

Table 16.1: Differences between civil and criminal negligence.

S.No	Features	Civil negligence	Criminal negligence
1.	Doctor's act	*Doctor's act is merely negligent.* He did not foresee any risk in his act. He is simply forgetful or careless. *Negligence is generally not culpable enough to attract criminal liability*	*Doctor's act is reckless.* He could foresee an unreasonable risk, yet went ahead with his act. *Recklessness is culpable enough to attract criminal liability*
2.	Damage	Damage to the patient is generally minor (e.g. there is a scar on face; deformity of a minor part, e.g. finger; patient was unable to attend office for a few days, etc.)	Damage to the patient is generally very gross (e.g. a wrong leg was amputated, or death was caused)
3.	Action of patient	Patient brings suit in a civil court seeking monetary compensation	Patient complains to the police [an organ of State], which brings and action against doctor
4.	Prosecuting party	Patient	State
5.	Prosecuting lawyer	Lawyer engaged by patient	Public prosecutor
6.	Case citation	*Patient versus doctor*	*State versus doctor*
7.	Trial by	Civil court (under tort law) or consumer forum (under the *Consumer Protection Act 1986*)	Criminal court
8.	Action by the court	The court asks doctor to pay monetary compensation. No imprisonment is given to the doctor	The doctor may be awarded fine as well as imprisonment by the court
9.	What needs to be proved	Damage Violation of law need not be proved	Specific violation of law resulting in damage
10.	Level of proof	There should be a *balance of probabilities* in favor of negligence (**>50%** probability). Less effort on part of patient to prove negligence	The doctor's guilt must be proved beyond reasonable doubt (**>99%**). Greater effort required to prove negligence. (That is why generally in damages of a minor nature, the patient may seek only civil compensation and may not go to police at all)
11.	Doctor's defenses	Informed consent and contributory negligence are good defenses	Informed consent and contributory negligence not good defenses

CHAPTER 16: Medicolegal Aspects of Lasers in Dermatological Practice

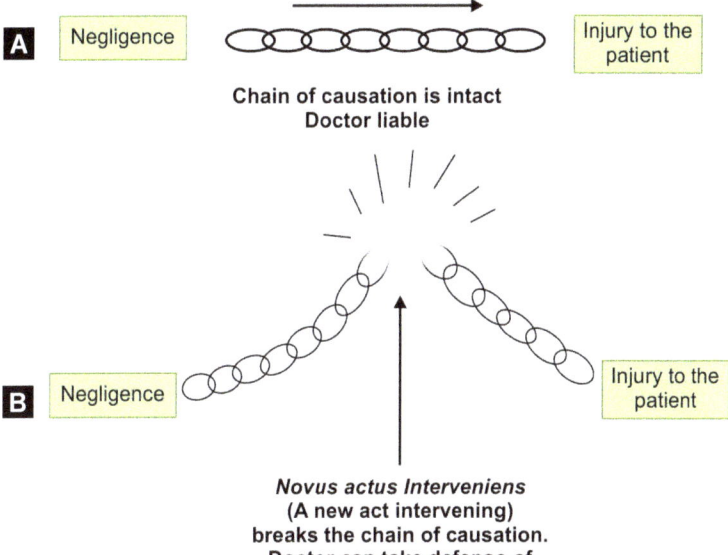

Figs. 16.5A and B: Concept of (A) proximate cause and (B) *novus actus interveniens*.

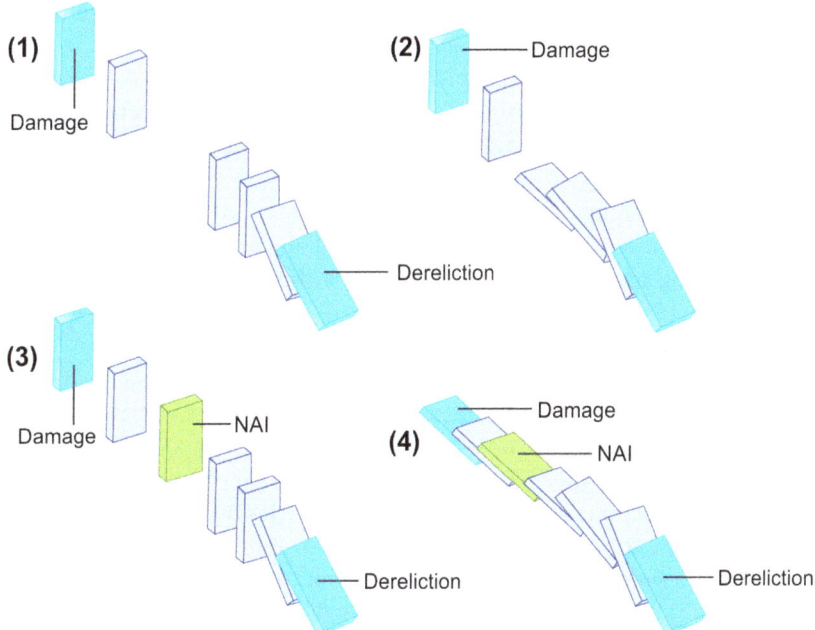

Fig. 16.6: Concept of proximate cause and *novus actus interveniens* as understood by falling dominoes. (1 and 2) Dereliction may not necessarily result in damage as shown here. (3 and 4) However, sometimes an unexpected event [*Novus Actus Interveniens* (NAI)] intervenes, causing the damage to occur.

electricity (an act of God) → Student cannot cram up → fails. Analysis – Student has to face consequences at two places – in the examination results (a stricter option, just like *criminal negligence*) and before his parents (a softer option, just like *civil negligence*) → His plea of NII (electricity failure on last night) will not help him pass the examination (loss of case in a stricter option), but he may perhaps convince his parents about his stand (a softer option).

5. *Examples*
   i. An myocardial infarction patient is under doctor's care since long → telephones doctor at 12 midnight that he is having severe chest pain → doctor agrees to come (duty established) → but does not take him seriously and gets busy in other affairs → patient phones again and again → doctor continues to ignore (dereliction) → at 3 am (i.e. after 3 hours) patient's wife phones that her husband's condition is worsening → doctor panics → sends an ambulance → instructs the driver to bring the patient back as fast as possible → as ambulance is coming back, it suffers a breakdown → No other alternative vehicle is available at that hour of night → for want of care, patient dies (damage) → wife sues doctor. Analysis - There was *duty, dereliction* and *damage*, but there was no direct causation. *Negligence (i.e. dereliction)* was *not the proximate cause of* death (*damage*). It was breakdown of the ambulance, which was completely unexpected and unforeseen. Plea of *NAI* may succeed.
   ii. Patient admitted to hospital treated with negligence → patient's condition starts getting worse → dengue breaks out in the hospital → patient dies of dengue → relative sues doctor. Analysis - same as above.
   iii. Patient being treated with negligence, develops a sudden complication necessitating an immediate operation → as patient is being prepared for operation, an earthquake occurs → operation cannot be performed → patient dies → relative sues doctor. Analysis - same as above.
   iv. Doctor D1 administers penicillin to patient P without testing for sensitivity → P suffers from anaphylaxis → immediately referred to a hospital H where he dies because of negligence of a different doctor D2 → *here negligence of D2 is NAI*, yet D1 can be successfully sued under section 304A Indian penal code (IPC) because NAI is not available for criminal negligence. However for compensation in the same case (civil negligence), D1 may succeed using this defense.
   v. Z stabs Y in the abdomen → Y is immediately taken to a doctor D → D is negligent in administering treatment → Y dies as a result → Z proves that Y could have been saved had there been no negligence → here medical negligence of D is NAI (as it was completely unexpected), yet Z cannot take the defense of NAI, because stabbing is criminal activity.

CHAPTER 16: Medicolegal Aspects of Lasers in Dermatological Practice

vi. A patient has mixed melasma, she comes to a laser center. The service provider promises a good result as the machine is US FDA approved. The patient develops persistent dyspigmentation. This is a classic case of negligence as in Indian skin melasma has consistently bad results and a US FDA approved laser is different from an FDA approved indication.

vii. A patient comes for leukocyte histamine release (LHR). She is investigated and there is an increase in the femoroacetabular impingement (FAI) and a high anti-Müllerian hormone (AMH). The patient is asked to take oral contraceptive pill (OCP) with spironolactone and told that the results will require a combination. The sessions are initiated and the patient is not happy with the results. Here there is no case made out as the patient had been told that the results would be better in combination with medical treatment.

6. Other ways that chain of causation may be broken: In tort law the chain of causation may be broken not only by natural events, but in 2 other ways:
    i. *By the claimant:* Best understood by a representative case. The claimant sustained an injury at work due to his employer's breach of duty. He strained his back and hips and his leg was prone to giving way. Whilst in this state he attempted to climb down a steep concrete staircase without a handrail unaided. He got part way down and felt his leg give way so he jumped 10 steps to the bottom. He suffered a fractured right ankle and was also left with a permanent disability. The defendant accepted liability for the injury sustained during his employment but disputed liability for further injuries resulting from the claimant's action in jumping down the stairs. It was held that the claimant's action amounted to an *NAI* because his action in attempting to climb the steps unaided knowing that his leg might give way was unreasonable. The defendant was therefore not liable for the injuries resulting from the incident on the stairs.
    ii. *By a third party:* Again best understood by a representative case. One Mr John was driving negligently in a tunnel → his car overturned in the tunnel → two police officers on motorcycles arrived at the scene → the senior officer instructed them both to ride their motorcycles to the other side of the tunnel and close the entrance to the tunnel as he had forgotten to close it earlier → they drove on the wrong side of the tunnel due to which one of the officers, Mr Knightly, had a head on collision with an oncoming vehicle driven by one Mr Cotton → Knightly sustained serious injuries → He brought an action against Mr John (whose initial negligence started the entire train of affairs), Mr Cotton and the senior officer who gave instructions to go to the other side of the tunnel. The main contentious point was whether Mr John remained liable or whether the actions of the other defendant's (Senior officer who gave instructions, Mr Cotton) and the claimant

amounted to an *NAI*. It was held that the senior officer's instructions and failure to close the entrance to the tunnel were negligent and broke the chain of causation; Mr John was thus not liable. The claimant was however entitled to full damages from the senior officer [*Knightley v John [1982] 1 WLR 349 (Court of Appeal)*].

HOW TO PREVENT MALPRACTICE CLAIMS?

An interesting insight into the types of complaints entertained in litigations in USA is given in Table 16.2. A few of them that can be of concern in India include deceptive trade practices, failure to properly hire, train, or supervise staff, failure to select appropriate laser and/or setting, not trained and/or certified to operate laser and failure to properly calibrate and maintain lasers.

We are adding one more to this list, which can be a valid cause of a civil suit, using non US FDA/CE approved lasers. With no certification in India, these are the certifications essential, which I dare say do not exist for most lasers sold.

Thus, prevention is better than facing malpractice claims. Following simple rules will help prevent malpractice claims to a great extent.

Patient Information and Documentation

Many malpractice claims arise due to lack of patient information, or sometimes inflated claims. Physicians should ensure that they themselves inform the patients and do not delegate the responsibility to nurses or paramedical staff. Informed consent must also be taken by dermatologists

Table 16.2: Common complaints in litigations in laser cases.

Cause of action	Specific allegations
Lack of informed consent	Failure to properly hire, train, or supervise staff
Fraud	Failure to properly perform treatment and/or operate laser
Loss of consortium	Failure to select appropriate laser and/or setting
Assault/battery	Failure to warn and/or inform of risk
Strict products liability	Failure to conduct test spot
Breach of contract	Not trained and/or certified to operate laser
Infliction of emotional distress	Failure to recognize and/or treat injury
Negligent misrepresentation	Failure to properly calibrate laser
Gross negligence	Failure to maintain laser
Recklessness	Failure to biopsy
Deceptive trade practices	Failure to supply goggles

themselves, and it must be written. A patient's signature on a preprinted consent form, which has not been preceded by a discussion with the physician, does not grant doctors free rein, and in the event of a legal dispute, such a form can be declared invalid. The optimal procedure consists of a thorough discussion, after which the patient is given a consent form to which handwritten additions are made as necessary. Detailed information should be provided about the diagnosis; the nature, extent, and process involved in the planned treatment; potential short- and long-term adverse effects; possible alternative treatments; and the costs to be expected. Rare concomitant effects, adverse effects, and risks should also be discussed if they are typical for the procedure in question.

Treatment should not be performed on the same day the discussion is held; patients should have the chance to make a decision without being pressured for time and without being affected by the psychological burden of the procedure awaiting them. Patient documentation should include information about discussions between the physician and patient, the preoperative diagnosis and histologic findings (to whatever degree present or necessary), the indication for laser treatment, test treatments, the kind of anesthesiology, the kind of laser and parameters of application, the results of treatment, and any concomitant reactions, adverse effects, and complications (intra- or postoperative, infections, late complications, etc.). Especially in the case of cosmetic procedures, additional photographic documentation is recommended. This is relevant from a forensic perspective, as well as being useful if the patient should question the success of the treatment.

Some clinicians prefer to write a risk, benefit and alternatives (RBA) note together with a written informed consent.

It is wise to seek informed consent for each type of laser that is operated by the physician. Each laser system functions in a unique fashion. The same laser created by various competitors may differ in terms of treatment settings and potential side effects. For this reason, establishing a relationship with the laser company for support is advantageous for the physician. Furthermore, ensuring that the medical device is FDA approved for patient therapy could minimize liability.

Though a detailed consent form is given in the online access of the book, we are detailing the essentials in a consent form, which can be remembered by the mnemonic LASER (Abel Torres et al.) (Table 16.3).

Training

Malpractice claims are mostly due to professional errors, which in turn, are due to lack of training and experience. Thus, training must be strengthened. The ideal method of ensuring thorough training is to establish teaching centers for laser treatment in qualified, certified offices or clinics. In such institutions, guidelines should be taught on topics including didactic,

Table 16.3: Ideal components of a consent form (mnemonic **LASERS**).

Liability waiver	A patient needs to be told that Laser procedures are not reimbursable and no other procedure will be shown in lieue of it !
Anesthesia type	There are risks associated with all types of anesthesia, including topical (see Chapter on Drugs)
Surveillance	Observations, outcomes and side effects on the postoperative record documents treatment course in the best interest of the patient
Expectations	A no guarantee clause should be emphasized as no indications has definite cures
Revocation of consent	Offer the option of letting the patient refuse treatment at any time especially if it alters outcome
Snapshot	Photographs are to be taken specifically for documenting results and are confidential unless specified

hands-on, and laser-specific clinical techniques. Standards of practice are sometimes handled as if they are top secret information. This should not be done; instead, they should be officially instructed and published. In the US and some other developed nations, an oral and written examination is a must for every dermatologist in practice. It serves as a rational and fair strategy to assess theoretical and practical proficiency objectively after a defined period of continuing education is completed. Sadly, in India, there is no such program. If such programs are started and widely followed, these may serve to reduce professional errors, and in turn, malpractice claims.

In case a physician is using lasers in dermatology, he must have dermatologic training in addition to laser-specific training.

Do not Make Unrealistic Claims

It has been seen that many malpractice claims originate as a result of failed patient expectations, which in the first place are raised very high almost to unrealistic levels. Some examples are *removal of 80-90% of the hair in 2-3 sessions* or *1064 nm Nd:YAG laser is superbly suited for removing moles and dark hyperpigmentation spots*. Experience has shown that whenever the patient has been given realistic assurances, the incidence of malpractice claims remains low.

Handling the Press

Proliferation of print and electronic media in India, has caused journalists to look around for cases to feed their 24 × 7 news channels. Medical malpractice cases, being inherently potential target rating point (TRP) enhancers are among the most hotly pursued stories by print and television journalists. If for example, a patient has been injured by laser treatment, the journalist would approach some top laser practitioners and would like to know their views on it. It would be wise for laser practitioners not to criticize their colleagues for two reasons—it is unethical to pass derogatory remarks against a colleague, and secondly, the case may be in court and any comments may cause an unduly adverse outcome in the case. The results of some surveys indicate that doctors need to be trained to handle the press.

HOW TO HANDLE A MALPRACTICE CLAIM IF IT DOES OCCUR?

Involvement in a lawsuit as a defendant may be in a civil or criminal case. Experience has shown that a vast majority of medical malpractice cases in India are civil cases, which is good news for doctors, because at most they would entail payment of damages and not imprisonment. A minority of cases (generally those in which death has occurred), are fought in the criminal court, in which there may be imprisonment to the doctor. However, there is no bar for a patient to go to a criminal court even for minor injuries (section 337 IPC) or most surprisingly even if no injury has occurred (section 336 IPC). The latter case may be unbelievable to some, but there is a distinct theoretical possibility of this occurring. The analogy is fast, reckless driving through a city. Even if no one is injured, the driver is still liable, because he could have caused injury by engaging in such a rash and negligent act. Similarly, if a doctor is rash and negligent in using lasers, and if a patient has ample proof of it, he can approach the court, even if no injury has occurred to him. Thankfully such situations are extremely rare.

It must be noted that a patient can sue for compensation in a consumer court only if he has paid fees to the doctor. If no professional fee has been paid, the patient cannot invoke a consumer court, but he can still approach a civil court under tort law. Generally, such cases drag on for years in India and are a cause of worry for doctors.

The most worrying cases are criminal cases, in which the patient complains to the police, and the police lodge a case against the doctor. In laser applications of dermatology, such cases are likely to be extremely rare, simply because grave laser injuries are virtually unknown, and as already stated, the patient generally would refrain from going to the police until and unless the injury is very grave and debilitating.

Countersuits

One way to deal with a suit is filing a countersuit. A countersuit is an action brought by a physician against the patient (the plaintiff in the original malpractice action), as a retaliation strategy. It is based on the maxim, *attack is the best form of defense*. This strategy works best, if the laser practitioner is sure that the malpractice claim is mala fide and unjust. The countersuit movement began in the mid-1970s with enthusiastic support by the medical profession in response to the dramatic rise in medical malpractice suits, many of which were perceived as lacking substantial merit. It must be remembered that courts would not take this approach very positively if the laser practitioner was actually at fault. They have rejected most countersuits, which were filed merely as an attacking policy. Courts follow a public policy interest in ensuring that injured parties have free and open access to the judicial system.

Alternative Dispute Resolution

A far simpler and better approach is alternative dispute resolution (ADR). It *refers to dispute resolution techniques that help plaintiffs and defendants resolve conflicts outside of the courtroom.* It is advantageous to both patients and doctors. Patient can save time from litigation and focus efforts on healing. Money saved on lawyers and court goes directly to the patient. Many hospitals in the US have embraced *early apology* programs, where physicians and hospital administrators reach out to the injured patient and express sympathy about the adverse event. This protects the natural doctor–patient relationship as well as encourages dialogue.

Mediation and Arbitration

The most popular ADR techniques are *mediation* and *arbitration*. They differ in both their binding nature and their formality. *Mediation is simple negotiation that is aided by an impartial mediator*. It is nonbinding, meaning that if a settlement cannot be reached, the plaintiff may pursue his claim in court. *Arbitration* is more court-like, with an arbiter hearing both sides much like a judge would. Similarly, there are rules for how and when to talk, and how to present evidence. Most importantly, it is binding, meaning that the judgment of the arbiter is final and litigation is not an option.

Mediation

Mediation has had excellent success where implemented, both in terms of cost-containment and satisfaction for both parties. From the plaintiff's perspective, mediation offers more flexibility than litigation, which only offers money as a remedy. Experience has shown that patients who come for laser cosmetic surgery are, by and large from upper echelons of society and often do not engage in litigation for money. Many sue for nonmonetary reasons, such as the desire for disclosure of information or the desire to hear an apology or explanation of what went wrong. In the US, for example, rather than just receiving money, some plaintiffs wish for a scholarship to be established in their family's name, or like their deceased's story told to incoming nurses or medical students to help prevent similar adverse events in the future.

Similar trends are appearing among the rich patients in India. For these reasons mediation often suits plaintiffs' needs better. Non-monetary aspects like the ones mentioned above are withheld in a litigious environment.

Arbitration

Arbitration is different from mediation. It is more acrimonious and expensive, being more trial-like than mediation. It is longer and more expensive than mediation, but much shorter and less expensive than court trials. Like court trials, arbitration can only offer money as a form of redress, eliminating the more creative and satisfying solutions offered in mediation.

Pretreatment Arbitration Agreement

Laser practitioners may want to undergo a pretreatment arbitration agreement. Under this arrangement, patients agree to arbitration as a condition of being seen in the first place. This has become an increasingly popular form of arbitration in the US. However, it suffers from the great disadvantage that it is awkward to discuss adversarial postures during the initial physician–patient visit itself.

Benefits of Mediation and Arbitration

Benefits of mediation and arbitration are almost 100% avoidance of litigation. Thus, these are very appealing to everyone alike—doctor, patient and even the insurer, as even a successful defense can cost a lot. There is a private and informal setting outside of the courtroom. In case of arbitration, the decision of arbiter is binding and there are no appeals processes. It occurs as scheduled and without delay, unlike many court cases. Damage awards tend to be more predictable and usually are more in line with settlement values than those afforded by court trials.

CONCLUSION

Laser cosmetic surgery can legally be done only by a person qualified in modern medicine and surgery. Any other person engaging in laser cosmetic surgery can only do so under supervision of a qualified dermatologist. If dermatologist is sure, the malpractice suit by the patient is mala fide, he can respond by filing a countersuit. If on the other hand, he knows he has been negligent, the best approach is mediation and arbitration.

Though varied medical specialties can be affected by litigations including plastic surgery, and otolaryngologists, we should be concerned about what plagues our own specialty. The take home messages, would be to be very cautious with certain procedures, like acne scars, photoaging procedures, pigmented (dermal) disorders and of course vascular disorders. The trend of combining multiple lasers in a single disorder, which had little sense except in photoaging, is a huge mistake and can actually lead to more litigations in case of complications. With very little concrete science on combination procedures, it is better not to intervene and remember with lasers the photographic evidence of complications can be persistent and in litiginous times can be a source of unnecessary censure and stress

BIBLIOGRAPHY

1. Abel Torres, Tejas Desai, Alpesh Desai, et al. Medicolegal issues (Documentation/Informed Consent). Nouri K (Ed.). Lasers in Dermatology and Medicine. London: Springer-Verlag Limited; 2011.
2. Greve B, Raulin C. Professional errors caused by lasers and intense pulsed light technology in dermatology and aesthetic medicine: Preventive strategies and case studies. Dermatol Surg. 2002;28(2):156-61.
3. Hammes S, Karsai S, Metelmann HR, et al. Treatment errors resulting from use of lasers and IPL by medical laypersons: Results of a nationwide survey. J Dtsch Dermatol Ges. 2013;11(2):149-56.
4. Jalian HR, Jalian CA, Avram MM. Common causes of injury and legal action in laser surgery. JAMA Dermatol. 2013;149(2):188-93.
5. Jalian HR, Jalian CA, Avram MM. Increased risk of litigation associated with laser surgery by nonphysician operators. JAMA Dermatol. 2014;150(4):407-11.
6. Svider PF, Carron MA, Zuliani GF, et al. Lasers and losers in the eyes of the law: Liability for head and neck procedures. JAMA Facial Plast Surg. 2014;16(4):277-83.

ANNEXURE 1: MEDICOLEGAL ASPECTS OF LASERS IN DERMATOLOGICAL PRACTICE

CONSUMER PROTECTION ACT

Consumer Protection Act 1986

[syn, CPA, COPRA] is a legal statute whose purpose is to provide for better protection of the interests of consumers.

Background

On 9th April 1985, the general assembly of United Nations at its 39th session adopted resolution no. 39/248, which recommended a set of guidelines for consumer protection. The Secretary General of the UN was authorized to persuade member countries to adopt these guidelines through policy changes or law. Following this, India passed Consumer Protection Act (CPA). *It came into force on 24 December, 1986, and was amended in 1991, 1993 and 2002.*

Salient Features

- *Aims and objectives:*
    - *To protect the interest of consumers* - of different commodities (e.g. TV, car) and services (e.g. banking, airline travel). It was seen that they paid but did not get quality goods or services. Before this Act, there was no forum, where the harassed consumer could appeal
    - *Medical services* - When the Act was passed in 1986, *medical services were not included in the Act. It was only after Supreme Court's VP Shantha's decision (please see below), that medical services were included in the Act.*
- *Some relevant definitions:*
    - *Consumer* - is any person who buys any goods or avails of any service by paying money *[section 2(1)(d)]*.
    - *Service* - is any person who buys any goods or avails of any service by paying money *[section 2(1)(d)]*.
- *Services included under the Act* – banking, financing insurance, transport, processing, supply of electrical or other energy, board or lodging or both, housing construction, entertainment, amusement, purveying of news or other information *[section 2(1)(o)]*.
- *Services excluded*:
    - Service provided *free of charge* (rationale – one cannot find fault with free service).

Box 16.3: Memory aid 1 – Services excluded from COPRA.

Free of charge
1. Free service
2. Contract of service [section 2(1)(o)]

- Service provided under a *contract* of *personal service* (rationale – the person providing service (servant) is under constant instructions and supervision from master. So master cannot find fault with his servant's service) [section 2(1)(o)] (Box 16.3).
- *Deficiency:* Means any fault, imperfection, shortcoming or inadequacy in the quality, nature and manner of performance which is required to be maintained by or under any law for the time being in force or has been undertaken to be performed by a person in pursuance of a contract or otherwise in relation to any service [section 2(1)(g)].

Consumer Disputes Redressal Agencies

1. There are three agencies:
    1. *District Forum (DF)* [section 9(a)]
    2. *State Commission* [section 9(b)]
    3. *National Commission (NC)* [section 9(c)].

Constitution and Jurisdiction

(i) District Forum
Consists of:
1. *President:* Serving or retired District Judge, appointed by the State Government on the recommendation of a *selection committee* consisting of the
    a. The president of the State Commission – Chairman
    b. Secretary, Law Department of the State – Member and
    c. Secretary, in-charge of the Department dealing with consumer affairs in the State – Member.

(ii) Two other members: One of these shall be a *woman.* They should be older than 35 years.

Should possess a bachelor's degree from a recognized university. Should be persons of ability, integrity and standing, and have adequate knowledge and experience of at least 10 years in dealing with problems relating to economics, law, commerce, accountancy, industry public affairs or administration. These same qualifications are also prescribed for members of State Commission and National Commission.

Significantly, the word *medicine* does not appear here. This point was raised by the IMA in *Indian Medical Association Vs. VP Shantha (1995)* (please see below). Members of State Commission and National Commission also need not *have adequate knowledge and experience* in medicine.

Every member holds office for a term of 5 years or up to the age of 65 year, whichever is earlier *(section 10)*
2. *Jurisdiction:* Up to claims of Rs. 20 lakhs *(section 11)*
3. *Powers:* For summoning and enforcing the attendance of any defendant or witness and examining the witness on oath and production of any document, etc. as evidence, the District Forum shall have the same powers as are vested in a civil court under Code of Civil Procedure, 1908 *[section 13(4)].*

(iii) State Commission
Consists of:
- *President:* Serving or retired Judge of a High court, appointed by the State Govt in consultation with the Chief Justice of High Court and on the recommendation of a selection committee.
- *Two or more other members:* Of which one shall be a woman. Other qualifications [including age] same as those for members of DF. Every member holds office for a term of 5 years or up to the age of 67 year, whichever is earlier. Members are eligible for re-appointment for another term of 5 years or up to the age of 67 year, whichever is earlier (section 16).

Jurisdiction:
- *Original jurisdiction*—between claims of ₹ 20 lakhs–1 crore (section 17).
- *Appellate jurisdiction*—appeals against the orders of District Forum.

(iv) National Commission
Consists of:
- *President:* Serving or retired Judge of the Supreme court, appointed by the Central Government in consultation with the Chief Justice of India and on the recommendation of a selection committee.
- Four or more other members—of which one shall be a woman. Other qualifications [including age] same as those for members of DF. There cannot be greater than 50% members from a judicial background. Every member holds office for a term of 5 years or up to the age of 70 years, whichever is earlier and shall not be eligible for reappointment. (section 20).

Jurisdiction:
- *Original jurisdiction*: Claims is greater than 1 crore
- *Appellate jurisdiction*: Appeals against the orders of any State Commission

Multiple benches—of National Commission and State Commission to function for speedy disposal of cases (Table 16.4).

Manner of Making Complaints

1. A complaint in relation to any goods sold or delivered or any service provided may be filed with a *DF* by
    a. The consumer. If consumer dies, his legal hair or representative
    b. Any recognized consumer association

Table 16.4: Comparison between various consumer forum agencies.

S.no.	Criteria	District Forum	State Commission	National Commission
1.	Total members	3	3	5
2.	Chairman	District Judge	High Court Judge	Supreme Court Judge
3.	Members	2 [1 of these must be a woman]	2 [1 of these must be a woman]	4 [1 of these must be a woman]
4.	Age of members including that of chairman	35–65 years	35–67 years	35–70 years
5.	Qualification of members	10 years experience in economics, law, commerce, accountancy, industry public affairs or administration	Same as in DF	Same as in DF
6.	Claims dealt with	Up to ₹ 20 lakhs	₹20 lakhs – 1 Crore	>1 Crore
7.	Jurisdiction	In district where dispute arose and claim is of above amount	• *Direct* – Claim is of above amount + dispute arose in concerned state; • *Appeal* – from district forum. Claim may be of any amount	• *Direct* – Claim is of above amount + dispute arose in any state except Jammu and Kashmir; • *Appeal*—from State and National Commission. Claim may be of any amount
8.	Time limit of filing original complaint	Within 2 years	Within 2 years	Within 2 years
9.	Time limit of filing appeal	-	Within 30 days of the order of District Forum	Within 30 days of the order of State Commission

    c. One or more consumers, where there are numerous consumers having the same interest, with the permission of the District Forum

    d. Central or the State Government. *Every complaint must be accompanied by a prescribed fee* (section 12).

The fee is payable in the form of crossed Demand Draft drawn on a nationalized bank or through a crossed Indian Postal Order drawn in favor of the Registrar of the State Commission and payable at the respective place where the State Commission or the National Commission is situated [Rule 9A(1) of *The Consumer Protection Rules, 1987]*.

Table 16.5: Fees payable for making complaints to the district forum.

S.no.	Value of goods or services and the compensation claimed [in ₹]	Amount of fee payable [in ₹]
	I. District Forum	
1.	Up to 1 lakh rupees–For complainants who are under the Below Poverty Line holding *Antyodaya Anna Yojana* Cards	Nil
2.	Up to 1 lakh rupees – For complaints other than *Antyodaya Anna Yojana* card holders.	100
3.	1 lakh - 5 lakhs	200
4.	5 lakh - 10 lakhs	400
5.	10 lakhs - 20 lakhs	500
	II. State Commission	
6.	20 lakhs - 50 lakhs	2000
7.	50 lakhs - 1 Crore	4000
	III. National Commission	
8.	> 1 Crore	5000

The concerned authority shall deposit the amount of fee so received into the *Consumer Welfare Fund* of the respective State and where such fund is not established, into the Receipt Account of the State Government and in the case of the National Commission, to the Consumer Welfare Fund of the Central Government *[Rule 9A(2)]* (Table 16.5).

The complainants who are under the Below Poverty Line shall be entitled for the exemption of payment of fee only on production of an attested copy of the *Antyodaya Anna Yojana* cards *[Rule 9A(3)]*.

2. *On receipt of a complaint* - The District Forum may allow the complaint to be proceeded with or rejected (after giving an opportunity to the complainant of being heard). Admissibility of the complaint shall ordinarily be decided within 21 days from the date on which the complaint was received *[section 12(3)]*.
3. *Frivolous or vexatious complaints* – are dismissed after recording the reasons in writing. The complainant may be asked to pay a cost of up to ₹ 10,000 to the opposite party *(section 26)*.

Procedure

1. Speedy trials:
    i. Every complaint is heard as early as possible and must preferably be decided within 3 months.
    ii. No adjournment are ordinarily granted by DF unless sufficient cause is shown and the reasons for grant of adjournment have been recorded in writing by the Forum [section 13(3A)].

2. If complaint refers to any service, the Forum shall refer a copy of such complaint to the opposite party directing him to give his version of the case within a period of 30 days. An extension of 15 days may be granted [section 13(2)(a)]. Notices may be served even by FAX [section 28(2)].
3. It is not necessary for parties to be represented by lawyers.
4. Every proceeding before the DF shall be deemed to be a judicial proceeding within the meaning of section 193 and 228 of IPC, and DF shall be deemed to be a civil court.
5. *Appeals against orders of District Forum:*
    i. Must be made to the State Commission within 30 days from the date of order.
    ii. If there was sufficient cause for appeal later than 30 days, State Commission can entertain it.
    iii. *Fees* - appellant must deposit 50% of amount ordered by DF or ₹ 25,000 whichever is less (section 15).
6. *Appeals against orders of State Commission*:
    i. Must be made to the National Commission within 30 days from the date of order.
    ii. If there was sufficient cause for appeal later than 30 days, National Commission can entertain it.
    iii. *Fees* - appellant must deposit 50% of amount ordered by SC or ₹ 35,000 whichever is less (section 19).
7. *Appeals against orders of National Commission*:
    i. National Commission is empowered to review its orders to avoid rush to the Supreme Court.
    ii. However even if review does not give relief to a party, the appeal must be made to the Supreme Court within 30 days from the date of order.
    iii. If there was sufficient cause for appeal later than 30 days, Supreme Court can entertain it
    iv. *Fees* - appellant must deposit 50% of amount ordered by SC or ₹ 50,000 whichever is less (section 23).
8. *Ensuring payment of compensation* – To ensure payment of compensation, the Consumer Courts (DF, SC, NC) can attach the property of the opposite party and dispose it to recover amount due to the complainant. District Collector would help the courts to recover this amount.
9. *Finality of orders* – If no appeal has been preferred against order of a DF, SC or NC, such order shall be final [section 24].

Limitation Period

The DF, the State Commission or the National Commission normally will not admit a complaint unless it is filed within 2 years from the date on which negligence was committed. But under special circumstances complaints after 2 years may be entertained if the Forum or Commission is satisfied that there is sufficient reason for doing so, and it must record in writing, the reasons for entertaining such late complaints *[section 24A]*.

Who is Covered Under COPRA

1. All doctors and hospitals who have charged for their services. Doctors and hospitals who have not charged can still be sued, but in *normal civil courts* under *tort law*. The pecuniary jurisdiction of district courts is ₹ 2 Crore (raised from ₹ 20 Lakh to 2 Crore in November 2012). Claims higher than this, must go to High Courts directly.
2. All doctors and hospitals (including Government hospitals, health centers, dispensaries, etc.) who perform *partial charitable services*, i.e. who charge from few patients only (rich) and other (poor) are not charged. All (both rich and poor) can get benefit under COPRA.

Who is Immune from COPRA

1. Doctors and hospitals [including Government hospitals] which are doing a *completely charitable servi*ce not charging anyone (i.e. neither rich nor poor are charged).
2. Hospitals charging a token amount for registration purpose only – It is *not payment* for the purposes of COPRA.

Criticisms

- Criticisms before inclusion of doctors under CPA—Please see VP Shantha case below
- Current criticisms—Please see Table 16.6.

Indian Medical Association Vs. VP Shantha (1995)

1. *Citation: Indian Medical Association Vs. VP Shantha & ORS. 1996 AIR 550; 1995 SCC (6) 651.*
2. *Facts:* VP Shantha's husband died as a result of medical negligence of Cosmopolitan Hospital, Kerala. VP Shantha claimed compensation under CPA 1986. The hospital claimed that doctors were not covered under CPA, as they were exempt under section 2(1)(o) of the CPA, 1986. Claim was however awarded by Kerala State Commission. The decision was upheld by National Commission. Cosmopolitan Hospital appealed but Indian Medical Association interjected as a third party, fearing an adverse decision against doctors.
3. *Issues:*
    i. *The foremost issue was whether or not doctors were covered under COPRA?* The contention of IMA was *that they were not covered*, which was clear from the fact that according to COPRA, members of DF, SC and NC should have adequate knowledge and experience

Table 16.6: Arguments for and against consumer courts.

S.no.	Arguments against Consumer courts	Arguments in favor of Consumer courts
1.	Civil courts are already there → consumer court is another type of civil court → hence we do not need consumer courts	Civil courts already present are slow. The general refrain in the country is "*criminal cases in this country are decided in decades; civil cases in generations*". Consumer courts are fast-track versions of civil courts
2.	Consumer courts are fast because they hurry through the cases → Thus all pros and cons of the case are not considered	There is no such evidence. Furthermore, the level of appeal is up to Supreme Court
3.	Doctors either do not take risky cases for fear of litigation, or order unnecessary tests in order to be doubly sure of diagnosis (defensive medicine). This has increased cost for patients.	There is no such evidence. Furthermore, the level of appeal is up to Supreme Court
4.	Since court fee is low any one can approach the court [frivolous complaints] → increases litigation; wastes valuable time and energy of doctor	Low fees in fact takes doors of justice closer to poorer people. Frivolous complaints are dealt with by heavy fines
5.	As there is no scope for testimony by medical experts, the Forum and Commission come to their own conclusions which may be wrong	This is not true. Medical evidence is allowed
6.	These courts have increased trust deficit between doctor and patient	Doctor need not mistrust his patient, if he pursues his profession honestly

in economics, law, commerce, accountancy, industry public affairs or administration. *The word medicine had been specifically left out*, which meant that legislature never intended doctors to be included under the Act. Even if one assumes that doctors are covered under the Act, the members cannot make an informed decision, since they are not qualified in medicine.

    ii. If at all doctors are covered under COPRA, whether, and in what circumstances, a medical practitioner can be regarded as rendering *service* under section 2(1)(o) of the CPA, 1986.

    iii. Whether the service rendered at a hospital or nursing home can be regarded as *service* under section 2(1)(o) of the Act.

4. *Existing law at the time:*
    i. Doctors were *not included* in CPA, since the *inclusionary provisions* of section 2(1)(o) (which defines service) specifically failed to mention their profession, while mentioning other professions such as banking, finance, insurance, etc.

CHAPTER 16: Medicolegal Aspects of Lasers in Dermatological Practice

  ii. *Section 2(1)(o) of CPA*, had *two exclusionary provisions. Service* did not include
    a. Service rendered free of charge and
    b. Service rendered under a *contract of personal service*. Doctors were excluded, because they were supposed to render a service under a *contract personal service*.
5. *Judges* - Agrawal, SC, Kuldip Singh, Hansaria BL – 3 judge Supreme Court Bench
6. *Lawyers for Indian Medical Association* - K Parasaran, Harish Salve, AM Singhvi, Krishnamani, S Balakrishnan
7. *Lawyer for VP Shantha* - Rajeev Dhavan
8. *Trial and Judgment* – Doctors *would be included* under CPA 1986 henceforth.
9. *Reasoning:*
    i. *On qualifications of members of various consumer forums*:
       a. It was not correct to say that since members of various consumer forums are not experts in medicine, they cannot deal with related matters. Quoting from Robin CA White's *The Administration of Justice*, 2nd Ed, pp. 345, the court said that lay adjudicators are in fact superior to professional judges in the application of general standards of conduct, in their notions of reasonableness, fairness and good faith and that they act as *an antidote against excessive technicality*.
       b. If it is presumed that members must have specialized knowledge in the field related to complaint, *then it would lead to impossible situations*. DF and St Comm. can have only 2 members besides president and NC can have 4. It meant that complaints of only 2 specialties could be dealt with at initial level.
       c. There is a safeguard of appeal against the orders. [Comment - The court however did not elaborate upon how this helps a non-expert in medicine to opine upon medical matters]
    ii. The Court specifically differentiated the meanings of *contract for service* and *contract of service*
       a. *Contract for service* – is a contract whereby one party undertakes to render services (such as professional or technical services) to another, in which the *service provider is not subjected to a detailed direction and control*. The provider exercises professional or technical skill and *uses his or her own knowledge and discretion*.
       b. *Contract of service* implies a relationship of master and servant and involves an *obligation to obey orders in the work to be performed and as to its mode and manner of performance*.
    iii. Doctor is a professional, and is thus *not subjected to a detailed direction and control of the patient*. A simple example (although not cited by court) is a *patient under anesthesia*; he is in no position to

Box 16.4: Memory aid 2 – Differences between contract for service and contract of service.

- **Contract for service** - Servant is NOT under *detailed direction and control* of master. Doctor is under a *contract for service*. *This type of contract is NOT exempt from the purview of CPA.*
- **Contract of service** - Servant is under *detailed direction and control* of master (Masters offers control). An ordinary sweeper is under a *contract of service*. *This type of contract is exempt from the purview of CPA.*

exercise any control over his surgeon. This is in sharp contrast to a domestic servant, who is unskilled and is under detailed direction and control of his master for every moment. Thus, doctor is under a 'contract for service' and not under a 'contract of service'. A domestic servant is under a '*contract of service*' (Box 16.4).

10. *Significance and Outcome* – Doctors were henceforth subject to the provisions of CPA
11. *Major criticisms*:
    i. *Double control* - Doctors are already under the supervisory control of MCI. They cannot behave like ordinary traders (e.g. advertisement, putting up large hoardings, employment of touts, taking favors from drug companies, etc.) as such acts would attract penal action by MCI. Still CPA treats them as traders. Thus, they get the worst deal from both.
    ii. *Relationship of trust* - Doctor-patient relationship is a *relationship of trust*. It must not be and cannot be controlled by legislation.
    iii. Doctors started resorting to defensive medicine, and the costs were ultimately passed on to the patients. Thus, it became lose-lose situation.

CHAPTER 17

Complications and their Management

Kabir Sardana, Ganesh S Pai

INTRODUCTION

There are very few studies that examine complications across different lasers. Most studies are focused on a particular device.

A recent study (Zelickson Z) that used the Manufacturer and User Facility Device Experience database (MAUDE) from 2006 to 2011 found that the most common cosmetic laser treatments with complications was hair removal. About 30% of laser surgery complications were due to user error, 20% device malfunction, and 4% due to patient error.

COMMON DEVICES AND THEIR COMPLICATIONS

Lumenis had the most (204) complications, followed by Candela (66), and Rhytec (65). The list of commonly reported devices causing side effects is given in Table 17.1. Intense pulsed light (IPL) devices had the most (142) complications, followed by plasma radiofrequency (RF) (65), and RF monopolar devices (59). The five most common complications were burns (36%), scarring (19.4%), pigmentation damage (8.5%), blistering (2.4%), and infection (8%). In darker skin types, postinflammatory hyperpigmentation (PIH) is by far the most important side effect.

A list of device-specific complications is given in Table 17.2. The IPL and the RF report the highest complications while the fractional devices and Q-switched (Qsw) lasers are safer. Notably the erbium-doped yttrium aluminum garnet laser (Er:YAG) has no complications reported which makes it the ideal laser in Indian skin type for ablative procedures.

With little by way of reporting, there is no database in India of the side effects, but the incidence would largely reflect the studies published.

OVERVIEW OF COMMON COMPLICATIONS

Pain

This is a universal feature of all laser procedures and a certain degree of interindividual variation is seen.

Table 17.1: A summary of complications of lasers.*

Device	Complications reported
IPL	142
Plasma devices	65
RF monopolar	59
CO_2	57
810 diode	39
1,064 nm Nd:YAG	37
755 nm alexandrite laser	29
NA fractional (NAFR)	21
Pulsed dye laser	15
Nd:YAG	6
Ablative fractional	3
RF (fractional, needle, suction)	2
Thulium	1
Fractional CO_2	
USG	

*(MAUDE): US Food and Drug Administration (FDA) manufacturer and user-facility device experience (Zelickson Z, et al.)
(Nd:YAG: neodymium-doped yttrium aluminum garnet lasers; IPL: intense pulsed light; RF: radiofrequency; USG: ultrasonography)

Table 17.2: A list of common side effects associated with common laser devices.*

Device	Common device complications
Intense pulsed light	Burn Blister Scar Pigmentation
Plasma resurfacing	Infection Scar Burn Pigmentation
Radiofrequency monopolar	Burn Blister Scar Pigmentation
Carbon dioxide	Scar Burn Pigmentation
810 diode	Burn Pigmentation Scar Blister

*(MAUDE): US Food and Drug Administration (FDA) manufacturer and user facility device experience

Prevention and Treatment

Cooling devices have played a large role in minimizing pain and optimizing treatment of specific lesions and are crucial in pigmented skin.

The use of anesthesia is important, though in some, it may not be required. For fractional lasers, we have found that pretreatment icepack cooling is adequate for most patients. This also has the added advantage of a modicum of cost saving for the patient. Some lasers [the pulsed dye laser (PDL)] often do not require pretreatment anesthesia. In some case, infiltration anesthesia may be required.

One protocol includes topical lidocaine or tetracaine application with another approach being a combination of hot compresses, topical lidocaine and oral anxiolytics (diazepam or ketorolac) for resurfacing procedures.

Erythema and Edema

They are both expected to occur and in fractional lasers, they are usually transient (Fig. 17.1). Some reasons for excessive edema include excess pulse stacking or passes, treatment of periocular areas, and use of high energy settings. Concomitant use of tretinoin is also a predisposing factor.

Prevention and Treatment

A simple method to resolve this is the use of post-treatment cold packs, head elevation and short-term use of topical steroids (Fucidin H^{TM}).

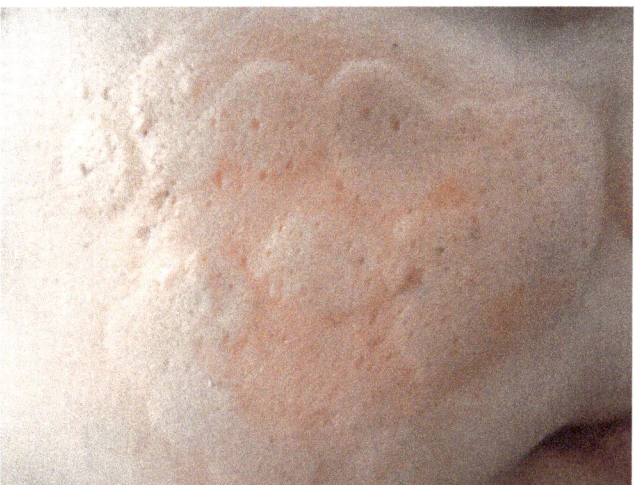

Fig. 17.1: Edema and erythema seen immediately after Er:Glass therapy for scars. Mild and reversible. Icepack suffices in most cases. A mild steroid can be used for 1–2 days to prevent postinflammatory hyperpigmentation.

Crusting and Vesiculation

Crusting and vesiculation are manifestations of epidermal damage in certain indications (Qsw lasers). It is bound to occur and the patient should be forewarned about it (Fig. 17.2). In fractional lasers, a certain degree of post-therapy "areal density" marks are also evident, which resolve in 3–5 days (Fig. 17.3).

Prevention and Treatment

- In most nonablative procedures, we usually give topical aloe vera gel (Jula™/Alokem 75™) or a bland nonsensitizing moisturizer (Cetaphil™/Physiogel™) with a topical steroid (Fucidin H™) and advise the patient not to remove the crust manually. Saline compresses are advised which help in rapid removal of the crust.
- For ablative procedures, a petrolatum-based preparation is advisable (Epiceram™, Eucerin™, Secalia™) with the use of a nonsensitizing antibiotic (Fucidin).
- Sunscreen (physical block) is advised till complete healing.

Purpura

Purpura results when there is damage to small vessels and subsequent extravasation of red blood cells. It is common following treatment with the PDL and is, in fact, a therapeutic end point when treating certain vascular lesions with short pulse durations and high fluences (so-called purpura-mode).

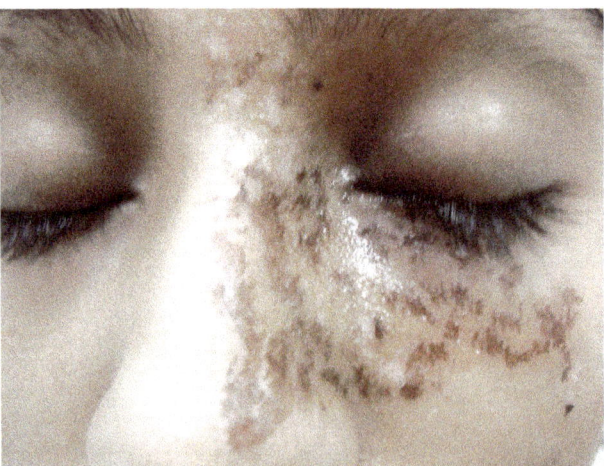

Fig. 17.2: A case of segmental lentigines post-Qsw Nd:YAG (day 2). Crusting is seen, and a bland moisturizer (petroleum jelly, Cetaphil™ cream, Alokem 75™ gel) is given till the crust falls off. Judicious sunscreen use is advised. (Qsw: Q-switched; Nd:YAG: neodymium-doped yttrium aluminum garnet)

CHAPTER 17: Complications and their Management **773**

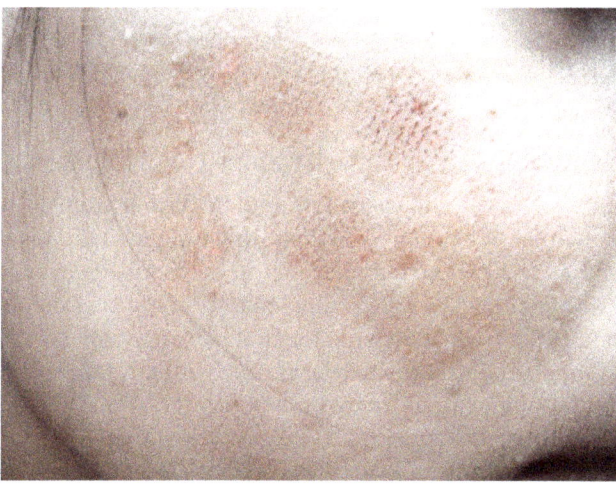

Fig. 17.3: Crusting seen corresponding to the microthermal zone (MTZ) patterns of a fractional Er:Glass (Lux Palomar). Mild and reversible. Sunscreen with a topical non-hydroquinone/tretinoin cream can be used for 14 days.

In case IPL is used for port-wine stains (PWS), a bruise-like appearance frequently occurs which can take 5–6 weeks to subside (Fig. 17.4) and is again part of the therapeutic response.

Prevention and Treatment

All patients should be off anticoagulant and antiplatelet agents at least 3–4 days prior to the planned procedure, which should be discussed with the physician.

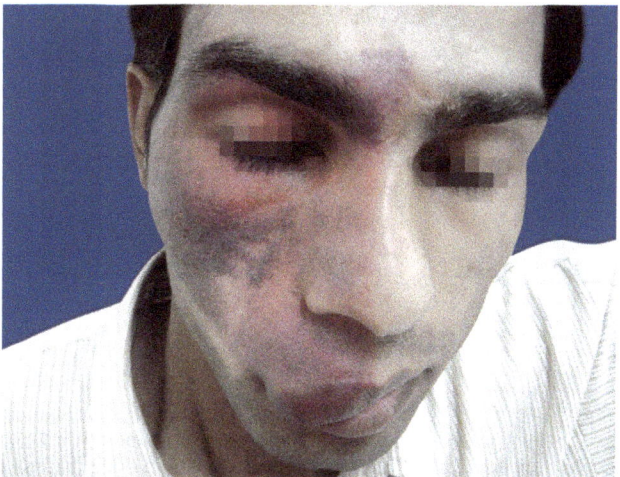

Fig. 17.4: A case of PWS treated with an IPL. Note the bruise-like darkening visible that precedes resolution. (IPL: intense pulsed light; PWS: port-wine stains)

Lowering fluence and increasing pulse duration (in the PDL) can help minimize purpura.

As PWS and hemangiomas cannot be effectively treated with nonpuruic parameters, patients should be aware of the potential of down-time.

Dyspigmentation or Postinflammatory Hyperpigmentation

Dyspigmentation can be transient or permanent and takes on two forms: hyperpigmentation or hypopigmentation. Hyperpigmentation is a common manifestation of postinflammatory change in the tissue. It generally appears 3-4 weeks postoperatively and spontaneously resolves over the next several months, though permanent hyperpigmentation can occur.

Hypopigmentation occurs when lasers inadvertently target melanin. Qsw lasers and IPL often cause a transient hypopigmentation during treatment due to the absorption of light by melanin and subsequent injury to individual melanosomes. Rarely, permanent hypopigmentation can appear 6-12 months after resurfacing procedures ("delayed hypopigmentation") due to thermal injury (Fig. 17.5).

In general, patients with dark or tanned skin have a greater risk of dyspigmentation. For such patients, treatment with lasers with shallower depths of penetration (i.e. shorter wavelengths and smaller spot sizes) confers greater injury to epidermal melanocytes and should be avoided.

Prevention and Treatment

Postinflammatory hyperpigmentation:
- Lasers with *longer* wavelengths and *larger* spot sizes should be used as the depth of penetration will be greater and risk of injury to epidermal

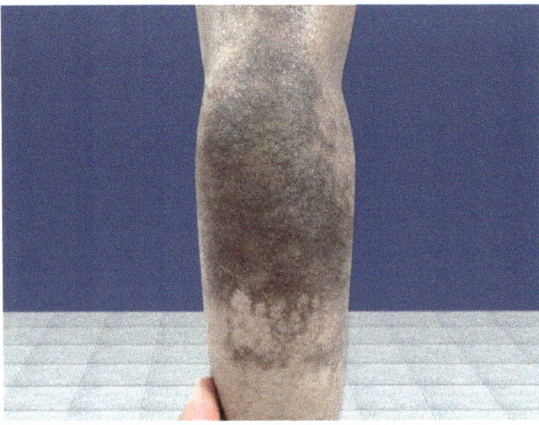

Fig. 17.5: A case of Becker's nevus treated with IPL. Note the hypopigmentation corresponding to the "footprint" of the probe. The nevus is usually difficult to treat by most lasers in Indian skin and thus a test spot is a good idea before aggressive therapy. (IPL: intense pulsed light)

melanocytes smaller. As a rule, a **test spot** and lower fluence should be used in pigmented skin.
- Though preoperative sunscreen and alpha-hydroxy acids or bleaching agents combined with a topical steroid may help, this has never been satisfactorily proved in any study, to prevent PIH. In fact, a prospective study of 100 patients undergoing CO_2 laser resurfacing found no significant difference in the incidence of PIH between patients pretreated 2 weeks with glycolic acid cream or combination of tretinoin and hydroquinone creams versus no treatment (West TB).
- In most nonablative procedures, we usually follow the following schedule:
    - First 7 days, a combination of aloe vera (Alokem 75™/Jula™ gel) in the morning with fucidin cream at night.
    - Second 7 days continue the aloe vera and add a non-hydroquinone or tretinoin cream at night. We prefer Brista™, Blise cream™, Golite cream™ or Lumivoid™. Another option often employed is a steroid antibiotic combination. Here, the relative potency must be understood. The common options are Fucidin H Fucibet and Flutibact. Flutibact ointment as per the American Classification contains fluticasone propionate ointment 0.005% which is a class 3 steroid similar to betamethasone valerate cream (class 3) which is a part of Fucibet hydrocortisone (class 6) a milder steroid which is a component of Fucidin H. It is inadvisable to use gentamicin or neomycin due to their allergenic potential or mupirocin acid as it may lead to resistance.
    - After 21 days, we stop the steroid and continue the use of the depigmenting cream.
    - A physical block sunscreen is preferred for the duration of posttreatment care.

Though we have discussed the demerits of using laser toning previously, it must be reemphasized that in Indian skin, it can cause perilous pigmentary alterations (Fig. 17.6)

Hypopigmentation: This is seen either while using a Qsw (Fig. 17.6), or as a consequence of overuse of topical steroids. For hypopigmentation, use of topical PUVA (psoralen and UVA light therapy) has been used to induce melanogenesis, so has been phototherapy (Mysore V). It is this author's opinion that the use of laser toning for melasma is best avoided as it can lead to unfortunate pigmentary alterations (Fig. 17.6).

In all cases, a test spot is a very useful tool as seen in the patient in Figure 17.7. Though the pigmentation resolved in this patient, it is a safe practice to forewarn the patient about the pigmentary sequelae.

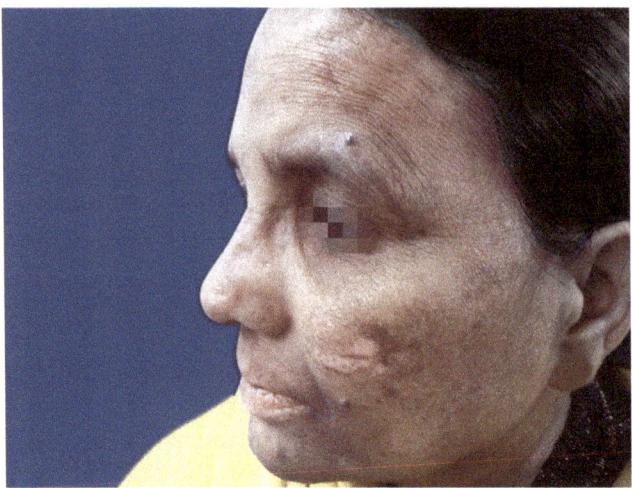

Fig. 17.6: A case of melasma treated with laser "toning" (Qsw Nd:YAG). Note the depigmentation and darkening of the melasma. (Qsw: Q-switched; Nd:YAG: neodymium-doped yttrium aluminum garnet)
Courtesy: Dr Shilpa Garg

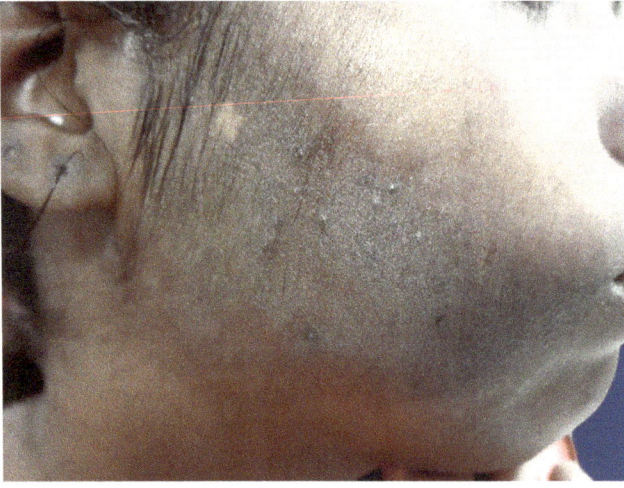

Fig. 17.7: A Becker's nevus, test spot with an Er:YAG laser. Note the hypopigmentation. The procedure was aborted. (Er:YAG: erbium-neodymium-doped yttrium aluminum garnet)

Scarring

Scarring is nowadays rare as it is seen mostly with ablative procedures, which are not done so commonly nowadays. The terminology in the literature can be confusing as some texts describe textural change where there is a change in the contour of the skin, truly differentiating it from a permanent scar.

Causes

The most likely cause of scar formation following laser treatment is excessive thermal injury to the treated tissue. Pulse stacking or multiple passes, high energy fluences or inadequate cooling can all precipitate thermal injury. Selection of an appropriate laser and use of the correct treatment parameters, for a given indication, is paramount in avoiding excessive tissue damage and scarring. Patients with a history of recent isotretinoin therapy, keloid scar formation or radiation therapy may be at increased risk for hypertrophic scar formation, following resurfacing procedures. Additionally, postoperative resurfacing complications, such as infection and contact dermatitis, may also lead to scarring. Treatment of certain anatomical locations, including the mandible, anterior neck and infraorbital areas are more likely to scar. Reduced laser parameters are recommended in these areas.

Prevention and Treatment

Some signs are useful indicators for impending scarring:
1. Marked erythema or graying of the epidermis during treatment may indicate significant damage and the need to discontinue treatment or adjust parameters.
    To avoid this, multiple test spots with varying fluences and/or pulse durations can be performed prior to treatment, particularly in patients with an increased risk of scarring.
2. Any sign of infection should be treated. We often use levofloxacin 750 mg a day before to 4 days after the laser intervention to avoid such complications. If infection is ruled out, prompt application or intralesional injection of corticosteroids can halt the progression of hypertrophic scars.

Intralesional steroids, 5-fluorouracil (5-FU) and laser therapy have proved beneficial in the treatment of hypertrophic scars. PDL treatment has been reported to improve the symptoms, pliability and color, and decrease the size of hypertrophic scars.

LASER-SPECIFIC COMPLICATIONS

Fractional Lasers

The side effects are mild, reversible and largely minor (*see* Figs. 17.1 and 17.3). Though it is believed that the ablative fractional lasers have more side effects, this has not been our experience (Sardana K, 2014). A retrospective evaluation of 961 successive 1,550 nm erbium-doped laser treatments in patients of various skin phototypes (I-V) was conducted by Graber EM et al., only 73 treatments (7.6%) resulted in development of complications. The most frequent complications were acneiform eruptions (1.87%) and herpes simplex virus outbreaks (1.77%). PIH, which occurred with increased frequency in patients with darker skin phototypes. Another study on Asian skin, (Vaiyavatjamai P et al.), where the 1,550 nm ytterbium/erbium fiber laser was used, found side effects in only six treatments (3.3%). The most common adverse event was PIH (2.2%), while acneiform eruption and desquamation were reported in 0.55%, equally. Although, none of the patients received herpes prophylaxis, there were no herpes outbreaks.

A summary of the side effects and their management is given in Tables 17.3 and 17.4. and an overview is given below:
- *Prolonged erythema:* This is seen when fractional techniques employ multiple passes, deep penetration, or pulse stacking. These can resolve within 3 months but persistent pinkness should be differentiated from the erythema that can be associated with developing hypertrophic scars.
- *Acne and milia:* Acne and milia are relatively common after fractional skin resurfacing, with 2–19% reported incidence. The likely cause is the use of occlusive ointment or moisturizers. In fact, in Indian environment with humidity, the unnecessary and enthusiastic use of moisturizers can be counterproductive in acne-prone skin. Also, sunscreen is an advice given to most patients, here a *matte finish* is better than lotions and other fancy bases.

A less occlusive moisturizer, use of aloe vera and use of moist gauze compresses with diluted white vinegar and water solution is a useful adjunct.
- *Postinflammatory hyperpigmentation:* A simple method to avoid this in Indian patients is to follow the cardinal rules of:
  i. Lower fluencies
  ii. Lower densities
  iii. Longer intervals between treatments utilized.

Any of these can lead to complications that may worsen the treated disorder (Fig. 17.8). The hyperpigmentation is self-limited and resolves with time (Fig. 17.9). Apart from sunscreens, numerous non-hydroquinone depigmentary agents are useful. Here, it must be noted that using a strong

Table 17.3: Complications reported with fractional lasers.

Mild	Prolonged erythema Acne, milia Delayed purpura Superficial erosions Contact dermatitis Recall phenomenon
Moderate	Infection Pigmentary alteration Anesthesia toxicity Eruptive keratoacanthomas
Severe	Hypertrophic scarring Ectropion formation Disseminated infection

Table 17.4: Complications and their management.*

Prolonged erythema (>1 month)	• Avoid use of irritating topical cream (hydroquinone/tretinoin) • Apply mild corticosteroid (Fucidin H) • Apply nonsteroidal anti-inflammatory agents (Clindamycin/metronidazole gel) • Topical vitamin C is a good option • LED photomodulation
Milia/acne exacerbation (>1 month)	• Discontinue occlusive dressings/ointments • It is best to use agents that are nonsticky (Sebamed Clear gel, Cetaphil™ cream) • Physical extraction of milia • Oral antibiotics for acne
Contact/allergic dermatitis	• Never use neomycin/gentamicin-based creams • Use nonsensitizing creams (Physiogel) • Topical/oral corticosteroids
Infection (1–14 days)	• Oral antibacterial/antiviral • Topical wound care (Fucidin)
Hyperpigmentation (1 month)	• Sunscreen (physical block) • Topical lighteners
Hypopigmentation (up to 6 months)	• Excimer laser • Topical photochemotherapy
Hypertrophic scar (1 month)	• Potent topical corticosteroid • Pulsed dye laser

*Brand names mentioned here are indicative only; does not indicate any commercial affiliations or endorsement
(LED: light-emitting diode)

exfoliant can be counterproductive and itself cause PIH. We have not seen hypopigmentation, but delayed hypopigmentation occurs more frequently after multipass CO laser resurfacing. Avoid the neck area as this is most prone to complications.

- *Infection:* Most infections associated with fractional skin resurfacing develop within the first week after treatment.

  Herpes simplex virus is the most common infection with fractional laser resurfacing, though we have not seen this very commonly. Some initiate antiviral 2 days before a procedure.

  Bacterial infection is a rarely seen complication while fungal infection if seen is predominantly composed of *Candida albicans* and can occur at a later postoperative period (7-14 days).

  Some authors recommend dilute acetic acid solution consisting of 1 tsp of white vinegar mixed with 2 cups of water, which inhibits the growth of fungal and gram-negative organisms.

- *Scarring:* This is an uncommon complications and is seen on the neck. The earliest pointer is localized erythema and induration at 2-4 weeks post-treatment.

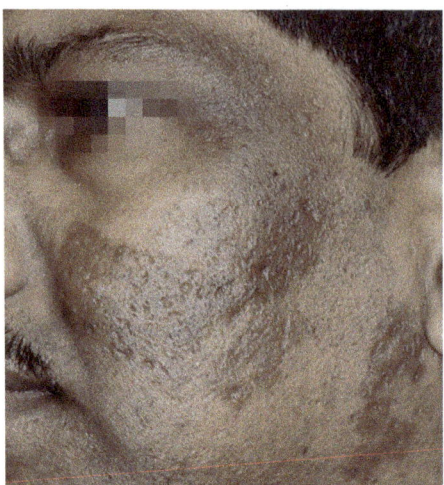

Fig. 17.8: Postinflammatory hyperpigmentation postfractional CO_2 after 1 month with worsening of scar. (Fractional CO_2: Energy used 22.5 mJ, density 10%-350 Hz; size 10). Ideally density of 5% would have reduced postinflammatory hyperpigmentation. (*Courtesy*: Dr Ganesh Pai)

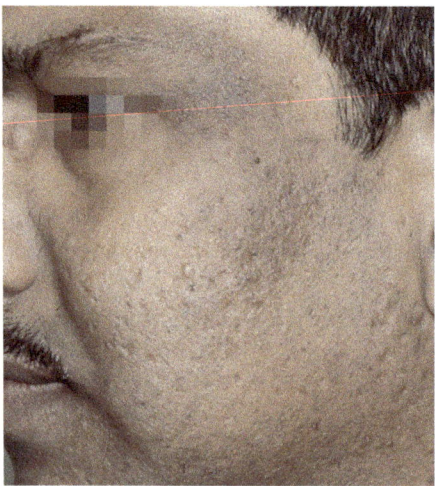

Fig. 17.9: Improvement of postinflammatory hyperpigmentation and scar after 6 months.

The neck is affected as the skin here is thin, there is a relative paucity of pilosebaceous units, as well as a different blood supply pattern in the neck in comparison to the face.

Other areas that can lead to scarring include the margin of the mandible and the lower eyelids. Previous radiation therapy and previous surgery is another cause for scarring.

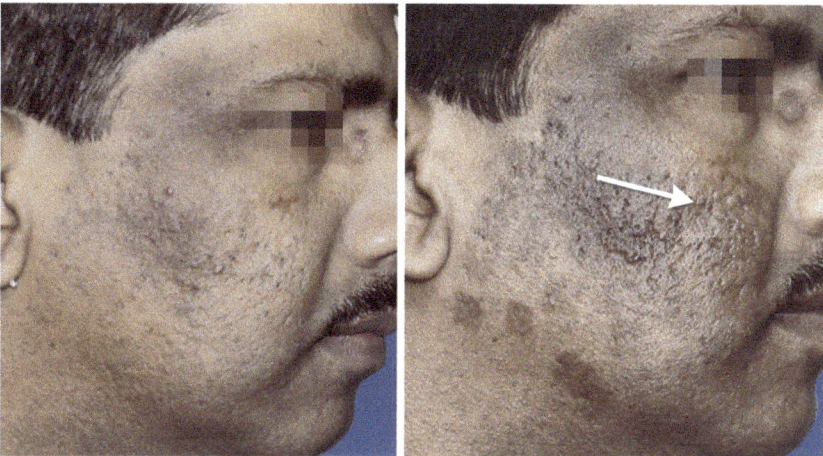

Fig. 17.10A: Concave scarring due to excess energy on right cheek. (*Courtesy*: Dr Ganesh Pai)

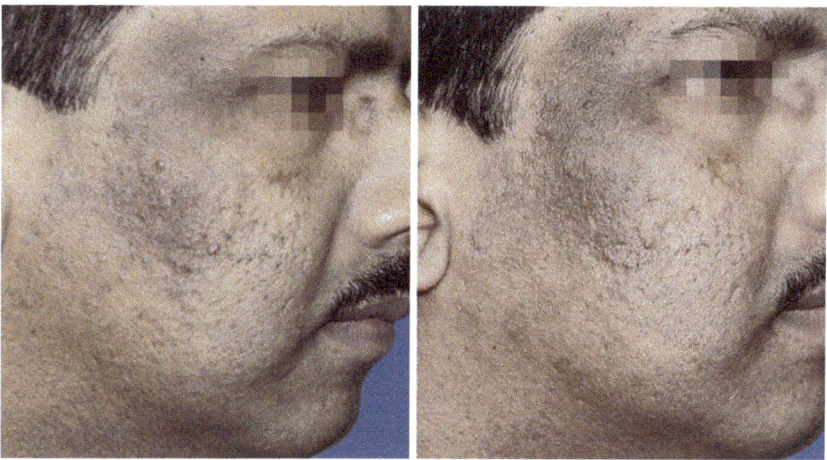

Fig. 17.10B: Disappearance of postinflammatory hyperpigmentation and partial improvement of concave scar. (*Courtesy*: Dr Ganesh Pai)

Occasionally, acne scar can aggravate due to inappropriate settings of the lasers (Figs. 17.10A and B).

LASERS FOR HAIR REMOVAL

This has been discussed in a previous chapter, thus a brief summary will be given here.

Hypertrichosis

Several studies have documented paradoxical hypertrichosis following laser hair removal. This primarily occurs after several treatments have been performed on the face and neck of female patients with darker skin types. The mechanism that triggers the conversion of these vellus to terminal hairs is unknown, but may be related to inflammation induced by the laser therapy itself. Management of this uncommon complication is with further photoepilation.

Leukotrichia

This is seen when patients are treated with long-pulsed neodymium-doped yttrium aluminum garnet (Nd:YAG) lasers. These lasers target melanin and penetrate deep enough to reach the hair follicle. With subtherapeutic fluence levels, follicular melanocytes may be destroyed in the absence of other follicular injury, resulting in leukotrichosis.

Reticulate Erythema

Persistent reticulate erythema has been described in at least 10 patients following hair removal with the diode laser (Lapidoth M). Pernio and perhaps other connective tissue diseases, as well as high energy fluences, seem to be potential risk factors.

Urticarial-like Plaques

Pruritic, urticarial-like plaques have been described following photoepilation. Unlike urticaria, however, lesions may last several days to weeks. Topical and oral corticosteroids and anti-histamines can be used for symptomatic relief.

Burns

These are commonly seen with the diode and IPL and with these systems, a preoperative, intraoperative and postoperative cooling is essential (Figs. 17.11A to C). Also, post-treatment, a steroid application for 3-5 days is advisable. In patients with an acne-prone skin, ice-pack cooling for 1-2 hours after therapy is another option.

LASERS FOR PIGMENTED LESIONS

Leukotrichia

Melanin, located in the epidermis, dermis, and follicular structures, is the primary chromophore targeted in the treatment of various pigmented lesions. Melanocytes within the hair follicle can be destroyed inadvertently

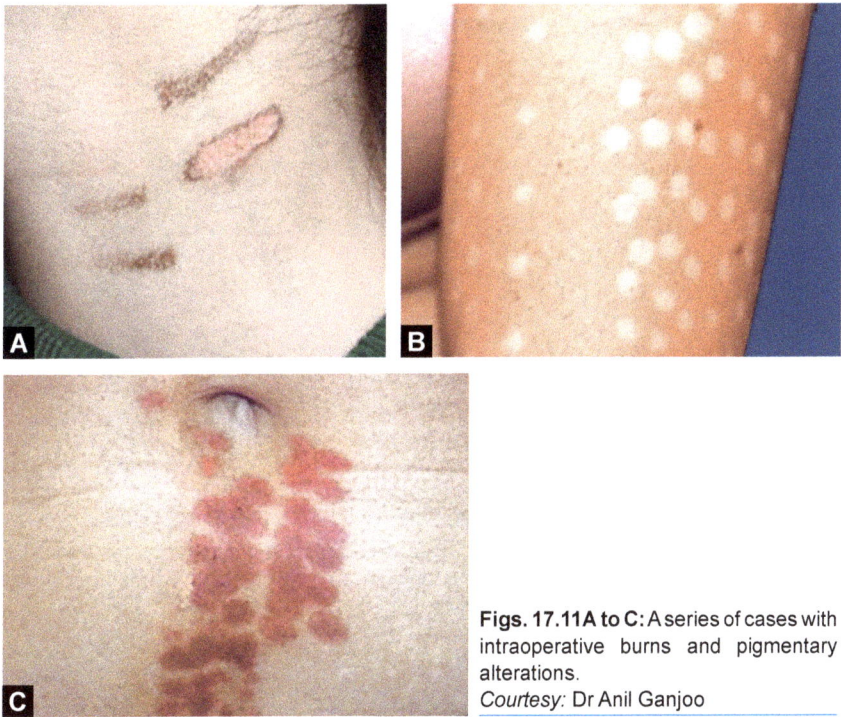

Figs. 17.11A to C: A series of cases with intraoperative burns and pigmentary alterations.
Courtesy: Dr Anil Ganjoo

when using high fluences and more deeply penetrating, longer wavelengths. Permanent leukotrichia can be the result. Limiting the fluences and selecting lasers with shorter wavelengths, if possible, will minimize this complication.

Tissue Splatter and Pinpoint Bleeding

Tissue splatter and pinpoint bleeding are expected side effects of treatment with Qsw lasers. When tissue targets are heated to destructive levels over nanosecond (Qs) pulse durations, particles can become aerosolized creating tissue splatter, and blood vessels can rupture leading to pinpoint bleeding and petechiae. Laser treatment through a water-based gel dressing (Fig. 17.12) minimizes tissue splatter and bleeding by acting as a heat sink and protecting the epidermis (Bernstein EF).

Pigmentary Alterations

In almost all cases, a transient hypopigmentation occurs as the Qsw lasers can impact on the normal epidermis. Luckily, the pigmentation resolves spontaneously in a few weeks (Fig. 17.13).

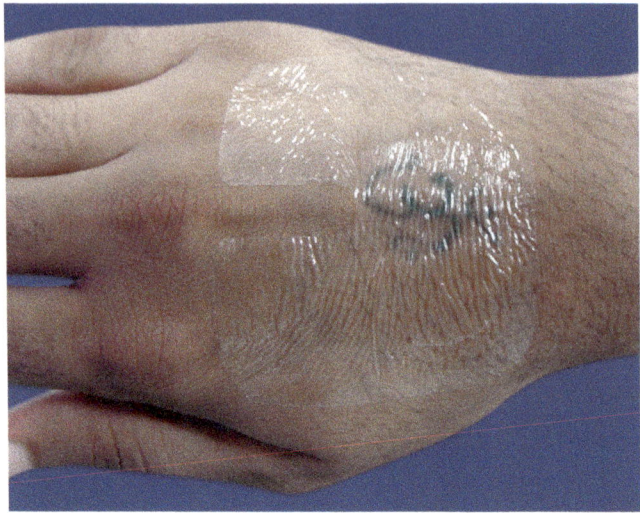

Fig. 17.12: Application of a transparent "Tegaderm" dressing before tattoo removal. This prevents tissue splatter but a slightly higher dose is required. The unique advantage is that this acts as a biological post-laser dressing.

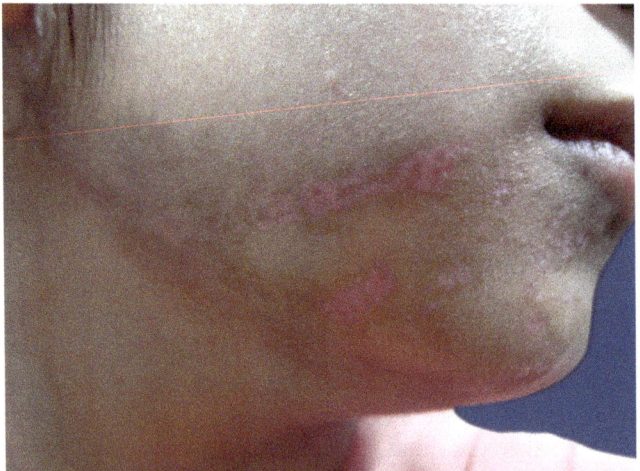

Fig. 17.13: A case of nevoid linear hypermelanosis after 1 week of treatment with a Qsw Nd:YAG (532 nm). The hypopigmentation is inevitable but transient. (Qsw: Q-switched; Nd:YAG: neodymium-doped yttrium aluminum garnet)

Tattoos

Allergic and Photoallergic Contact Dermatitis

During laser treatment of tattoos, pigment is released from intra- to extracellular sites exposing these antigens to the immune system. Rarely, a type-IV hypersensitivity reaction or photoallergic reaction to the components in the pigment can develop. Cinnabar, found in "red" tattoo pigment, is the most common contact allergen, while cadmium, which is found in "yellow" tattoo pigment, is the most frequent photoallergen. Those who have a contact dermatitis to pigment often give a history of pruritus and raised red areas over their tattoo sites. In photodermatitis, this reaction is heightened when exposed to sunlight.

Ablative resurfacing procedures can be used for tattoo removal with less risk of mounting an allergic response. However, a localized allergic reaction has been reported to become generalized following CO_2 laser removal of a tattoo.

Combustion

Treatment of tattoos that contain combustible material should be avoided. Sparks and incipient pox-like scars occur after Qsw Ruby laser treatment of a traumatic tattoo. If the composition of the pigment is unknown, a biopsy and/or test spot should be performed to help elucidate the material.

Paradoxical Tattoo Darkening

Paradoxical darkening of certain tattoo pigments has been reported with Qsw laser treatments. The exact mechanism is unknown, but the reduction of ferric oxide to ferrous oxide may play a role. Titanium dioxide may also be implicated in paradoxical darkening through a similar mechanism.

Ferrous oxide is found in some red, orange, peach or other skin-colored pigments and titanium dioxide is found in white pigments, often used alone or in conjunction with other colors to brighten them. As such, specific areas of tattoos containing these colors should undergo spot testing prior to full treatment with a Qsw laser. Once paradoxical darkening has occurred, correction can be difficult. Repeated laser treatments have been successful, as well as ablative resurfacing procedures.

LASERS FOR VASCULAR LESIONS

Reticulated Purpura

Purpura is a common, and usually expected side effect of the PDL. Often a reticulated pattern of purpura develops after treatment due to the Gaussian distribution of energy of each laser pulse. Overlapping pulses by 18% can minimize this complication.

Some uncommon complications are depicted in Figures 17.14 and 17.15.

ABLATIVE LASERS

As full face resurfacing is rarely done, the side effects are hardly reported. With Er:YAG, almost no side effects are seen. With the CO_2 laser, infections, textural alterations, PIH, and scarring may be seen (Figs. 17.16 and 17.17).

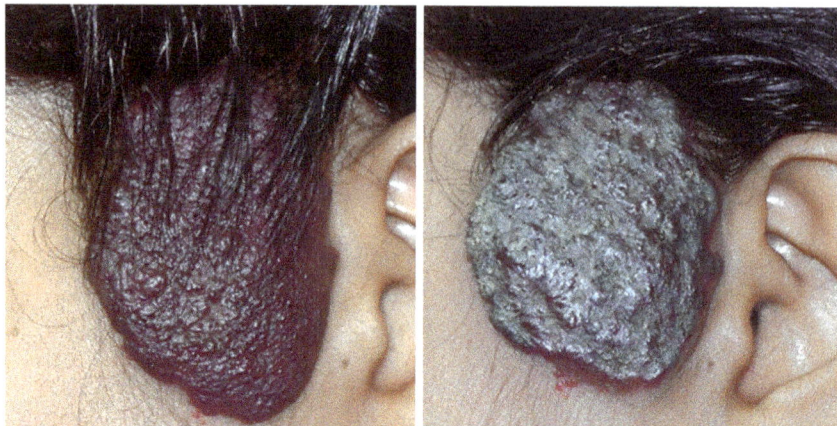

Fig. 17.14A: Hemangioma—Alma Dye-VL pulse duration 12 ms, repetition rate 1 Hz, spot size 3 cm^2, fluence 15 J/cm^2, cooling 100%, light source—pulsed light spectrum 500–600 nm.

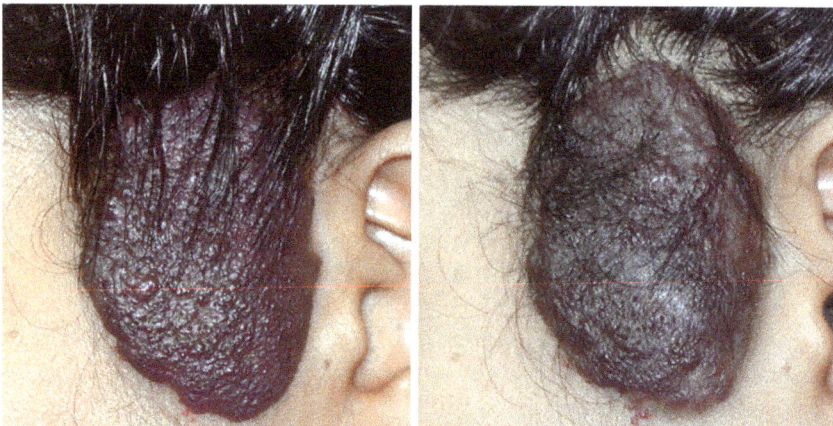

Fig. 17.14B: Shrinkage after 10 days.

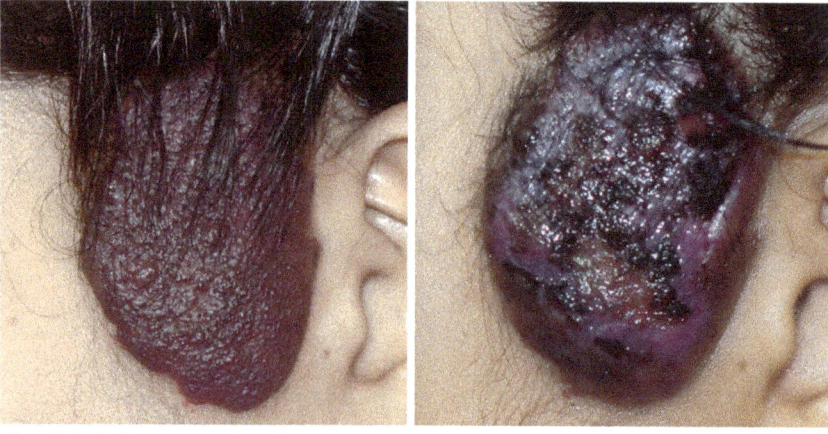

Fig. 17.14C: Repeat session after 3 months.

CHAPTER 17: Complications and their Management   **787**

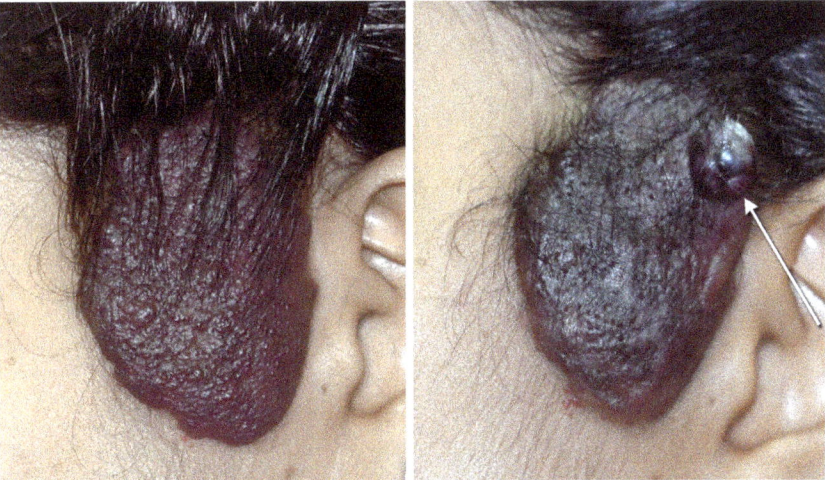

Fig. 17.14D: Resultant granuloma pyogenicum is an unpredictable outcome. Subsequently, hemangioma had to excised.

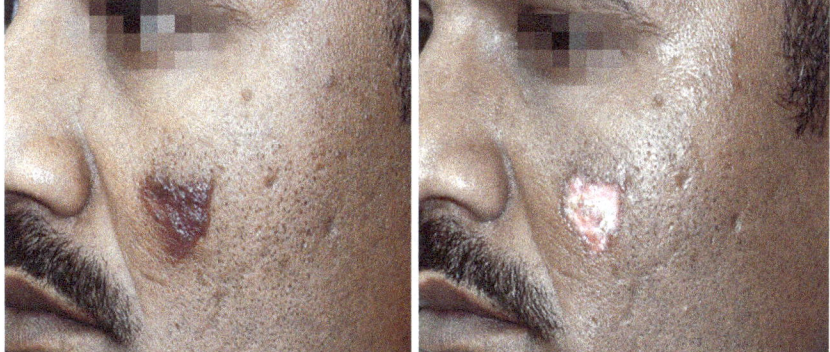

Fig. 17.15: Hemangioma on left cheek ablated by long pulse Nd:YAG 1064 laser. Absence of cooling leads to deep scar. As melanocyte and water compete with hemoglobin as target tissue, cooling of tissue prior to laser surgery ensures only hemoglobin is targeted and scarring is minimized.

CONCLUSION

Laser-induced complications are largely preventable, except pigmentary alterations in pigmented skin. But a simple rule that this author follows is not to replicate results reported in literature in fair skin types with lasers that have a short wavelength (Qsw Ruby or Alex) as they are most prone to pigmentary alterations as the epidermal pigment competes with the laser. The triad of consent, test spot, and pre- and post-photography is crucial. Methods of cooling, both device based and extrinsic with a good postoperative care are essential. A list of checklists and postoperative care is provided in the online

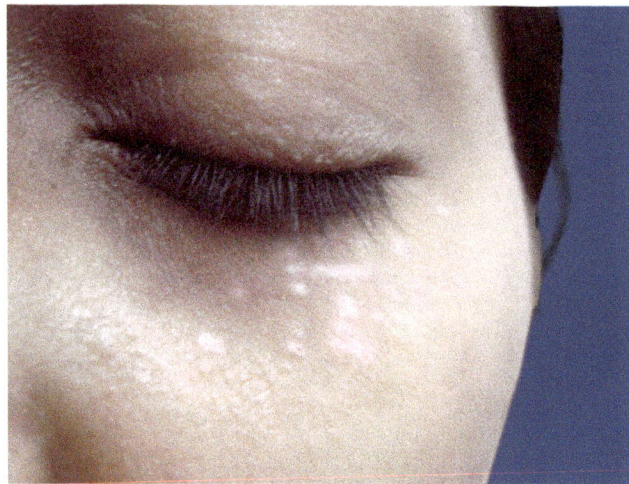

Fig. 17.16: Postoperative view of a syringoma case after pulsed CO_2 laser. Note the hypopigmentation corresponding to the syringoma which tend to persist for 1–2 months.

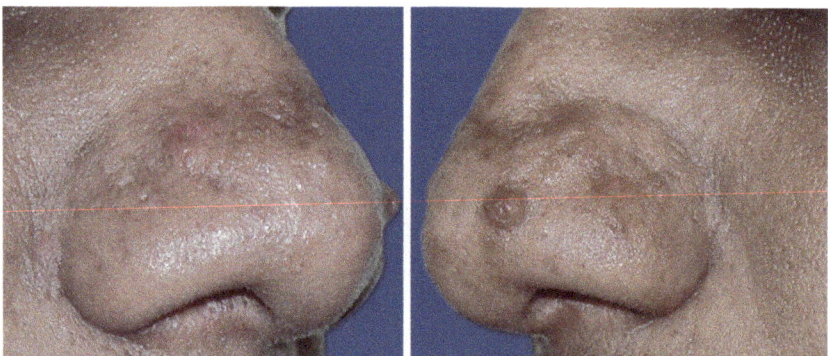

Fig. 17.17A: Rhinophyma prior to fractional CO_2.

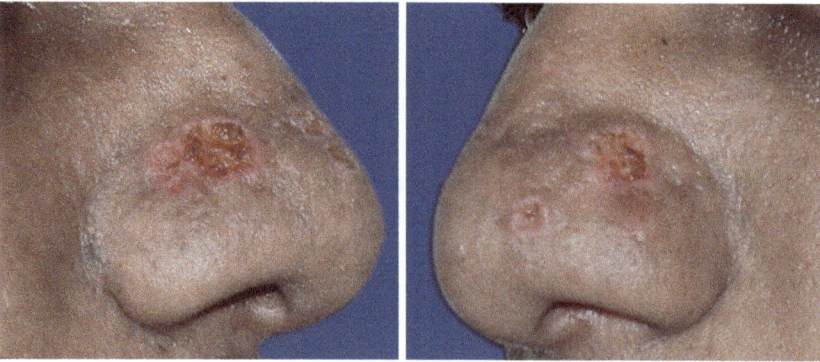

Fig. 17.17B: Excess energy applied to hypertrophic area (Day 7). Ideal energy should have been 20 mJ, 300 Hz, density 10%, 3 passes (Equipment used UltraPulse Lumenis). (*Courtesy*: Dr Ganesh Pai)

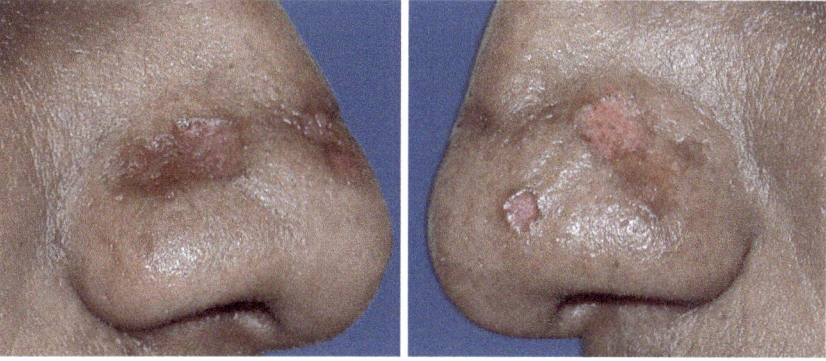

Fig. 17.17C: Day 20: Resultant depressed scarring.

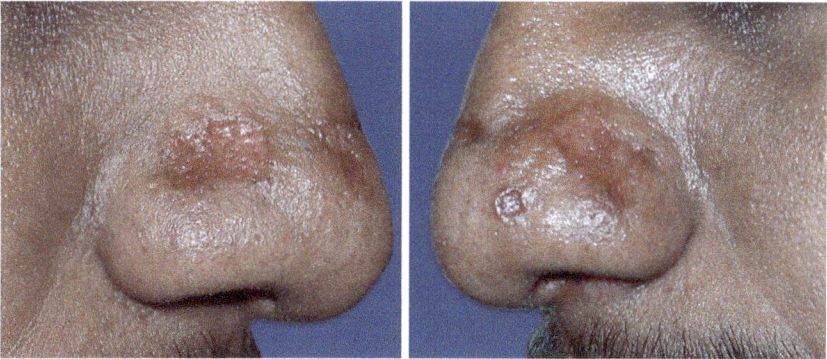

Fig. 17.17D: Reasonable recovery after 2 years.

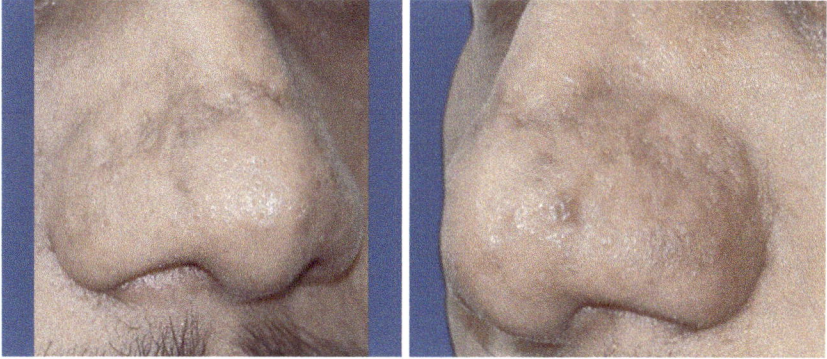

Fig. 17.17E: Reasonable recovery at the end of follow-up.

section of the book which can obviate and preempt most laser-induced complications. The consent form provided in the online section takes into account most of the legal possibilities and help to negate any medicolegal issues (*see* **Chapter 16**), if they do happen.

BIBLIOGRAPHY

1. Bernstein EF. Laser treatment of tattoos. Clin Dermatol. 2006;24:43-55.
2. Graber EM, Tanzi EL, Alster TS. Side effects and complications of fractional laser photothermolysis: Experience with 961 treatments. Dermatol Surg; 2008;34(3):301-5.
3. Lapidoth M, Shafirstein G, Ben Amitai D, et al. Reticulate erythema following diode laser-assisted hair removal: A new side effect of a common procedure. J Am Acad Dermatol. 2004;51:774-7.
4. Mysore V, Anitha B, Hosthota A. Successful treatment of laser induced hypopigmentation with narrowband ultraviolet B targeted phototherapy. J Cutan Aesthet Surg. 2013;6(2):117-9.
5. Sardana K, Manjhi M, Garg VK, et al. Which type of atrophic acne scar (Ice-pick, Boxcar, or Rolling) responds to nonablative fractional laser therapy? Dermatol Surg. 2014;40(3):288-300.
6. Vaiyavatjamai P, Wattanakrai P. Side effects and complications of fractional 1550-nm erbium fiber laser treatment among Asians. J Cosmet Dermatol. 2011;10(4):313-6.
7. West TB, Alster TS. Effect of pretreatment on the incidence of hyperpigmentation following cutaneous CO_2 laser resurfacing. Dermatol Surg. 1999;25:15-7.
8. Zelickson Z, Schram S, Zelickson B. Complications in cosmetic laser surgery: A review of 494 food and drug administration manufacturer and user facility device experience reports. Dermatol Surg. 2014;40(4):378-82.

Index

Page numbers followed by *b* refer to box, *f* refer to figure, *fc* refer to flowchart, and *t* refer to table.

A

Abdomen
   and flanks, lower anterior 471*f*
   lower 450
Ablative fractional
   laser 179, 242*f*, 248, 281, 294, 313, 424, 608, 609, 612
      treatment 313
   resurfacing 236, 252, 259, 262, 277
      lasers 534, 539
      types of 252
Ablative lasers 34, 36*t*, 50, 78*f*, 157, 169, 180, 192, 242*f*, 267*f*, 306, 492, 541, 581, 663, 713, 734, 785
   advent of 50
   indications of 86*t*, 87*t*
   limitations of 82
   major 70
   thermal damage of major 74*f*
   traditional 242*t*
      skin resurfacing 434
   treatment 76, 85
Ablative radiofrequency, fractional 256
Ablative technologies, common 31
Abnom's macule 188
Absorption 26
   coefficient 19
   low-fat 466
   spectra 19*f*
   spectrum 18, 19
Abundant pilosebaceous units 44*f*
Acanthosis 508
   dual laser toning 510*f*
Acne 87, 489, 540, 572, 778
   exacerbation 779
   keloidalis nuchae 91
   prone skin 378
   therapy 573*t*
   vulgaris 577*f*
Acne scars 78, 84, 281, 283*f*, 289*t*, 429, 494, 516, 516*f*, 520, 523*f*, 524*f*, 525*f*, 529
   classification of 517*t*
   deep 430
   medical therapy for 517
   mild 430
   moderate 430
   reduction, technique of 529*f*
   resurfacing fractional laser in 287*t*

Acneiform eruption 507
Acoustic shock wave therapy 233
Acquired benign melanocytic nevi, laser in treatment of 167*fc*
Acquired bilateral nevus 188
Acquired generalized hypertrichosis, causes of 357
Acquired localized hypertrichosis, causes of 357
Acquired melanocytic nevi 145, 163
Actinic cheilitis 86, 87, 91, 92*f*, 127
   step-by-step approach 91
Actinic keratosis 87, 300, 304
Actinic telangiectasia 331
Adenoma sebaceum 84, 87, 104, 331
Adenosine triphosphate 628*f*
   production 626
Adipocyte 455
   absorption spectrum 466*t*
   removal 456
Adipolysis 567
Adipose tissue stores triglycerides 456
Adjacent epidermis skin, level of 90*f*
Adjunctive techniques 505
Adrenal hyperplasia, congenital 359, 360
Adrenal hypersecretion 358
Aesthetic medicine 700
Aesthetic practice, radiofrequency in 421*b*
AFR *See* Ablative fractional laser
Aged skin 483
Alexandrite laser 149, 346, 368, 733
Allergic contact dermatitis 784
Allergic dermatitis 779
Allergic reactions 210
Alma Accent 448
Alopecia 314, 625, 628*f*
   areata 314, 620*t*, 626
   chemotherapy-induced 626
   nonscarring 626
Alpha-hydroxy acid lotions 594
Alphastria 551
Amateur tattoo 200, 211*f*
Amelanotic melanoma 657
Amelioration 309
American Academy of Dermatology 745
American Academy of Facial Plastic and Reconstructive Surgery 736
American Society for Lasers in Medicine and Surgery 745

American Society of Aesthetic Plastic Surgery 387
Aminoamides 77
Aminoester 77
Aminolevulinic acid 30, 383
Amiodarone 192
Amorphous carbon 39
Amyloidosis, macular 196
Anabolic steroids 360
Anagen 354
Anderson and Parrish's theory 132
Androgen
  creams 358
  metabolism 358
  secreting tumor 356
Androgenetic alopecia 625, 630
Anesthesia 76, 569
  toxicity 778
Angiokeratoma 87, 331, 647, 649*f*, 650*f*
Angiolymphoid hyperplasia 598
  treatment of 598
Angioma, treatment of 646*f*
Anorexia nervosa 357
Anti-angiogenesis 336
Antibiotic cream, application of 587
Anticoagulant therapy 689
Antidepressants 452
Anti-inflammatory properties 550
Anxiety level 316
Appearance-enhancing scarring 459
Appendageal tumors 127
Arbitration 757
Argon
  dye lasers 661
  laser 329, 341, 535
Asclepion laser technologies 205*f*
Atrophic acne scars, treatment of 521
Atrophic chickenpox scar, laser treatment of 88*f*
Atrophic scars, deep 293*f*
Autologous noncultured cell 312
Axillae 355
Azelaic acid 616
Azidothymidine 192

B

Backscattered light 27
Bacterial infection 689, 779
Bactroban ointment 115
Baker's phenol peel 63
Balanitis xerotica obliterans 86, 87, 125
Bare optical fibers 674
Basal cell carcinoma 95, 663
Basal layer 324
Basic radiofrequency system classification 394*t*
Beam profile 15, 327

Becker's nevus 78, 80*f*, 84, 142, 144, 145, 147, 150, 159, 160*f*-162*f*, 198, 309, 357, 624, 774*f*, 776*f*
  removal of 308
  therapy of 625
  treatment of 160*f*
Bella contour 448
Benign disorders 578
Biomodulation 567
Bipolar electrodes 36
Bipolar fractional radiofrequency 400
Bipolar radiofrequency 384, 395*f*, 397, 401*f*, 402, 411, 448
  device 406
  system 394
  vacuum-assisted 398
Birds-eye view of plethora 695
Black amateur tattoo 220*f*, 232*f*
Bleomycin 519, 598
Blepharochalasia 300
Blood
  perfusion 550
  vessel 17*f*
Bloodless dermis 29
Blue nevus 144, 146
Blue rubber bleb nevi 331
Body contouring
  devices 448*b*, 458*b*
  nonsurgical 448
Body mass index 452, 565
Botox 669
Botulin toxin injection 670*f*
Botulinum neurotoxin 670*f*
Botulinum toxin 271, 671*f*, 682
Bowen's disease 87, 664
Boxcar atrophic acne scars, large 285*f*
Boxcar scars 269*f*, 282, 285, 516*f*, 518, 520*f*
  deep 282, 518
  shallow 282, 517, 518
  superficial 315, 520
Bruising 442
Bulges 450
Burn 76, 742, 782
  debridement 87
Burn scar 544
  dyschromia 539
  stiffness of 539
Burst mode 387

Index **793**

C

Cadmium
  red 202
  selenide 202
  sulfide 202
  yellow 202
Café-au-lait macule 84, 142, 144, 147, 150, 155
  follicular melanocytic component of 157
Café-au-lait patches 146
Café-au-lait spot 200
CAH *See* Congenital adrenal hyperplasia
Calcipotriol 196
CALM *See* Café-au-lait macule
Camper's fascia 460
Candida albicans 779
Cannula 569
Capillary malformations 331
Carbon dioxide 10, 11*f*, 18, 20*f*, 29, 31, 35*f*, 36, 50, 93, 184, 204, 205, 205*f*, 209, 226, 227*f*, 232*f*, 238*f*, 424, 482, 493, 495, 504, 536, 578, 582, 586, 593, 612, 656, 663, 683, 735*f*
  fractional laser 34*f*
  pulsed 665*f*
Carbon dioxide laser 51, 80, 82, 125, 342, 585, 634, 644
  ablation 93
  therapy, fractional 311
  clinical aspects of 61
  fractional 254, 311, 613*f*, 639
  tissue effect of 14*f*
  principles of 52
  types of 53
Carbonization 60*f*
Cardiovascular disease 456
Casalis green 202
Catagen 354
Cavernous hemangiomas 320
Cell suspension transplantation 312
Cellulaze 467
Cellulite 387, 406, 407, 447, 450, 451, 454, 557, 567
  grading of 453*t*
  management of 558*t*
  presence of 453*f*
  process of 452
  therapeutic modalities for 454*t*
  tissue 453*f*
  treatment of 452, 454
Central nervous system-related disorders 357
Central vigilance commission 726
Cetaphil cream 317
Cetuximab 358
Chemical lipolysis 448
Chemical peels 616
Chemotherapy, topical 665

Cherry angiomas 87, 331, 346, 348, 641, 644
Chickenpox 540
  scar 88, 89*f*
Chill tip cooling 363
Cholesterol deposition disorders 104
Chondrodermatitis nodularis helices 125
Chromium oxide 202
Chromophore 241, 322*f*, 361, 379, 449
  absorption spectra of 45
  water, primary 259*f*
Cinnabar 202
Civil and criminal negligence 747*f*, 748*t*
Cleansing gel 372
Clinician's eyewear 381
Clobetasol propionate cream 311
Clomiphene 358
Club-hair 354
CO_2 laser *See* Carbon dioxide laser
Coagulates collagen fibers 466
Coagulative necrosis, small zones of 436
Cobalt aluminate 202
Cobb syndrome 331
Cocoa butter 551
Cold
  exposure 472
  steel surgery 91, 93
Collagen 21
  contraction of 127, 427
  induction 305
  stimulation 449
Collateral tissue 24
Colloid 369
  milium 314
Color blind 38, 390
Combination laser therapy 482
  drawbacks of 497
Combo suction 448
Common laser
  devices 770*t*
  used in dermatology 29*f*
Complete blood count 475
Component-wise therapy 486
Concave scar, partial improvement of 781*f*
Condylomata acuminata 83, 87, 116
Confluent thermal damage 265
Connective tissue 454
Consequent tissue 68*f*
Consumer disputes redressal agencies 760
Consumer Protection Act 759
Contact dermatitis 778, 779
Continuous wave 9, 278, 387, 593
Contraceptive pill 452

Contrary heat 80
Control over laser usage, lack of 724
Conventional laser 5*f*
　toning 501
Cooling devices 704
CoolLipo 448
Copper
　salts 202
　vapor laser 598
Corticoid therapies, chronic 689
Corticosteroids 594
　topical 381, 598
Cosmetic
　industry 434
　machine 716
　tattoo darkening 210
　vaginal surgery 687
　vulvar surgery 687
Crest syndrome 331
Criminal negligence 746, 750
Crow's-feet area 413
Cryogen sprays 363
Cryolipolysis 473*f*, 474, 478, 568*f*
　cup, medium 474
　mechanism of 472*f*
　preoperative counseling 478
　procedure 478
　selective 471
Cryoprobe, application of 473*f*
Cryosurgery 93
Cryotherapy 580, 598, 600
Cutaneous amyloidosis, localized 603
Cutaneous blood vessels, selective
　　　photothermolysis of 42
Cutaneous disease 115
Cutaneous vascular lesions 320
Cutis marmorata telangiectasia congenital 653*f*
Cyclosporine 358
Cymedics cryo cryolipolysis 568*f*
Cynosure 467
　photogeniaca V laser 327*f*
Cysts 578
Cytoplasm 504
Cytoplasmic retraction 466

D

Darier's disease 114, 598, 599
Dark hyperpigmentation spots 754
Dark skin types, laser in 380
Deka system 254
Dental implants 431
Deoxycholate 567
Deoxyhb 29
Deoxyribonucleic acid 628*f*
Dermablate 252*f*
Dermabrasion 63, 93, 600
Dermal bands 283*f*

Dermal damage 242
Dermal disorders 56*f*, 71, 86, 149, 163
Dermal epidermal junction 22, 23, 116, 611
Dermal growths, number of 104
Dermal injury, creation of 77
Dermal lesions 87
Dermal melanocytosis 142
　congenital 190
Dermal melanophores 500
Dermal necrosis 54
Dermal nevi 87, 101
Dermal pigmentation 430
Dermal pigmented lesions 147, 199
Dermal septa, denaturation of 562*f*
Dermal static pigmented lesions 41
Dermal tumors, benign 86, 87
Dermatology, technologies use in 37*f*
Dermatomyositis 599, 602
Dermatoses 281, 607
Dermis 127, 459
Dermoepidermal junction 227, 419
Designing laser center 707
Dexamethasone 358
Diazoxide 358
Diet 456, 682
Digital photography 707
Dimple severity 479
Diode 672, 579
　laser 5, 250, 368, 448, 466, 594, 634, 639, 655
　　fiber 674
　　　wavelengths 33
　systems, modern 733
Direct phototoxicity 511
Discoid lupus erythematosus 602
Disseminated granuloma annulare 314
Disseminated infection 778
Distal lateral onychomycosis 636*f*
Down's syndrome 599
Doxycycline 192
Drug
　and anesthesia 706
　causing hirsutism 358*b*
　delivery, fractional 314
Drug-induced hyperpigmentation 192
Dry skin 430
Dual laser toning 501, 505, 508
Dual pulse laser toning 501
Dual-wavelength laser system 649
Dye laser 5
　pulsed 8*f*, 9, 29, 204, 209, 236, 331, 346, 485-487, 534-537, 547, 548, 551, 552, 555, 573, 583, 586, 612, 618, 644, 648, 651, 655, 713, 771
Dynamic pigmented lesions 608
Dyschromia 281
Dyspareunia 688, 691*f*, 693*f*
Dyspigmentation 125, 774

Index **795**

E

Earlobe keloids 120
    step-by-step approach 120
Eccrine 104
    gland tumors 106*f*
Ectropion formation 778
Eczema 599
Edema 771, 771*f*
    severe 317
Eflornithine, role of 378
Elastin 388
Elastosis perforans serpiginosa 599
Electrical conductivity 391
Electrical energy 397
Electrical field 390
Electrical safety 381
Electrical stimulation 567
Electrolysis 76
Electronic medical record 7
Electro-optical synergy 384, 486
Electrosurgery 93, 583, 600, 644
Electrosurgical device 387
Elevated scar, laser treatment of 90*f*
Emotional distress 742
Encephalitis 357
Endoscopic thoracic sympathectomy 670
Energy 6, 261, 390, 569
    and depth, correlation of 261
    based devices 566, 567, 673
    device-assisted liposuction 448
    devices, fractional 494
    modalities 276
    per pulse 139
    pulse duration 8*f*
Eosinophilia 598
    treatment of 598
Ephelides 144, 147, 158
Epidermal cooling 381
Epidermal dermal
    junction 79, 130
    separation 591
Epidermal disorders 71, 86, 134*f*, 150
Epidermal growth factor 626
Epidermal injury 227
Epidermal lesions 735*f*
Epidermal necrotic debris, microscopic 242, 244, 309
Epidermal nevus 86, 87, 95, 96*f*, 99*f*, 127, 590
Epidermal pathology 273
Epidermal pigmentation 430
Epidermal pigmented lesions 147
Epidermal tumors 86
Epidermis 22, 79, 130, 324, 362
    fraction of 241
    pigmented 149
    removal of 69
    total ablation of 242*f*
    whitening of 582*f*

Epithelial dysplasia 83
Epithelioma adenoides cysticum 578
ER:YAG See Erbium-doped yttrium aluminum garnet
Erbium laser 251
    resurfacing 76
Erbium peel 125
Erbium:yttrium aluminum garnet 70*f*, 82, 85, 173, 204, 205, 205*f*, 209, 225, 226, 227*f*, 229*f*
    laser 66, 77, 82, 223*f*, 255
        ablation 93
        bleeding 82
        noise level 82
        plume 82
        resurfacing 129
        systems 260
Erbium:yttrium scandium gallium garnet laser 424
    resurfacing 75
Erbium-doped yttrium aluminum garnet 20*f*, 29, 31, 35*f*, 36, 495, 495*f*, 534, 534, 548, 569, 578, 579, 582, 583, 586, 593, 596*f*, 612, 663, 712
    depiction of 688*f*
    laser 5, 424, 622*f*
        Alma's fractional 255
        minimal thermal damage of 74*f*
        modulated 67*t*
        pulsed 74
        short-pulsed 541
        treatment 493
        treatment guidelines for 84*t*
    palomar fractional 254
    system, modified 66*f*
Erosions, superficial 778
Erythema 373*f*, 504, 552, 684, 742, 771, 771*f*
    background 348
    dyschromicus pigmentosus 194
    macular 575*f*
    postoperative 82
    prolonged 778, 779
    reticulate 782
Erythematous scars 331
Erythematous shallow boxcar scars 520*f*
Erythrocyte 22, 324
Erythroplasia of Queyrat 87, 664, 665*f*
Estrogen antagonists 358
Ethnic skin 243
Excimer laser 714
    indications of 621
    light 621*t*

Excimer system 619
Excisional surgery 118
Exilis Elite 405
Exophytic lesions 58
Exophytic scars 84
Exploded cells, solid residue of 58
Extension rhytides 300
External nonfocused ultrasound 461
Extracorporeal shockwaves 562
Extrafacial port-wine stain 492
Eye
    injury 742
    protection 372, 381
Eyeliner tattoos 87
Eyewear 381

F

Face 377
    lower 419
Facial erythema 331, 343*b*
    diffuse 343
Facial hair, whitening of fine 507
Facial muscle twitching 445
Facial pores 683*t*
    enlarged 679, 680*f*
Facial rejuvenation 684
Facial telangiectasia 343
Facial tips 383
Facial tissue 43*f*
Famciclovir 77
Far infrared systems 31
Fat 23, 450, 472, 563, 567
    cell destruction 567
    excess 447, 451
    loss 567
    reduction 448, 557
    tissue 112
    treatment of 480
Fatty liver, acute 307
Fatty tissue, cryolysis of 472
FDA *See* Food and Drug Administration
Femoroacetabular impingement 751
Ferric hydrate 202
Ferric sulfate 202
Ferrous ferricyanide 202
Fibroblast growth factor 626
Fibrous septae, cutting superficial 567
Fillers 88
Fine wrinkles 281
Fire protection 381
Fitzpatrick skin
    phenotypes 384
    type 369
Flaps hair reduction, reconstructive 356

Flashlamp-pumped pulsed dye laser 326, 595
Fluences, lower 449
Fluorouracil 518, 538
Focal hyperhidrosis, primary 667*b*
Follicular melanocytes 157
Follicular stem cells 354
Folliculitis, chronic 539
Fractional lasers 43, 136, 172, 174*f*, 180, 182, 184, 243, 246*t*, 265*f*, 267*f*, 270*f*, 272*f*, 278, 281*f*, 298, 199*t*, 300, 301, 301*t*, 307, 310, 311*b*, 330, 520, 535, 536, 539, 542, 552, 714, 734, 777, 778*t*
    ablative 242*t*
    effect of 283*f*, 516*f*
    future of 314
    nonablative 242*t*
    therapy 244*f*
    treatment 258
Fractional photothermolysis 34, 241, 245, 245*t*, 330
    fundamental principles of 315
    intraoperative
        procedure 271
        steps 316
    management 270
    patient selection 315
    pearls 318
    pitfalls 318
    postoperative
        care 317
        instructions 275
    predictable side effects 276
    preoperative evaluation 270
    procedure 317
    scientific logic 241
    side effects 276
    step-by-step approach 315
    treatment principles 266
Fractional radiofrequency 398
    systems 399*t*, 408
Fractional ruby laser 173
Fractional skin ablation 387
Fractional technology 34, 303
    classification of 245
Fractional thulium laser 173, 257
Fraxel repair 543
Freckles 38, 146
Frequency electromagnetic radiation 458
Fresnel equation 3
Frictional melanosis 508

Fucidin 115, 131
Functional aspiration controlled electrothermal stimulation 407
Fungal vaginal infection 689
Fusarium solani spp 638, 638*f*

G

Gallium-aluminum-arsenid 661
Gallium-arsenide 661
Ganglion ablation, multiple 671
Gas lasers 5
Gaussian beam 16*f*
 profile 138
Gaussian curve 77
Gaussian distribution 13
Gel application 372
Genital lichen planus 125
Genital warts 597
Genitourinary syndrome of menopause 686, 687*b*, 691*f*, 693*f*
Glogau photoaging classification 299*t*
Glomus tumors 331, 650
Glycerol 227
Glycolic acid 551, 681
 peel 524
Goodman baron scale 523*f*, 524*f*
Grafts 88
Granuloma 212
 annulare 600
  treatment of 600*t*
 faciale 87, 125, 600
  management of 600
 pyogenicum 787*f*
 telangiectaticum 345
Gray hair, number of 379
Gustatory hyperhidrosis 671*f*
Gustatory phantom sweat 671
Gynecological cancers, post-treatment for 688

H

Hailey-Hailey disease 114, 118, 601
Hair 356
 acquired hypertrichosis 357
 anatomy 354
 bulb 16
 bulge 16
 coarseness 369
 color 369, 370*t*, 384
 dark terminal 355*f*
 disorders 624
 gray 374*f*, 375*f*
 in anagen phase, percentage of 355*t*
 laser for fine 379
 light 362
 long 378
 persisting long 378*f*
 physiology 354
 pigmented 362
 predominant 375*f*
 removal of nonpigmented 379
 shaft 16
 thickness 370*t*
 transplants 120
Hair follicle 44, 354, 361, 681
 excessive genetic sensitivity of 358
 photothermal destruction of 361
Hair growth 627*t*
 cycle 354
Hair reduction 356, 364, 365
 lasers for 353, 380*f*, 732
 male 356
 technologies 378*f*
Hair removal 361, 364, 742, 744*f*
 calibration 371
 devices for 365, 366*t*
 intraoperative 371
 laser for 353, 594, 714, 781
 pearls 377
 pitfalls 377
 postoperative 372
 postprocedure care 372
 procedure 368, 371
 safety issues 381
 side effects 375
 sitting 373*f*
 special situations 378
 standard precautionary measures 381
 test patch 371
 topical anesthesia 371
Halogen lamps, deeply penetrating 30
Heat conduction, superior 427
Heat diffusion 26
Heat shock proteins 629
Heat-coagulated collagen fibers 466
Helium-neon 661
Hemangioma 122*f*, 314, 331, 349, 786*f*
 laser in 340, 343*b*
 laser used for 341
 mixed-type 331
 superficial 331
Hemoglobin 20, 322*f*, 484, 485
Hepatitis
 B 76
 C 76
Hereditary hemorrhagic telangiectasia 331
Hereditary multiple glomus tumors 650
Herpes labialis 77

Herpes simplex
  infection 270, 316
  reactivation 507
Herpes viral infection, active 689
Hidrocystomas 104
HIFU *See* High intensity focused ultrasound
High intensity focused ultrasound 434, 455, 461
  system 463
High-frequency focused ultrasound energy devices 458
High-intensity focused
  radiofrequency 411
  ultrasound 567, 570, 673, 678, 735*f*
Hirsutism 356, 357, 358*fc*
Histiocytoma 114
HIV *See* Human immunodeficiency virus
Hori's macules 188, 243
Hori's nevus, treatment of 489
Hormones 452
Horner's syndrome 671
Human epidermis, selective destruction of 132
Human hair follicle 41
Human immunodeficiency virus 76
Human melanocytes 500
Human papillomavirus
  development of 115
  infection 689
Human skin contains hair follicles 353
Human terminal hair follicles 362
Hyaluronic acid 489
  injections 521
Hybrid laser 329
  systems 329
Hydrated chromium sesquioxide 202
Hydroquinone 179, 270, 615
  monobenzylether of 622
Hyperemia 539
Hyperhidrosis 667, 668*f*, 669*t*, 672*t*, 673
  disease severity score 678
Hyperkeratotic debris, remove thickened 115
Hyperpigmentation 146, 375, 375*f*, 779
Hyperplasia, sebaceous 87, 104, 108, 582, 583*f*
Hypertrichosis 162, 357, 782
Hypertrophic scars 238*f*, 282, 331, 369, 430, 518, 520*f*, 532, 536-539, 547, 778, 779
  formation 270
Hypodermal adipocytes, denaturation of 562*f*
Hypodermal tissue, stimulation of 562*f*
Hypopigmentation 487, 775, 779, 784*f*
  delayed 774
Hypothyroidism 357
Hypotrophy 688

I

Iatrogenic tattoos 236
Ibuprofen 270

Ice pack 364
  predominantly 269*f*
  scars 282, 284, 518, 521*f*, 522
  deep 286, 516*f*
Idiopathic elastosis perforans serpiginosa 599
Imiquimod 229, 598, 665
  topical 660
Immune system, impaired 689
Immunization, site of 357
Indian skin types 510
Infection 742, 778, 779
  active 431
Inflammation 472
Inflammatory disorders 598
Inflammatory wound healing 437
Infraorbital hyperpigmentation 191
Infraorbital pigmentation 107
Infrared wavelength 573
Intense focused ultrasound 256
Intense pulsed light 24, 144, 151, 173, 180, 300, 322, 368, 487, 515, 539, 551, 573, 608, 611*f*, 612, 618, 651, 714, 733, 769, 770
Interferon 358
International Society of Aesthetic Plastic Surgeons 700
Interstitial laser lipolysis 465
Intradermal mesotherapy 562
Intralesional injection 660
Intraurethral wart 117*f*, 597*f*
IPL *See* Intense pulsed light
Iron oxide 202
Irradiated tissue, heating of 32
Irreversible corneal burns 367
Isotretinoin 76

J

Jacques notes 28
Japanese skin 505
Junctional nevus 80*f*, 87, 100, 144
Juvenile dermatomyositis 357

K

Keloid 120, 532, 536-538, 547, 548
  acne scars 517
  history of 198, 316
  larger 120
  laser for 532
Keloidal scar 522
Keloidal tendency 431
Keratinocytes 147, 500
Keratoacanthomas 778
Keratoderma 125
Keratosis pilaris 594
  atrophicans 594

Ketorolac 270
Kirby-Desai scale 208*f*
Klippel-Trenaunay syndrome 331
Koebnerizing disease 128
Koenen tumors 578
Kojic acid 616
Kraurosis vulvae 125
KTP *See* Potassium titanyl phosphate

L

Labia majora
   three thermiva treatments of 691*f*
   treatment of 693*f*
   vulvar laxity of 692*f*
Labial melanotic macules 153, 154*f*
Lactic acid 594
Laser 5, 184, 190, 195, 579, 598, 617, 644, 648, 651, 655, 658, 672, 712
   ablation, pulsed 33*f*
   and aesthetic practice, advantages of 701*b*
   and energy devices 485*t*, 672, 682
   and intense pulsed light 741
   and light
      based treatments 608
      therapy 608
   and liposuction 467
   and melanocyte grafting 621
   basics of 3
   beam types of 16*f*
   clinic, layout plan of 708*f*
   combination of 169, 184, 225, 335
   complications of 770*t*
   density of 263
   dependent factors 215
   diode 483
   emits 361
   energy, divergence of 44*f*
   exposure duration 7
   genesis 489
   in pigmented skin, modulation of 46
   legal ramifications of maintenance of 725
   lipectomy 448
   lipolysis 448, 466, 715
   medicolegal aspects of 741
   mid-infrared 30, 300
   mode of action of 634
   monotherapy 520
   nanosecond 165
   parameters 5, 115
   penetration depth of 46
   physics 608
   pigmented 182
   pulse 31
      duration of 39, 46
      width of 8*f*
   responsive disorders, miscellaneous 572
   settings and tissue effect, variations in 55
   skin resurfacing 285
   source 370*t*
   specific complications 777
   surgery 744
   systems, several 504
   tattoo removal 234*t*
   technologies 435
   tissue
      effects of 7*f*
      interface, manipulation of 227
   treatment 181, 211*f*, 234, 552, 658
   types of 586, 600
   use of 728
   vis-à-vis disorder 663
   wavelength 135, 186
Laser and energy-based
   devices 379
   technologies 1
Laser-assisted
   delivery systems 547
   drug delivery 610
   hair removal 41, 361
   lipolysis 465
      procedure of 474
   liposuction 476*f*, 477*f*
Laser beam 210*f*
   interaction, simulation of 4*f*
Laser burns 742
   deep 376*f*
   superficial 376*f*
Laser center
   aesthetics of 729
   air conditioning 703
   device maintenance 703
   emergency protocols 705
   facility 701
   power supply 703
   rooms 702
   safety protocols 704
   staff training 705
   startup mini checklist 707*b*
Laser device 622, 694, 705
   low-intensity 661
Laser hair
   reduction 125, 353, 374*f*, 378, 379
      indications of 356
      principles of 361
      results of 365
   removal 353, 361, 362*t*, 376*f*
      advances in 382

Laser machine 383
  settings 502
Laser sweat ablation 673-675, 676f
  technique of 674
Laser therapy 271, 492, 534t, 583, 585, 594, 598, 600, 618
  for scars, principles of 547b
Laser tissue interaction 3, 26f, 67, 132
  fundamental principles of 45
  practical applications of 38
Laser toning
  in dermatology 500
  in melasma 504
  side effects of 507
  types of 500
Laser-assisted liposuction
  advantages of 478
  limitations of 478
Laxity 563
Lead chromate 202
LED See Light-emitting diode
Leg vein 346, 742
  treatment 490
Lens cataracts 367
Lentigines 38, 78, 146, 147, 150, 243, 281
  spilus 84
Lentiginosis, segmental 151f
Lentigo 144
Leser-Trélat, sign of 579
Lesion
  color of 184, 334
  depth of 334
  morphology of 334
  pigmented 40, 132, 144, 684, 742
  site of 333
  superficial 87
Less pigment selective lasers 136
Leukocyte histamine release 751
Leukoderma 511
  laser for inducing 622
Leukotrichia 782
Levofloxacin 270
Lichen planus 194
  pigmentosus 145, 147, 194, 195f, 508
Lichen sclerosus et atrophicus 125
Lichen sclerosus 86, 87, 601, 689
Lidocaine
  allergy 270, 316
  toxicity 371
Light and heat generation, absorption of 26
Light-based devices 465
Light cryotherapy 583
Light devices, types of 4
Light-emitting diode 454, 484, 487, 536, 557, 562, 567, 612, 630, 779
  phototherapy 505

Light source
  and massage 454
  practical applications for 331b
  wavelength of 321
Light therapy 645
Lipid crystallization 472
LipoLite 448
Lipolysis 567
Lipoprotein, high density 584
Liposonix 448, 463
Liposuction 448
  procedure 569t
  ultrasound assisted 448
  water-assisted 448
Low-frequency focused ultrasound 461
Low-level laser therapy 455, 567, 570, 625, 627, 628, 630, 715
  basic science of 626
Lumenis system 543
Lupus erythematosus 125, 602
Lymphangioma 86
  circumscriptum 121
Lymphatic drainage 567
Lymphatic tumors 59f
Lymphedema 357
Lymphocircumscriptum, preoperative photograph of 122f

M

Macular port-wine stain 331
Malachite green 202
Malignant disorders 662
Manganese violet 202
Massage devices 457, 458
Medical shaping devices 567t
Meladine 383
Melanin 20, 29, 322f, 379, 484, 485
  absorbs light 361
  absorption 39, 40
    coefficient of 133f
  curtain 20
  lack of 369
  paucity of 369
  relative sparing of 256
  shuttle 309
Melanocytes 147, 164, 172, 500
Melanocytic nevi 38, 100, 101f, 164f
  congenital 168
  macular congenital 169
Melanophores 500
Melanosome 22, 164, 324
  smaller 17f
Melasma 23, 86, 144, 145, 149, 150, 171, 172, 172f, 174, 174f, 176t, 180, 243, 257, 281, 306, 429, 504, 508, 607, 608, 613t, 774f
  dual laser toning 509f
  lasers used 306

Index **801**

mechanism of action 306
pigment removal 505
with aging 488
Melasma
  laser in 612
  modified 179
  treatment of 307, 611*f*
Membranes, disruption of 466
Mercury sulfide 202
Mesotherapy 448
Metabolic disorders 452
Metal implants 431
Methemoglobinemia 371
Metoclopramide 358
Microcannula 466
Microcannular technique 569*f*
Microfractional systems 254
Microneedle radiofrequency, fractional 676
Microneedling radiofrequency 424, 567, 673
  devices 410*t*, 425
  procedure 416
  systems 408
Microthermal zone 43*f*, 242*f*, 495
  treatment 424
Milia 126, 778, 779
Millisecond devices 150
Millisecond domain pulses 168
Minocycline 192
  pigmentation 193
Minoxidil 358
Miradry microwave sweat ablation 677
Mobile laser unit 705
Mohs surgery 662
Molluscum contagiosum 595, 597
Mongolian spots 190, 191
Monochromatic excimer light 620
Monopolar configurations 36
Monopolar devices 395, 396, 400, 402
Monopolar radiofrequency 277, 395*f*, 448
  procedure 412
  system 394, 396, 405
Motor nerve paresis 442
Mottled pigmentation 487
MTZ *See* Microthermal zone
Multiple-drilling method 106
Multipolar radiofrequency
  devices 460
  system 394
Multipulsed laser 324
Muscle 567
  tone 567
Musculoaponeurotic system
  contraction, superficial 463
  superficial 256, 437, 437*f*
Mycosis fungoides 665
Myocardial infarction 750
Myxoid cysts 104

N

NAFR *See* Nonablative fractional resurfacing
Nail
  disorders 634
  matrixectomy 118
    anesthesia 118
    pearls 119
    pitfalls 119
    step-by-step approach 118
Nanofractional radiofrequency 407, 427, 432
  basis of 425
  depth of penetration of 426*f*
Nanofractional technology 426*f*
Narrowband ultraviolet B, treatment with 312
Nd:YAG *See* Neodymium-doped yttrium aluminum garnet
Near infrared lasers 328
Neck rejuvenation 419
Necrobiosis lipoidica 602
Neodymium:yttrium aluminum garnet 164, 328, 535
  laser 536
Neodymium-doped yttrium aluminum garnet 5, 20*f*, 27, 29, 30, 35*f*, 36, 205, 205*f*, 218*f*, 238*f*, 353, 465, 485, 487, 501, 534, 548, 573, 586, 600, 612, 625, 633, 635, 645*b*, 656, 663, 668*f*, 672, 673, 713, 776, 784*f*
  frequency-doubled 203
  laser 237*f*, 250, 346, 366, 374*f*, 380*f*, 634, 770
    Q-switched frequency doubled 733
    treatment 237*f*, 238*f*
  long pulsed 636, 645, 732, 782
  short-pulse 636
Neoplasm 742
Neurofibromas 87, 104, 105, 105*f*, 579, 580*f*
Nevocellular nevus 144
Nevoid linear hypermelanosis 784*f*
Nevus
  comedonicus 95, 95*f*
  compound 87, 100, 144
  congenital 142, 146
  hard 590, 590*f*
  lighter 165
  morphological classification
    of hard 590*f*
    of soft 590*f*
  of Ito 142, 144, 183
  spilus 144, 146, 147, 150, 153, 154*f*, 155*f*
Nevus lipomatosus superficialis 591, 593*f*
  pathology of 592
Nevus of Ota 144, 146, 150, 183, 184, 187*f*
  color of 20, 186
  laser used for 185*t*

Nevus sebaceous 100
    pearls 100
    pitfalls 100
    step-by-step approach 100
New age diode lasers 733*f*
New fractional devices and technology 255
Nodular amyloidosis 603
Nodules 442
Noise reduction 709
Nonablative fractional
    laser 179, 242*f*, 246, 281, 487, 611*f*, 613, 618, 734
    resurfacing 204, 245, 262, 277, 298, 307, 314, 534, 539
Nonablative lasers 34, 36*t*, 242*f*, 306, 542
Nonacne scars 302*t*
Non-Asian skin types 257
Nondistensible scars 519, 521*f*
Nonearlobe keloids 120
Non-facial hair colors 384
Nonfocused ultrasound devices 458
Noninvasive body 447
    contouring
        and lipolysis 447
        contraindications 456
        indications 456
Noninvasive labia tissue tightening 420
Noninvasive vaginovulval tightening 686
Non-melanoma skin cancer 315
Nonmelanoma skin cancer, low-risk 663
Nonpedunculated pyogenic granuloma 658
Nonsegmental vitiligo, treatment of 312
Nonselective laser injury 361
Nonsteroidal nonhydroquinone 318
Nonthermal stress 462
Normal-mode ruby lasers 157, 161, 168, 169, 308
Nose, fibrous papule of 578
Nova-pulse 53
Novel laser therapy 221
Novus actus interveniens 749*f*
Nozzle effect 58

O

Obesity 451
    platform 468, 470*f*
        machine 468*f*
Ocular metal, placement of 316
Oculoplastic surgery 743*f*
Ohm's law 390
Olive oil 551
Onabotulinum toxin 669
Onychomycosis 634, 636*f*
    treatment of 635*t*
Optical energy 397
Optical penetration 323
    depth 259

Optimum fluence 363
Oral
    contraceptives 358
    corticosteroids 598
    florid papillomatosis 125
    glycopyrrolate 669
    isotretinoin 270
    oxybutynin 669
    retinoid 598
        therapy 76
Orange-peel 451
Orgasmic dysfunction 420, 686
Ota-like macules 188
Otolaryngology 743*f*
Ower fluence 199
Oxyhemoglobin 321

P

Paget's disease 664
    extramammary 664
Pain 769
    free lasers 382
    tolerance 316
Paintbrush technique 78, 97*f*, 122*f*
Palmoplantar hyperhidrosis 670*f*
Palomar medical technologies 250
Pancreatic carcinoma 108
Panniculitis, anatomic depth of 472
Papillary dermis 96, 130, 622*f*
    bleed 582*f*
    invasion 596*f*
    level of 99*f*, 170*f*, 180
    lower 79, 130
Papular scar 518, 521*f*, 522
Paradoxical hair stimulation 376
Paradoxical hypertrichosis 628
Paradoxical ink darkening 212
Parapsoriasis 665
Patches 358
PCOS *See* Polycystic ovary syndrome
PDL *See* Pulsed dye laser
Peak power 139
Pedunculated pyogenic granuloma 658
Peels 505
Pelleve device 413
Pelleve system 405
Pelleve treatment probe 414*f*
Pelvic pressure 692*f*
Penetration depth 13, 15, 28, 392
Penicillamine 358
Penile papules 106, 314
Perfluorodecalin, topical 229
Perioral area 77
Periungual wart 116, 117
Persistent erythema 375
    post-retinoid therapy 652*f*

Persistent reticulate erythema 782
Petechiae, minute 507
Petroleum jelly 772*f*
Phenol, topical 659
Phenytoin 358
Phosphatidylcholine 567
Photoacoustic toning pulse 500
    mode 501
Photoaging-associated mottled pigmentary lesions 180
Photoallergic contact dermatitis 784
Photobiostimulation 626
Photodamage skin 297, 299*t*
    classification of 484*t*
    mild-to-moderate 281
Photodynamic therapy 300, 329, 361, 383, 536, 575, 663
Photo-induced wrinkles 281
Photopneumatic devices 575
Photosensitizing drugs 369
Phototherapy 196, 665
Photothermal
    ablation 31
    coagulation 32
Photothermolysis 245*t*
    principle of selective 18
    subcellular selective 500
    selective 18, 41, 52, 132, 245, 361
Phthalocyanine dyes 202
Pico lasers 171
Picosecond 191, 591
    laser 13, 136, 139, 141, 150, 157, 184, 257, 608, 609
        operation 140*f*
    pulse 142*f*
    technology 143*t*
Pigment laser 169
Pigment nonselective lasers 136
Pigment selective lasers, highly 136, 138
Pigment specific lasers 203
Pigmentary aberration 243
Pigmentary alteration 281, 778, 783
    undesired 215
Pigmentary clearance 308
Pigmentary disorder 308, 489, 607, 742
Pigmented lasers, treatment by 144*f*
Pigmented lesions
    laser for 782
    selective photothermolysis of 40
    treatment approach of 198
Pigmented skin 132
Pinhole technique 106
Pinpoint bleeding 130, 783
Pitted scars 532
Pixilated injury 34
Planning laser clinic 728
Plantar wart 115, 127

Plasma skin regeneration 75
Plastic surgery 743*f*
Platelet-rich plasma 551
Pneumatic skin flattening 382
Pockels cell 12
Poems syndrome 357
Poikiloderma 281
    of civatte 310, 331, 344, 617
Polka-dot technique 220
Pollogen regenxl 448
Polycystic ovarian
    disease 358, 368
    disorders 379
    syndrome 359, 360
Polymethylmethacrylate 211
Polypropylene glycol 227
Poor healing, risks of 128
Popsicle panniculitis 471
Porcine model 63
Porokeratosis 125
Port-wine stain 15, 330, 492, 714, 773
    infantile 331
    treatment of 320
Post-acne hyperpigmented macules 510*f*
Postburn scarring 508, 511*f*
Postinflammatory depigmentation 237*f*
Postinflammatory hyperpigmentation 27, 38, 133, 182, 270, 314, 316, 369, 381, 487, 518, 608, 615, 616*f*, 679, 771*f*, 774, 778, 780*f*, 781*f*
    signs of 251
Postinflammatory pigmentation 508
Post-laser burn 375*f*
Post-traumatic scar 89, 301, 546*f*
Potassium
    hydroxide 597
    titanyl phosphate 328, 341, 485, 573, 601, 653
        laser 300, 328, 485, 644
        pulsed 322
Power density 6
Power-assisted liposuction 448
Pregnancy-induced hypertension, risk of 307
Pregnant and lactating women, laser in 381
Premalignant disorders 662
Prescars 533, 543
Progestins 358
ProLipo 448
Prophylactic antibiotic course 270
Prophylactic antiviral medications 270
Propionibacterium acnes 572, 573, 575, 576
Protease activated receptor-2 611*f*
Proteus syndrome 331
Protocadamus laser system 252*f*
Proximal nail block 119*f*
Pseudocontinuous lasers 9

Pseudofolliculitis 379, 631
  barbae 633
    prevention of 632*t*
    treatment of 633
  treatment for 379
Pseudo-picosecond lasers 222
Psoriasis 125, 604, 620*t*, 689
PTP *See* Photoacoustic toning pulse
Pulse 73
  duration 63, 70, 86, 139, 186, 219, 260, 320
    effect 393
    low-medium 57
  frequency 259
  interval 63
  lasers, long 157
  long 9
  nanosecond 142*f*
  number 259
  profile 15
  stacking 343
  to-pulse mode 501
  variable 67
    square 218
    width 135, 324
Pulsed dye laser 302
  use of 597*t*
Punch excision 88
Pure laser devices 466
Purists 482
Purpura 348, 442, 772
  reticulate 785
PWS *See* Port-wine stain
Pyogenic granuloma 120, 121*f*, 331, 345, 349, 657, 658*b*, 659*f*
  pearls 121
  pitfalls 121
  recurrent 658
  step-by-step approach 121

Q

QS Alex *See* Q-switched alexandrite
QSND:YAG *See* Q-switched neodymium-doped yttrium aluminum garnet
QSRL *See* Q-switched ruby laser
Q-switched alexandrite 201, 205, 216, 504
  laser 190, 617, 623, 733
Q-switched beam, single 501
Q-switched devices 150

Q-switched laser 9, 41, 133, 135, 137, 141-143, 147, 150, 156, 159, 166, 183, 184, 191, 216*t*, 218, 220, 221, 482, 608, 637, 713, 769
  monotherapy with 163
Q-switched modes 505
Q-switched neodymium-doped yttrium 232*f*
  aluminum garnet 159*f*, 204, 205, 213*f*, 216, 226, 227, 229*f*, 491
  aluminum garnet laser 733
  machine 138*f*
  use of 636*f*
Q-switched ruby 143, 149, 163
  laser 132, 138, 184, 201, 205, 216, 490, 733
  tattoo star for melasma 175*f*

R

Radiation dermatitis 331
Radiofrequency 535, 551, 676, 683, 690, 715
  bipolar 395*f*
  device 62, 454
    classification of 402*t*
    types of 394
  energy
    devices 457, 458
    pulse 401
  system 394
  technology 35
  vacuum-assisted 463
  waves 388*f*
Randomized control trial 179, 572, 627, 683
Rapamycin, mammalian target of 338
Rapid skin regeneration, process of 34*f*
Rapid tattoo removal technique 123, 222, 226*f*, 227*f*
Recalcitrant melasma, treatment of 250
Red blood cell 324
Red tattoo reactions 87
Reflectance confocal microscopy 553
Regen tripolar radiofrequency 407
Rejuvenation 281, 430
  technologies for 35*f*
Reserpine 358
Residual macular erythema 574*f*
Residual thermal
  damage 31, 54, 58, 59, 61, 68
    extent of 261
  injury, excessive 81
Resurfacing techniques, types of 78
Retinal damage 367
Retinal injury 199
Retinoids 616, 665
  topical 369, 517
Rhinophyma 87, 92, 788*f*
  background 92
  level of difficulty 94
  pearls 94

pitfalls 94
step-by-step approach 93
treat 93
Rhytides 243, 301
   mild 487
   moderate 487
Richly pigmented skin 368
Rolling technique 264
Rosacea 331, 344, 429, 489, 654*f*
   dual laser toning 511*f*
   pretreatment image of 344*f*
RTR *See* Rapid tattoo removal
Ruby laser 5

S

Sarcoidosis 602, 603
Saturable absorber 12
Scalp 355
Scars 86, 87, 212, 488, 534*t*, 742, 776, 779
   atrophic 519, 532, 533, 540, 547, 548
   bridge 522
   deep 269*f*
   depressed 519
   distensible 519, 522
      retraction 519
   flat 84
   laser for 532
   management of 534, 535*t*
   morphological type of 282*t*, 518*t*
   nonacne 301
   partial amelioration of 554*f*
   predominantly rolling 284*f*
   rolling 282, 283, 283*f*, 293*f*, 428*f*, 429*f*, 519
   sarcoidosis 603
   shouldering 530*f*
   surgical 301, 544
   therapy for individual 522*b*
   treatment of 282
      paradigms 302
   types of 294*f*, 532
   undulated 519
Schizophrenia 357
Scleroderma 602, 689
Sclerotherapy 657, 658
Sebaceous gland 19, 44, 573
   tumors, benign 583
Sebaceum 84
Sebamed clear gel 317
Seborrheic keratoses 38, 86, 87, 107, 108*f*, 144, 147, 159, 579, 581
Seborrheic melanosis 508
   dual laser toning 509*f*
Selective photothermolysis, theory of 320
Semiconductor laser material 19*f*
Senile angiomas 641
Sequential multimodal laser protocol 684
Serum androgen-binding proteins 358

Sessile lesions 106
Sessions, number of 186
Sexual dysfunction 688
Sharplan silk laser 54
Short pulse, high-power 32*f*
Sienna 202
Silicone gel 551
Single spot technique 78, 151*f*, 643*f*
Single vessel technique 643*f*
Skin 4*f*, 526
   abdominal 44*f*
   appendages, lack of 76
   cooling 325, 363
      procedures, use of 262
   disorders, treatment of 424
   dyspigmentation 128
   elasticity 680
   fraction of 173
   hydration 550
   hyperpigmentation of 192
   laxity of 38, 281, 407, 447
   needling, laser equivalent of 282
   pigmentation of 125
   pigmented 82, 149, 210, 212
   poikilodermatous 344
   preparations, alcohol-based 381
   rejuvenation 508
      dual laser toning 509*f*
   scars, chemical reconstruction of 318, 518, 519
   texture 281
   tightening 313, 387, 449
      lipolysis with 488
   tumors 87
      benign 83
   type 135, 186, 212, 270, 278, 334, 370*t*
Slight tissue discoloration 58
Small-molecule drugs 315
SmartLipo 448
Smooth shapes 467
Soft epidermal nevi 99*f*, 590*f*
Soft nevus 590
Soft tissue ablation 32*f*
Solar elastosis 281
Solar keratoses 87
Solar lentigines 87
Solid-state lasers 5
Solta device 254
Sonablate 200 435
Soprano ice laser 367*f*
   handpiece of 383*f*
South-east Asian skin type 362
Speckled lentiginous nevus 153
Speckled white frost, presence of 528*f*
Spider angiomas 348, 644
Spider angiomata 331

Spider nevi 641
Split face trial 179
Split lesion tattoo removal 227*f*
Spot 84
    laser resurfacing 90
    size 13, 139, 186, 218, 234, 323, 325
        larger 186, 218, 427
    vaporization 83
Spot-by-spot technique 643*f*
Squamous cell carcinoma 87, 95, 657, 663
Stamping technique 264*f*
Starch iodine test 676*f*
Static epidermal pigmented lesions 41
Static mode 251
Steatocystomas 109
Steroid 665
    acne 574*f*, 576*f*
Steroid antibiotic cream 373
Stimulates lymphatic drainage 468
Stimulates mitochondrial transport chain 626
Stimulates wound healing 626
Stratum corneum damage 242
Stress 452
    relaxation time theory 139
Stretch marks 419, 550
    laser for 532
Striae 305, 551*t*
    alba 305, 550*f*
        repigmentation 305
    color of 555*f*
    distensae 281, 331, 550, 550*f*, 553*f*, 555*f*
    rubrae 550*f*
    surface topographical depiction of 554*f*
    therapies 556
Sturge-Weber syndrome 331
Subcutaneous fat 19, 387, 454
    layer 459
        measurement of 568*f*
        reduction 455
Subdermal radiofrequency sweat ablation thermiDry 677
Subphotothermolytic fluence 504
Subsurface lasers 715
Suction devices 457
Suction liposuction 466
Suction massage 448
Sun protection 381, 615
Superficial actinic porokeratosis, recalcitrant disseminated 314
Superpulse 18*f*
    carbon dioxide 253*f*
    laser 52
    mode 11*f*, 122*f*
    technology 9
Suture ligation 660
Synergie esthetic massage system 454
Syneron eMax 448
Syringocystadenoma papilliferum 104
Syringomas 78, 84, 87, 104, 106, 106*f*, 788*f*
Systemic disease, sign of 356
Systemic hormonal replacement therapy 687
Systemic therapy 594

T

Tacrolimus 598
Tamoxifen 358
Tap water iontophoresis 668
Tapid tattoo removal 202, 226, 227*f*, 229*f*, 491
Tattoo 25, 132, 198, 201, 214*f*, 223*f*, 281, 742, 784
    artists, pigments used by 202*b*
    color of 210, 224*f*
    complete removal of 232*f*
    darkening of 235
    darkening, paradoxical 785
    dependent factors 207
    depth of 202, 208
    dirt 200
    double 236
    dye, composition of 211
    emergent removal of 236
    iatrogenic 236
    in pigmented skin 236
    laser for black-red 213*f*
    multicolored 206*f*, 226*f*, 235
    particle, size of 207
    professional 200
        black 214*f*
    recalcitrant 235*t*
    selective photothermolysis of 39
    star 137
    traumatic 236
    types of 201*t*, 210
Tattoo ink
    lightening scores 225
    nonresponsive 215
Tattoo pigment 205*t*
    host removal of 210
    laser
        induced resolution of 204
        used for 212*t*
Tattoo removal 123, 201, 203, 209, 216*t*
    enhance 210*f*
    laser used for 204*fc*, 205*f*
    modifications for 221

technique
    modified 232*f*
    to enhance 124*f*
    variables affecting 207
TCA See Trichloroacetic acid
Telangiectasia 331, 348, 487, 651, 684
    laser for 343*b*
    macularis eruptiva perstans 653*f*
    nonvisible 487
    treatment of 654*f*
Telangiectatic rosacea 508
Telogen 354
    effluvium 626
Temperature elevation 26
Tensile strength 680
Terminal hair 354, 358
Tethered fibrotic bands 283
Tethered rolling scars 293*f*
Therapeutic machine 716
Thermabrasion 60
Thermage 400, 448
Thermal damage time 16
Thermal devices 458
Thermal injury
    microscopic columns of 241
    range of 73
Thermal kinetic selectivity 17
Thermal relaxation time 7, 10, 21, 22, 165, 259, 324*t*, 387
Thick black hair on chin 355*f*
Thick hair 362
    skin 362
Thin hair 362, 363, 368
Thumb 86
    rule 62, 126, 144, 163
        deep dermal 86
Tissue
    ablation 80, 396
    change, sequence of 57*f*
    collagen 567
    cooling of 32
    destruction, localized 584
    effects 11*f*, 53*f*, 73
    fluence 32*f*
    interactions 3
    levels 73
    penetration 20*f*
    sculpting 69
    soldering 661
    splatter 783
    technologies 53
    tightening 448
        nonsurgical 439
    types of 391
    water 241
    welding 661

Titanium 214
    dioxide 202, 214, 785
Titanium:sapphire laser 223
Toe nail, ingrowing 118
Transcutaneous temperature controlled radiofrequency device 688*f*
Traumatic scar 319*f*
    preoperative view of 303*f*
Treating melasma, option for 512
Tretinoin 551
    cream 529
Triactive device 468
Triacylglycerol 456
Triamcinolone 540*f*, 545*f*
Tribeam machine 502, 502*f*
Trichloroacetic acid 524, 584
    peel 63, 523*f*, 524, 528*f*
Trichoepithelioma 87, 104, 109, 110*f*, 578
Trichophyton rubrum 634, 638
Tripolar radiofrequency 404
    system 394
Trofolastin 551
Tumescent liposuction 450
Tumor 578
    benign 11*f*, 104
    sebaceous 104

U

Ulceration 742
Ulthera 448
    system 438
Ultherapy mechanism of action 437
Ultracavitators 461
Ultrapulse 18*f*
    carbon dioxide 225, 253*f*, 588*f*
        procedure of 587*f*
    laser 52, 53, 62
    lumenis 788*f*
    mode 83
Ultrashape, third-generation 463
Ultrashort acting radiant heat effect 500
Ultrashort laser 13
Ultrasonography 770
Ultrasound skin tightening 448
Ultraviolet B phototherapy 604
Unipolar devices utilize 458
Unipolar fractional radiofrequency 399
Unipolar radiofrequency 404
    device 406, 460
Upper face 440
    contouring 440
Upper lip 355
Upper papillary dermis 491*f*
Upper reticular dermis 79, 130
Urinary incontinence 689
    mild-to-moderate 688
Urogenital atrophy 686

Urticaria, physical 507
Urticarial-like plaques 782
UV See Ultraviolet

V

Vacuum apparatus 406
Vaginal atrophy 686, 688
Vaginal bleeding 693*f*
Vaginal laxity 686, 688
Vaginal rejuvenation 686, 688*f*
Vaginal relaxation 686, 688
Vaginal sensitivity, low 688
Vaginitis, atrophic 686
Vaporization 115
    mode 57
Vascular component 486
Vascular conditions 86
Vascular disorders 641
Vascular endothelial growth factor 331, 629
Vascular growths 86
Vascular indications 490
Vascular laser 182, 320, 330, 488, 713, 736
    practical application for 331*b*
Vascular lesions
    laser for 785
    without purpura, treatment of 42*f*
Vascular specific pulsed dye laser therapy 539
Vascular tumors 59*f*
Velashape systems 459, 468
Velasmooth 557
    action of 560*f*
    handpiece 459*f*
    systems 459
    technology 559
Vellus hair 358
    follicles, terminalization of 628
Verrucae 83, 86, 87
    plana 596*f*
    vulgaris 83
Versa pulse 137
Videomicroscopy 334
Viral diseases 76
Viral disorders 595, 597*t*
Virally-mediated diseases, treating 117
Virilization 356
Visible light technologies 24
Visual analog scale 225
Vitiligo 310, 311*b*, 619, 620*t*, 621*t*, 689

    nonsegmental 312
    patch 123*f*
    surgery 122
    treatment of 311
Vulval rejuvenation 688*f*, 690
Vulvar surgery 420
Vulvovaginal atrophy 686

W

Wart 115, 331
    common 116, 597
    tissue bubbles 117
Waterlogged cotton-thread appearance 65
Weight loss treatments 566*t*
White hair 379
Wider single pulse 324
Wound
    laser
        for acute 661
        for chronic 661
    size of 258
        macrowound 258
        microwound 258
Wound care 82
    dressings 82
    post 82
Wound healing 73
    process 438*t*
Wrinkles 125

X

Xanthelasma 84, 87, 104, 109, 111*f*, 112*f*, 584, 585
    palpebrarum 585
        treatment of 586*t*
    with modalities, management of 113*fc*
Xanthoma disseminatum 114

Y

Yellow coal tar dyes 202
YSGG laser *See* Yttrium-scandium-gallium-garnet laser
Yttrium-aluminum-garnet 518
    flashlamp-pumped 66
Yttrium-scandium-gallium-garnet lasers 136

Z

Zeltiq 448
    coolsculpt 473
Zerona 448
Zidovudine 192
Zinc oxide 202
Zoon's balanitis 86, 87, 125, 662, 663

EU GSPR Authorised Reprsentative
Logos Europe, 9 rue Nicolas Poussin
1700, La Rochelle, France
Phone: +33 (0) 6 67 93 73 78
E-mail: contact@logoseurope.eu

www.ingramcontent.com/pod-product-compliance
Ingram Content Group UK Ltd.
Pitfield, Milton Keynes, MK11 3LW, UK
UKHW060933280126
467427UK00003B/13